Study Guide for
Goldfrank's
Toxicologic Emergencies, 11th Edition

Editors

Rana Biary
Mary Ann Howland
Silas W. Smith
Richard S. Weisman
Neal A. Lewin
Lewis R. Goldfrank
Robert S. Hoffman

New York/Chicago/San Francisco/Athens/London/Madrid/Mexico City/
Milan/New Delhi/Singapore/Sydney/Toronto

ISBN 978-1-260-47502-9
MHID 1-260-47502-6

Notice

Medicine is an ever-changing science. As new research and clinical experience broaden our knowledge, changes in treatment and drug therapy are required. The authors and the publisher of this work have checked with sources believed to be reliable in their efforts to provide information that is complete and generally in accord with the standards accepted at the time of publication. However, in view of the possibility of human error or changes in medical sciences, neither the authors nor the publisher nor any other party who has been involved in the preparation or publication of this work warrants that the information contained herein is in every respect accurate or complete, and they disclaim all responsibility for any errors or omissions or for the results obtained from use of the information contained in this work. Readers are encouraged to confirm the information contained herein with other sources. For example and in particular, readers are advised to check the product information sheet included in the package of each drug they plan to administer to be certain that the information contained in this work is accurate and that changes have not been made in the recommended dose or in the contraindications for administration. This recommendation is of particular importance in connection with new or infrequently used drugs.

This book was set in Kepler Std by KnowledgeWorks Global Ltd.
The editor was Kay Conerly.
The production supervisor was Catherine Saggese.
Project management was provided by Revathi Viswanathan, KnowledgeWorks Global Ltd.

This book is printed on acid-free paper.

Library of Congress Control Number: 2022941497

Contents

Editors

Rana Biary, MD
Assistant Professor of Emergency Medicine
Ronald O. Perelman Department of Emergency Medicine
New York University Grossman School of Medicine
Attending Physician, Emergency Medicine Bellevue Hospital Center
    and New York University Langone Health
Consultant, New York City Poison Control Center
New York, New York

Mary Ann Howland, PharmD, DABAT, FACCT
Clinical Professor of Pharmacy
St. John's University College of Pharmacy and Health Sciences
Adjunct Professor of Emergency Medicine
Ronald O. Perelman Department of Emergency Medicine
New York University Grossman School of Medicine
Bellevue Hospital Center
Senior consultant in residence
New York City Poison Control Center
New York, New York

Silas W. Smith, MD, FACEP, FACMT
JoAnn G. and Kenneth Wellner Clinical Associate Professor of
    Emergency Medicine
Ronald O. Perelman Department of Emergency Medicine
New York University Grossman School of Medicine
Chief, Division of Quality, Safety, and Practice Innovation
Attending Physician, Emergency Medicine
Bellevue Hospital Center and New York University Langone Health
Consultant, New York City Poison Control Center
New York, New York

Richard S. Weisman, PharmD, DABAT, FAACT
Professor of Pediatrics and Medical Education
Associate Dean for Admissions & Enrollment
University of Miami Miller School of Medicine
Director, Florida Poison Control Center – Miami
Miami, Florida

Neal A. Lewin, MD, FACEP, FACMT, FACP
Druckenmiller Professor of Emergency Medicine and Medicine
Ronald O. Perelman Department of Emergency Medicine
New York University Grossman School of Medicine
Director, Didactic Education Emergency Medicine Residency
Attending Physician, Emergency Medicine and Internal Medicine
Bellevue Hospital Center and New York University Langone Health
New York, New York

Lewis R. Goldfrank, MD, FAAEM, FACCT, FACEP, FACMT, FACP
Herbert W. Adams Professor of Emergency Medicine
Ronald O. Perelman Department of Emergency Medicine
New York University Grossman School of Medicine
Attending Physician, Emergency Medicine
Bellevue Hospital Center and New York University Langone Health
Medical Director, New York City Poison Control Center
New York, New York

Robert S. Hoffman, MD, FACCT, FRCP Edin, FEAPCCT
Professor of Emergency Medicine and Medicine
Ronald O. Perelman Department of Emergency Medicine
New York University Grossman School of Medicine
Attending Physician, Emergency Medicine Bellevue Hospital Center
    and New York University Langone Health
Consultant, New York City Poison Control Center
New York, New York

Contributors

Timothy Charles Backus, DO
Assistant Program Director
Emergency Medicine Residency
Mohawk Valley Health System
Utica, New York

Emily T. Cohen, MD
Assistant Professor
Ronald O. Perelman Department of Emergency Medicine at
    NYU Grossman School of Medicine
Consultant, New York City Poison Control Center
New York, New York

Philip DiSalvo, MD
Emergency Medicine
Carle Foundation Hospital
Urbana, illinois

Arie Francis, MD
Clinical Assistant Professor
Department of Emergency Medicine
Renaissance School of Medicine
Stony Brook University
Stony Brook, New York

Emma Furlano, MD
Assistant Professor
Department of Emergency Medicine
Albany Medical College
Albany, New York

Sarah Mahonski, MD
Clinical Assistant Professor
Department of Emergency Medicine at SUNY Upstate Medical University
Syracuse, New York

Joshua Trebach, MD
Clinical Assistant Professor
Division of Medical Toxicology and Department of Emergency Medicine
University of Iowa
Iowa City, Iowa

Josh Wang, MD, FRCPC
Assistant Professor, McGill University
Emergency Physician, McGill University Health Centre
Consultant, Centre anti-poison du Québec
Québec, Canada

Preface

In response to reader feedback, we have returned to the concept of an independent study guide, now partnered to the 11th edition of our text, *Goldfrank's Toxicologic Emergencies*. This study guide is focused on critical issues raised by the physicians, nurses, pharmacists, and students who comprise multidisciplinary toxicology teams all over the world.

In this new study guide you will find 1,400 unique multiple-choice questions arranged according to chapters of the Goldfrank's text. The answers to each question are annotated and referenced. We believe that these changes enable the reader to use this book as a rigorous self-assessment workbook independent of our text.

At the same time, we believe that the value of this book is enhanced by using it in conjunction with the Goldfrank's text, leading to greater intellectual enrichment. We hope that the workbook will assist you in improving your knowledge and critical skills to serve your patients more successfully and your students with more wisdom. We wish you well in your studies of toxicology.

Rana Biary
Mary Ann Howland
Silas W. Smith
Richard S. Weisman
Neal A. Lewin
Lewis R. Goldfrank
Robert S. Hoffman

Historical Principles and Perspectives

QUESTIONS

1.1. *Toxicology* is derived from the word *toxikon*. What does the word *toxikon* mean?
- A. Death
- B. An evil curse
- C. The poison into which arrowheads are dipped
- D. Poisons of animal, vegetable, or mineral origin
- E. Judicial punishment

1.2. What xenobiotic causes "saturnine gout?"
- A. Arsenic
- B. Antimony
- C. Chromium
- D. Lead
- E. Thallium

1.3. Which of the following options was the poison of choice used by the ancient Greeks to execute criminals and dissidents such as Socrates?
- A. Digitalis leaf
- B. Arsenic
- C. Poison hemlock
- D. Strychnine
- E. Heroin

1.4. Who is often credited with developing the concept of dose-response in toxicology?
- A. Maimonides
- B. Paracelsus
- C. Galen
- D. Ambroise Pare
- E. Theodore Wormley

1.5. The Marsh test was developed to detect which of the following xenobiotics?
- A. Aconite
- B. Arsenic
- C. Heroin
- D. Strychnine
- E. Cocaine

1.6. In the late 19th century, which of the following options was recommended for the treatment of opioid addiction?
- A. Heroin
- B. Chloral hydrate
- C. Caffeine
- D. Cocaine
- E. Strychnine

1.7. In 1775, Sir Percivall Pott described the first cancer that was linked to an occupational exposure. What cancer was associated with being a chimney sweep?
- A. Lung
- B. Skin
- C. Scrotal
- D. Kidney
- E. Leukemia

1.8. Poisoning from which of the following xenobiotics precipitated the first US federal regulatory legislation that specifically addressed household exposures?
- A. Petroleum distillates
- B. Opiates
- C. Strychnine
- D. Pesticides
- E. Caustics

1.9. The therapeutic use of Elixir of Sulfanilamide-Massengill led to more than 100 deaths. Which xenobiotic was responsible for these deaths?
A. Ethylene glycol
B. Diethylene glycol
C. Propylene glycol
D. Glycerol
E. Benzyl alcohol

1.10. What xenobiotic was implicated in two wars between England and China in the mid-19th century?
A. Arsenic
B. Aconite
C. Caffeine
D. Strychnine
E. Opium

ANSWERS

1.1. Answer: C. The term *toxicology* is derived from two Greek terms: *toxicos* ("bow") and *toxicon* ("poison into which arrowheads are dipped"). Cave paintings of arrowheads and spearheads reveal that these weapons were crafted with small depressions at the end that might have held poison.

American Heritage Dictionary. 2nd college ed. Boston: Houghton Mifflin; 1991.

1.2. Answer: D. Saturnine gout is associated with lead toxicity. Elevated concentrations of uric acid predispose to gout. It is believed that lead inhibits the renal excretion of uric acid, thus favoring the formation of urate crystals. Another theory posits that the accumulation of guanine, a purine nucleic acid, secondary to the inhibition of gaunine deaminase (guanase) by the presence of lead, also contributes to this form of gout. Lead toxicity occurred in noblemen of the Roman Empire as well as British aristocracy because of lead contamination during the manufacturing of wine. In fact, the instructions explicitly called for the use of lead vessels since copper rust negatively altered the flavor.

Nriagu JO. Saturnine gout among Roman aristocrats. Did lead poisoning contribute to the fall of the Empire? *N Engl J Med.* 1983;308:660-663.

1.3. Answer: C. Poison hemlock was the official poison used by the Greeks and was employed in the execution of Socrates.

Ober WB. Did Socrates die of hemlock poisoning? *NY State Med J.* 1977;77:254-258.

1.4. Answer: B. Paracelsus' study of the dose-response relationship is usually considered the beginning of the scientific approach to toxicology. He was the first to emphasize the chemical nature of toxins. He underscored the need to differentiate between the therapeutic and toxic properties of chemicals when he stated in his Third Defense, "What is there that is not poison? All things are poison and nothing

[is] without poison. Solely the dose determines that a thing is not poison."

Deichmann WB, et al. What is there that is not poison? A study of the Third Defense by Paracelsus. *Arch Toxicol.* 1986;58:207-213.

1.5. Answer: B. The Marsh test was first used in a trial in 1839 to convict Madame Marie Lafarge in the poisoning of her husband using arsenic.

Smith S. Poisons and poisoners through the ages. *Med Leg J.* 1952; 20:153-167.

1.6. Answer: D. During the latter part of the 19th century, cocaine was enthusiastically recommended as a treatment for opioid addiction. In 1884, Sigmund Freud wrote *Uber Cocaine* advocating cocaine as an opium and morphine addiction cure and as a treatment for fatigue and hysteria.

Karch SB. The history of cocaine toxicity. *Hum Pathol.* 1989;20: 1037-1039.

1.7. Answer: C. Historically, chimney sweeps were young boys who climbed down chimneys to clean them. The boys had prolonged exposure to tar and soot, which led to an increased risk of scrotal cancer. The etiologic carcinogenic compounds are the polyaromatic hydrocarbons, including benzo[*a*]pyrene, contained in coal tar. Percivall Pott first identified the causal association between chimney sweeps and this form of scrotal squamous cell carcinoma, making it the first reported occupational cancer.

Hunter D. *The Diseases of Occupations.* 6th ed. London: Hodder & Stoughton; 1978.

1.8. Answer: E. The Federal Caustic Poison Act of 1927 was the first federal legislation specifically addressing household poisoning. The legislative efforts were led by Dr. Chevalier Jackson, an otolaryngologist who showed that unintentional exposures to household caustics were an increasingly frequent cause of severe gastrointestinal burns. The Act mandated that lye- and acid-containing products clearly display a "poison" warning label.

> Taylor HM. A preliminary survey of the effect which lye legislation has had on the incidence of esophageal stricture. *Ann Otolaryngol Rhinol Laryngol.* 1935;44:1157-1158.

1.9. Answer: B. In September and October 1937, more than 100 deaths were associated with the use of one of the early sulfa preparations, Elixir of Sulfanilamide-Massengill, which contained 72% diethylene glycol as the vehicle for drug delivery. Little was known about diethylene glycol toxicity at the time, and many cases of acute kidney injury and death occurred. As a result of this catastrophe, animal drug testing was mandated by the Food, Drug, and Cosmetic Act of 1938 to avoid similar tragedies in the future. Unfortunately, diethylene glycol would continue to be sporadically used in other countries as a medicinal diluent, resulting in additional deaths in South Africa (1969), India (1986), Nigeria (1990), Bangladesh (1990-1992), Argentina (1992), Haiti (1995), India (1998), Panama (2006), and Nigeria (2008-2009).

> Geiling EHK, Cannon PR. Pathological effects of elixir of sulfanilamide (diethylene glycol) poisoning: A clinical and experimental correlation - final report. *JAMA.* 1938;111:919-926.

1.10. Answer: E. In 1839, the first opium war was waged between China and Great Britain. Opium was grown in British-colonized India and exported to China. The British were reluctant to give up their flourishing drug trade, despite widespread Chinese protests calling for the discontinuation of this practice. This led to a war, led by Britain, to maintain a right to sell opium. In 1853, a second war was waged, with the British demanding even more concessions, including the complete legalization of opium in China. As a result, opioid use was endemic in China during the 19th century.

> Sapira JD. Speculations concerning opium abuse and world history. *Perspect Biol Med.* 1975;18:379-398.

Toxicologic Misfortunes and Catastrophes in History

2

2.1. In 1986, nearly 2,000 villagers and their animals were found dead near Lake Nyos in Cameroon. Many people died in their sleep. What was the cause of this toxicologic disaster?
A. CO_2
B. Phosphine gas
C. CO
D. Sulfuric acid
E. Methyl isocyanate

2.2. In 1984, Union Carbide, a chemical company, suffered a gas leak that led to the liberation of 40 metric tons of methyl isocyanate in Bhopal, India. What was the most common presenting symptom in survivors?
A. Seizures
B. Blindness
C. Respiratory depression
D. Chloracne
E. Diarrhea

2.3. In 1952, smog in London was responsible for about 4,000 deaths. This eventually led to the passing of the 1956 Clean Air Act by the British parliament. What toxin contributed to the deaths?
A. Carbon dioxide
B. Carbon monoxide
C. Sulfur dioxide
D. Dioxin
E. Chlorine

2.4. In 994 AD, 40,000 people died in Aquitania, France, because of an outbreak that caused excruciating burning extremity pain and eventually gangrene of the extremities. Some people manifested hallucinations. What was the cause of this event?
A. Colchicine
B. Ergot
C. Arsenic
D. Thallium
E. Atropine

2.5. In Turkey, between 1955 and 1959, 4,000 cases of porphyria cutanea tarda were diagnosed. Families presented with kara para (black sore). Breastfed babies presented with pemba yara (pink sore) with a mortality of about 95%. What xenobiotic led to this outbreak?
A. Hexachlorophene
B. Hexachlorobenzene
C. Dioxin
D. Ergotamine
E. Benzyl alcohol

2.6. In Epping, England, an outbreak occurred due to exposure to methylene dianiline. What organ was primarily affected?
A. Heart
B. Lungs
C. Liver
D. Kidney
E. Skin

2.7. In Japan, an outbreak of a disease known as Itai-Itai, or "ouch-ouch," led to bony pain as well as osteomalacia. What metal is associated with this syndrome?
A. Cobalt
B. Chromium
C. Cadmium
D. Copper
E. Thallium

2.8. The daughters of women who were treated with diethylstilbesterol (DES) for threatened miscarriages are at risk for developing what type of cancer?
A. Lung cancer
B. Clear cell vaginal cancer
C. Breast cancer
D. Renal cancer
E. Hepatic angiosarcoma

2.9. The eosinophilia-myalgia syndrome was associated with which of the following xenobiotics?
A. Pyridoxine
B. Melatonin
C. Niacin
D. L-tryptophan
E. Folate

2.10. A serious radiation incident occurred in 1987 in Brazil when 244 people were exposed to a radiation source found in a junkyard. The radiation was emitted by an isotope of which of the following elements?
A. Iodine
B. Thallium
C. Cesium
D. Uranium
E. Plutonium

ANSWERS

2.1. Answer: A. Lake Nyos in Cameroon is a volcanic crater lake. In 1986, a large bubble of carbon dioxide erupted. Approximately 1,700 humans died from asphyxiation in the area directly surrounding the lake.

> Baxter PJ, et al. Lake Nyos disaster, Cameroon, 1986: The medical effects of large scale emission of carbon dioxide? *BMJ*. 1989;298:1437-1441.

2.2. Answer: B. Methyl isocyanate is used in the manufacture of polyurethane foam and plastics, among many other products. In this chemical plant, methyl isocyanate was the intermediate chemical in the production of carbamate pesticides. Chronic occupational exposure is associated with asthma from a sensitization and stimulation to protein-isocyanate conjugates. Methyl isocyanate is very reactive on direct contact with liquids, resulting in eye pain, lacrimation, photophobia, and corneal ulcerations. This explains why many patients in Bhopal presented with blindness. Methyl isocyanate is also a mitochondrial toxin, inhibiting complex 1 and acting as a weak uncoupler. Unlike with cyanide toxicity, the deaths are not instantaneous, but instead occur within a few hours of the exposure. Autopsies performed on the victims of Bhopal showed that the predominant cause of death was acute respiratory distress syndrome (ARDS).

> Mehta PS, et al. Bhopal tragedy's health effects. A review of methyl isocyanate toxicity. *JAMA*. 1990;264:2781-2787.

2.3. Answer: C. Air pollution increases morbidity and mortality, especially as the world has become more industrialized. At certain times in history, as pollution worsened, a thermal inversion occurred, trapping the smog closer to the ground and leading to worsening respiratory symptoms, particularly in people with underlying reactive airways diseases. Similar events occurred in the Meuse Valley, Belgium, in 1930, Donora, Pennsylvania, in 1948, and London in 1952. Sulfur dioxide is the most significant component of smog causing these symptoms.

> Logan WPD. Mortality in the London fog incident, 1952. *Lancet*. 1953;1:336-338.

2.4. Answer: B. Outbreaks of ergotamine poisoning occurred as early as 994 AD in Aquitana, France. Their presentation was called "St. Anthony's Fire" as their pain was described as burning and excruciating. People who improved made pilgrimages to the shrine of St. Anthony. These outbreaks occurred secondary to the fungus *Claviceps purpura*, which infects rye and leads to the production of ergotamine, histamine, and lysergic acid. The painful extremities are due to peripheral vasospasm.

> Merhoff GC, et al. Ergot intoxication: Historical review and description of unusual clinical manifestations. *Ann Surg*. 1974;180:773-779.

2.5. Answer: B. These diagnoses were only made in families who had eaten wheat that was distributed by the government solely for planting. This syndrome was eventually linked with the ingestion of wheat treated with the fungicide hexachlorobenzene.

> Schmid R. Cutaneous porphyria in Turkey. *N Engl J Med*. 1960;263:397-398.

2.6. Answer: C. Methylene dianiline toxicity is also known as Epping jaundice. In 1965, a truck carrying both flour and methylene dianiline had an unintentional spill that resulted in the methylene dianiline admixing with the flour. Eighty-four people presented with influenzalike illness, right upper quadrant pain, and jaundice. Liver biopsies demonstrated cellular infiltration and cholestasis. The vast majority of patients survived and had normalization of their liver function within 2-4 weeks. A generation of follow-up failed to reveal any obvious link between the poisoning and longstanding health effects.

Kopelman H, et al. The Epping jaundice. *Br Med J.* 1966;5486: 514-516.

2.7. Answer: C. Between 1939 and 1954, 200 people who lived along the Jintsu River developed this painful constellation of symptoms. Cadmium contaminated the local water supply used for rice cultivation, the community's food staple.

Anonymous. Cadmium pollution and Itai-itai disease. *Lancet.* 1971; 1:382-383.

2.8. Answer: B. Diethylstilbestrol (DES) daughters are women who were born to mothers who were given DES while they were pregnant. They are prone to developing clear cell vaginal and cervical cancers as early as their teenage years. Diethylstilbestrol mothers are the women themselves who were prescribed DES. They were at an increased risk of developing breast cancer.

Herbst AL, et al. Adenocarcinoma of the vagina. Association of maternal stilbestrol therapy with tumor appearance in young women. *N Engl J Med.* 1971;284:878-881.

2.9. Answer: D. Between 1989 and 1990 an epidemic of eosinophilia-myalgia developed in more than 1,500 people who had taken L-tryptophan. These patients presented with sclerodermalike features and eosinophilia. All affected patients had ingested tryptophan produced by a single manufacturer. That manufacturer introduced a new process involving genetically altered bacteria to improve tryptophan production. A contaminant produced by this process is suggested as the etiology of this syndrome.

Vargas J, et al. The cause and pathogenesis of the eosinophilia-myalgia syndrome. *Ann Intern Med.* 1992;116:140-147.

2.10. Answer: C. In 1987, in Goiania, Brazil, 244 people were exposed to Cesium-137 when an abandoned radiotherapy unit was opened in a junkyard. One hundred four people showed evidence of internal contamination, 28 had local radiation injuries, and eight developed acute radiation syndrome. There were at least four deaths.

Oliveria AR, et al. Medical and related aspects of the Goiania accident: An overview. *Health Phys.* 1991;60:17-24.

Initial Evaluation of the Patient: Vital Signs and Toxic Syndromes

3

QUESTIONS

3.1. A 19-year-old man presents to the emergency department after an intentional overdose. Which of the following ingestions would explain his blood pressure of 60/20 mmHg and heart rate of 142 beats/min?
A. Clonidine
B. Digoxin
C. Morphine
D. Nifedipine
E. Nadolol

3.2. Which of the following xenobiotics causes respiratory stimulation?
A. Opioids
B. Salicylates
C. Flunitrazepam
D. Propofol
E. Secobarbital

3.3. A 19-year-old man presents to the emergency department with confusion. He is hallucinating and picking at objects. His heart rate is 156 beats/min, his blood pressure is 178/98 mmHg, and his temperature is 100.6 °F (38.1 °C). On physical examination, his mucous membranes are dry and he has a palpable distended bladder. Which of the following antidotes is associated with a shorter hospital length of stay in this patient?
A. Naloxone
B. Cyproheptadine
C. Physostigmine
D. Flumazenil
E. Dantrolene

3.4. Bradycardia is most characteristic of which of the following ingestions?
A. Phenylpropanolamine
B. Iron
C. Isoniazid
D. Diphenhydramine
E. Phencyclidine

3.5. Chronic exposure to which of the following toxic inhalants causes an increase in the incidence of hypertension?
A. Nitrates
B. Carbon disulfide
C. Carbon monoxide
D. Sulfur dioxide
E. Methane

3.6. A 26-year-old woman is brought into the emergency department after being found confused at a party. Her vital signs are blood pressure: 168/90 mmHg; heart rate: 167 beats/min; respiratory rate: 25 breaths/min; rectal temperature: 108.9 °F (42.7 °C). Her examination is remarkable for lower extremity rigidity with sustained clonus. What is the most important intervention that should be undertaken in the care of this patient?
A. Initiation of a 30 mL/kg bolus of crystalloid fluid
B. Administration of broad-spectrum antibiotics
C. Administration of cyproheptadine
D. Cooling measures using the misting and fanning technique
E. Immediate placement of patient in an ice bath

3.7. A 35-year-old man presents to the emergency department following an intentional overdose. On examination, he is bradycardic to 38 beats/min, tachypneic to 42 breaths/min, and has diffuse expiratory wheezing throughout his lung fields. He also has significant lacrimation, vomiting, diarrhea, and is weak. The patient is immediately decontaminated. Which of the following antidotes should be administered as part of his treatment?
A. Naloxone
B. Flumazenil
C. Pralidoxime
D. Dantrolene
E. Cyproheptadine

3.8. A 19-year-old woman presents to the emergency department after being found near drug paraphernalia on the street. On examination, she is unresponsive to stimulation with constricted pupils. She has a heart rate of 50 beats/min, a blood pressure of 90/45 mmHg, a respiratory rate of 12 breaths/min, and an oxygen saturation of 98% on room air. Which of the following therapies is indicated in the management of this patient?
A. Oxygen via a facemask
B. Naloxone

C. Flumazenil
D. Physostigmine
E. Supportive measures alone

3.9. The anticholinergic and sympathomimetic toxidromes share many signs and symptoms. Which of the following is more characteristic of anticholinergic toxicity alone?
A. Tachycardia
B. Hypertension
C. Elevated temperature
D. Diaphoresis
E. Urinary retention

3.10. A 27-year-old man presents to the emergency department with nausea, vomiting, and anxiety. His blood pressure is 150/80 mmHg, and his heart rate is 90 beats/min. On examination, he is yawning and has significant piloerection. Which of the following medications will best relieve his symptoms?
A. Naloxone
B. Methadone
C. Lorazepam
D. Flumazenil
E. Metoprolol

ANSWERS

3.1. Answer: D. Digoxin, nadolol, and morphine cause bradycardia in overdose. Clonidine initially causes tachycardia before a persistent bradycardia develops; however, patients usually have an increase in blood pressure during the initial stimulatory phase. Nifedipine is a calcium channel blocker that increases the heart rate and vasodilates to produce the combination of hypotension and tachycardia.

> Weiner DA. Calcium channel blockers. *Med Clin North Am.* 1988; 72:83-115.

3.2. Answer: B. Opioids depress respirations by stimulation of the μ_2 receptors. Flunitrazepam, propofol, and secobarbital are GABA agonists that produce central nervous system depression. In overdose, salicylates produce stimulation of the respiratory center, causing both tachypnea and hyperpnea.

> Milhorn DE, et al. Effects of salicylate and 2,4 dinitrophenol on respiration and metabolism. *J Appl Physiol.* 1982;53:925-929.

3.3. Answer: C. This patient is presenting with an anticholinergic toxidrome. This toxidrome consists of delirium,

hypertension, tachycardia, an elevated temperature, dilated and minimally reactive pupils, decreased peristalsis, urinary retention, and dry skin and mucous membranes. Physostigmine is a carbamate that is capable of penetrating the blood-brain barrier and is used to treat anticholinergic toxicity. While physostigmine does not lead to a reduction in mortality, it is associated with a shorter length of stay in the hospital and a reduction in both imaging and procedures performed. In patients whose electrocardiogram shows a QRS interval that is less than 100 msec and no contraindications to its use, physostigmine is an appropriate antidote to use in anticholinergic toxicity.

> Burns MJ, et al. A comparison of physostigmine and benzodiazepines for the treatment of anticholinergic poisoning. *Ann Emerg Med.* 2000;35:374-381.

3.4. Answer: A. Phencyclidine and diphenhydramine cause tachycardia in overdose. Iron and isoniazid either will not change heart rate or will cause an increase in heart rate as the patient becomes hypotensive or develops a metabolic acidosis. Phenylpropanolamine is a pure alpha-adrenergic agonist. As blood pressure increases, patients often develop a reflex bradycardia.

Horowitz JD, et al. Hypertensive response induced by phenylpropanolamine in anorectic and decongestant preparations. *Lancet.* 1980;1:60-61.

3.5. Answer: B. Chronic occupational exposure to carbon disulfide causes an acceleration of atherosclerotic heart disease with an increase in both coronary artery disease and hypertension. Chronic exposure to sulfur dioxide causes an increase in chronic obstructive pulmonary disease and coronary artery disease. The nitrates cause an increase in headaches and orthostatic hypotension. Chronic low-level exposure to carbon monoxide causes an array of neuropsychiatric symptoms.

Partanen T. Coronary heart disease among workers exposed to carbon disulfide. *Br J Ind Med.* 1970;27:313-325.

3.6. Answer: E. The most critical intervention in the management of this patient is rapid cooling. While historically it was taught that misting and fanning is an appropriate way to cool patients, in reality, it is not a fast enough method. Patients need to be cooled as quickly as possible, ideally within 20 minutes of arrival at a healthcare facility. The best way to achieve this is through ice water immersion. The patient should be cooled until their core temperature has dropped to approximately 101 °F (38.3 °C), at which point they should be removed from the ice bath as it is common for patients' temperatures to continue to drop. Addressing hyperthermia should take precedence over all other interventions. If airway management is necessary, that occurs concurrently and should not delay cooling.

Simon HB. Hyperthermia. *N Engl J Med.* 1993;329:483-487.

Armstrong LE, et al. Whole-body cooling of hyperthermic runners: Comparison of two field therapies. *Am J Emerg Med.* 1996;14:355-358.

3.7. Answer: C. This patient is presenting with signs and symptoms consistent with a cholinergic toxidrome. Atropine is indicated in patients who have muscarinic symptoms, and enough atropine should be administered to dry respiratory secretions. Pralidoxime, or 2-PAM, is another antidote that is used in the treatment of cholinergic toxicity. 2-PAM helps to regenerate acetylcholinesterase. It is particularly helpful in patients who develop nicotinic symptoms, as atropine is an antimuscarinic and will not be effective in the treatment of the nicotinic symptoms.

Taylor P. Anticholinesterase agents. In: Hardman JG, et al., eds. *Goodman and Gilman's The Pharmacological Basis of Therapeutics.* 9th ed. New York, NY: Macmillan; 1996:100-119.

3.8. Answer: E. This patient is presenting with an opioid toxidrome. However, her respiratory rate is greater than 8 breaths/min and her oxygen saturation is 98%. There is no indication to give naloxone therapy at this time. Naloxone is indicated in patients who either have a respiratory rate that is less than 8 breaths/min or who have shallow breathing and have a significantly elevated PCO_2. Oxygen should not be administered prophylactically to patients who present following an opioid overdose as they are dependent on their hypoxic respiratory drive. If a patient's oxygen saturation begins to drop following an opioid overdose, the treatment would be ventilation and naloxone administration, not just oxygen.

Yealy DM, et al. The safety of prehospital naloxone administration by paramedics. *Ann Emerg Med.* 1990;19:902-905.

3.9. Answer: E. It would be impossible to differentiate between a patient who is sympathomimetic from one who is anticholinergic based on vital signs alone. While both toxidromes will lead to pupillary dilation, the pupils are minimally reactive in anticholinergic toxicity and completely reactive in sympathomimetic toxicity. Patients with anticholinergic toxicity have dry mucous membranes and urinary retention. Diaphoresis is present in patients who have sympathomimetic toxicity.

Goldfrank L, et al. Anticholinergic poisoning. *J Toxicol Clin Toxicol.* 1982;19:17-25.

3.10. Answer: B. This patient is presenting with opioid withdrawal. Patients in opioid withdrawal have an elevated blood pressure and an elevated heart rate, and they are often anxious with dilated pupils. They also have vomiting and diarrhea with increased peristalsis. Piloerection and yawning are typical of opioid withdrawal. Administration of 10 mg of intramuscular methadone is a safe and effective therapy in patients who present with acute opioid withdrawal.

Su MK, et al. Low dose intramuscular methadone for acute mild to moderate opioid withdrawal syndrome. *Am J Emerg Med.* 2018;36: 1951-1956.

Principles of Managing the Acutely Poisoned or Overdosed Patient

4

QUESTIONS

4.1. A 27-year-old man with a history of opioid use disorder presents to the emergency department unresponsive and cyanotic with a respiratory rate of 4 breaths/minute. What is the first priority in the management of this patient?
A. Ensuring adequate airway positioning and providing bag valve mask ventilation
B. Endotracheal intubation
C. 100% oxygen by non-rebreather mask
D. Administration of naloxone either intramuscularly or intravenously
E. Arterial blood gas

4.2. Which of the following interventions is acceptable as empiric therapy for a patient who presents to the emergency department with altered mental status?
A. Physostigmine
B. Flumazenil
C. Forced diuresis
D. Urinary alkalinization
E. Thiamine

4.3. A 24-year-old man presents to the emergency department with altered mental status. He has a rectal temperature of 106.2 °F (41.2 °C). How should this patient's temperature be lowered?
A. Ice packs to the axillae and groin
B. Immediate immersion in an ice bath
C. A towel soaked with rubbing alcohol placed on his forehead and chest
D. Administration of 20 mg/kg of rectal acetaminophen
E. No indication to actively cool this patient until temperature exceeds 107 °F (41.2 °C)

4.4. A 22-year-old man presents to the emergency department following an intentional ingestion. Which of the following physical examination findings is more consistent with an underlying neurological disorder as compared to a toxicologic etiology?
A. Asymmetric pupillary examination
B. Bilaterally fixed and dilated pupils
C. Bilateral lower extremity clonus
D. Ascending painful neuropathy
E. Generalized tonic-clonic seizure

4.5. A 72-year-old man presents to the emergency department following an intentional overdose of his oral sulfonylurea. He is hypoglycemic to 15 mg/dL (0.83 mmol/L). How many milliliters of 10% dextrose are needed to ensure that he gets a 50-gram bolus of dextrose?
A. 50 mL
B. 100 mL
C. 200 mL
D. 500 mL
E. 1,000 mL

4.6. A 27-year-old man presents to the emergency department with altered mental status that is attributed to alcohol intoxication. His initial ethanol concentration is 320 mg/dL (69.5 mmol/L). Five hours later, the team is concerned that he is still not awake and are planning on performing imaging and laboratory evaluations. Which of the following ethanol concentrations would be within the range of his expected repeat ethanol concentration?
A. 0 mg/dL
B. 50 mg/dL (10.9 mmol/L)
C. 100 mg/dL (21.7 mmol/L)
D. 200 mg/dL (43.4 mmol/L)
E. 300 mg/dL (65.1 mmol/L)

4.7. Which of the following interventions is a first-line therapy for a hypotensive patient with clear lungs and an unknown overdose?
A. Fluid challenge
B. Cardiac inotrope
C. Vasopressor
D. Whole blood
E. Glucagon

4.8. Naloxone administration is indicated in patients who exhibit which of the following findings?
A. Tramadol-associated seizures
B. Nausea and vomiting following administration of morphine
C. Unresponsiveness following an unknown ingestion
D. Respiratory depression of an unknown etiology
E. Hearing loss after chronic opioid use

4.9. Which of the following statements is correct regarding the management of a poisoned patient in her third trimester of pregnancy?
A. Activated charcoal is contraindicated in pregnancy
B. Shock is easier to identify in pregnant patients than patients who are not pregnant
C. Hypotension improves if a pregnant patient is laid flat on her back
D. Hyperbaric oxygen therapy is indicated at lower carboxyhemoglobin levels as compared to non-pregnant patients
E. N-acetylcysteine should not be given in pregnancy

4.10. A 26-year-old man presents to the emergency department with altered mental status, tachypnea, and hyperpnea following a known ingestion of aspirin. He has a serum blood glucose concentration of 90 mg/dL (5 mmol/L). Which of the following interventions is immediately indicated?
A. Immediate endotracheal intubation
B. Acetazolamide administration to achieve urine alkalinization
C. Sedation with midazolam to treat the patient's agitation
D. Dextrose, 1 g/kg bolus
E. Continuous kidney replacement therapy

ANSWERS

4.1. Answer: A. Ensuring adequate airway positioning, appropriate oxygenation, and ventilation is always the priority in the management of any patient. This should never be delayed for any laboratory evaluation or antidote administration. Furthermore, in patients who present following an opioid overdose, administering bag valve ventilation prior to administration of naloxone minimizes the incidence of acute respiratory distress syndrome (ARDS).

Mills CA, et al. Cardiovascular effects of fentanyl reversal by naloxone at varying arterial carbon dioxide tensions in dogs. *Anesth Analg.* 1988;67:730-736.

4.2. Answer: E. Thiamine is an exceptionally safe medication and is reasonable to administer to all patients who present with altered mental status. Patients who have Wernicke encephalopathy will improve after thiamine administration. Administration of physostigmine in the absence of antimuscarinic toxicity causes muscarinic toxicity characterized by salivation, urination, defecation, and possibly severe bradycardia or asystole. Flumazenil is a competitive benzodiazepine antagonist. It should not be administered to patients with unknown or unclear overdoses as it precipitates withdrawal seizures in benzodiazepine-dependent patients. Forced diuresis is not efficacious and causes pulmonary and cerebral edema. Empiric urinary alkalinization puts patients at an increased risk of hypokalemia, resultant electrocardiographic changes, and dysrhythmias.

Reuler JB, et al. Wernicke's encephalopathy. *N Engl J Med.* 1985;312: 1035-1037.

4.3. Answer: B. Hyperthermia is associated with significant mortality, regardless of etiology. Patients who have core temperatures greater than 105 °F (40.6 °C) should be cooled immediately as rapid cooling results in improved outcomes. In heatstroke victims, cooling within 1 hour resulted in 5% mortality, but mortality rose to 18% when cooling required more than 1 hour. The fastest way to cool hyperthermic patients is by immersing them in an ice bath until they reach a temperature of 101 °F (38.3 °C).

Knochel JP. Environmental heat illness: An eclectic review. *Arch Intern Med.* 1974;133:841-863.

4.4. Answer: A. Asymmetric findings, such as this patient's pupillary examination, make a toxicologic etiology very unlikely and warrant further evaluation for an underlying neurologic disorder. While it would be possible to have asymmetric pupils following a topical administration of certain eyedrops (for example, ones with antimuscarinic properties), this does not typically occur after an ingestion.

Bilaterally fixed and dilated pupils occur with antimuscarinic toxicity; bilateral lower extremity clonus occurs with serotonin toxicity; an ascending painful neuropathy occurs with thallium poisoning; and generalized tonic-clonic seizures develop following both overdose and withdrawal of many xenobiotics.

Tokuda Y, et al. Pupillary evaluation for differential diagnosis of coma. *Postgrad Med J.* 2003;79:49-51.

4.5. Answer: D. The correct dose of dextrose in patients who are hypoglycemic is 0.5-1 gram/kg. Adults who are hypoglycemic are usually treated with 25-50 grams of 50% dextrose in water (D50). Occasionally, however, there are shortages of D50, and alternative formulations are necessary. By definition, 10% dextrose is equal to 10 grams of dextrose in 100 mL of water; therefore, 500 mL is needed to administer 50 grams.

https://www.fda.gov/drugs/drug-shortages/search-list-extended-use-dates-assist-drug-shortages. Accessed July 4, 2021.

4.6. Answer: D. The metabolism of ethanol is fairly constant between 15 and 30 mg/dL/hour (3.3-6.5 mmol/L/hour). This patient, therefore, should have metabolized somewhere between 75 and 150 mg/dL (16.3-32.6 mmol/L), which would put his expected concentration between 170 and 245 mg/dL (36.9-53.2 mmol/L). Patients who are still unarousable at 3-4 hours after initial assessment should be evaluated for other causes that lead to change in mental status, including an underlying intracranial process.

Brennan DF, et al. Ethanol elimination rates in an ED population. *Am J Emerg Med.* 1995;13:276-280.

4.7. Answer: A. Multiple physiologic mechanisms exist for the hypotension that occurs following an overdose and include decreased cardiac output, relative hypovolemia, and decreased peripheral vascular resistance. The initial treatment is isotonic saline infusion. If hypotension or shock continues despite a fluid challenge or if the patient is unable to tolerate a fluid challenge, an antidote, a vasopressor, or an inotrope is often indicated.

Benowitz NL, et al. Cardiopulmonary catastrophes in drug overdosed patients. *Med Clin North Am.* 1979;63:267-297.

4.8. Answer: D. Naloxone is indicated in patients who have respiratory depression following an opioid overdose. It is reasonable to try a dose of naloxone in patients who have an unknown ingestion and respiratory depression. Seizures that occur following tramadol overdose respond to benzodiazepines. Nausea and vomiting are not an indication to administer naloxone. Naloxone is not indicated in patients who are only unresponsive with no respiratory depression.

While hearing loss and tinnitus occur in patients following both acute and chronic opioid use, the treatment is to stop the opioid, not to administer naloxone.

Pasternak GW. Pharmacological mechanisms of opioid analgesics. *Clin Neuropharmacol.* 1993;16:1-18.

4.9. Answer: D. Maternal carboxyhemoglobin levels do not accurately reflect fetal carboxyhemoglobin or tissue carbon monoxide concentrations; therefore, hyperbaric oxygen therapy is indicated at lower levels in pregnant woman. Activated charcoal is not contraindicated in pregnancy; however, caution regarding the volume administered is warranted to ensure that the patient does not vomit and aspirate the activated charcoal. The primary concern should be for the health of the mother and a lifesaving antidote should not be withheld. Cardiac output and total blood volume increase throughout pregnancy; therefore, signs of shock manifest later than they would in a woman who is not pregnant. Rolling a patient to her left side would remove vena caval compression from the gravid uterus, permitting more blood return to the heart.

Goldstein DP. Carbon monoxide poisoning in pregnancy. *Am J Obstet Gynecol.* 1965;92:526-528.

Koren G, et al. A multicenter, prospective study of fetal outcome following accidental carbon monoxide poisoning in pregnancy. *Reprod Toxicol.* 1991;5:397-403.

4.10. Answer: D. Patients who present with salicylate toxicity and have altered mental status could have neuroglycopenia, a condition where their serum glucose does not correspond with the central nervous system glucose. It is reasonable to trial a bolus of dextrose to see if a patient's mental status improves. Tachypnea and hyperpnea alone are not an indication to intubate a patient who has salicylate toxicity; in fact, caution is needed prior to intubation as acidemia worsens salicylism. While acetazolamide causes urinary alkalinization, it also leads to a decrease in the serum pH, which should be avoided in patients who have aspirin toxicity. Sedation also leads to a drop in the serum pH and should be done carefully; if sedation is needed for placement of a hemodialysis catheter, ketamine is a reasonable option. If dialysis is indicated, intermittent hemodialysis is far superior to continuous kidney replacement therapy in the management of aspirin toxicity.

Thurston JH, et al. Reduced brain glucose with normal plasma glucose in salicylate poisoning. *Clin Invest.* 1970;49:2139-2145.

Kuzak N, et al. Reversal of salicylate-induced euglycemic delirium with dextrose. *Clin Toxicol.* 2007;45:526-529.

Techniques Used to Prevent Gastrointestinal Absorption

5

QUESTIONS

5.1. A 27-year-old woman presents to the hospital 3.5 hours after an intentional overdose of salicylates. She is awake and alert with marked tachypnea and hyperpnea. What method of gastrointestinal decontamination is most reasonable in this scenario?
A. Orogastric lavage
B. Activated charcoal
C. Induced emesis
D. Whole bowel irrigation
E. Gastric decontamination should not be performed

5.2. Which of the following cathartics does not lead to life-threatening fluid and electrolyte disturbances and is therefore reasonably safe to administer in large amounts?
A. Sodium sulfate
B. Sodium phosphate
C. Magnesium sulfate
D. Sorbitol
E. Polyethylene glycol electrolyte lavage solution (PEG-ELS)

5.3. Which of the following options would be most completely adsorbed by 100 g of activated charcoal?
A. 100 tablets of 325 mg aspirin
B. 100 tablets of 200 mg sustained-release theophylline
C. 100 tablets of 500 mg L-dopa
D. 100 mL of 30% ethanol
E. 200 mg of potassium cyanide

5.4. Which of the following options is true of activated charcoal and oral N-acetylcysteine (NAC) interactions?
A. Activated charcoal adsorbs NAC in vitro but does not actually decrease bioavailability
B. Activated charcoal adsorbs NAC and decreases bioavailability, but not to a clinically significant degree
C. A clinically significant decrease in NAC bioavailability is demonstrated due to activated charcoal, but this is overcome by increasing NAC dosage
D. The need to use activated charcoal and NAC concomitantly is an absolute indication for the use of IV NAC
E. Well-controlled clinical studies show that the interaction between NAC and activated charcoal is of no significance

5.5. A 30-year-old man presents to the hospital 2 hours following an intentional overdose of acetaminophen. What therapy is indicated at this time?
A. Immediate administration of N-acetylcysteine (NAC)
B. Obtain an acetaminophen concentration and plot it on the Rumack-Mathew nomogram
C. Perform an orogastric lavage
D. Administer a single dose of activated charcoal
E. Transfer to psychiatry if the reported ingestion is less than 150 mg/kg

5.6. A 36-year-old woman presents to the hospital 35 minutes following an intentional ingestion of immediate-release diltiazem. On her initial abdominal examination, surgical scars are noted, and further history reveals that she had bariatric surgery performed. Which of the following therapies is contraindicated?
   A. Orogastric lavage
   B. Extracorporeal membrane oxygenation
   C. High-dose insulin euglycemia therapy
   D. Norepinephrine
   E. Multiple-dose activated charcoal

5.7. Syrup of ipecac is no longer routinely recommended in the management of poisoned patients due its significant side effect profile. Patients who chronically abused syrup of ipecac were at risk of developing what disease process?
   A. Cardiomyopathy
   B. Pneumonitis
   C. Rhabdomyolysis
   D. Lung cancer
   E. Chloracne

5.8. Which of the following options is the most reasonable initial dose of activated charcoal?
   A. 200 g
   B. 100 g
   C. 50 g

   D. A 10:1 ratio (10 times the amount ingested by history)
   E. 0.5-1 g/kg

5.9. A 65-year-old patient receives a large intravenous dose of aminophylline in error. Activated charcoal is recommended due to which of the following properties of this xenobiotic?
   A. High protein binding
   B. Large volume of distribution
   C. Enterohepatic recirculation
   D. Enteroenteric recirculation
   E. It forms concretions

5.10. A 27-year-old man presents to the emergency department for further management of drug package ingestion. Which of the following options is an indication to perform surgery on a patient who is a body packer?
   A. More than 50 packages in the gastrointestinal tract
   B. Respiratory depression requiring naloxone
   C. A negative urine drug screen that turns positive for cocaine
   D. Antimuscarinic toxicity
   E. Further history reveals the patient is a body stuffer not a body packer

ANSWERS

5.1. Answer: B. Although this patient presented greater than 1 hour after an ingestion, studies have demonstrated that in 60% of patients who presented later than an hour following ingestion, residual drug contents were still present in their stomachs. In the setting of large overdoses, there is delayed gastric emptying as well as pylorospasm. Autopsies of patients who died several hours after overdose still demonstrated pill fragments in the gastrointestinal tract. This patient is awake and alert and would be able to drink the activated charcoal. Since salicylates form concretions, an additional dose of activated charcoal would be reasonable. Although an awake lavage is possible, many clinicians have not performed an orogastric lavage, and the risks of an endotracheal intubation in this patient would be much higher than the potential benefit of an orogastric lavage 3.5 hours after an overdose. Induced emesis is no longer used routinely in the treatment of overdose patients. Whole bowel irrigation is used for patients who are "body packers," who have lead chips in their gastrointestinal tract, who overdose on iron and lithium, and who overdose on certain extended-release formulations of medication. It is not indicated in this patient.

Miyauchi M, et al. Evaluation of residual toxic substances in the stomach using upper gastrointestinal endoscopy for management of patients with oral drug overdose on admission: A prospective, observational study. *Medicine (Baltimore)*. 2015;94:e463.

Livshits Z, et al. Retained drugs in the gastrointestinal tracts of deceased victims of oral drug overdose. *Clin Toxicol*. 2015;53:113-118.

5.2. Answer: E. Large volumes of polyethylene glycol electrolyte lavage solution (PEG-ELS) are used as part of whole bowel irrigation as it does not lead to fluid and electrolyte disturbances. All the other listed options are associated with life-threatening fluid and electrolyte disturbances, with rare cases of death reported.

Martin R, et al. Fatal poisoning from sodium phosphate enema: A case report and experimental study. *JAMA*. 1987;257:2190-2192.

Smilkstein MJ, et al. Magnesium levels after magnesium containing cathartics. *J Toxicol Clin Toxicol*. 1988;26:51-65.

Farley TA. Severe hypernatremia after use of an activated charcoal-sorbitol suspension. *J Pediatr*. 1986;109:719-722.

5.3. Answer: E. Using the concept of an ideal activated charcoal-to-drug ratio of 10:1, it is evident that the amounts in A, B, and C would exceed the capacity of this activated charcoal dose. The same is true of the ethanol, but particularly since ethanol is so rapidly absorbed from the gastrointestinal tract. Cyanide salts are often thought not to be adsorbed to charcoal, but in fact, they are adsorbed at a much lower affinity (1 g activated charcoal: 35 mg KCN). Despite the low affinity, a 100:1 activated charcoal-to-drug ratio would be effective for cyanide salts.

Anderson AH. Experimental studies on the pharmacology of activated charcoal: I. Absorption power of charcoal in aqueous solutions. *Acta Pharmacol.* 1947;2:68-78.

Lass W. Therapy of acute oral poisonings by organic solvents: Treatment by activated charcoal in combination with laxatives. *Arch Toxicol.* 1980;4(suppl):406-409.

Neuvonen PJ, Olkkola KT. Effect of purgatives on antidotal efficacy of oral activated charcoal. *Hum Toxicol.* 1986;5:255-263.

5.4. Answer: B. When enough subjects are used, activated charcoal studies confirm N-acetylcysteine (NAC) adsorption and decreased bioavailability. Indirect evidence, however, strongly suggests that the interaction is of probably no concern in most circumstances. Definitive studies have not been done, but there is no evidence that the efficacy of oral NAC is diminished when activated charcoal is used. Intravenous NAC completely negates any relevant effect of oral activated charcoal on NAC kinetics.

Ekins BR, et al. The effects of activated charcoal on N-acetylcysteine absorption in normal subjects. *Am J Emerg Med.* 1987;5:483-487.

Spiller HA, et al. A prospective evaluation of the effect of activated charcoal before oral N-acetylcysteine in acetaminophen overdose. *Ann Emerg Med.* 1994;23:519-523.

5.5. Answer: D. In patients who present following an acute acetaminophen overdose with a known time of ingestion, the Rumack-Mathew nomogram should be used to guide treatment decisions. The nomogram, however, begins at 4 hours post ingestion and is not used to predict toxicity before then. Therefore, we recommend that a 4-hour concentration be drawn and that concentration be plotted on the nomogram. Since the patient presented early, it is recommended to administer a single dose of 1 g/kg of oral activated charcoal to adsorb some of the drug in the gastrointestinal tract, with the hope that this will drop the concentration below the nomogram treatment line. Since N-acetylcysteine (NAC) is very safe and effective, there is no need to perform an orogastric lavage on this patient. Furthermore, the success of NAC approaches 100% if it is given prior to 8 hours; therefore, there is no reason to initiate NAC, and it is safe to wait for a 4-hour concentration to make treatment decisions. This patient presented following an intentional ingestion. It is not enough to rely on the reported dose; a concentration should be checked prior to the decision to transfer any patient to psychiatry.

Buckley NA, et al. Activated charcoal reduces the need for *N*-acetylcysteine treatment after acetaminophen (paracetamol) overdose. *J Toxicol Clin Toxicol.* 1999;37:753-757.

5.6. Answer: A. Diltiazem overdoses are life-threatening, and in most situations if a patient presents this soon after overdose, orogastric lavage is recommended. However, bariatric surgery poses an increased risk of perforation given the altered gastric anatomy, and therefore, orogastric lavage is contraindicated in this patient.

Layton GM, et al. Gastrointestinal decontamination considerations in weight loss surgery patients. *Clin Toxicol.* 2015;53:702.

Personne M, Westberg US. Gastric decontamination in poisoned patients operated for bariatric surgery. *Clin Toxicol.* 2014;52:412.

5.7. Answer: A. Syrup of ipecac was formerly recommended as standard treatment for children who ingested toxic substances at home and was readily available without a prescription. However, it was abused by patients who suffered from bulimia. In addition to electrolyte abnormalities, patients who abuse ipecac chronically are at risk for developing cardiomyopathy, dysrhythmias, and dying. The toxin in ipecac that is responsible is emetine. The US Food and Drug Administration (FDA) rescinded the recommendation for the nonprescription use of ipecac in 2003.

Friedman EJ. Death from ipecac intoxication in a patient with anorexia nervosa. *Am J Psychiatry.* 1984;141:702-703.

5.8. Answer: E. The optimum dose of activated charcoal is the largest dose that is safely tolerated, 0.5-1 g/kg. Two hundred grams in one dose exceeds any patient's tolerance. Fifty or 100 g might be appropriate in an adult but could be excessive in a child, especially as the larger volume is a risk for vomiting. Using the activated charcoal:drug ratio is a useful concept to be aware of when greater initial or repeat dosing is needed. It is not logical to use doses of activated charcoal less than 0.5-1 g/kg for small ingestions when a larger activated charcoal dose is generally well tolerated.

Olkkola KT. Effect of charcoal-drug ratio on antidotal efficacy of oral activated charcoal in man. *Br J Clin Pharmacol.* 1985;19:767-773.

5.9. Answer: D. In certain xenobiotics, activated charcoal enhances elimination through interruption of either the enteroenteric or the enterohepatic recirculation. The entire effect of activated charcoal takes place in the gastrointestinal tract. Oral activated charcoal is not absorbed through the wall of the gastrointestinal tract, but rather passes straight through the gut unchanged. To be adsorbed to activated charcoal, the xenobiotic must be dissolved in the gastrointestinal liquid phase and be in physical contact with the activated charcoal. Theophylline ophylline undergoes enteroenteric recirculation, and when activated charcoal is administered orally, it functions as gut dialysis. In one study, the area under the curve and half-life of aminophylline were reduced by 46% and 49% respectively following multiple-dose activated charcoal administration.

Berlinger WG, et al. Enhancement of theophylline clearance by oral activated charcoal. *Clin Pharmacol Ther*. 1983;33:351-354.

5.10. Answer: C. Body packers are patients who transport large amounts of well-manufactured drug packages. Most of these patients are managed safely with whole bowel irrigation until the packages are all passed. Indications to surgically remove the packets include signs of a cocaine package leakage or a small bowel obstruction. If the package contains an opioid, management with naloxone alone is acceptable. However, given the significant toxicity caused by a ruptured cocaine package with no known antidote, signs of a leaking package, such as a conversion to a positive urine drug screen, prompts surgical consultation. There is no specific number of packages that mandates surgical intervention. Often, patients will ingest an antimuscarinic xenobiotic to slow gastric motility so as not pass the packages prematurely; antimuscarinic toxicity is not an indication to perform surgery. Body stuffers usually ingest a small amount of drug to avoid detection by law enforcement agents. They are managed symptomatically and typically do not need surgical intervention.

Traub SJ, et al. Body packing—the internal concealment of illicit drugs. *N Engl J Med*. 2003;349:2519-2526.

Principles and Techniques Applied to Enhance Elimination

6

QUESTIONS

6.1. High-flux hemodialysis, using membranes with larger pores and surface area, effectively enhances clearance for xenobiotics up to what size?
   A. 15 Daltons (Da)
   B. 150 Da
   C. 1,500 Da
   D. 15,000 Da
   E. 150,000 Da

6.2. A 56-year-old man is brought to the hospital with confusion and somnolence. He has anuric kidney failure, with a serum lithium concentration of 5.9 mmol/L. His last dose of lithium was 3 days prior to presentation and he did not take more than his prescribed dose. After a 4-hour session of high-efficiency hemodialysis, his lithium concentration is 2.3 mmol/L. If the concentration is checked again 2 hours later, which of the following concentrations would be expected?
   A. 0 mmol/L
   B. 1.4 mmol/L
   C. 2.3 mmol/L
   D. 3.5 mmol/L
   E. 7.2 mmol/L

6.3. Which of the following xenobiotics would most likely reduce absorption if given shortly following an acute overdose of lithium carbonate?
   A. Prussian blue
   B. Activated charcoal
   C. Cholestyramine
   D. Fuller's earth
   E. Sodium polystyrene sulfonate

6.4. Three patients from a hemodialysis unit present to the emergency department simultaneously with nausea, emesis, and elevated methemoglobin levels. What might have prevented their presentation?
   A. Slowing the rate of dialysis
   B. Running dialysate fluid over activated charcoal
   C. Replacing cellulose membranes with polysulfone
   D. Pretreating the patients with corticosteroids
   E. Flushing the dialysis membrane with 0.9% sodium chloride

6.5. Which of the following characteristics would make a toxin most amenable to removal with hemodialysis?
   A. Small volume of distribution, low protein binding, high water solubility
   B. Small volume of distribution, high protein binding, high water solubility
   C. Small volume of distribution, low protein binding, low water solubility
   D. Large volume of distribution, low protein binding, high water solubility
   E. Large volume of distribution, low protein binding, low water solubility

6.6. If a 60-kg man ingests 2,400 mg of a cyclic antidepressant with a volume of distribution (Vd) of 40 L/kg, what would his expected serum concentration be?
   A. 10 ng/mL
   B. 100 ng/mL
   C. 1 mcg/mL
   D. 10 mcg/mL
   E. 100 mcg/mL

6.7. The patient in question 6.6 undergoes 4 hours of intermittent hemodialysis, resulting in a clearance of the drug of 200 mL/min. What percentage of the initial dose did the hemodialysis session remove?
A. 2%
B. 10%
C. 20%
D. 50%
E. 100%

6.8. What is the change to the urinary excretion of salicylates when urine pH increases from 6.5 to 7.5?
A. Decrease by 50%
B. No change
C. Increase by 100%
D. Increase by 400%
E. Increase by 800%

6.9. In comparison to conventional hemodialysis, the Molecular Adsorbents Recirculation System (MARS) or the Prometheus system is better suited to remove toxins with what characteristic?
A. High volume of distribution
B. High protein binding
C. Large molecular weight
D. Low water solubility
E. High lipophilicity

6.10. A 1-month-old girl is brought to the emergency department after ingestion of methyl salicylate. Her serum concentration on presentation is 85 mg/dL. If standard treatment fails, what other modality would be reasonable?
A. Plasmapheresis
B. Molecular Adsorbents Recirculation System (MARS)
C. Single-pass albumin dialysis
D. Forced diuresis
E. Exchange transfusion

ANSWERS

6.1. Answer: C. Although most xenobiotics susceptible to enhanced clearance by hemodialysis are less than 1,000 Da, high-flux hemodialysis employs modern membranes capable of effective removal of larger compounds, such as vancomycin (1,449 Da).

Decker BS, et al. Vancomycin pharmacokinetics and pharmacodynamics during short daily hemodialysis. *Clin J Am Soc Nephrol.* 2010;5:1981-1987.

6.2. Answer: D. Shortly after cessation of intermittent hemodialysis, lithium concentrations in patients with chronic toxicity are expected to rise slightly, as lithium redistributes from the extravascular space into the blood. This "rebound" is seldom worrisome, as it represents drug leaving more toxicologically susceptible compartments. After 3 days, it is unlikely that lithium would continue to be absorbed, making it unlikely to rise above the initial concentration.

Amdisen A, Skjoldborg H. Haemodialysis for lithium poisoning. *Lancet.* 1969;2:213.

6.3. Answer: E. Sodium polystyrene sulfonate reduces lithium absorption; however, it is associated with hypokalemia and is not routinely recommended. While the other choices are used to reduce absorption in other poisonings, there is no role for Prussian Blue, activated charcoal, cholestyramine, or Fuller's earth in the management of patients with lithium overdose.

Ghannoum M, et al. Successful treatment of lithium toxicity with sodium polystyrene sulfonate: A retrospective cohort study. *Clin Toxicol (Phila).* 2010;48:34-41.

6.4. Answer: B. Chloramine forms when chlorine in municipal water supplies complexes with nitrogenous compounds and causes gastrointestinal symptoms, hemolytic anemia, and methemoglobinemia. To avoid chloramine toxicity in dialysis patients who are exposed to high volumes of municipal water, redundant beds of activated charcoal are typically required to purify dialysate water.

Ward DM. Chloramine removal from water used in hemodialysis. *Adv Ren Replace Ther.* 1996;3:337-347.

6.5. Answer: A. In order for a toxin to be dialyzable, a significant portion must remain within the blood compartment for a reasonable period of time after exposure (low volume of distribution) and have a high water solubility. Protein binding must generally be low, though some protein-bound toxins become more amenable to removal when binding sites are saturated at high serum toxin concentrations, such as valproic acid.

Hicks LK, McFarlane PA. Valproic acid overdose and haemodialysis. *Nephrol Dial Transplant.* 2001;16:1483-1486.

Kielstein JT, et al. Efficiency of high-flux hemodialysis in the treatment of valproic acid intoxication. *J Toxicol Clin Toxicol.* 2003;41:873-876.

6.6. Answer: C. The formula for estimation of maximum concentration by ingested dose is given by:

$$\text{Concentration} = \text{Dose (mg)}/(\text{Vd [L/kg]} \times \text{Patient weight [kg]})$$
$$= 2{,}400 \text{ mg}/(40 \text{ L/kg} \times 60 \text{ kg})$$
$$= 2{,}400 \text{ mg}/2{,}400 \text{ L}$$
$$= 1 \text{ mg/L}$$
$$= 1 \text{ mcg/mL}$$

Garella S. Extracorporeal techniques in the treatment of exogenous intoxications. *Kidney Int.* 1988;33:735-754.

6.7. Answer: A. This question highlights the ineffectiveness of dialysis for a toxin with a large volume of distribution. If hemodialysis results in a clearance of 200 mL/min of the toxin, and the serum concentration is 1 microg/mL, then for 4 hours:

$$1 \text{ mcg/mL} \times 200 \text{ mL} \times 240 \text{ min} = 48 \text{ mg removed}$$
$$48 \text{ mg}/2400 \text{ mg} = 2\%$$

Garella S. Extracorporeal techniques in the treatment of exogenous intoxications. *Kidney Int.* 1988;33:735-754.

6.8. Answer: D. Elimination of weak acids, including salicylates, is enhanced by alkalinization of the urine. At an alkaline urine pH, weak acids are in the ionic form, reducing tubular reabsorption. Volume overload, hypernatremia, and hypokalemia are possible complications of urine alkalinization by sodium bicarbonate infusion, but effective alkalinization to 7.5 from 6.5 increases urinary excretion fourfold.

Proudfoot AT, et al. Does urine alkalinization increase salicylate elimination? If so, why? *Toxicol Rev.* 2003;22:129-136.

6.9. Answer: B. Both MARS and the Prometheus system include human albumin in the dialysate solution to capture and remove protein-bound compounds. While typically used as a bridge to transplant in cases of liver failure, such as that resulting from acetaminophen or amatoxin poisoning, their use is also described in case reports for early toxin removal.

Kantola T, et al. Early molecular adsorbents recirculating system treatment of Amanita mushroom poisoning. *Ther Apher Dial.* 2009;13: 399-403.

6.10. Answer: E. Exchange transfusion is reasonable in small children, especially in facilities that are unable to perform hemodialysis. In addition to successfully being used for severe salicylism in pediatric patients, exchange transfusion is also employed for toxins that are large (>10,000 Da) or highly protein bound.

Manikian A, et al. Exchange transfusion in severe infant salicylism. *Vet Hum Toxicol.* 2002;44:224-227.

Laboratory Principles

QUESTIONS

7.1. Which laboratory technique is most commonly used to detect the presence of a toxic alcohol?
   A. Atomic absorption
   B. Gas chromatography
   C. Thin-layer chromatography
   D. Gas chromatography + mass spectrometry
   E. Immunoassay

7.2. The gold standard for confirmation of drugs of abuse in urine is an analysis performed using which of the following techniques?
   A. Immunoassay
   B. Gas chromatography + mass spectrometry
   C. Atomic absorption spectrophotometry
   D. Thin-layer chromatography
   E. High-performance liquid chromatography

7.3. A 26-year-old man presents to the emergency department with generalized tonic-clonic seizures. In which of the following ingestions should a quantitative concentration be obtained?
   A. Isoniazid
   B. Phencyclidine
   C. Theophylline
   D. Isopropyl alcohol
   E. Benzodiazepines

7.4. Which of the following statements regarding the analysis of drugs in body fluids is correct?
   A. False-positive results are more common than false-negative results
   B. Gas chromatography + mass spectroscopy should always be used, if available
   C. A confirmed positive finding on a toxicology screen confirms the diagnosis of poisoning
   D. The sensitivity of thin-layer chromatography is extremely high
   E. Immunoassays provide both high sensitivity and high specificity

7.5. Comparable ethanol concentrations will be present in which pairs of specimens?
   A. Serum and whole blood
   B. Serum and urine
   C. Serum and plasma
   D. Serum and breath
   E. Serum and saliva

7.6. Regarding high-performance liquid chromatography (HPLC), which of the following options is true?
   A. The column temperature is not regulated
   B. The operating costs are much lower in comparison to gas chromatography
   C. Compounds are separated based on volatility
   D. Compounds are separated based on solubility
   E. Compounds are separately based on viscosity

7.7. A 22-year-old woman presents to the emergency department unconscious with respiratory depression and miotic pupils. Naloxone 0.04 mg is administered intravenously and the patient's respiratory effort improves. A urine drug screen is obtained and it demonstrates no opioids. Which of the following xenobiotics best explains her presentation?
A. Codeine
B. Hydrocodone
C. Hydromorphone
D. Diacetylmorphine
E. Fentanyl

7.8. A 3-year-old boy presents to the emergency department for evaluation of a cough and shortness of breath. A urine drug screen is sent unintentionally, and the results are positive for phencyclidine (PCP). Which of the following xenobiotics is the best explanation for this result?
A. Diphenhydramine
B. Albuterol
C. Prednisone
D. Ipratropium
E. Phencyclidine

7.9. An 84-year-old woman presents to the emergency department with ataxia and nystagmus. She has a known past medical history of a seizure disorder and is prescribed phenytoin. Her dosage has not changed. A serum concentration is obtained, and it is within a therapeutic range. Which of the following is the likely explanation for her symptoms?
A. Hypoalbuminemia
B. Tricyclic antidepressant ingestion
C. Acetaminophen ingestion
D. Hypermagnesemia
E. Opioid withdrawal

7.10. Which analyte and laboratory method are **incorrectly** matched?
A. Digoxin: Immunoassay
B. Lead: Atomic absorption spectrometry
C. Carbamazepine: Immunoassay
D. Phenothiazines: Thin-layer chromatography
E. Isopropanol: Flame emission photometry

ANSWERS

7.1. Answer: B. Gas chromatography (GC) separates, identifies, and quantitates methanol, acetone, ethanol, ethylene glycol, and isopropanol. In a closed system, these alcohols are sufficiently volatile to be present in easily measurable concentrations in the air space (headspace) above a liquid specimen. A portion of this headspace is injected into a gas chromatography for analysis. Laboratories that do not have GC equipment often measure serum ethanol by manual or automated spectrophotometric methods that use alcohol dehydrogenase.

Burtis C, et al., eds. *Tietz Textbook of Clinical Chemistry and Molecular Diagnostics*. 5th ed. St. Louis, MO: Elsevier; 2012:832-888.

7.2. Answer: B. When urine drug testing is regulated by federal law, quantitative confirmation by gas chromatography + mass spectrometry (GC-MS) must be completed before a verified positive test result can be reported.

Department of Health and Human Services, Substance Abuse and Mental Health Services Administration. Mandatory guidelines and proposed revisions to mandatory guidelines for federal workplace drug testing programs. *Fed Reg.* 2015;80:28101-28151.

7.3. Answer: C. In patients with a suspected theophylline overdose, serum theophylline concentrations influence the decision to begin or maintain hemodialysis. Concentrations of the other xenobiotics will not lead to a change in management of the patient, which is based on the patient's signs and symptoms.

Shannon MW. Predictors of major toxicity after theophylline overdose. *Ann Intern Med.* 1993;119:1161-1167.

7.4. Answer: E. Proficiency testing data suggest that false-negative rates in toxicology testing are typically 10 to 30%, while false-positive rates are 0 to 10%. Gas chromatography + mass spectroscopy is relatively slow, expensive, and excessive in many instances. A consistent clinical presentation provides adequate confirmation for most results of medical testing, particularly if performed by immunoassays. Immunoassays have the sensitivity to detect nanomolar quantities, as in the case of digoxin assays, and also show excellent specificity when focused on a specific drug rather than a drug class. The sensitivity of thin-layer chromatography is typically around 0.5 to 1 mg/L, compared with 0.1 mg/L or less for other chromatographic approaches or immunoassays. Confirmed positives document the presence of a drug, but do not necessarily establish the presence of clinical toxicity.

> Osterloh JD. Utility and reliability of emergency toxicologic testing. *Emerg Med Clin North Am.* 1990;8:693-723.

7.5. Answer: C. Ethanol is dissolved in the water of body fluids and its concentration at equilibrium will be proportional to the water content. Serum and plasma both have a water content of 93% and will have comparable alcohol concentrations. Urine has a higher water content, and ethanol concentrations are likewise higher by 5-7%. Additionally, the urine concentration will be determined by the average ethanol concentration in the serum over the time of urine formation, rather than the serum concentration at time of urine collection. This leads to a higher urine/serum ratio during times when ethanol concentration is declining. Although saliva has a higher water content than plasma, salivary concentrations are typically 4-6% lower than serum concentrations, presumably reflecting incomplete equilibration. Breath ethanol is measured in g/210 L of breath. The amount of ethanol in 210 L of breath is approximately equal to the amount in 100 mL of whole blood. Because of the lower water content of red cells, whole blood ethanol concentration is about 13% lower than serum ethanol.

> Caplan YH. Blood, urine and other fluid and tissue specimens for alcohol analysis. In Garrott JC, ed. Medicolegal Aspects of Alcohol, 3d ed. Tucson, Lawyers and Judges Publishing, 1996, pp. 137-150.

> Morton MH, Dubowski KM. Breath as a specimen for analysis for ethanol and other low molecular weight alcohols. In: Garrott JC, ed. *Medicolegal Aspects of Alcohol.* 3rd ed. Tucson, AZ: Lawyers and Judges Publishing; 1996:171-180.

7.6. Answer: D. Column temperature is tightly regulated in gas chromatography as well as HPLC. HPLC is significantly more expensive to obtain and operate. Gas chromatography relies on volatility of a substance to determine the retention time. HPLC requires at least some solubility in the solvent of choice. The retention time of HPLC will be higher the more hydrophobic the substance is, in addition to its size and weight.

> Burtis C, et al, eds. *Tietz Textbook of Clinical Chemistry and Molecular Diagnostics.* 5th ed. St. Louis, MO: Elsevier; 2012:266-295.

7.7. Answer: E. Synthetic opioids, such as fentanyl, methadone, and meperidine have limited cross-reactivity with the standard opiate immunoassays. As much of the opioid supply in the United States contains synthetic opioids, it is important to rely on the history and physical examination in the management of these patients and not on a urine drug screen result.

> Reisfield GM, Bertholf RL. "Practical guide" to urine drug screening clarified. *Mayo Clin Proc.* 2008;83:848-849.

7.8. Answer: A. False positives on the PCP assay occur with xenobiotics that are structurally similar such as diphenhydramine, dextromethorphan, ketamine, and tramadol.

> Moeller KE, et al. Clinical interpretation of urine drug tests: What clinicians need to know about urine drug screens. *Mayo Clin Proc.* 2017;92:774-796.

7.9. Answer: A. This patient is exhibiting signs of phenytoin toxicity despite a therapeutic concentration. Phenytoin is highly protein bound (up to 90% at therapeutic concentrations). It is the free drug, however, that is responsible for toxicity. In hypoalbuminemia there is less protein available, and therefore, there is more free phenytoin. Patients also develop signs of phenytoin toxicity if another drug that binds even more strongly to albumin is ingested and thus displaces the phenytoin off the protein, causing signs of toxicity.

> Olanow CW, et al. The effects of salicylate on the pharmacokinetics of phenytoin. *Neurology.* 1981;31:341-342.

7.10. Answer: E. Isopropanol is typically quantitated by gas chromatography. Flame emission photometry is typically used to determine the concentration of lithium in body fluids.

> Burtis C, et al, eds. *Tietz Textbook of Clinical Chemistry and Molecular Diagnostics.* 5th ed. St. Louis, MO: Elsevier; 2012:266-295.

Principles of Diagnostic Imaging

QUESTIONS

8.1. Chronic exposure to which of the following xeno-biotics causes a decrease in bone density on plain radiographs?
A. Corticosteroids
B. Fluoride
C. Lithium carbonate
D. Calcium carbonate
E. Lead

8.2. An 80-year-old woman presents to the hospital with severe left-sided lower extremity pain. A radiograph demonstrates a mid-shaft transverse fracture of her femur. Which of the following medications best explains her presentation?
A. Ibuprofen
B. Calcium carbonate
C. Omeprazole
D. Prednisone
E. Alendronate

8.3. Which of the following inhaled xenobiotics causes coughing, wheezing, and diffuse airspace filling on chest radiograph?
A. Carbon monoxide
B. Ozone
C. Nitrogen dioxide
D. Carbon dioxide
E. Particulate fumes of zinc

8.4. Which of the following hydrocarbons is the most radiopaque?
A. Methylene chloride
B. Methylbromide
C. Dichloromethane
D. Trichloroethylene
E. Carbon tetrachloride

8.5. A chest radiograph is ordered on a 76-year-old man who is prescribed procainamide. Which of the following findings is an adverse effect of this medicine?
A. Hilar adenopathy
B. Diffuse patchy infiltrates
C. Fine reticular interstitial pattern
D. Pleural effusions
E. Mesothelioma

8.6. A 29-year-old man presents to the hospital after he was shot in the arm with a lead bullet. A radiograph demonstrates that the bullet is in the soft tissue of the forearm. Which of the following management strategies is indicated?
A. Surgical removal of the bullet
B. Oral succimer
C. Intramuscular dimercaprol (BAL)
D. Calcium disodium ethylenediaminetetraacetic acid (EDTA)
E. Local wound care

8.7. A 50-year-old man presents to the emergency department with painful, hypertrophic nodules in his bilateral wrists and knees. He reports that he was inhaling a chemical recreationally for several years while at work. Radiographic imaging of the affected joints suggests a diagnosis. Which of the following inhalants is most likely responsible?
A. Isobutyl nitrite
B. Carbon tetrachloride
C. Toluene
D. Difluoroethane
E. N-hexane

8.8. An 86-year-old woman presents to the emergency department with a chief complaint of shortness of breath and fever. A chest radiograph is performed and demonstrates fine interstitial and alveolar infiltrates. The symptoms began approximately 9 days following the initiation of a new medication. Which of the following is the most likely cause?
A. Nitrofurantoin
B. Ciprofloxacin
C. Bumetanide
D. Ibuprofen
E. Doxorubicin

8.9. Exposure to which of the following xenobiotics leads to cerebellar atrophy on magnetic resonance imaging (MRI)?
A. Lithium carbonate
B. Cadmium
C. Manganese
D. Methylmercury
E. Magnesium

8.10. An 89-year-old man presents to the emergency department with abdominal pain. A computed tomography (CT) of his abdomen demonstrates a new hepatic malignancy as well as multiple punctate opacities in the liver, spleen, and lymph nodes. Which of the following xenobiotics best explains this patient's findings?
A. Iron
B. Acetaminophen
C. Amitriptyline
D. Thorium dioxide
E. Thallium

ANSWERS

8.1. Answer: A. Chronic corticosteroid use frequently causes osteoporosis with resultant insufficiency fractures, most commonly vertebral body compression fractures. Chronic corticosteroid therapy is also associated with avascular necrosis, most frequently involving the femoral head and humeral head. The purported mechanism is increased fat deposition in the medullary cavity with resultant diminished blood flow. Avascular necrosis results in medullary lucencies followed by reparative sclerosis and skeletal collapse. Other causes include alcoholism, sickle cell disease, Caisson disease (dysbarism), and trauma. Fluorosis is associated with increased bone density. Lead toxicity causes a transverse metaphyseal band in the immature skeleton.

Mankin HJ. Nontraumatic necrosis of bone (osteonecrosis). *N Engl J Med.* 1992;326:1473-1479.

Neustadter LM, Weiss M. Medication-induced changes of bone. *Semin Roentgenol.* 1995;30:88-95.

8.2. Answer: E. A transverse, mid-shaft fracture of the femur is an atypical type of femur fracture. When it occurs, however, this fracture is associated with bisphosphonate use. Bisphosphonates supress bone turnover and fracture healing. While other medications are associated with osteopenia and increased risk of fracture, bisphosphonates are the only medication on this list that cause atypical fractures.

Schilcher J, et al. Bisphosphonate use and atypical fractures of the femoral shaft. *N Engl J Med.* 2011;364:1728-1737.

8.3. Answer: C. Delayed onset of diffuse airspace filling is characteristic of inhalation injury caused by a low water-soluble irritant gas such as nitrogen dioxide. The gas itself is nonirritating and so it is inhaled without the victim being aware of it. In the aqueous environment of the lung, it is converted into a highly irritating acid that is responsible for delayed onset of symptoms and radiographic findings. Carbon monoxide and carbon dioxide are a chemical asphyxiant and a simple asphyxiant, respectively, and cause hypoxia without radiographic abnormalities. Zinc oxide causes a delayed-onset influenza-like syndrome, usually without radiographic abnormalities.

Behrman AJ. Welders. In: Greenberg MI, et al, eds. *Occupational, Industrial and Environmental Toxicology.* St. Louis, MO: Mosby–Year Book; 1997:303-309.

Dee P, Armstrong P. Inhalational lung diseases. In: Armstrong P, et al, eds. *Imaging of Diseases of the Chest.* 2nd ed. St. Louis, MO: Mosby–Year Book; 1995:426-460.

8.4. Answer: E. Although knowing the atomic numbers of the constituent atoms in a molecule usually does not permit prediction of its radiopacity, for these simple molecules, the one with the greatest number of chlorine atoms (atomic number 17) will be the most radiopaque. If enough carbon tetrachloride is ingested, it is visible in the stomach on an abdominal radiograph if performed soon after the ingestion. It will most likely be visible on an upright radiograph because this will cause layering of the hydrocarbon in the stomach and produce a sharp horizontal border.

Dally SL, et al. Diagnosis of chlorinated hydrocarbon poisoning by x-ray examination. *Br J Ind Med*. 1987;44:424-425.

8.5. Answer: D. Procainamide is a common cause of the drug-induced lupus syndrome. Pleural effusions are often the major clinical manifestation. Fever, myalgias, and arthralgias are also common. More serious systemic lupus involvement, such as kidney or central nervous system disease, is uncommon. Pericardial effusions also sometimes occur. Patchy infiltrates occur only rarely. Medication-induced hilar adenopathy is associated with phenytoin.

Fraser RO, et al. *Diagnosis of Diseases of the Chest*. 3rd ed. Philadelphia, PA: Saunders; 1991:2417-2479.

Miller WT. Pleural and mediastinal disorders related to drug use. *Semin Roentgenol*. 1995;30:35-48.

8.6. Answer: E. Lead that is in soft tissues is not usually systemically absorbed, and therefore, there is no toxicologic indication to surgically remove the bullet or to initiate chelation. Surgical removal is indicated if either the bullet or any fragments are in the joint space, as the acidic environment of the synovial fluid causes absorption of lead.

DeMartini J, et al. Lead arthropathy and systemic lead poisoning from an intraarticular bullet. *AJR Am J Roentgenol*. 2001;176:1144.

8.7. Answer: D. These radiograph findings are consistent with skeletal fluorosis, a sequela of inhalation of fluorinated hydrocarbons like 1,1-difluoroethane. Patients develop painful nodules in bones and joints and decreased joint mobility. Periostitis deformans, which is exuberant periosteal new bone formation, is a characteristic radiographic finding of fluorosis.

Wang Y, et al. Endemic fluorosis of the skeleton: Radiographic features in 127 patients. *AJR Am J Roentgenol*. 1994;162:93-98.

Bruns BR, Tytle T. Skeletal fluorosis. A report of two cases. *Orthopedics*. 1988;11:1083-1087.

8.8. Answer: A. There are a very large number of causes of interstitial lung disease, and their radiographic appearance includes a fine or coarse reticular pattern or a nodular pattern. Many of the disorders causing a reticular pattern also lead to multifocal ill-defined airspace filling. Hypersensitivity pneumonitis is a delayed-type allergic reaction to an ingested or inhaled allergen. The most common medication causing hypersensitivity pneumonitis is nitrofurantoin. Clinical signs generally begin 1–2 weeks into the course of therapy.

Armstrong P, et al. *Imaging of Diseases of the Chest*. 2nd ed. St. Louis, MO: Mosby–Year Book; 1995:426-460, 461-483.

Fishman AP. *Pulmonary Diseases and Disorders*. 2nd ed. New York, NY: McGraw-Hill; 1988:667-674, 793-811, 1465-1474.

Reed JC. *Chest Radiology: Plain Film Pattern and Differential Diagnosis*. 3rd ed. St. Louis, MO: Mosby-Year Book; 1991.

8.9. Answer: D. Ingestion of toxic quantities of organic mercury results in a variety of severe neurologic disorders including developmental delay, cortical blindness, and movement disorders. Magnetic resonance imaging (MRI) reveals atrophy of the cerebellum as well as the calcarine cerebral cortex. Chronic alcoholism and solvent vapor exposure also cause diffuse cerebral atrophy and cerebellar atrophy.

Davis LE, et al. Methylmercury poisoning: Long-term clinical radiological, toxicological, and pathological studies of an affected family. *Ann Neurol*. 1994;35:680-688.

Lexa FJ. Drug-induced disorders of the central nervous system. *Semin Roentgenol*. 1995;30:7-17.

8.10. Answer: D. Thorium dioxide, an historic radiocontrast agent also known as thorotrast, was used as angiographic contrast until 1947, when it was found to cause hepatic malignancies. The radioactive isotope of thorium has a half-life of 400 years. It accumulates in the reticuloendothelial system and remains there for the life of the patient. The characteristic radiographic appearance includes multiple punctate opacities in the liver, spleen, and lymph nodes. Patients who were exposed to thorium dioxide prior to its removal still present with hepatic malignancies.

Bensinger TA, et al. Thorotrast-induced reticuloendothelial blockade in man. Clinical equivalent of the experimental model associated with patent pneumococcal septicemia. *Am J Med*. 1971;51:663-668.

Velasquez G, et al. Thorium dioxide: Still around. *South Med J*. 1985; 78:743-745.

Pharmacokinetic and Toxicokinetic Principles

9

QUESTIONS

9.1. Lithium and digoxin are best described by which of the following models?
A. Zero-compartment kinetics
B. One-compartment kinetics
C. Two-compartment kinetics
D. Michaelis-Menten kinetics
E. Andover-Martin kinetics

9.2. A 3-year-old, 10-kg girl ingests 10 mL of a 100% methanol solution. If the volume of distribution (Vd) for methanol is 0.6 L/kg, what is the predicted peak methanol concentration (assuming instantaneous distribution, no elimination, and a methanol specific gravity of 1)?
A. 16.7 mg/dL
B. 167 mg/dL
C. 167 mg/mL
D. 1.67 mg/L
E. 1.67 mg/dL

9.3. Phenytoin elimination is best characterized by which of the following processes?
A. Michaelis-Menten kinetics
B. Zero-order kinetics
C. First-order kinetics
D. Linear-order kinetics
E. None of the above

9.4. Pharmacodynamics characterizes which of the following processes?
A. Absorption across semipermeable membranes
B. Distribution kinetics
C. Concentration and clinical effects
D. Metabolic rates and processes
E. Elimination rates and processes

9.5. A 65-year-old, 60-kg man is taking 0.25 mg of digoxin daily to control his atrial fibrillation. Approximately 80% of the oral dose is absorbed. His steady-state digoxin concentration is 0.8 ng/mL. What is the patient's clearance of digoxin each day?
A. 50 L/day
B. 100 L/day
C. 150 L/day
D. 250 L/day
E. 300 L/day

9.6. Where does the phase I oxidative process of alcohol dehydrogenation primarily occur?
A. Mitochondria
B. Cytosol
C. Colonic microflora
D. Golgi apparatus
E. Phospholipid membrane of the gastrointestinal (GI) tract

9.7. A 77-year-old man presents after ingesting his entire bottle of nitroglycerin. Which of the following effects would be expected to develop in this patient?
A. Hypotension
B. Altered mental status
C. Diarrhea
D. Cardiogenic shock
E. No effect

9.8. Which of the following characteristics of a xenobiotic would make it amenable to being removed by hemodialysis?
A. A low volume of distribution
B. High protein binding
C. Large molecular weight
D. A high LogP
E. A high LogD

9.9. A 22-year-old man has an acetaminophen concentration of 150 mcg/mL (992 micromol/L) at 4 hours after an intentional ingestion and a concentration of 37.5 mcg/mL (248 micromol/L) at 16 hours. What is the acetaminophen half-life in this patient?
A. 2 hours
B. 3 hours
C. 4 hours
D. 6 hours
E. 12 hours

9.10. An 82-year-old man presents to the emergency department with nystagmus and ataxia. He is prescribed phenytoin as a treatment for his seizure disorder. His measured phenytoin concentration is 15 mcg/mL. His albumin is 2 g/dL. What is this patient's corrected phenytoin concentration?
A. 18 mcg/mL
B. 20 mcg/mL
C. 25 mcg/mL
D. 30 mcg/mL
E. 35 mcg/mL

ANSWERS

9.1. Answer: C. Lithium and digoxin are best characterized by two-compartment kinetics. In two-compartment kinetics, a xenobiotic is distributed instantaneously to a highly perfused central compartment and then is more slowly distributed to a peripheral (often intracellular) compartment. Therefore, blood concentrations obtained shortly after the dose are higher than those drawn after distribution is complete and do not correlate with toxicity (central nervous system for lithium and the heart for digoxin).

Jaeger A, et al. Toxicokinetics of lithium intoxication treated by hemodialysis. *J Toxicol Clin Toxicol.* 1985;23:501-517.

Knox E, Dopheide J. Chapter 12: Lithium. In: Beringer P, ed. *Winter's Basic Clinical Pharmacokinetics.* 6th ed. Philadelphia, PA: Wolters Kluwer; 2018:358-370.

Boro M. Chapter 10: Digoxin. In: Beringer P, ed. *Winter's Basic Clinical Pharmacokinetics.* 6th ed. Philadelphia, PA: Wolters Kluwer; 2018: 281-319.

9.2. Answer: B. The predicted peak concentration would be 167 mg/dL. This 10-kg girl ingested 10 mL of 100% (100 g/100 mL) methanol. It will be distributed in 6,000 mL (10 kg × 600 mL/kg), which is 60 dL.

Using the formula: Dose/Vd = Cp

$$(10 \text{ mL} \times 100 \text{ g}/100 \text{ mL} \times 1{,}000 \text{ mg}/1 \text{ g})$$
$$\div (6{,}000 \text{ mL} \times 1 \text{ dL}/100 \text{ mL}) = 167 \text{ mg/dL}$$

Beringer P, Winter M. Chapter 1: Pharmacokinetic processes and parameters. In: Beringer P, ed. *Winter's Basic Clinical Pharmacokinetics.* 6th ed. Philadelphia, PA: Wolters Kluwer; 2018:3-58.

9.3. Answer: A. Phenytoin is metabolized by enzymes that become saturated at concentrations just above the therapeutic range. As the dose increases, there is a disproportionate increase in serum concentration. At steady state, doubling the dose will more than double the serum concentration. This phenomenon is characteristic of Michaelis-Menten kinetics.

Winter M. Chapter 14: Phenytoin. In: Beringer P, ed. *Winter's Basic Clinical Pharmacokinetics.* 6th ed. Philadelphia, PA: Wolters Kluwer; 2018: 398-445.

9.4. Answer: C. Pharmacodynamics is the investigation of the relationship of drug concentration to clinical effects.

Woosley RL. Pharmacokinetics and pharmacodynamics of antiarrhythmic agents in patients with congestive heart failure. *Am Heart J.* 1987;114: 1280-1285.

9.5. Answer: D. At steady state, the amount of drug entering the system equals the amount of drug leaving the system, and the ratio is the resultant serum concentration. The amount of digoxin going into (and out of) the system is 80% of 0.25 mg (80% × 250 mcg × 1,000 ng/mcg) or 200,000 ng/24 h. Clearance is the theoretical volume of blood cleared of drug or, in this case, digoxin, each day. Therefore, 200,000 ng/24 h divided by the concentration at steady state (0.8 ng/mL = 800 ng/L) = (200,000 ng/24 h)/800 ng/L = 250 L/day. Clearance is conventionally reported as volume per unit of time.

Shargel L, et al. Drug elimination and clearance. In: *Applied Biopharmaceutics and Pharmacokinetics*. 5th ed. New York, NY: McGraw-Hill; 2005:131-160.

9.6. Answer: B. Alcohol dehydrogenation is a phase I reaction and is primarily located in the cytosol of hepatic cells and in select extrahepatic metabolic cells. Phase I reactions are a preparative metabolism. Alcohol dehydrogenase reduces alcohols. The location of the enzymes are important, especially if they form reactive metabolites, which then accumulate at the site of metabolism and cause local toxicity.

Parkinson A. Biotransformation of xenobiotics. In: Klaassen C, ed. *Casarett & Doull's Toxicology: The Basic Science of Poisons*. 5th ed. New York, NY: McGraw-Hill; 1996:113-186.

9.7. Answer: E. The first-pass effect refers to the process where venous drainage from the stomach and the intestine delivers orally administered medication to the liver via the portal vein. This venous drainage allows hepatic metabolism to occur before the xenobiotic reaches the systemic circulation. Nitroglycerin is not administered orally due to a significant first-pass effect. Patients who overdose on nitroglycerin orally do not usually develop any toxic symptoms.

Pond SM, Tozer TN. First-pass elimination. Basic concepts and clinical consequences. *Clin Pharmacokinet*. 1984;9:1-25.

9.8. Answer: A. For a xenobiotic to be dialyzable, it should have a low volume of distribution. Hemodialysis is unlikely to be effective for xenobiotics with a volume of distributions >1 L/kg as most of the xenobiotics will not be in the serum compartment. Other properties that would be needed for a xenobiotic to be able to be dialyzed include low protein binding, as only unbound xenobiotics cross the dialysis membrane; a small molecular size; and water solubility (low LogP and low LogD).

Ghannoum M, et al. Use of extracorporeal treatments in the management of poisonings. *Kidney Int*. 2018;94:682-688.

9.9. Answer: D. The patient's serum acetaminophen concentration has fallen by 50% every six hours. Half-life is defined as the time required for a xenobiotic's concentration to decline by 50%. At 10 hours (Six hours after the first concentration of 150 mcg/mL [992.3 micromol/L]), this patient's concentration would be 75 mcg/mL (496.2 micromol/L) and then, at 16 hours (12 hours after the first concentration), 37.5 mcg/mL (248.1 micromol/L). An alternate method to approach this is: Half-life = 0.693/ke. ke = (ln Cp_1 – ln Cp_2/$(t_2 - t_1)$ = (ln 150 – ln 37.5)/(16 – 4) = 0.1155 h^{-1} and 0.693/0.1155 h^{-1} = 6 h.

Prescott LF, et al. Plasma-paracetamol half-life and hepatic necrosis in patients with paracetamol overdosage. *Lancet*. 1971;1:519-522.

9.10. Answer: C. Phenytoin is a xenobiotic where the effects are significantly influenced by changes in the concentration of plasma albumin as only free phenytoin is active. When albumin concentrations are in normal range, approximately 90% of the phenytoin is bound to albumin. As the albumin concentration decreases, more phenytoin is free and able to cause toxicity. There are different equations, and all provide an approximate concentration. An accepted equation is:

$$\text{Cp interpreted} = \frac{\text{Cp observed}}{[(0.25^* \times \text{Alb (in g/dL)}] + 0.1}$$

When Alb = 2 and Cp = 15 mg/L, then

$$\text{Cp interpreted} = \frac{15 \text{ mg/L}}{(0.25^* \times 2) + 0.1} = 25 \text{ mg/L}$$

*Some use an adjustment factor of 0.275 for CrCl >20 mL/min and 0.2 for CrCl <20 mL/min; no adjustment is necessary for Alb >3.2 g/dL

Cheng W, et al. Predictive performance of the Winter-Tozer and derivative equations for estimating free phenytoin concentration. *Can J Hosp Pharm*. 2016;69:269-279.

https://www.mdcalc.com/phenytoin-dilantin-correction-albumin-renal-failure#evidence. Accessed June 2, 2021.

Chapter

Chemical Principles

10.1. Which of the following common acids is the strongest?
   A. Carbonic acid (H_2CO_3)
   B. Hydrochloric acid (HCl)
   C. Sulfurous acid (H_2SO_3)
   D. Acetic acid (CH_3CH_2OH)
   E. Hydrocyanic acid (HCN)

10.2. The metabolism of which of the following molecules would be directly affected after the treatment of an unknown toxic alcohol ingestion with fomepizole?
   A. CH_3CHO
   B. $H_2C=O$
   C. CH_3CH_2OH
   D. CH_3-CO-CH_3
   E. HCOOH

10.3. Which of the following options is true of halogens?
   A. In their elemental form, they are strong reducing agents
   B. All hydrogen halides, except hydrogen chloride (HCl) ionize nearly completely in water
   C. Bromine is the most electronegative
   D. Most hydrogen halides are strong acids
   E. Of the hydrogen halides, hydrogen fluoride (HF) is the strongest acid

10.4. Which of the following options explains the mechanism of toxicity of arsenate?
   A. Substitution for phosphate in the mitochondria
   B. Inhibition of neuronal voltage-sensitive calcium channels
   C. Alteration of DNA methylation
   D. Inhibition of astrocyte uptake of cysteine
   E. Arsenate behaves biologically in a manner similar to potassium

10.5. Which of the following statements about metals is correct?
   A. Heavy metals do not create free radicals
   B. The mercuric form of mercury is less toxic than the mercurous form
   C. Elemental lead is toxic
   D. Lead ions replace calcium in certain physiologic processes
   E. Trivalent arsenate is less toxic than pentavalent arsenite

10.6. Which group of elements on the periodic table has the most members?
   A. Alkali metals
   B. Alkaline earth metals
   C. Transition metals
   D. Halogens
   E. Inert gases

10.7. Which of the following antidotes is a racemate composed of two pharmacologically active optic isomers?
A. N-acetylcysteine
B. Atropine
C. Flumazenil
D. Glucose
E. Naloxone

10.8. A shoemaker presents to a neurologist's office with a peripheral neuropathy. The neuropathy is a mixed sensorimotor neuropathy with loss of reflexes. The weakness is more pronounced in the distal extremities and worse in his legs than in his arms. Which of the following is responsible for his toxicity?
A. C_6H_{14}
B. C_6H_6
C. CO
D. CH_3OH
E. $C_2H_6O_2$

10.9. The serine residue in the active site of acetylcholinesterase attacks which location on acetylcholine?

A. A
B. B
C. C
D. D
E. All of the sites

10.10. Which of the following reactions best describes the formation of chloramine gas?
A. $NH_4^+ + HOCl \rightarrow H^+ + H_2O + NH_2Cl$
B. $Cl_2 + H_2O \rightarrow 2HCl + \{O\}$ (where $\{O\}$ is nascent oxygen)
C. $N_2 + 3H_2O \rightarrow H_2NO_3 + 2H_2$
D. $O_2 + Fe^{2+} \rightarrow Fe^{3+} + O_2^-$
E. $SO_2 + H_2O \rightarrow H_2SO_3$

ANSWERS

10.1. Answer: B. Acidity and alkalinity are determined by the number of available H^+ ions. Strong acids ionize almost completely in aqueous solution, and very little of the parent compound remains. Weak acids reach an equilibrium between parent and ionized forms and thus do not alter the pH to the same degree as a similar quantity of a strong acid (hydrochloric > sulfurous > acetic > carbonic > hydrocyanic).

Higton A, et al. *Access to Chemistry*. London, United Kingdom: Royal Society of Chemistry; 1999:260-262.

10.2. Answer: C. Only the metabolism of an alcohol (in this case, ethanol) would be blocked by the administration of a competitive inhibitor of alcohol dehydrogenase. The other molecules are aldehydes (A, acetaldehyde and B, formaldehyde), a ketone (D, acetone), and a carboxylic acid (E, formic acid).

McMartin KE, et al. Kinetics and metabolism of fomepizole in healthy humans. *Clin Toxicol*. 2012;50:375-383.

10.3. Answer: D. All hydrogen halides, except for HF, ionize nearly completely in water to release H^+ and are considered strong acids. HF ionizes poorly and is considered a weak acid. In their elemental form, halogens carry the suffix (*-ine*). Halogens are strong oxidizing agents. Because they are highly electronegative, they readily form halides. Halides are much less reactive than their elemental form and are reducing agents.

Higton A, et al. *Access to Chemistry*. London, United Kingdom: Royal Society of Chemistry; 1999:53-54.

10.4. Answer: A. The toxicity of certain metals is predicted based on their location in the periodic table. Arsenate (pentavalent arsenic) will substitute for phosphate in the mitochondrial production of adenosine triphosphate (ATP), creating adenosine monoarsenate and therefore interfering with oxidative phosphorylation. Choices B and C describe different mechanisms by which lead causes toxicity. Choice D contributes to methylmercury toxicity. Thallium behaves in a manner similar to potassium because both have similar ionic radii.

Huang R-N, Lee T-C. Cellular uptake of trivalent arsenite and pentavalent arsenate in KB cells cultured in phosphate-free medium. *Toxicol Appl Pharmacol*. 1996;136:243-249.

10.5. Answer: D. Lead, in its Pb^{2+} form, is absorbed in place of Ca^{2+} and replaces Ca^{2+} in certain systemic processes, eventually leading to neurotoxicity. Elemental lead itself is not toxic, but it develops a coat of lead oxide or carbonate, which is toxic when exposed to air or water. Some heavy metals create free radicals through Fenton chemistry. The mercurous form is less toxic than the mercuric form of mercury. The trivalent arsenate form is more toxic than the pentavalent form.

Lidsky TI, Schneider JS. Lead neurotoxicity in children: Basic mechanisms and clinical correlates. *Brain*. 2003;126:5-19.

10.6. Answer: C. The transition metals are the largest group of elements in the periodic table. Unlike the alkaline and alkaline earth metals, most other metallic elements are neither soluble nor reactive.

Fluck E. New notations in the periodic table. *Pure Appl Chem.* 1988;60:431-436.

10.7. Answer: B. Atropine is a mixture of D- and L-hyoscyamine, which are both antimuscarinics, whereas only D-glucose, (-)-naloxone, and L-N-acetylcysteine are pharmacologically active antidotes. Flumazenil is achiral.

Kentala E, et al. Intramuscular atropine in healthy volunteers: A pharmacokinetic and pharmacodynamic study. *Int J Clin Pharmacol Ther Toxicol.* 1990;28:399-404.

10.8. Answer: A. This patient has a peripheral neuropathy from an occupational exposure to n-hexane. The chemical formulas for the other choices are as follows: B is benzene, C is carbon monoxide, D is methanol, and E is ethylene glycol.

Rizzuto N, et al. n-hexane polyneuropathy. An occupational disease of shoemakers. *Eur Neurol.* 1980;19:308-315.

10.9. Answer: A. The nucleophilic serine residue on acetylcholinesterase attacks the electrophilic carbon that forms the carbon-oxygen double bond on acetylcholine, cleaving off choline. The serine-acetyl complex then is rapidly hydrolyzed, regenerating the serine residue.

Taylor P. Anticholinesterase agents. In: Hardman JG, et al, eds. *Goodman and Gilman's The Pharmacological Basis of Therapeutics.* 9th ed. New York, NY: Macmillan; 1996:100-119.

10.10. Answer: A. Ammonia added to hypochlorous acid (bleach) forms chloramine gas (A). Chlorine dissolved in water liberates both acid and nascent oxygen, which is a potent oxidizer (B). Oxygen generates superoxide and other free radicals in the presence of transition metal catalysts such as iron (D). Sulfur dioxide forms sulfurous acid when exposed to water (E). Nitrogen (C) is inert and does not dissolve well in water; nitrous acid is not formed.

Hattis RP, et al. Chlorine gas toxicity from mixture of bleach with other cleaning products—California. *MMWR.* 1991;40:619-629.

Ryrfeldt A, et al. Free radicals and lung disease. *Br Med Bull.* 1993; 49:588-603.

Biochemical and Metabolic Principles

QUESTIONS

11.1. Which of the following options is a phase I biotransformation reaction?
A. Sulfation
B. Glucuronidation
C. Carboxylation
D. Conjugation with glutathione
E. Transluminal P-glycoprotein transport

11.2. A 72-year-old man presents to the emergency department with a new facial droop and ipsilateral hemiparesis. The patient had an ischemic stroke three weeks prior to this presentation and was prescribed aspirin and clopidogrel at that time. Which of the following cytochrome (CYP) 450 polymorphisms is responsible for the lack of efficacy of his antiplatelet medication?
A. CYP3A4
B. CYP2D6
C. CYP2E1
D. CYP2C19
E. CYP2C9

11.3. Which of the following xenobiotics causes injury at the site of its metabolic transformation?
A. Cyanide
B. Succinylcholine
C. Salicylate
D. Carbon tetrachloride
E. 1-Methyl-4-phenyl-1,2,3,6-tetrahydropyridine (MPTP)

11.4. Which of the following statements about phase II reactions is true?
A. Decreased availability of glutathione limits the rate of detoxification of both acetaminophen and bromobenzene
B. Phase II reactions decrease the polarity of xenobiotics
C. Phase II reactions are primarily oxidation-reduction reactions
D. The products of phase II biotransformation reactions are highly toxic
E. Phase II enzymes result in addition of sulfhydryl, hydroxyl, or carboxyl groups to xenobiotics

11.5. Which of the following xenobiotics is associated with an uncoupling of oxidative phosphorylation?
A. Hydrogen sulfide
B. Sodium fluoroacetate
C. Dinitrophenol
D. Ricin
E. Carbon tetrachloride

11.6. A 3-week-old boy is brought into the emergency department apneic. As part of his resuscitation, naloxone is administered, and the baby's breathing improves. The mother states that she had recently started a new pain medication after breaking her wrist. Which of the following cytochrome (CYP) 450 polymorphisms is responsible for this infant's presentation?
A. CYP3A4
B. CYP2D6
C. CYP2E1
D. CYP2C19
E. CYP2C9

32

11.7. A 56-year-old woman presents to the emergency department with significant hematomas to her scalp, eyelids, left flank, and buttock. She has a history of factor V Leiden deficiency for which she is prescribed warfarin. She is compliant with her warfarin and notes that her international normalized ratio (INR) has been around 2.5 for the last 3 years. Her INR today is greater than 6. Which of the following additions explains the patient's supratherapeutic INR?
A. Grapefruit juice
B. Phenobarbital
C. Phenytoin
D. St. John's wort
E. Rifampicin

11.8. Which of the following statements about biotransformation reactions is true?
A. The majority of the metabolites produced by phase I biotransformation of lipophilic xenobiotics are water soluble and readily excretable
B. Phase I biotransformation of a xenobiotic is always a mechanism for detoxification
C. The metabolism of ethanol to acetaldehyde is a phase II reaction
D. CYP2E1 has a higher Michaelis constant (Km) for ethanol than alcohol dehydrogenase, making it less likely to be involved in the metabolism of ethanol in most individuals
E. Most phase I biotransformation enzymes are highly specific with regard to which substrates they act upon

11.9. A 52-year-old man presents to the emergency department with myalgias and tea-colored urine. He is diagnosed with rhabdomyolysis. His past medical history includes hyperlipidemia for which he is prescribed simvastatin. Which new medication led to the patient's current presentation?
A. Itraconazole
B. Dexamethasone
C. Rifampin
D. Carbamazepine
E. Phenobarbital

11.10. A 27-year-old man presents to the emergency department with a depressed mental status and pinpoint pupils. His friends report that he has been abusing loperamide. What other medication did this patient take to increase the opioid effects of loperamide?
A. Phenytoin
B. Rifampin
C. Carbamazepine
D. St. John's wort
E. Quinidine

ANSWERS

11.1. Answer: C. Sulfation, glucuronidation, and conjugation with glutathione are phase II reactions that occur after modification of the substrate by phase I reactions. Phase I reactions result in the addition of more reactive groups such as hydroxyl, amino, carboxyl, or sulfhydryl groups to lipophilic molecules. Transluminal transport by transporter proteins, such as P-glycoprotein, is often referred to as a phase III reaction.

Krishna DR, Klotz U. Extrahepatic metabolism of drugs in humans. *Clin Pharmacokinet.* 1994;26:144-160.

11.2. Answer: D. CYP2C19 is responsible for converting clopidogrel into a pharmacologically active platelet inhibitor. Patients with loss-of-function variants are more likely to experience thrombotic events. CYP2C19 is also responsible for the metabolism of many benzodiazepines.

Shuldiner AR, et al. Association of cytochrome P450 2C19 genotype with the antiplatelet effect and clinical efficacy of clopidogrel therapy. *JAMA.* 2009;302:849-857.

Karazniewicz-Lada M, et al. The influence of genetic polymorphism of CYP2C19 isoenzyme on the pharmacokinetics of clopidogrel and its metabolites in patients with cardiovascular diseases. *J Clin Pharmacol.* 2014;54:874-880.

11.3. Answer: D. Carbon tetrachloride causes in situ hepatic injury in the zone 3 areas of the liver, where it is metabolized. Of the others, only MPTP requires metabolic transformation to exert its toxicity, which occurs following transport of the metabolite into dopaminergic neurons and not at the site of its synthesis.

> Brent JA, Rumack BH. Role of free radicals in toxic hepatic injury: II. Are free radicals the cause of toxin induced liver disease? *J Toxicol Clin Toxicol.* 1993;31:173-196.

11.4. Answer: A. Both acetaminophen and bromobenzene are metabolized by phase I reactions to highly reactive metabolites that have significant toxicity when glutathione availability is limited. Phase II reactions are conjugation reactions that increase the polarity (and water solubility) and result in detoxification in most cases.

> Zamek-Gliszczynski MJ, et al. Integration of hepatic drug transporters and phase II metabolizing enzymes: Mechanisms of hepatic excretion of sulfate, glucuronide, and glutathione metabolites. *Eur J Pharm Sci.* 2006;27:447-486.

11.5. Answer: C. Xenobiotics that uncouple oxidative phosphorylation lead to a decrease in ATP production. Due to oxygen consumption being uncoupled from ATP production, the energy that normally is used to form ATP is instead released as heat. Dinitrophenol and pentachlorophenol, another uncoupler, are associated with severe hyperthermia and death.

> Proudfoot AT. Pentachlorophenol poisoning. *Toxicol Rev.* 2003;22:3-11.

11.6. Answer: B. Codeine is inactive and needs to be metabolized by CYP2D6 to form morphine. This infant developed toxicity because codeine is excreted in the breast milk. Furthermore, patients who are ultrarapid metabolizers with CYP2D6 have up to 13 copies of the gene and therefore develop very toxic concentrations of morphine. This scenario is made worse if the mother is a poor metabolizer of codeine and therefore, does not appreciate the opioid effects of the drug.

> Lundqvist E, et al. Genetic mechanisms for duplication and multiduplication of the human CYP2D6 gene and methods for detection of duplicated CYP2D6 genes. *Gene.* 1999;226:327-338.

11.7. Answer: A. This patient is presenting with an elevation of her INR despite no adjustments to her warfarin dosage. Grapefruit juice is a CYP3A4 inhibitor and leads to supratherapeutic INRs. Other CYP3A4 inhibitors include clarithromycin, erythromycin, ketoconazole, and goldenseal. Answer choices B-E are all CYP3A4 inducers and would lower the INR.

> Conney AH. Induction of drug-metabolizing enzymes: A path to the discovery of multiple cytochromes P450. *Annu Rev Pharmacol Toxicol.* 2003;43:1-30.

11.8. Answer: D. Although phase I biotransformation increases the water solubility of many toxins, they remain relatively lipophilic and often require phase II conjugation for excretion. Most of these enzymes are not highly selective, altering many different substrates within broad classes. The metabolism of ethanol to acetaldehyde is a phase I oxidation reaction. The higher Km for ethanol of CYP2E1 makes alcohol dehydrogenase the primary enzyme for metabolizing ethanol in nontolerant persons.

> Guegenrich FP. Catalytic selectivity of human cytochrome P450 enzymes: Relevance to drug metabolism and toxicity. *Toxicol Lett.* 1994;70:133-138.

11.9. Answer: A. Simvastatin is primarily biotransformed by CYP3A4. Itraconazole is a specific and potent inhibitor of CYP3A4. Addition of this medication increases the risk of developing rhabdomyolysis from simvastatin.

> Abernethy DR, Flockhart DA. Molecular basis of cardiovascular drug metabolism: Implications for predicting clinically important drug interactions. *Circulation.* 2000;101:1749-1753.

11.10. Answer: E. Loperamide is a P-glycoprotein substrate and quinidine is a P-glycoprotein inhibitor. When large doses of quinidine are co-ingested with loperamide, it overwhelms the capacity of the P-glycoprotein, and therefore loperamide enters the CNS causing toxicity. Choices A-D are all P-glycoprotein inducers.

> Daniulaityte R, et al. "I just wanted to tell you that loperamide WILL WORK": A web-based study of extra-medical use of loperamide. *Drug Alcohol Depend.* 2013;130:241-244.

> Ho RH, Kim RB. Transporters and drug therapy: Implications for drug disposition and disease. *Clin Pharmacol Ther.* 2005;78:260-277.

Fluid, Electrolytes, and Acid–Base Principles

QUESTIONS

12.1. Which of the following xenobiotics is associated with the development of diabetes insipidus (DI)?
A. Tramadol
B. Lactulose
C. Lithium
D. Cyclophosphamide
E. Amiloride

12.2. Which of the following xenobiotics is associated with a high anion gap metabolic acidosis?
A. Inorganic sulfur
B. Digoxin
C. Nitrates
D. Organic mercury
E. Acetazolamide

12.3. A 56-year-old man is brought into the hospital minimally responsive. His serum ethanol concentration obtained by an enzyme-based assay is undetectable. His pH is 7.28 with an anion gap of 24 mEq/L. His serum osmolality is 285 mOsm/kg with an osmol gap of 7.0 mOsm/kg. His osmol gap is repeated 20 minutes later and is essentially unchanged. Confirmatory testing via gas chromatography demonstrates a methanol concentration of 80 mg/dL (24.97 mmol/L). What is the best explanation for the normal osmolality despite a measurable concentration of methanol?
A. Methanol is ionized at physiological pH
B. The measurement was obtained by boiling point elevation
C. The analysis was done on incorrectly labeled specimens

D. The analysis equipment was not calibrated prior to use
E. The measurement was obtained by freezing point depression

12.4. A 71-year-old woman is admitted to the hospital for further management of a *Pseudomonas aeruginosa* urinary tract infection. She is treated with intravenous carbenicillin. Her blood work is notable for a potassium of 2.5 mEq/L. Her preadmission potassium was within normal limits. What is the best explanation for this patient's new hypokalemia?
A. Analysis interference by carbenicillin resulting in a falsely low serum potassium
B. Carbenicillin acts as a nonabsorbable anion promoting potassium loss at the distal convoluted tubule of the kidney
C. Carbenicillin leads to decreased reabsorption of potassium secondary to activity at the thick ascending limb of the kidney
D. Carbenicillin has chelating properties and binds to potassium
E. Carbenicillin causes severe alkalosis, which leads to intracellular shift of potassium out of the serum

12.5. Which of the following xenobiotics is associated with hyponatremia?
A. Glycyrrhizic acid
B. Sorbitol
C. Glycerol
D. Amphotericin
E. Foscarnet

12.6. A 30-year-old woman presents to the emergency department with severe spasticity and "seizurelike" movements of her upper and lower extremities. Her sensorium is clear. She has a history of chronic malabsorption requiring total parental nutrition. Which electrolyte abnormality best explains her symptoms?
   A. Hyponatremia
   B. Hyperkalemia
   C. Hypermagnesemia
   D. Hypocalcemia
   E. Hypercalcemia

12.7. A 52-year-old man presents to the hospital with a high anion gap (24 mEq/L) metabolic acidosis and is found to have an osmol gap of 15 mOsm/kg. Which of the following options is the most likely diagnosis?
   A. Methanol intoxication
   B. Alcoholic ketoacidosis
   C. Sepsis
   D. Kidney failure
   E. Any of the above

12.8. A 4-week-old boy presents to the emergency department with lethargy and persistent vomiting. His basic metabolic panel demonstrates an increased creatinine. A kidney ultrasound reveals hyperechoic medulla bilaterally. Which of the following xenobiotics led to this presentation?
   A. Ethanol
   B. Furosemide
   C. Vitamin D
   D. Acetaminophen
   E. Ibuprofen

12.9. Which of the following xenobiotics causes hyperkalemia?
   A. Furosemide
   B. Heparin
   C. Theophylline
   D. Toluene
   E. Insulin

12.10. Which of the following xenobiotics is associated with hypermagnesemia?
   A. Theophylline
   B. Ethanol
   C. Furosemide
   D. Amphotericin
   E. Lithium

ANSWERS

12.1. Answer: C. Of the listed answer choices, only lithium is associated with nephrogenic diabetes insipidus (DI). Patients with DI present with polyuria and polydipsia, and often, the urine volumes exceed 30 mL/kg/day. In nephrogenic DI, desmopressin will have no significant effect. Treatment for nephrogenic DI includes thiazide diuretics, prostaglandin inhibitors, or amiloride.

Vokes TJ, Robertson GL. Disorders of antidiuretic hormone. *Endocrinol Metab Clin North Am.* 1988;17:281-299.

12.2. Answer: A. Inorganic sulfur causes a high anion gap metabolic acidosis that is likely unrelated to the generation of hydrogen sulfide. It results from excess sulfate in patients with kidney dysfunction. Digoxin and organic mercury do not commonly cause acid–base abnormalities. Acetazolamide causes a normal anion gap (nongap) metabolic acidosis. Excessive nitrates (NO_3) lower the anion gap because of an interference with the determination of chloride.

Schwartz SM, et al. Sublimed (inorganic) sulfur ingestion. A cause of life-threatening metabolic acidosis with a high anion gap. *Arch Intern Med.* 1986;146:1437–1438.

12.3. Answer: B. Given the elevated methanol concentration, an elevated osmol gap would be expected. This discrepancy is due to an analytical error caused by incorrect protocols used to measure osmolality. The measurement should have been performed using freezing point depression. Methanol has a low boiling point (approximately 150 °F or 65.6 °C). Therefore, a falsely normal osmolality is expected if boiling point elevation is used to determine the osmolality because the methanol would be gone before the plasma began to boil.

Hammerling J. A review of medical errors in laboratory diagnostics and where we are today. *Lab Med.* 2012;57:41-44.

Eisen TF, et al. Serum osmolality in alcohol ingestions: Differences in availability among laboratories of teaching hospital, nonteaching hospital, and commercial facilities. *Am J Emerg Med.* 1989;7:256-259.

12.4. Answer: B. Carbenicillin and other penicillin salts are very soluble at physiologic pH. Carbenicillin becomes a nonreabsorbable anion and causes a negative transtubular potential, thereby enhancing passive excretion of potassium from the distal tubule of the kidney.

Brunner FP, Frick PG. Hypokalaemia, metabolic alkalosis, and hypernatraemia due to "massive" sodium penicillin therapy. *Br Med J.* 1968;4:550-552.

12.5. Answer: A. Glycyrrhizic acid (found in imported licorice) produces hyponatremia through a mineralocorticoid effect. Amphotericin and foscarnet are associated with diabetes insipidus. Sorbitol and glycerol produce hypernatremia largely through volume depletion.

Edwards CRW. Lessons from licorice. *N Engl J Med.* 1991;325:1242-1243.

Farese RV, et al. Licorice induced hypermineralocorticoidism. *N Engl J Med.* 1991;325:1223-1227.

12.6. Answer: D. Hypocalcemia, hypokalemia, and hypomagnesemia cause acute tetany. This patient's malabsorption led to her hypocalcemia and resultant symptoms.

Edmondson JW, et al. Tetany: Quantitative interrelationships between calcium and alkalosis. *Am J Physiol.* 1975;228:1082-1086.

12.7. Answer: E. In addition to the toxic alcohols (such as methanol and ethylene glycol), liver failure, kidney failure, sepsis, shock, and the ketoacidoses are all associated with an elevated osmol gap. This is one of the major limitations of using this test in patients with unknown causes of metabolic acidosis.

Inaba H, et al. Serum osmolality gap in postoperative patients in intensive care. *Lancet.* 1987;1:1331-1335.

Schelling JR, et al. Increased osmolal gap in alcoholic ketoacidosis and lactic acidosis. *Ann Intern Med.* 1990;113:580-582.

Sklar AH, Linas SL. The osmolal gap in renal failure. *Ann Intern Med.* 1983;98:481-482.

12.8. Answer: C. This patient is presenting with hypercalcemia and resultant nephrocalcinosis. Severe hypercalcemia occurs with repeated exposure to vitamin D. Treatment involves discontinuing the vitamin D and intravenous hydration and, in severe cases, adding calcitonin and pamidronate.

Koul PA, et al. Vitamin D toxicity in adults: A case series from an area with endemic hypovitaminosis D. *Oman Med J.* 2011;26:201-204.

Khadgawat R, et al. Acute vitamin D toxicity in an infant. *Clin Pediatr Endocrinol.* 2007;16:89-93.

12.9. Answer: B. Heparin produces hyperkalemia through the suppression of aldosterone. Furosemide causes hypokalemia due to its effect on the distal convoluted tubule of the kidney. Toluene is associated with a profound hypokalemia produced by a distal renal tubular acidosis. Theophylline and albuterol move potassium intracellularly through stimulation of the beta-adrenergic receptor. Insulin is used for the treatment of hyperkalemia because it moves potassium intracellularly with glucose.

Oster JR, et al. Heparin-induced aldosterone suppression and hyperkalemia. *Am J Med.* 1995;98:575-586.

12.10. Answer: E. Xenobiotic-induced hypermagnesemia is rare, especially in patients with normally functioning kidneys. Xenobiotics that cause hypermagnesemia include lithium, magnesium-containing antacids, magnesium-containing cathartics, and magnesium salts. Theophylline produces hypomagnesemia through activation of the beta-adrenergic receptor. Ethanol is associated with renal magnesium wasting and poor gastrointestinal absorption. Furosemide (and the other loop diuretics) cause renal wasting of magnesium. Amphotericin produces a distal renal tubular acidosis with magnesium wasting.

Brass EP, Thompson WL. Drug-induced electrolyte abnormalities. *Med Toxicol.* 1982;24:207-228.

Neurotransmitters and Neuromodulators

13

QUESTIONS

13.1. A 22-year-old man being treated for tuberculosis presents in status epilepticus. What is the mechanism of action of the drug that is causing his seizures?
A. Inhibition of inhibition at the gamma-aminobutyric acid (GABA)$_B$ receptor
B. Impairment of pyridoxal-5′-phosphate (PLP) production
C. Binding at the picrotoxin site on GABA$_A$
D. Noncompetitive GABA$_A$ antagonism
E. Central adenosine antagonism

13.2. A 26-year-old woman is bitten on the hand by a dark spider with a red hourglass shape on its abdomen. One hour later, she develops sweating on her palms and soles. She presents to the emergency department and is found to be hypertensive to 195/104 mmHg. What is the mechanism by which this spider's toxin is causing the described effects?
A. Upregulation of catechol-O-methyltransferase (COMT) enzymatic activity
B. Competitive inhibition of membrane norepinephrine reuptake transporter (NET)
C. Increased exocytosis of vesicular norepinephrine (NE)
D. Noncompetitive inhibition of NET
E. Increased synthesis of NE

13.3. Which of the following neurotransmitters is responsible for self-termination of seizures?
A. Serotonin
B. Dopamine
C. Adenosine
D. Norepinephrine
E. Gamma-aminobutyric acid (GABA)

13.4. A 3-year-old boy presents to the emergency department somnolent after ingesting one of his grandfather's medications. He is bradycardic to 45 beats/min and hypotensive to 60/30 mmHg. His examination is also remarkable for miotic pupils and respiratory depression. Which of the following receptors mediates the central nervous system depression in this patient?
A. Beta$_2$-adrenergic
B. Imidazoline
C. Gamma-aminobutyric acid (GABA)$_A$
D. Alpha$_2$-adrenergic
E. Acetylcholine muscarinic

13.5. Which one of the following options causes the release of acetylcholine from nerve endings?
A. Black widow spider venom
B. Botulinum toxin
C. Cocaine
D. Clonidine
E. Diphenhydramine

13.6. A 37-year-old man presents after ingesting a substance from an antique medication bag. He is awake; however, he has frequent tonic-clonic movements of his arms and legs. These movements are made worse when he is startled. Which of the following neurotransmitters is antagonized by this toxin?
A. Serotonin
B. Glutamate
C. Adenosine
D. Dopamine
E. Glycine

13.7. Which of the following options produces seizures through antagonism at the GABA$_A$ receptor complex?
  A. Domoic acid
  B. Baclofen
  C. Penicillin
  D. Muscimol
  E. Carbamazepine

13.8. Which of the following xenobiotics inhibits dopamine-beta-hydroxylase?
  A. Propranolol
  B. Disulfiram
  C. Clonidine
  D. Mescaline
  E. Chlorpromazine

13.9. A 24-year-old, 37-week-pregnant woman presents to the emergency department after having a generalized tonic-clonic seizure at home. A magnesium infusion is ordered as part of her therapy; however, a medication error occurs, and she develops paralysis. What is the proposed mechanism of her paralysis?
  A. Stimulation of acetylcholine release
  B. Inhibition of acetylcholine release
  C. Stimulation of the glycine receptor
  D. Inhibition of the glycine receptor
  E. Depolarizing muscular blockade

13.10. A 22-year-old man presents to the emergency department somnolent after an intentional overdose of phenibut. On which receptor does phenibut act?
  A. Gamma aminobutyric acid (GABA)$_A$
  B. GABA$_B$
  C. Mu opioid
  D. Kappa opioid
  E. Glycine

ANSWERS

13.1. Answer: B. Isoniazid (INH) inhibits the conversion of glutamate to gamma aminobutyric acid (GABA) by glutamate decarboxylase, which requires PLP as a cofactor. INH competes with pyridoxine for binding to pyridoxine phosphokinase, which impairs PLP production. The mechanism in answer A is the purported mechanism of seizures in baclofen overdose. Alpha-thujone, the active component in wormwood oil, and cicutoxin both bind noncompetitively to GABA$_A$. Methylxanthines cause adenosine antagonism.

Miller J, et al. Acute isoniazid poisoning in childhood. *Am J Dis Child.* 1980;134:290-292.

13.2. Answer: C. Although all the mechanisms listed would increase noradrenergic tone, alpha-latrotoxin, from the black widow spider described here, specifically works by increasing exocytosis of norepinephrine.

Allen C. Arachnid envenomations. *Emerg Med Clin North Am.* 1992;10:269-298.

13.3. Answer: C. Adenosine is released with excitatory neurotransmitters such as glutamate. Adenosine stimulates presynaptic A$_1$ receptors to inhibit Ca^{2+} influx, limits release of neurotransmitters, and binds to postsynaptic A$_1$ receptors to hyperpolarize the neuron.

Eldridge FL, et al. Role of endogenous adenosine in recurrent generalized seizures. *Exp Neurol.* 1989;103:179-185.

13.4. Answer: D. Stimulation of imidazoline receptors by clonidine contributes to hypotension and bradycardia. Clonidine's stimulation of alpha$_2$-adrenergic receptors produces CNS depression as well as sympatholytic effects. Clonidine does not bind to the other listed receptors.

Dominiak P. Historic aspects in the identification of the I$_1$ receptor and the pharmacology of imidazolines. *Cardiovase Drugs Ther.* 1994; 8(suppl):21-26.

Lowry JA, Brown JT. Significance of the imidazoline receptors in toxicology. *Clin Toxicol.* 2014;52:454-469.

13.5. Answer: A. Black widow spider venom causes release of acetylcholine from nerve endings. Botulinum toxins prevent release of acetylcholine. Clonidine indirectly prevents acetylcholine by stimulating presynaptic alpha$_2$-adrenergic receptors on cholinergic nerve endings. Diphenhydramine blocks muscarinic acetylcholine receptors.

Baba A, Cooper JR. The action of black widow spider venom on cholinergic mechanisms in synaptosomes. *J Neurochem.* 1980;34:1369-1379.

13.6. Answer: E. Strychnine antagonizes the inhibitory effect of glycine at Cl$^-$ channel glycine receptors. Strychnine has no major action on the other listed neurotransmitters.

Betz H, et al. The vertebrate glycine receptor protein. *Biochem Soc Symp.* 1986;52:57-63.

13.7. **Answer: C.** Penicillin directly antagonizes gamma-aminobutyric acid (GABA) binding and blocks the Cl⁻ channel to prevent Cl⁻ influx in response to GABA. Baclofen binds to $GABA_B$ receptors. Domoic acid produces convulsions through actions at glutamate receptors. Muscimol activates $GABA_A$ receptors. Carbamazepine produces convulsions through antagonism of adenosine receptors.

Fujimoto M, et al. Dual mechanisms of $GABA_A$ response inhibition by beta-lactam antibiotics in the pyramidal neurones of the rat cerebral cortex. *Br J Pharmacol.* 1995;116:3014-3020.

Tsuda A, et al. Effect of penicillin on GABA-gated chloride ion influx. *Neurochem Res.* 1994;19:1-4.

13.8. **Answer: B.** Inhibition of dopamine-beta-hydroxylase results in less norepinephrine release in response to nerve ending depolarization or actions of indirectly acting sympathomimetics. In the setting of hypotension from a disulfiram-ethanol interaction, dopamine would be expected to have little benefit.

Eneanya DI, et al. The actions and metabolic fate of disulfiram. *Annu Rev Pharmacol Toxicol.* 1981;21:575-596.

13.9. **Answer: B.** Magnesium inhibits presynaptic acetylcholine release at the neuromuscular junction, likely by inhibiting calcium influx into the nerve endings. In patients who develop paralysis following a magnesium overdose, intravenous calcium therapy should be administered as an antidote.

Swartjes JM, et al. Management of eclampsia: Cardiopulmonary arrest resulting from magnesium sulfate overdose. *Eur J Obstet Gynecol Reprod Biol.* 1992;47:73-75.

13.10. **Answer: B.** Beta-phenyl-gamma-aminobutyric acid, or phenibut, is structurally similar to baclofen. It activates the $GABA_B$ receptor.

McCabe DJ, et al. Phenibut exposures and clinical effects reported to a regional poison center. *Am J Emerg Med.* 2019;37:2066-2071.

Withdrawal Principles

QUESTIONS

14.1. What characteristic best describes a "withdrawal syndrome"?

A. Greater amounts of a xenobiotic are required to achieve a given effect

B. A physiologic derangement in response to **decreasing** concentrations of a xenobiotic

C. Xenobiotic use resulting in impairment of social, occupational, or other important areas of functioning

D. Onset of a characteristic set of symptoms only after abrupt, complete cessation of heavy xenobiotic use

E. Persistence of a characteristic set of symptoms for greater than 1 day following cessation of xenobiotic use

14.2. What feature is unique to a withdrawal syndrome in comparison to a post toxicity syndrome?

A. Resolution with supportive care alone

B. Compulsive drug-seeking behavior

C. A shift in the dose-response curve to the right

D. The discontinued (or a closely related) xenobiotic is taken to relieve symptoms

E. The continued use of a xenobiotic despite adverse consequences

14.3. Which physiologic adaptation to ethanol explains the "kindling" hypothesis of withdrawal?

A. *N*-Methyl-D-aspartate (NMDA) receptor upregulation

B. Increased gamma aminobutyric acid $(GABA)_A$ receptor sensitivity

C. Substitution of $GABA_A$ $alpha_4$ subunits for $alpha_1$ subunits

D. Neurosteroidal modulation of GABA receptors

E. NMDA receptor downregulation

14.4. Baclofen withdrawal and baclofen overdose share which of the following features?

A. Anxiety

B. Somnolence

C. Diaphoresis

D. Tremor

E. Seizures

14.5. Discontinuation of which of the following xenobiotics causes a withdrawal syndrome?

A. Calcium channel blockers

B. Methamphetamine

C. Cocaine

D. Naloxone

E. Paroxetine

14.6. Which of the following best describes alcohol withdrawal seizures?

A. They are usually partial complex

B. They usually progress to status epilepticus

C. The almost never recur

D. They are usually brief

E. They are always accompanied by signs of withdrawal

14.7. A 61-year-old woman is admitted to the intensive care unit and is being sedated with dexmedetomidine. Seven days later, she is extubated and dexmedetomidine is tapered over 8 hours. Her heart rate at the time of discontinuation is 90 beats/min and her blood pressure is 135/90 mmHg. Three hours later, she becomes agitated, her heart rate increases to 115 beats/min, and her blood pressure is 190/120 mmHg. What is the most appropriate intervention at this time?

   A. Lorazepam
   B. Midazolam
   C. Metoprolol
   D. Clonidine
   E. Haloperidol

14.8. Which of the following options best describes benzodiazepine withdrawal?

   A. It occurs up to several days after cessation of benzodiazepines
   B. It does not respond to barbiturates
   C. It is characterized by seizures, miosis, tachycardia, piloerection, and agitation
   D. It is associated with thiamine deficiency
   E. It is almost always benign

14.9. Opioid withdrawal shares which of the following characteristics with ethanol withdrawal?

   A. High rate of concurrent infections
   B. Fever
   C. Piloerection
   D. Tachycardia
   E. High mortality rate

14.10. Which of the following is a manifestation of nicotine withdrawal?

   A. Diarrhea
   B. Depression
   C. Increased heart rate
   D. Muscle relaxation
   E. Anorexia

ANSWERS

14.1. Answer: B. Every withdrawal syndrome requires a preexisting compensatory physiologic adaptation to the continuous presence of a xenobiotic or decreasing concentrations of that xenobiotic below some threshold necessary to prevent physiologic derangement. Choice A best describes tolerance. Choice C is characteristic of a substance use disorder. Choice D is incorrect because withdrawal develops with any decrease in prolonged xenobiotic use. Choice E is incorrect because there is no absolute time frame of duration of symptoms attached to *Diagnostic and Statistical Manual of Mental Disorders,* fifth edition (DSM-5) diagnosis of withdrawal syndromes

American Psychiatric Association. *Diagnostic and Statistical Manual of Mental Disorders.* 5th ed. Washington, DC: American Psychiatric Association; 2013.

14.2. Answer: D. For the purposes of defining a unifying pathophysiologic pattern, withdrawal syndromes are those in which (1) there is a characteristic withdrawal syndrome for the xenobiotic, or (2) the same (or a closely related) xenobiotic is taken to relieve withdrawal symptoms. Choice A distinguishes post toxicity syndromes from withdrawal syndromes. Choices B and E define severe substance use disorders. Choice C is the definition of physiologic tolerance.

American Psychiatric Association. *Diagnostic and Statistical Manual of Mental Disorders.* 5th ed. Washington, DC: American Psychiatric Association; 2013.

14.3. Answer: A. The *N*-methyl-D-aspartate (NMDA) subtype of glutamate receptor increases in number and function as a result of exposure to ethanol due to epigenetic modifications. This, coupled with decreased activity of gamma-aminobutyric acid (GABA)$_A$ receptors, leads to progressive worsening of withdrawal. Choices B and C are the opposite effects of long-term exposure to ethanol. Choice D is the mechanism by which C occurs.

Haugbol SR, et al. Upregulation of glutamate receptor subtypes during alcohol withdrawal in rats. *Alcohol Alcohol.* 2005;40:89-95.

14.4. Answer: E. Baclofen withdrawal and overdose both produce seizures. The mechanism is unclear, but it is believed to occur due to its role as a gamma-aminobutyric acid (GABA)$_B$ agonist. GABA$_B$ receptors function as both presynaptic autoreceptors and postsynaptic inhibitory receptors.

Ogata N. Pharmacology and physiology of GABA$_B$ receptors. *Gen Pharmacol.* 1990;21:395-402.

14.5. Answer: E. Of these xenobiotics, the abstinence syndrome that develops from paroxetine discontinuation is the only one that would be treated by resuming treatment with paroxetine or another selective serotonin reuptake inhibitor (SSRI), thus meeting the definition for a withdrawal syndrome. Drug discontinuation syndrome is used to describe the withdrawal syndrome caused by the discontinuation of an SSRI. The remainder of the xenobiotics listed do not generate a withdrawal syndrome.

Nielsen M, et al. What is the difference between dependence and withdrawal reactions? A comparison of benzodiazepines and selective serotonin re-uptake inhibitors. *Addiction.* 2012;107:900-908.

14.6. Answer: D. Alcohol withdrawal seizures are usually brief, generalized tonic-clonic seizures with a short postictal period and occasionally are the first and only sign of withdrawal.

Victor M, Brausch C. The role of abstinence in the genesis of alcoholic epilepsy. *Epilepsia.* 1967;8:1-20.

14.7. Answer: D. Dexmedetomidine, like clonidine, acts as a central and peripheral presynaptic alpha$_2$-adrenergic agonist. It also causes a withdrawal syndrome that is identical to clonidine withdrawal, with hypertension, tachycardia, and agitation. Clonidine is used to treat dexmedetomidine withdrawal.

Weber MD, et al. Acute discontinuation syndrome from dexmedetomidine after protracted use in a pediatric patient. *Paediatr Anaesth.* 2008;18:87-88.

14.8. Answer: A. Benzodiazepine withdrawal occurs up to 10-14 days after cessation of drugs with active metabolites and is similar to alcohol withdrawal in its presentation.

Thiamine and magnesium have little role unless a deficiency is first identified. Phenobarbital is an excellent choice for this condition.

Robinson GM, et al. Barbiturate and hypnosedative withdrawal by a multiple oral phenobarbital loading dose technique. *Clin Pharmacol Ther.* 1981;30:71-76.

14.9. Answer: D. Tachycardia, mild hypertension, mild diaphoresis, and agitation are characteristics that the two withdrawal states share. Without intensive supportive care and benzodiazepines, ethanol withdrawal carries a high mortality rate. Naturally occurring opioid withdrawal is treated on an outpatient basis in all but the rarest circumstances and is rarely associated with life-threatening complications.

Victor M, Adams RD. The effect of alcohol on the nervous system. *Res Publ Assoc Res Nerv Ment Dis.* 1953:32:526-533.

14.10. Answer: B. Nicotine withdrawal produces a general dysphoria. Antidepressants are used in the treatment of this withdrawal. Withdrawal symptoms also include constipation, agitation, and increased appetite. Heart rate falls by an average of 9 beats/min due to reduced catecholamine concentrations.

Hughes JR, et al. Nicotine withdrawal versus other drug withdrawal syndromes: Similarities and dissimilarities. *Addiction.* 1994;89: 1461-1470.

Cardiologic Principles I: Electrophysiologic and Electrocardiographic Principles

15

QUESTIONS

15.1. A 25-year-old man presents to the emergency department after a syncopal episode at home. His heart rate is 38 beats/min and his blood pressure is 88/52 mm Hg. On physical examination, he is ataxic, has paresthesias in all four extremities, and has reversal of hot and cold sensation. His history reveals a recent ingestion of fish. What site on the alpha subunit of the sodium channel does the xenobiotic he was exposed to act on?
A. Site 1
B. Site 3
C. Site 4
D. Site 5
E. Site 6

15.2. A 52-year-old man is being evaluated in the emergency department for an episode of loss of consciousness. An electrocardiogram is performed and demonstrates bidirectional ventricular tachycardia (VT). Which of the following processes is a possible explanation for this abnormal rhythm?
A. Aconitine toxicity
B. Hypokalemia
C. Catecholaminergic excess
D. Procainamide toxicity
E. Chloroquine toxicity

15.3. A 22-year-old woman presents to the emergency department following an intentional ingestion of loperamide. Loperamide acts on which of the following channels and causes prolongation of what portion of the electrocardiogram?
A. Potassium channel that conducts I_{Kr}; QT interval
B. Potassium channel that conducts I_{Kr}; QT interval
C. Potassium channel that conducts I_{Kr}; QRS complex
D. D11 subunit of the voltage-sensitive sodium channel; QRS complex
E. L-type calcium channel; PR interval

15.4. Which of the following opioids is associated with QRS complex prolongation in overdose?
A. Heroin
B. Morphine
C. Meperidine
D. Propoxyphene
E. Diphenoxylate

15.5. A 5-year-old boy presents to the emergency department in cardiac arrest after he was exposed to chloral hydrate. Which of the following mechanisms best explains this patient's presentation?
A. Increased adrenergic release
B. Sensitization of the myocardium to catecholamines
C. Atrial ventricular conduction defects
D. Intraventricular conduction delays
E. Hypoxia

15.6. A 34-year-old woman presents to the emergency department with oropharyngeal burns, severe dermal pain, and an electrocardiogram that demonstrates significant QT interval prolongation. Which of the following caustic ingestions best explains this patient's presentation?

A. Hydrochloric acid
B. Hydrofluoric acid
C. Potassium permanganate
D. Sulfuric acid
E. Sodium hydroxide

15.7. Which of the following xenobiotics would be safe to administer to an agitated patient who has a documented prolonged QT interval?

A. Droperidol
B. Haloperidol
C. Olanzapine
D. Midazolam
E. Quetiapine

15.8. A 22-year-old woman presents to the emergency department after an intentional overdose of her friend's medication. An electrocardiogram is performed, demonstrating a wide notched P wave. Which of the following medications best explains her presentation?

A. Lorazepam
B. Quinidine
C. Metoprolol
D. Diltiazem
E. Diphenhydramine

15.9. Chronic use of which of the following xenobiotics is associated with a Brugada electrocardiographic pattern?

A. Acetaminophen
B. Digoxin
C. Lithium
D. Sotalol
E. Hydrochlorothiazide

15.10. A 38-year-old woman presents to the emergency department with fatigue. Her electrocardiogram demonstrates marked QT interval shortening. Toxicity from which of the following xenobiotics best explains her presentation?

A. Methadone
B. Aspirin
C. Hydrofluoric acid
D. Amitriptyline
E. Cholecalciferol

ANSWERS

15.1. Answer: D. Brevotoxins and ciguatoxins bind to site 5 of the alpha-subunit of the sodium channel. Mu-conotoxins, saxitoxin, and tetrodotoxin bind to site 1. Scorpion alpha-toxins and sea anemone toxins bind to site 3. Scorpion beta-toxins bind to site 4. Delta-conotoxins bind to site 6.

Keating MT, Sangoinetti MC. Molecular and cellular mechanism of cardiac arrhythmias. *Cell.* 2001;104:569-580.

15.2. Answer: A. Aconitine, usually obtained from traditional Chinese medication or from the monkshood plant, causes a bidirectional VT. Bidirectional VT is also rarely associated with severe cardioactive steroid toxicity and results from alterations of intraventricular conduction, junctional tachycardia, and aberrant intraventricular conduction or alternating ventricular pacemaker.

Smith SN, et al. Bidirectional ventricular tachycardia resulting aconite poisoning. *Ann Emerg Med.* 2005;45:100-101.

15.3. Answer: B. Loperamide inhibits the potassium channel that conducts the delayed rectifier I_{Kr} current, specifically the human ether-a-go-go–related gene (hERG) alpha subunit of this channel and leads to QT interval prolongation. Potassium channel blockade prolongs the QT interval and not the QRS complex duration or the PR interval.

Eggleston W. et al. Loperamide abuse associated with cardiac dysrhythmia and death. *Ann Emerg Med.* 2017;69:83-86.

15.4. Answer: D. Propoxyphene is metabolized in the liver to norpropoxyphene, which has less analgesic effect, a much longer half-life, and local anesthetic properties like those of the class I antidysrhythmics. The marked QRS widening and dysrhythmias associated with propoxyphene toxicity respond to hypertonic sodium bicarbonate.

Stork CM, et al. Propoxyphene-induced wide QRS complex dysrhythmia responsive to sodium bicarbonate—a case report. *J Toxicol Clin Toxicol.* 1995;33:179–183.

Whitcomb DC, et al. Marked QRS complex abnormalities and sodium channel blockade by propoxyphene reversed with lidocaine. *J Clin Invest.* 1989;84:1629-1636.

15.5. Answer: B. The cardiovascular toxicity of chloral hydrate, inhalational anesthetics, and halogenated solvents results from sensitization of the myocardium to catecholamine activity. A beta-adrenergic antagonist, such as esmolol, is the preferred antidysrhythmic for atrial or ventricular dysrhythmias that occur in this setting.

Graham SR, et al. Overdose with chloral hydrate: A pharmacological and therapeutic review. *Med J Aust.* 1988;149:686-688.

15.6. Answer: B. An electrocardiogram (ECG) assists in diagnosing certain unknown exposures, especially when they are associated with electrolyte disturbances. Significant hydrofluoric acid (HF) ingestions lead to profound hypocalcemia and a resultant prolonged QT interval. Other ECG findings associated with HF ingestions include findings consistent with hyperkalemia. ECG findings in HF are often reliable indicators of systemic toxicity.

Wrenn KD, et al. The ability of physicians to predict electrolyte deficiency from the ECG. *Ann Emerg Med.* 1990;19:580-583.

Greco RJ, et al. Hydrofluoric acid-induced hypocalcemia. *J Trauma.* 1988;28:1593-1596.

15.7. Answer: D. Of the listed options, midazolam is the safest xenobiotic to administer to a patient who is acutely agitated with a concomitant prolonged QT interval. All the other xenobiotics are associated with QT interval prolongation and would place a patient at an increased risk of a resultant dysrhythmia.

Ray WA, et al. Atypical antipsychotic drugs and the risk of sudden cardiac death. *N Engl J Med.* 2009;360:225-235.

15.8. Answer: B. A wide notched P wave suggests delayed conduction across the atrial septum and is characteristic of quinidine poisoning.

Dubin, D. Rapid Interpretation of EKG's. Fifth Edition. Cover Publishing Company. Tampa, USA. 1996. p 299.

15.9. Answer: C. The Brugada electrocardiographic pattern is characterized by terminal positivity of the QRS complex and ST-segment elevation in the right precordial leads. This pattern is found in some patients who have a mutation of the genes that code for the alpha subunit of the sodium channel. A similar pattern sometimes occurs in patients who are poisoned by sodium channel blocking xenobiotics. This pattern is also associated with lithium toxicity.

Wright D, Salehian O. Brugada-type electrocardiographic changes induced by long-term lithium use. *Circulation.* 2010;122:e418-e419.

15.10. Answer: E. Toxicity from cholecalciferol, or vitamin D, leads to hypercalcemia. Hypercalcemia causes shortening of the ST segment through enhanced calcium influx during the plateau phase of the cardiac cycle, speeding the onset of repolarization. This effect leads to shortening of the QT interval.

de Paula ALT, et al. Exogenous intoxication by non-prescribed use of vitamin D, a case report. *BMC Geriatr.* 2020;20:221.

Cardiologic Principles II: Hemodynamics

QUESTIONS

16.1. A 22-year-old man goes to an herbalist and purchases a natural aphrodisiac. He consumes the substance and then presents to the emergency department with anxiety. His blood pressure is 172/98 mmHg and his heart rate is 145 beats/min. Which of the following xenobiotics led to his presentation?
A. Water hemlock
B. Veratridine
C. Yohimbine
D. Grayanotoxin
E. Aconitine

16.2. A 35-year-old woman presents to the emergency department hypotensive and bradycardic following an intentional ingestion. Which of the following xenobiotics would lead to this type of presentation?
A. Chlorpromazine
B. Amitriptyline
C. Glutethimide
D. Sotalol
E. Nifedipine

16.3. An increase in both blood pressure and pulse rate would be expected immediately following an overdose with which of the following xenobiotics?
A. Nifedipine
B. Phenylpropanolamine

C. Bretylium
D. Theophylline
E. Practolol

16.4. A 28-year-old man presents to the emergency department in cardiac arrest. Following defibrillation, he has return of spontaneous circulation and an electrocardiogram reveals that he has a Brugada pattern. The addition of which of the following xenobiotics to his medication regimen likely contributed to his cardiac arrest?
A. Amitriptyline
B. Acetaminophen
C. Nitroglycerin
D. Dabigatran
E. Diazepam

16.5. Which of the following mechanisms best explains how beta adrenergic antagonist toxicity leads to hypotension?
A. Decreased stimulation of adenylate cyclase by G_s proteins and resultant decrease in the production of cAMP
B. Inhibition of L-type calcium channels
C. Inhibition of phosphodiesterase enzyme
D. Activation of the hydrolysis of phosphatidyl inositol 4,5-bisposhpate (PIP$_2$) to 1,2-diacylglycerol (DAG) and inositol triphosphate (IP$_3$)
E. Decreased central sympathetic outflow

16.6. A 65-year-old man presents to the emergency department following in intentional overdose of aconitine. Which of the following mechanisms best explain his bradycardia?
- A. Enhancement of vagal tone
- B. Intracellular sodium overload with resultant alterations in calcium handling
- C. Direct depressant effect on the cardiac pacemaker
- D. Decreased sympathetic outflow to the heart
- E. Inhibition of phosphodiesterase enzyme

16.7. Which of the following choices leads to hypotension partly because of volume depletion?
- A. *Datura stramonium*
- B. Diltiazem
- C. Clonidine
- D. Hydralazine
- E. Iron

16.8. Which of the following options is the only truly reliable means to assess whether a patient will respond to a fluid bolus?
- A. Central venous pressure
- B. Ultrasonography of the inferior vena cava
- C. Neck vein distension
- D. Orthostatic vital sign monitoring
- E. Administration of a fluid bolus

16.9. A 34-year-old man presents to the emergency department with chest pain, an elevated temperature to 101.5 °F (38.6 °C) and persistent tachycardia. A bedside echocardiogram reveals a very diminished ejection fracture. His blood work demonstrates an elevated serum troponin. The patient has not overdosed on any of his medications. Which of the following xenobiotics could explain his presentation?
- A. Clozapine
- B. Nicardipine
- C. Alprazolam
- D. Doxycycline
- E. Methadone

16.10. A 16-year-old boy with a history of attention deficit hyperactivity disorder (ADHD) presents to the emergency department with a depressed mental status and pinpoint pupils. His vital signs are: blood pressure, 82/40 mmHg; heart rate, 38 beats/min; respiratory rate, 8 breaths/min; SpO$_2$, 92% on 2 L of oxygen; temperature, 96.2 °F (35.7 °C); and glucose, 73 mg/dL (4.1 mmol/L). Which of the following options would be the best first-line vasopressor option in this patient?
- A. Dopamine
- B. Epinephrine
- C. Milrinone
- D. Norepinephrine
- E. Phenylephrine

ANSWERS

16.1. Answer: C. Yohimbine is an indole alkylamine alkaloid from the West African yohimbe tree. It is an alpha$_2$ adrenergic antagonist (the opposite effect of clonidine). Adverse effects include anxiety, headache, confusion, seizures, coma, tachycardia, hypertension, QRS widening, and priapism. It is used in some cultures to enhance sexual performance. Water hemlock contains cicutoxin, which inhibits GABA receptors. Veratridine, grayanotoxin, and aconitine are sodium channel openers, which produce bradycardia.

Giampreti A, et al. Acute neurotoxicity after yohimbine ingestion by a body builder. *Clin Toxicol.* 2009;47:827-829.

16.2. Answer: D. Sotalol is a class III antidysrhythmic that also has beta adrenergic antagonist properties. Overdose of a class III antidysrhythmic prolongs the QT interval and leads to an increased risk of dysrhythmias, including torsade de pointes. Overdose of sotalol also presents with features suggestive of beta adrenergic antagonist toxicity, including bradycardia and hypotension.

Reith DM, et al. Relative toxicity of beta blockers in overdose. *J Toxicol Clin Toxicol.* 1996:34:273-278.

16.3. Answer: C. Bretylium initially results in increased norepinephrine release from sympathetic neurons and inhibition of subsequent uptake. Bretylium causes transient hypertension, tachycardia, and increased dysrhythmias through this norepinephrine release.

Leatham EW, et al. Class III antiarrhythmics in overdose. Presenting features and management principles. *Drug Safety.* 1993;9:450-462.

16.4. Answer: A. Brugada syndrome is a congenital cardiac channelopathy that predisposes to sudden cardiac death. Brugada syndrome is characterized by an atypical right bundle branch pattern with a characteristic cove-shaped ST-segment elevation in leads V1 to V3 of the electrocardiogram. Certain xenobiotics, such as vagotonic medications, class I antidysrhythmics, or sodium channel blockers, unmask an underlying Brugada pattern on the electrocardiogram. In this patient, it was the addition of amitriptyline that likely precipitated an unstable rhythm.

BrugadaDrugs.org. Safe drug use and the Brugada syndrome. http://www.brugadadrugs.org/. Accessed July 7, 2021.

16.5. Answer: A. Beta adrenergic antagonist overdose results in decreased stimulation of adenylate cyclase by G_s proteins, decreased production of cAMP, decreased activation of the cAMP-dependent kinases, and ultimately decreased Ca^{2+} release.

Levitzki A, et al. The signal transduction between beta-receptors and adenylyl cyclase. *Life Sci.* 1993;52:2093-2100.

16.6. Answer: B. Aconitine, derived from the monkshood plant, is a sodium channel activator and causes bradycardia due to intracellular sodium overload with resultant alteration in calcium handling.

Chan TY. Aconite poisoning. *Clin Toxicol.* 2009;47:279-285.

16.7. Answer: E. Intravascular volume depletion in toxic exposures occurs through gastrointestinal losses (iron, theophylline), insensible losses, diaphoresis (cocaine, organic phosphorus compounds, theophylline), urinary losses (theophylline), interstitial redistribution (iron), and vascular dilatation (iron, theophylline).

Thomson J. Ferrous sulphate poisoning. *Br Med J.* 1950;1:645-646.

16.8. Answer: E. While central venous pressure monitoring, ultrasonography of the inferior vena cava, neck vein distension, and orthostatic vital sign monitoring are used as modes of hemodynamic monitoring, the only truly reliable means to assess whether a patient will respond to fluids is by administering a trial fluid bolus. An alternate test that provides helpful information is a passive leg-raising test, which functionally gives the patient a fluid bolus to assess the adequacy of fluid resuscitation without adding to the whole-body volume status. The test is performed by having the patient sit upright in a semi-recumbent position at about 45 degrees. The head is then lowered to the recumbent position and the legs are raised about 45 degrees. This transiently increases the circulatory volume by 130-300 mL. This is a good predictor of hemodynamic response to a fluid bolus in critically ill patients without actually administering fluids.

Carsetti A, et al. Fluid bolus therapy: Monitoring and predicting fluid responsiveness. *Curr Opin Crit Care.* 2015;21:388-394.

Lafanechère A, et al. Changes in aortic blood flow induced by passive leg raising predict fluid responsiveness in critically ill patients. *Crit Care Lond Engl.* 2006;10:R132.

16.9. Answer: A. Clozapine is an atypical antipsychotic that requires a special registry in order to prescribe it in the United States. Two potentially life-threatening effects are agranulocytosis and myocarditis. Clozapine myocarditis includes at least one of the following symptoms and/or signs of cardiac dysfunction: chest pain, influenzalike symptoms, persistent tachycardia, and signs of heart failure. Patients also require at least one of the following diagnostic abnormalities: elevated serum troponin, echocardiographic evidence of systolic dysfunction, and electrocardiographic changes involving T-wave inversion or greater than 1 mm ST-segment deviation in at least two contiguous leads.

Miller DD. Review and management of clozapine side effects. *J Clin Psychiatry.* 2000;61(suppl 8):14-17.

Youssef DL, et al. Incidence and risk factors for clozapine-induced myocarditis and cardiomyopathy at a regional mental health service in Australia. *Australas Psychiatry.* 2016;24:176-180.

16.10. Answer: D. This patient is presenting following a clonidine overdose. It is reasonable to start with naloxone as a first line antidote, especially as this patient has both a depressed mental status and respirations. If a vasopressor is still needed, norepinephrine is the best of the listed vasopressors to treat this patient. Dopamine is an indirect vasopressor and inotrope and therefore is not an ideal option. While epinephrine is reasonable, it is less effective at reversing the imidazoline-induced central sympatholysis at the locus coeruleus. Milrinone is a phosphodiesterase inhibitor and causes undesirable peripheral vasodilation. Phenylephrine does not directly improve inotropy.

Anderson RJ, et al. Clonidine overdose: Report of six cases and review of the literature. *Ann Emerg Med.* 1981;10:107-112.

Dermatologic Principles

17

QUESTIONS

17.1. A 25-year-old woman presents to the hospital with a rash that looks like linear streaks of erythema only in sun-exposed areas. Which of the following foods could have caused this rash?
A. Apple
B. Banana
C. Cilantro
D. Parsnip
E. Carrot

17.2. A 37-year-old woman presents to the emergency department with a rash on her right cheek and forehead that developed approximately 24 hours after she went on a hike in the forest. The rash is itchy with some small overlying blisters. Which of the following options is the best way to treat her rash?
A. Low-potency corticosteroid cream
B. Medium-potency corticosteroid cream
C. High-potency corticosteroid cream
D. A corticosteroid ointment
E. Topical corticosteroids under occlusion

17.3. Which of the following options is the xenobiotic most commonly associated with allergic contact dermatitis?
A. Bacitracin
B. Anthralin
C. Silver sulfadiazine
D. Polymyxin
E. Neomycin

17.4. A 39-year-old woman has a known history of hypersensitivity to poison ivy. Exposure to which of the following substances would the lead to a similar reaction?
A. Cashew nuts
B. Bergamot orange
C. Neomycin
D. Henna
E. Parabens

17.5. What is the most significant factor that determines the percutaneous absorption of a chemical?
A. Concentration
B. Molecular size
C. pH
D. Lipid solubility
E. Water solubility

17.6. A 27-year-old man presents to the emergency department with a diffuse, edematous rash associated with facial edema. His vital signs are notable for a fever to 102.3 °F (39.1 °C). His alanine aminotransferase (ALT) is 700 IU/L (11.6 ukat/L). Which of the following medications led to his presentation?
A. Sertraline
B. Ondansetron
C. Diazepam
D. Aspirin
E. Carbamazepine

17.7. A 42-year-old man presents with a rash that was initially erythematous streaks. As it is healing, it is becoming hyperpigmented. An astute clinician diagnoses him with a flagellate dermatitis. What is the likely cause of the rash?
A. Shiitake mushrooms
B. Carbamazepine
C. Heparin
D. Vancomycin
E. Minocycline

17.8. A 62-year-old man is being evaluated in the clinic for a rash that resembles severe acne vulgaris. His rash is predominantly in the malar and mandibular regions. Exposure to which substance explains his presentation?
A. Amiodarone
B. Bleomycin
C. Phenol
D. 2,3,7,8-Tetrachlorodibenzodioxin
E. Topiramate

17.9. Skin decontamination using water is contraindicated in which of the following exposures?
A. Potassium hydroxide dust
B. Hydrochloric acid
C. Hydrofluoric acid
D. Phenol liquid
E. Zinc dust

17.10. A 68-year-old man is sent to the hospital for evaluation of his discolored skin. His primary physician is concerned that the patient is jaundiced. On physical examination, the patient has white sclera. As an intravenous catheter is being placed, the nurse notes that the discoloration improves as the area is cleaned with an alcohol swab. Which of the following is the likely culprit?
A. Acetaminophen toxicity
B. Hypercarotenemia
C. Sulfhemoglobin
D. Argyria
E. Excess vitamin A

ANSWERS

17.1. Answer: D. This patient has phytophotodermatitis, which occurs because of sun exposure to skin that was in contact with furocoumarins. Phytotoxic dermatitis is caused by several different substances, including lime, parsnip, fig, celery, and fragrance materials.

Morison WL. Clinical practice. Photosensitivity. *N Engl J Med.* 2004;350:1111 1117.

17.2. Answer: A. In cases of poison ivy, low-potency corticosteroid preparations should be used to treat steroid-responsive dermatitis on areas of thin skin, as on the face, or intertriginous skin, like the groin and axilla. The risk of acneiform eruption, striae, telangiectasia, petechiae, and atrophy increases with higher potency corticosteroids and corticosteroids under occlusion. Ointments are messy and promote acneiform eruptions in areas with high concentrations of sebaceous glands.

Grevelink SA, et al. Effectiveness of various barrier preparations in preventing and/or ameliorating experimentally produced toxicodendron dermatitis. *J Am Acad Dermatol.* 1992;27:182-188.

17.3. Answer: E. Neomycin is the most common cause of medication-related contact dermatitis. Bacitracin is the most common topical medication causing anaphylactic reactions.

Leyden JJ, Kligman AM. Contact dermatitis to neomycin sulfate. *JAMA.* 1979;242:1276-1278.

17.4. Answer: A. Urushiol, which comes from plants species of the genus *Anacardiaciae*, causes a type IV hypersensitivity reaction. *Rhus* dermatitis and *Toxicodendron* dermatitis are two other names used to describe the rash caused by urushiol. In addition to poison ivy, other members include poison sumac, cashew nuts, *Ginkgo* tree, mango, and the Japanese lacquer tree.

Stoner JG, Rasmussen JE. Plant dermatitis. *J Am Acad Dermatol.* 1983;9:1-15.

17.5. Answer: D. While all these factors are significant, a chemical's lipid solubility has the greatest influence on absorption through the skin.

Wester RC, Maibach HI. In vivo percutaneous absorption: Critical factors in transdermal transport. In: Marzulli FN, Maibach HI, eds. *Dermatoxicology.* 4th ed. New York, NY: Hemisphere; 1991:1-36.

17.6. Answer: E. This patient is presenting with drug-induced hypersensitivity syndrome (DIHS). This was formerly called drug reaction with eosinophilia syndrome (DRESS). It is characterized by a triad of fever, skin eruption, and internal organ involvement. Aromatic antiepileptics, such as phenobarbital, carbamazepine, and phenytoin, are typical causes. If a patient develops DIHS from one of these antiepileptics, there is a risk of cross-reaction with the other aromatic antiepileptics. Allopurinol, dapsone, lamotrigine, and sulfonamide antibiotics also cause DIHS. The most important intervention is to discontinue the offending drug. If there is cardiac or pulmonary involvement, systemic corticosteroids should be given.

Knowles SR, Shear NH. Recognition and management of severe cutaneous drug reactions. *Dermatol Clin*. 2007;25:245-253.

17.7. Answer: A. Flagellate dermatitis was initially reported to be caused by bleomycin. However, it is also caused by the ingestion of raw or undercooked shiitake mushrooms. The rash is attributed to lentinan, which is found in shiitake mushrooms as well as some chemotherapeutics.

Hamer S, Rabindranathnambi R. A wide-spread flagellate dermatitis. *BMJ Case Rep*. 2013;2013:bcr2012007682.

17.8. Answer: D. This patient is presenting with chloracne, which is caused by halogenated aromatic chemicals. The classic exposure is dioxin (2,3,7,8-tetrachlorodibenzodioxin), however, other xenobiotics such as polychlorinated biphenyls and 2,4-dichlorophenoxyacetic acid also cause this.

Zugerman C. Chloracne. Clinical manifestations and etiology. *Dermatol Clin*. 1990;8:209-213.

17.9. Answer: E. Exposure to the dusts of certain metals, including zinc, strontium, titanium, sulfur, all of the Group I elements (sodium, potassium, etc), and pure magnesium will ignite on contact with water. Instead, the metal should be removed with forceps, gauze, or towels and stored in mineral oil.

https://cameochemicals.noaa.gov/chemical/4814. Accessed April 13, 2021.

17.10. Answer: B. Hypercarotenemia occurs in patients who take supplements that contain carotene. This patient's yellow-tinged skin spares his sclera, which is an important way to differentiate between true jaundice and hypercarotenemia. Furthermore, the yellow discoloration is removed with an alcohol swab. Patients who have hypercarotenemia also appear well and do not have any other stigmata of liver disease.

Takita Y, et al. A case of carotenemia associated with ingestion of nutrient supplements. *J Dermatol*. 2006;33:132-134.

Gastrointestinal Principles

QUESTIONS

18.1. A 72-year-old woman presents to the emergency department with 6 hours of constant retrosternal chest pain. It is worse when she swallows. Her cardiac evaluation and a computed tomography (CT) scan of her chest are within normal limits. Which of the following medications best explains her symptoms?
A. Acetaminophen
B. Alendronate
C. Diphenhydramine
D. Zolpidem
E. Morphine

18.2. A 6-year-old boy is brought into the emergency department immediately after he had a witnessed button battery ingestion. An abdominal radiograph demonstrates that the button battery is in the stomach. He is currently asymptomatic. Which of the following options is the best next step in his management?
A. Endoscopic removal within 2 hours
B. Endoscopic removal within 24 hours
C. Surgical consultation for laparoscopic foreign body removal
D. Whole bowel irrigation
E. Expectant management and allow spontaneous passage of the battery

18.3. Which of the following statements regarding the effects of ethanol on the gastrointestinal (GI) tract is true?
A. Ethanol-induced lesions occur after acute ingestions of ethanol at concentrations of 1%
B. Ethanol-induced erosive gastritis is a minor cause of GI hemorrhage

C. Ethanol increases the secretion of gastric juices
D. Ethanol decreases gastric mucosal permeability
E. Ethanol-induced diarrhea is partly due to increased transit time

18.4. The major toxicity associated with eating oxalate-containing plants such as *Dieffenbachia spp.* includes which of the following findings?
A. Hypocalcemia
B. Kidney failure
C. Pain and swelling of the mouth and tongue
D. Constipation
E. Peptic ulcers

18.5. Ingestion of which of the following caustic xenobiotics results in oral pain, ulcerations, pulmonary complications, and the formation of a pharyngeal pseudomembrane?
A. Sodium hydroxide
B. Concentrated hydrochloric acid
C. Concentrated hydrofluoric acid
D. Paraquat
E. Ethanol in greater than 40% concentrations

18.6. Which of the following xenobiotics is associated with a dry mouth?
A. Caustics
B. Carbamates
C. Tetrodotoxin
D. Protease inhibitors
E. Hastily swallowed drug packets

18.7. A 65-year-old man presents to the emergency department after not having had a bowel movement in more than 7 days. He has a history of metastatic prostate cancer with painful bony metastasis. Which of the following medications would be the best therapy for his constipation?
A. Physostigmine
B. Flumazenil
C. Oxybutynin
D. Senna
E. Methylnaltrexone

18.8. A 27-year-old man presents to his dentist for further evaluation of gingival hyperplasia. Which of the following medications is implicated in causing this finding?
A. Acetaminophen
B. Carbamazepine
C. Digoxin
D. Topiramate
E. Aspirin

18.9. A 76-year-old woman presents to the emergency department for further evaluation of a left-sided hip fracture. Which of the following medications is associated with an increased risk of developing fracture?
A. Aspirin
B. Digoxin
C. Omeprazole
D. Colchicine
E. Acetaminophen

18.10. A 3-year-old girl presents to the emergency department after eating an unknown quantity of pyrinuron. The product was in her grandmother's attic and was sold under the brand name Vacor. Which of the following toxicities would be expected following this ingestion?
A. Diabetic ketoacidosis
B. Ascending paralysis
C. Wrist drop
D. Trigeminal neuralgia
E. Uncontrolled seizures

ANSWERS

18.1. Answer: B. This patient is presenting with post-pill esophagitis. Alendronate, a type of bisphosphonate, causes a chemical esophagitis and occasionally severe ulceration. To decrease the risk of developing an esophagitis, patients should be instructed to be sitting up when taking this medication, should ensure that they drink plenty of liquids with the pills, and must remain upright for at least 30 minutes after taking the medication. Other at-risk medications include risedronate, ibandronate, doxycyline, and potassium chloride.

de Groen PC, et al. Esophagitis associated with the use of alendronate. *N Engl J Med.* 1996;335:1016-1021.

18.2. Answer: E. Esophageal button batteries cause significant mucosal injury within 2-4 hours and perforation within 6 hours. All suspected esophageal button batteries should undergo endoscopic removal within 2 hours. Button batteries that are in the stomach in asymptomatic patients are managed expectantly, with the button battery being allowed to pass sponatenously.

Litovitz T, et al. Emerging battery-ingestion hazard: Clinical implications. *Pediatrics.*2010;125:1168-1177.

Sharpe SJ, et al. Pediatric battery-related emergency department visits in the United States, 1990-2009. *Pediatrics.* 2012;129:1111-1117.

Leinwand K, et al. Button battery ingestion in children: A paradigm for management of severe pediatric foreign body ingestions. *Gastrointest Endosc Clin N Am.* 2016;26:99-118.

Mubarak A, et al. Diagnosis, management, and prevention of button battery ingestion in childhood: An ESPGHAN position paper. *J Pediatr Gastroenterol Nutr.* 2021;73:e29.

18.3. Answer: C. Ethanol increases the secretion of gastric juices reduces the transmucosal potential difference allowing for back-diffusion of hydrogen ions, and increases mucosal permeability. Ethanol concentrations as low as 8% are associated with gastrointestinal (GI) lesions. In some series, ethanol-induced erosive gastritis, with or without concomitant use of salicylates, accounts for 45-90% of upper GI hemorrhages. Ethanol causes diarrhea through several mechamisms, including decreased transit time, decreased pancreatic function, and decreased disaccharidase activity.

Geall MG, et al. Profile of gastric potential difference in man. Effects of aspirin, alcohol, bile, and endogenous acid. *Gastroenterology.* 1970;58:437-443.

Nalin DR, et al. Cannabis, hydrochlorhydria and cholera. *Lancet.* 1978;2:859-861.

18.4. Answer: C. Oxalate-containing plants, particularly *Dieffenbachia spp.* (dumbcane), cause local irritation, which results in pain and edema of the mouth and tongue. On occasion, the effects are severe enough to cause death. As it is almost impossible to ingest significant amounts of oxalate-containing plants, systemic problems such as hypocalcemia and kidney failure do not occur. Diarrhea, not constipation, occurs because of an ingestion. Peptic ulcers are not described with *Dieffenbachia spp.* ingestion.

Altin G, et al. Severe destruction of the upper respiratory structures after brief exposure to a *Dieffenbachia* plant. *J Craniofac Surg.* 2013;24: e245-e247.

18.5. Answer: D. Paraquat ingestions result in lip, tongue, and pharyngeal pain and ulceration. Systemic complications include acute respiratory distress syndrome (ARDS), pneumothorax, liver and kidney failure, dysrhythmias, shock, coma, and convulsions. A unique feature of paraquat is the formation of a pseudomembrane in the pharynx, resembling diphtheria. Of the other items listed, ingestion of concentrated hydrofluoric acid and concentrated hydrochloric acid are associated with severe systemic effects in addition to the local damage, but none are associated with a pseudomembrane.

Stephens DS, et al. Pseudodiphtheria. *Ann Intern Med.* 1981;94:202-204.

18.6. Answer: D. Dry mouth, also known as xerostomia, is an adverse effect of certain xenobiotics and is associateed with dental decay. Protease inhibitors cause xerostomia in as many as 7% of patients. The list of other xenobiotics that do this is quite extensive; however, common causes include xenobiotics that have anticholinergic effects. Cholinergic agents, such as organic phosphorous compounds and carbamate insecticides, lead to drooling and salivation. Caustics and tetrodotoxin are also associated with drooling, as is partial obstruction from foreign bodies.

Abdollahi M, et al. Current opinion on drug-induced oral reactions: A comprehensive review. *J Contemp Dent Pract.* 2008;9:1-15.

Diz Dios P, Scully C. Adverse effects of antiretroviral therapy: Focus on orofacial effects. *Expert Opin Drug Saf.* 2002;1:307-317.

18.7. Answer: E. Patients with chronic pain who are prescribed opioid medication are at risk of developing severe constipation, leading to abdominal pain, bowel obstruction, and perforation. Peripherally acting mu opioid receptor antagonists, such as methylnaltrexone, help to treat opioid-induced constipation without the risk of percipitating dangerous and uncomfortably opioid withdrawal.

Argoff CE, et al. Consensus recommendations on initiating prescription therapies for opioid-induced constipation. *Pain Med.* 2015;16:2324-2337.

18.8. Answer: D. Gingival hyperplasia is an overgrowth of the gums around the teeth. It is an uncommon condition, but is associated with several xenobiotics. Medications implicated in causing this finding include phenytoin, cyclosporine, lithium, phenobarbital, valproic acid, calcium channel blockers, and topiramate.

Abdollahi M, et al. Current opinion on drug-induced oral reactions: A comprehensive review. *J Contemp Dent Pract.* 2008;9:1-15.

18.9. Answer: C. Proton pump inhibitors, such as omeprazole, lead to hypochlorhydria or achlorhydria. Hypochlorhydria is the reduction of gastric acid while achlorhydria is the absence of gastric acid. By raising the pH of the stomach, proton pump inhibitors lead to impaired calcium absorption and thereby increase the risk of fractures. Proton pump inhibitors are also associated with bacterial overgrowth, atrophic gastritis, *Salmonella* and *Vibrio cholerae* infections, gastric carcinoma, and impaired magnesium absorption.

Vakil N. Prescribing proton pump inhibitors: Is it time to pause and rethink? *Drugs.* 2012;72:437-445.

18.10. Answer: A. Pyrinuron (*N*-3 pyridylmethyl-*N'* 4 nitrophenyl urea, PNU), sold under the brand name Vacor, leads to beta islet cell destruction with resultant hyperglycemia. Patients are at risk of developing diabetic ketoacidosis. Vacor was a rodenticide that was available between 1975 and 1979. Vacor structurally resembles streptazocin and alloxan.

Schum TR, Lachman BS. Effects of packaging and appearance on childhood poisoning. Vacor rat poison. *Clin Pediatr.* 1982;21:282-285.

Genitourinary Principles

QUESTIONS

19.1. A 62-year-old-man from California presents to the hospital for further evaluation of his infertility. On history, he tells you that he was a farmer in the 1970s. Which of the following is a soil fumigant associated with testicular toxicity?
A. 1,2-Dibromo-3-chloropropane
B. Carbaryl
C. Yohimbine
D. Cantharidin
E. Sildenafil

19.2. An 18-year-old man presents to the hospital after using yohimbine for sexual enhancement. Which of the following options best explains the mechanism of action of yohimbine?
A. Anticholinergic activity
B. Alpha$_1$ adrenergic antagonism
C. Alpha$_2$ adrenergic agonism
D. Alpha$_2$ adrenergic antagonism
E. Beta$_2$ adrenergic agonism

19.3. An 18-year-old man presents to the emergency department with an episode of loss of consciousness following an ingestion of an aphrodisiac. His vital signs are: blood pressure, 110/80 mmHg; heart rate, 35 beats/min; respiratory rate, 14 breaths/min; and oxygen saturation, 100% on room air. His blood work is notable for a potassium of 5.8 mEq/L. Which of the following treatments should be administered?
A. Calcium chloride
B. Dimercaptosuccinic acid (DMSA)
C. Clonidine
D. Methylene blue
E. Digoxin-specific antibody fragments

19.4. A 16-year-old woman presents to the emergency department with hepatotoxicity. Two days prior to her presentation, she took a xenobiotic at home to induce an abortion. Which of the following abortifacients would best explain her presentation?
A. Blue cohosh
B. Cantharidin
C. Pulegone
D. Trichosanthin
E. Mifepristone

19.5. Which of the following options is responsible for cyclophosphamide-induced hemorrhagic cystitis?
A. Pulegone
B. Acrolein
C. 1,2-Dibromo-3-chloropropane
D. Cantharidin
E. Trichosanthin

19.6. A 67-year-old man is concerned that his vision is blue-green tinged. On medication reconciliation, which xenobiotic might explain his presentation?
A. Sildenafil
B. Nitrofurantoin
C. Nitroglycerin
D. Tamsulosin
E. Trazadone

19.7. A 26-year-old man presents to the emergency department with multiple episodes of hematemesis. During his resuscitation, a Foley catheter is inserted and significant hematuria is found. A friend reports that he had ingested a product he thought would enhance his sexual performance. Which of the following xenobiotics best explains his presentation?
A. Rock Hard
B. Poppers
C. Yohimbine
D. Ginseng
E. Spanish fly

19.8. A 19-year-old man presents to the emergency department several times for symptoms of cysititis. He has also developed colicky abdominal pain. A computed tomography (CT) scan of his abdomen is performed and demonstrates generalized bladder wall thickening as well as ureteric wall thickening and enhancement. What explains his symptoms?
A. Marijuana
B. Ketamine
C. Cocaine
D. Amphetamine
E. *Amanita muscaria*

19.9. A 33-year-old woman is being evaluated by her psychiatrist because her current antidepressant medication has led to sexual dysfunction. Which of the following antidepressants would be a reasonable alternate medication regimen?
A. Fluoxetine
B. Bupropion
C. Escitalopram
D. Citalopram
E. Amitriptyline

19.10. An 83-year-old man presents to the emergency department for evaluation of new-onset kidney failure. A bedside sonogram demonstrates a very distended bladder. A Foley catheter is inserted with return of 2.5 L of urine. Which medication led to his presentation?
A. Disopyramide
B. Lorazepam
C. Tamsulosin
D. Lidocaine
E. Aspirin

ANSWERS

19.1. Answer: A. In 1977, a study of Californian pesticide workers exposed to dibromochloropropane (DBCP) showed an increased incidence of male infertility due to oligospermia and azospermia. DBCP was banned by the Environmental Protection Agency (EPA) for use in the United States in 1979.

Biava CG, et al. The testicular morphology of individuals exposed to dibromochloropropane. *Exp Molec Pathol.* 1978;29:448-458.

Whorton MD, Foliart DE. Mutagenicity, carcinogenicity, and reproductive effects of dibromochloropropane (DBCP). *Mutat Res.* 1983;123:13-30.

19.2. Answer: D. Yohimbine is an alpha$_2$ adrenergic antagonist with cholinergic activity used to treat erectile dysfunction.

Owen JA, et al. The pharmacokinetics of yohimbine in man. *Eur J Clin Pharmacol.* 1987;32:577-582.

19.3. Answer: E. Rock Hard, an aphrodisiac that is intended to be applied topically, contains steroids from the bufadienolide class (toad venom), which are similar in both structure and toxicity to digoxin. Digoxin-specific antibody fragments are demonstrated to be effective treatments for human and animal toxicity from bufotoxins. However, as there are structural differences between the two cardioactive steroids, higher doses of digoxin-specific antibody fragments are needed.

Brubacher JR, et al. Treatment of toad venom poisoning with digoxin-specfic Fab fragments. *Chest.* 1996;110:1282-1288.

19.4. Answer: C. Pulegone, the ketone in pennyroyal oil, is a direct hepatotoxin. Fulminant hepatic failure occurs after ingestion of 2 oz of pennyroyal oil. The mechanism of toxicity includes glutathione depletion; therefore, patients suspected of overdosing on pennyroyal should be treated with *N*-acetylcysteine. Blue cohosh contains methylcytosine and leads to nausea, vomiting, and salivation. Cantharidin, also known as Spanish fly, has vesicant activity that causes gastrointestinal hemorrhage. Trichosanthin, commonly known as snake gourd, inhibits protein synthesis and decreases human chorionic gonadotropin (HCG) and progesterone concentrations. Mifepristone causes nausea, vomiting, abdominal pain, and vaginal bleeding.

Buechel DW. Pennyroyal oil ingestion: Report of a case. *J Am Osteopath Assoc.* 1983;2:793-794.

Sullivan JB, et al. Pennyroyal oil poisoning with hepatotoxicity. *JAMA.* 1979;242:2873-2874.

19.5.   Answer: B. Up to 46% of patients receiving cyclophosphamide develop hemorrhagic cystitis. Acrolein is a metabolite of cyclophosphamide that damages the urothelium. Acrolein also develops from treatment with ifosfamide. The hemorrhagic cystits should be treated with mesna.

Droller MJ, et al. Prevention of cyclophosphamide-induced hemorrhagic cystitis. *Urology.* 1982;20:256-258.

Klein FA, Smith MJV. Urinary complications of cyclophosphamide therapy. *South Med J.* 1983;76:1413-1416.

19.6.   Answer: A. Sildanefil causes weak phosphodiesterase 6 inhibition in the retina, which leads to blurred vision, increased light perception, and transient blue-green vision.

Goldstein I, et al. Oral sildenafil in the treatment of erectile dysfunction. Sildanefil Study Group. *N Engl J Med.* 1998;338:1397-1404.

19.7.   Answer: E. Spanish fly is the common name for cantharidin, which is derived from the blister beetle. Cantharidin has vesicant activity and causes gastrointestinal hemorrhage, blister formation in the lower urinary tract, kidney failure, vaginal bleeding, electrocardiographic changes, and disseminated intravascular coagulation (DIC). Neurologic symptoms are rare. Rock Hard is the common name for a substance that contains bufotoxin and leads to cardioactive steroid toxicity. Poppers contain amyl nitrite and cause methemoglobinemia. Yohimbine is an alpha$_2$ adrenergic antagonist and causes hypertension and tachycardia. Ginseng leads to gastrointestinal distress, seizures, and vaginal bleeding.

Karras DJ, et al. Poisoning from "Spanish fly" (Cantharidin). *Am J Emerg Med.* 1996;14:478-483.

19.8.   Answer: B. Chronic ketamine use is associated with the development of ketamine cystitis, leading to severe bladder inflammation, and eventually causes upper urinary tract damage. The underlying etiology is believed to be ketamine metabolites. The mainstay of therapy is to ensure abstinence from further ketamine use.

Mason K, et al. Ketamine-associated lower urinary tract destruction: A new radiological challenge. *Clin Radiol.* 2010;65:795-800.

Middela S, Pearce I. Ketamine-induced vesicopathy: A literature review. *Int J Clin Pract.* 2011;65:27-30.

19.9.   Answer: B. Antidepressants, especially selective serotonin reuptake inhibitors (SSRIs), often lead to sexual dysfunction. The treatment includes either decreasing the dosage of the causative medication or changing to an alternate medication with less sexual side effects. Bupropion alone was as effective as fluoxetine in treating depression and was associated with less sexual side effects.

Coleman CC, et al. A placebo-controlled comparison of the effects on sexual functioning of bupropion sustained release and fluoxetine. *Clin Ther.* 2001;23:1040-1058.

19.10.   Answer: A. This patient's kidney failure occurred as a result of his urinary retention. While the most common cause of urinary retention in older men is from benign prostatic hyperplasia, certain medication also contribute. Scopolamine patches and other antimuscarinics are commonly implicated as causes of new urinary retention. However, other medications, including the antidysrhythmics, such as disopyramide, procainamide, and quinidine also cause urinary retention.

Fontanarosa PB, Roush WR. Acute urinary retention. *Emerg Med Clin North Am.* 1988;6:419-437.

Hematologic Principles

QUESTIONS

20.1. A 32-year-old man presents to the emergency department for further evaluation of aplastic anemia. He was recently started on an antiepileptic medication. Which of the following xenobiotics likely contributed to his aplastic anemia?
A. Valproic acid
B. Carbamazepine
C. Topiramate
D. Lacosamide
E. Phenytoin

20.2. Which of the following statements best explains why neonates are at particular risk for hypoxic injury?
A. They are generally anemic
B. The volume of distribution of many xenobiotics is altered in neonates
C. The persistence of fetal hemoglobin impairs oxygen unloading
D. The tidal volume of neonates is much smaller
E. The immature liver is less able to detoxify various toxins

20.3. A 2-year-old girl is brought to her pediatrician due to a concern of decreased activity and vigor. She has laboratory studies performed that demonstrate a hemoglobin of 8.5 g/dL. Which of the following moth-repellents is most likely to cause this laboratory abnormality?
A. 1,4-Dichlorobenzene (paradichlorobenzene)
B. Camphor

C. Naphthalene
D. Menthol
E. Red cedar wood

20.4. Which of the following statements is true regarding benzene toxicity?
A. The primary route of exposure is transcutaneous
B. None of the metabolites are excreted in the urine
C. Exposure results in thrombocytosis
D. Toxic metabolites are formed in the bone marrow
E. Exposure results in acute lymphocytic leukemia

20.5. A 37-year-old man presents to the emergency department with shortness of breath and increasing fatigue over the past several months. He has no melena, hematochezia, coffee-ground emesis, or chest pain. His vital signs are: blood pressure, 135/70 mmHg; heart rate, 122 beats/min; respiratory rate, 22 breaths/min; temperature, 98.6 °F (37 °C); and oxygen saturation, 97%. He appears pale, his lungs are clear to auscultation, his abdomen is soft and nontender, and his stool has no occult blood. His complete blood cell count demonstrates a white blood cell count (WBC) of 7.2×10^9/L, hemoglobin 6.5 g/dL, hematocrit 19.5%, platelet count 270×10^9/L, mean corpuscular volume 82 fL (normal 76-100 fL), mean corpuscular hemoglobin 29 pg (normal 27-31 pg), lymphocytes 34%, segmented neutrophils 56%, eosinophils 2.7%, basophils 0.5%, monocytes 4%, and reticulocyte count <0.2%. Which of the following medications is the most likely cause?
A. Carbamazepine
B. Clozapine
C. Phenytoin
D. Phenobarbital
E. Ibuprofen

20.6. A 22-year-old man presents to the emergency department after he is bitten by a crotaline (pit viper) snake. His initial blood work demonstrates thrombocytopenia. What would the remainder of his coagulation panel demonstrate?

A. Elevated prothrombin time (PT), normal partial thromboplastin time (PTT), abnormal thrombin time, normal fibrinogen

B. Elevated PT, elevated PTT, abnormal thrombin time, abnormal fibrinogen

C. Elevated PT, elevated PTT, abnormal thrombin time, normal fibrinogen

D. Normal PT, normal PTT, abnormal thrombin, abnormal fibrinogen

E. Normal PT, normal PTT, normal thrombin, normal fibrinogen

20.7. Chloramphenicol toxicity is characterized by which of the following statements?

A. The development of aplastic anemia is inevitable in all patients who develop anemia following exposure

B. Aplastic anemia usually occurs within 5 months of exposure to chloramphenicol

C. Toxicity to bone marrow is based on an immune mechanism

D. Affected bone marrow cells are morphologically normal when viewed with an electron microscope

E. Recovery following the onset of aplastic anemia occurs in about 25% of patients

20.8. Which of the following statements describing ionizing radiation is correct?

A. Rapidly proliferating cells are at the greatest risk of injury

B. A significant exposure will result in anemia almost immediately

C. Inflammation is the most significant harmful effect

D. One of the most sensitive indicators of an acute recent exposure is the platelet count

E. It is not known to result in hematologic malignances

20.9. Which of the following statements best describes the mature erythrocyte?

A. It is 90% hemoglobin by dry weight

B. It relies only on aerobic metabolism

C. It has no mechanism to protect itself from oxidative attack

D. It replaces hemoglobin lost to senescence

E. It forms 2,3-diphosphoglycerate (2,3-DPG) in the red cell prior to the loss of the red cell nucleus

20.10. Which of the following statements is most accurate with regard to glucose-6-phosphate dehydrogenase (G6PD) deficiency?

A. Women are more commonly affected than men

B. Hemolysis occurs following exposure to strong reducing agents

C. As red cells age, the activity of G6PD increases

D. Measurement of G6PD activity is inaccurate following a hemolytic episode

E. G6PD is an autosomal dominant trait

ANSWERS

20.1. Answer: B. There are many xenobiotics that are associated with aplastic anemia. Of the antiepileptic medications, carbamazepine, felbamate, and levetiracetam are all associated with aplastic anemia. The other antiepileptics listed here do not cause aplastic anemia.

Franceschi M, et al. Fatal aplastic anemia in a patient treated with carbamazepine. *Epilepsia.* 1988;29:582-583.

20.2. Answer: C. Fetal hemoglobin has a greater affinity for oxygen than hemoglobin A. This confers an advantage in utero as the fetus competes effectively with maternal hemoglobin. It is a disadvantage after birth as oxygen unloading at tissue sites is impaired.

Lukens J. Blood formation in the embryo, fetus and newborn. In: Lee RG, Bithell TC, Foerster J, et al, eds. *Wintrobe's Clinical Hematology.* 9th ed. Philadelphia, PA: Lea & Febiger; 1993:79-100.

20.3. Answer: C. Naphthalene causes hemolysis. Patients with G6PD deficiency are particularly susceptible, but if enough is ingested, anyone hemolyzes. Camphor is associated with both central nervous system toxicity, such as seizures, and gastrointestinal symptoms. 1,4-Dichlorobenzene (paradichlorobenzene) toxicity is less severe than that of camphor and naphthalene. While hemolytic anemia is reported, it is much less common. It has a Group 2B (possible carcinogen) International Agency for Research on Cancer classification. Paradichlorobenzene is associated with a leukoencephalopathy when abused chronically. Menthol has a low toxicity profile limited to case reports; it rarely causes ataxia, nystagmus, and altered mental status. Red cedar wood causes respiratory symptoms in susceptible patients.

Dela Cruz M, et al. Hemolytic crisis following naphthalene mothball Ingestion in a 21-month-old patient with glucose-6-phosphate dehydrogenase (G6PD) deficiency. *Case Rep Pediatr.* 2019;2019:1092575.

20.4. Answer: D. While transcutaneous absorption of benzene does occur, the most significant route of exposure is pulmonary. Benzene is metabolized by hepatic mixed-function oxidase. Phase I metabolites (phenol and hydroquinone) are substrates for phase II reactions. The products of phase II metabolism, as well as *trans-trans*-muconic acid, are excreted in the urine. The oxidative metabolites formed in the liver are transported in the blood to the bone marrow, where a mixed-function oxidase produces metabolites that are toxic to the bone marrow. Thrombocytosis and acute lymphocytic leukemia are not typical of benzene poisoning.

Ganousis LG, et al. Cell-specific metabolism in mouse bone marrow stroma: Studies of activation and detoxification of benzene metabolism. *Mol Pharmacol.* 1992;42:1118-1125.

Seaton MJ, et al. In vitro conjugation of benzene metabolites by human liver: Potential influence of interindividual variability on benzene toxicity. *Carcinogenesis.* 1995;16:1519-1527.

20.5. Answer: C. This patient has a pure red cell aplasia (PRCA), which is an uncommon condition in which erythrocyte precursors are absent from an otherwise normal bone marrow. Of these listed medications, only phenytoin causes PRCA. Azathioprine and isoniazid are also associated with pure red cell aplasia. All five answer choices listed are also associated with agranulocytosis, but this patient's white blood cell count is normal.

Thompson DF, Gales MA. Drug-induced pure red cell aplasia. *Pharmacotherapy.* 1996;16:1002-1008.

20.6. Answer: B. All the listed coagulation markers would be abnormal due to an array of venom components including C-type lectinlike proteins, metalloproteinases, serine proteases, and phospholipases A_2.

Boyer LV, et al. Recurrent and persistent coagulopathy following pit viper envenomation. *Arch Intern Med.* 1999;159:706-710.

20.7. Answer: B. Both anemia and aplastic anemia develop after chloramphenicol use. Patients with anemia generally recover following the cessation of chloramphenicol exposure, but patients who develop aplastic anemia typically die. Aplastic anemia usually occurs within 5 months of exposure to chloramphenicol. Electron microscopic abnormalities include disordered mitochondria and an increased density of the mitochondrial matrix.

Yunis AA. Chloramphenicol toxicity: Induced bone marrow suspension. *Semin Hematol.* 1973;10:225-234.

20.8. Answer: A. Ionizing radiation directly damages cellular DNA, preventing cellular replication. It affects the most rapidly dividing cells. Cells that do not divide (mature red cells, neutrophils, and platelets) will be unaffected by an exposure but are not replaced by the bone marrow. While inflammation is probably a significant effect of radiation exposure, direct damage to DNA is the most significant effect. Patients who survive an exposure are at increased risk of the development of hematologic malignancies.

Fliedner TM, et al. Blood cell changes after radiation exposure as an indicator for hemopoietic stem cell function. *Bone Marrow Transplant.* 1988;3:77-84.

Ichimaru M, et al. Incidence of aplastic anemia in A-bomb survivors. Hiroshima and Nagasaki, 1946-1967. *Radiat Res.* 1972;49:461-472.

20.9. Answer: A. The red blood cell's (or erythrocyte) primary function is oxygen transport. The mature erythrocyte is densely packed with hemoglobin, which constitutes approximately 90% of the dry weight of the erythrocyte. The erythrocyte relies on both aerobic and anaerobic metabolism. The red cell has multiple enzymatic mechanisms to protect itself from oxidative attack, including NADH methemoglobin reductase and NADPH-dependent methemoglobin reductase. The erythrocyte produces 2,3-DPG as a by-product of aerobic respiration. As it lacks a nucleus, it cannot replace lost proteins.

Telen MJ. The mature erythrocyte. In: Lee RG, Bithell TC, Foerster J, et al, eds. *Wintrobe's Clinical Hematology.* 9th ed. Philadelphia, PA: Lea & Febiger, 1993, pp. 101–133.

Reiter CD, et al. Cell-free hemoglobin limits nitric oxide bioavailability in sickle-cell disease. *Nat Med.* 2002;8:1383-1389.

20.10. Answer: D. G6PD is encoded on the X chromosome, so it more commonly affects men. Hemolysis occurs following an exposure to an oxidizing agent. The activity of G6PD decreases as red cells age. The measurement of the activity of G6PD will not be accurate following an episode of hemolysis, as the cells with the least activity are hemolyzed selectively.

Frank JE. Diagnosis and management of G6PD deficiency. *Am Fam Physician.* 2005;72:1277-1282.

Hepatic Principles

QUESTIONS

21.1. Pyrrolizidine alkaloids cause what kind of liver injury?
A. Steatosis caused by mitochondrial dysfunction
B. Acute hepatocellular necrosis
C. Vanishing bile duct syndrome
D. Sinusoidal obstruction syndrome
E. Cirrhosis

21.2. How does hypervitaminosis A cause liver injury?
A. Activation of stellate cells, which causes hepatic fibrosis
B. Autoimmune injury, which causes cholestasis
C. Impairment of beta-oxidation of fatty acids, causing microvesicular steatosis
D. Development of an angiosarcoma after repeated exposure
E. Acute hepatocellular necrosis

21.3. A 27-year-old woman dies after a massive overdose of prenatal vitamins. Which hepatic zone would be expected to show the most severe injury on autopsy?
A. Zone 1
B. Zone 2
C. Zone 3
D. Zone 4
E. Zone 5

21.4. Acute intraperitoneal hemorrhage is associated with hepatoxicity caused by which of the following drugs?
A. Chlorpromazine
B. Anabolic steroids
C. Tetracycline
D. Isoniazid
E. Erythromycin

21.5. An aspartate aminotransferase (AST) of 5000 IU/L is most consistent with hepatic injury caused by which of the following options?
A. Acute extrahepatic obstruction of the common bile duct
B. Acute alcoholic hepatitis
C. Hepatotoxicity due to chronic treatment with methotrexate
D. Acute hepatic injury due to acetaminophen toxicity
E. Infiltrative liver disease

21.6. A 32-year-old man with a past medical history of human immunodeficiency virus (HIV) presents to the emergency department with 2 days of malaise, vomiting, diarrhea, and a rash. He is febrile to 101.2 °F (38.4 °C). He was recently started on a new HIV medication 6 weeks prior to presentation. Which human leukocyte antigen (HLA) is associated with his presentation?
A. HLA-B*5701
B. HLA-B27
C. HLA-A*3101
D. HLA-DRB1*07
E. HLA-DQA1*02

21.7. A 12-year-old boy with a past medical history of a seizure disorder presents to the emergency department because he had an elevated ammonia concentration on his routine outpatient blood analysis. He is entirely asymptomatic at this time. Which of the following explains his hyperammonemia?
A. Impairment of the urea cycle enzyme ornithine transcarbamylase
B. Stimulation of carbamyl phosphate synthetase
C. Accumulation of *N*-acetyl-*p*-benzoquinoneimine
D. Acute extrahepatic obstruction of the common bile duct
E. Initiation of lipid peroxidation by free radicals

21.8. Which of the following options is a risk factor for the development of hepatotoxicity from isoniazid (INH)?
A. Male gender
B. Young age
C. Use as an isolated therapy
D. Alcohol use disorder
E. Treatment with pyridoxine

21.9. The hepatotoxicity caused by oral amiodarone most closely resembles hepatotoxicity caused by which of the following?
A. Ethanol
B. Acetaminophen
C. Iron
D. Carbon tetrachloride
E. *Amanita phalloides*

21.10. Hypoglycin A induces a type of hepatic injury that is most similar to which of the following substances?
A. Acetaminophen
B. Ethanol
C. Iron
D. Zidovudine
E. Chlorpromazine

ANSWERS

21.1. Answer: D. Pyrrolizidine alkaloids injure the endothelium of the hepatic venous system causing intimal thickening, edema, and nonthrombotic obstruction. Plant species that contain these alkaloids include *Symphytum* spp (comfrey tea), *Heliotrope* spp (India/Afghanistan, cereal mixed with seeds), *Senecio* spp (South Africa, ragwort), and *Crotalaria* spp (Jamaica, "bush teas").

Yeong ML, et al. Hepatic veno-occlusive disease associated with comfrey ingestion. *J Gastrenterol Hepatol.* 1990;5:211-214.

21.2. Answer: A. Vitamin A is a fat soluble vitamin stored in stelate cells. Reactive oxygen species derived from lipid peroxidation, reduced NADPH, and apoptotic cells activate stellate cells leading to cirrhosis. Drugs most commonly involved in autoimmune liver injury are nitrofurantoin and minocycline. The mechanism of valproic acid liver injury is impairment of beta-oxidation of fatty acids. Vinyl chloride exposure leads to the development of angiosarcoma. Hepatocellular necrosis is the mechanism of injury of many xenobiotics, most notably acetaminophen.

Geubel AP, et al. Liver damage caused by therapeutic vitamin A administration: Estimate of dose related toxicity in 41 cases. *Gastroenterology.* 1991;100:1701-1709.

21.3. Answer: A. Uptake of iron from the gastrointestinal tract primarily injures zone 1, which is anatomically adjacent to the portal veins and carries blood with higher O_2 content. This is also referred to as periportal necrosis. Iron ions disrupt critical cellular processes, such as mitochondrial oxidative phosphorylation, disrupting the synthesis of ATP.

Gleason WA, et al. Acute hepatic failure in severe iron poisoning. *J Pediatrics.* 1979;95:138-140.

21.4. Answer: B. Anabolic steroids are associated with the development of blood-filled cavities in the liver, a condition called "peliosis hepatis." These cavities rupture, causing hemoperitoneum.

Bagheri SA, Boyer JL. Peliosis hepatis associated with androgenic-anabolic steroid therapy. *Ann Intern Med.* 1974;81:610-618.

21.5. Answer: D. The AST rarely rises above 1000 IU/L in cases of extrahepatic bile duct obstruction and rarely rises above 300 IU/L in hepatitis related to ethanol. Methotrexate causes indolent hepatitis, leading to cirrhosis without dramatic elevations of hepatocellular enzymes. Acute massive hepatocellular injury by acetaminophen causes very significant elevation of the AST.

Lee WM. Drug-induced hepatotoxicity. *N Engl J Med.* 1995;333:1118-1127.

21.6. Answer: A. This patient is presenting with a hypersensitivity reaction to abacavir. HLA-B*5701 is significantly associated with hypersensitivity reactions to abacavir. The US Food and Drug Administration (FDA) recommends HLA screening for patients being started on a few select medications such as abacavir. HLA-A*3101 is associated with hypersensitivity reactions after taking carbamazepine. Both HLA-DRB1*07 and HLA-DQA1*02 are associated with drug-induced liver injury (DILI) after taking ximelagatran. HLA-B27 predisposes to the development of agranulocytosis in patients exposed to levamisole.

Mallal S, et al. HLA-B*5701 screening for hypersensitivity to abacavir. *N Engl J Med*. 2008;358:568-579.

21.7. Answer: A. This patient is presenting with asymptomatic hyperammonemia in the setting of therapeutic valproic acid use. This is caused by selective impairment of the urea cycle enzymes ornithine transcarbamylase or carbamyl phosphate synthetase by pentanoic acid metabolites. Oral supplementation with L-carnitine is usually indicated in these cases.

Thomas KL, et al. Valproic acid-induced hyperammonemia and minimal hepatic encephalopathy prevalence among psychiatric inpatients. *Ann Clin Psychiatry*. 2016;28:37-42.

21.8. Answer: D. Alcohol use disorder is a risk factor for the development of hepatotoxicity from isoniazid. Other risk factors include female gender, increasing age, and co-administration with rifampin. The hepatotoxicity is multifactorial and occurs directly through hepatotoxic metabolites, such as hydroxylamine, hydrazine, and acetylhydrazine, and indirectly through apoptosis and steatosis.

American Thoracic Society, Centers for Disease Control and Prevention, Infectious Diseases Society of America. Treatment of tuberculosis. *MMWR Morb Mortal Wkly Rep*. 2003;52:1-72.

21.9. Answer: A. Amiodarone-induced hepatoxicity is dose-dependent and most closely resembles alcoholic hepatitis. Amiodarone-induced hepatitis causes steatosis and Mallory bodies, and there is a risk that patients will progress to cirrhosis. Biopsies of amiodarone-induced hepatoxicity also reveal lamellated intralysosomal phospholipid inclusion bodies.

Lee WM. Drug-induced hepatotoxicity. *N Engl J Med*. 1995;333: 1118-1127.

21.10. Answer: D. Zidovudine, an antiretroviral, causes microvascular steatosis. It also causes a metabolic acidosis with an elevated lactate concentration. The hepatic injury from both hypoglycin A and zidovudine is secondary to a failure of energy production by the mitochondria.

Day L, et al. Mitochondrial injury in the pathogenesis of antiretroviral-induced hepatic steatosis and lactic acidemia. *Mitochondrion*. 2004;4:95-109.

Neurologic Principles

QUESTIONS

22.1. Asymmetric (focal) neurologic findings are found with which of the following overdoses?
A. Amphetamine
B. Diazepam
C. Glyburide
D. Haloperidol
E. Phenytoin

22.2. Transient ataxia and ophthalmoplegia are described in Nigerian patients who ingested the larvae of the moth *Anaphe venata* as a source of protein. Which of the following causes best explains their physical examination findings?
A. Thiamine deficiency
B. Excess copper
C. Lead poisoning
D. Arsenic poisoning
E. Chronic selenium deficiency

22.3. A 53-year-old man presents to the emergency department with pain to the muscles of his arms and legs. A creatinine phosphokinase is elevated. Which of the following choices contributed to this patient's presentation?
A. Acetaminophen
B. Zolpidem
C. *Amanita muscaria*
D. Susumber berries
E. Atorvastatin

22.4. A 36-year-old woman presents to the emergency department with bilateral extremity weakness. On physical examination, she is unable to raise either her arms or legs up against gravity. She has a history of an eating disorder with frequent binging and purging episodes. She recently ingested a large amount of an over-the-counter laxative. Which of the following medications would be helpful in the treatment of her paralysis?
A. Calcium gluconate
B. Thiamine
C. Methylnaltrexone
D. Pyridoxine
E. Botulinum antitoxin

22.5. A pyridoxine overdose most commonly causes which of the following findings?
A. Proximal weakness secondary to myopathy
B. Marked atrophy caused by demyelination of peripheral nerve fibers
C. Diffuse loss of reflexes secondary to an acute axonopathy
D. Ataxia caused by sensory neuronopathy
E. Autonomic instability caused by interference with transmission at the neuromuscular junction

22.6. Which of the following xenobiotics is most likely to produce permanent Parkinson disease?
A. Droperidol
B. Thioridazine
C. Thiothixene
D. Clozapine
E. 1-Methyl-4-phenyl-1,2,3,6-tetrahydropyridine

22.7. In the 1990s, there was an outbreak of patients who developed sudden-onset severe myalgias after ingesting a dietary supplement. Which of the following was most likely to appear as a laboratory finding?
A. Elevated liver function tests
B. Elevated creatine kinase MB (CK-MB) fraction
C. Depressed thyroid function tests
D. Eosinophilia on complete blood count (CBC)
E. Increased blood urea nitrogen (BUN) and creatinine

22.8. Which of the following mechanisms best explains how *Clostridium tetani* travels from point of entry to the central nervous system (CNS) following initial infection?
A. Blood-borne via *C. tetani* bacteremia
B. Lymphatics
C. Myelin sheath
D. Axon
E. Attachment of exotoxin to red blood cells

22.9. An 8-year-old girl who recently immigrated from West Africa presents to the emergency department for further evaluation of a spastic paralysis, bilateral optic atrophy, and bilateral sensorineural deafness.

Which of the following xenobiotics best explains her presentation?
A. Linamarin
B. Carbon monoxide
C. Pyridoxine
D. Colchicine
E. Nitrous oxide

22.10. A 26-year-old man presents to the emergency department with lethargy after he "used a lot" of cocaine. He awakes only with repeated stimulation; however, he moves both his arms and legs. His heart rate is 41 beats/min, and his respiratory rate is 12 breaths/min. A computed tomography (CT) scan of his brain is performed and demonstrates no acute findings. Which of the following interventions should be performed on this patient?
A. Admission for placement of a pacemaker
B. Administration of atropine
C. Administration of calcium gluconate
D. Administration of naloxone
E. Supportive measures alone

ANSWERS

22.1. Answer: C. Although toxic-metabolic causes of altered consciousness are characterized by an absence of focality, hypoglycemia sometimes presents with asymmetric findings, suggesting a structural lesion when, in fact, none is present. The pathophysiology is unknown.

> Wallis WE, et al. Hypoglycemia masquerading as cerebrovascular disease (hypoglycemic hemiplegia). *Ann Neurol*. 1985;18:510-512.

> Spiller HA, et al. Hemiparesis and altered mental status in a child after glyburide in gestion. *J Emerg Med*. 1998;16:433-435.

22.2. Answer: A. The larvae of the moth *Anaphe venata* contain thiaminase, which renders patients thiamine deficient. The outbreaks of ataxia and opthalmoplegia consistent with Wernicke encephalopthy were seasonal and consistent with availability of the larvae. Patients improve following thiamine supplementation.

> Adelmolekun B, Ibikunle FR. Investigation of an epidemic of seasonal ataxia in Ikare, Western Nigeria. *Acta Neurol Scand*. 1994;90:309-311.

22.3. Answer: E. This patient is presenting with a myopathy as a result of atorvastatin use. Statins, which are 3-hydroxy-3-methylglutaryl-coenzyme A (HMG-CoA) reductase inhibitors,

cause myalgias, cramping, myositis, and rhabdomyolysis. This is likely a result of either impared cholesterol synthesis in myocytes or diminished production of regulatory proteins such as ubiquinone or GTP-binding proteins required for mitochondrial function.

> Rosenson RS. Current overview of statin-induced myopathy. *Am J Med*. 2004;116:408-416.

22.4. Answer: A. This patient is presenting with hypermagnesmia in the setting of a large ingestion of magnesium citrate in an attempt to purge. With large enough ingestions, patients develop hypermagnesemia, despite normal kidney function. Magnesium inhibits presynaptic acetylcholine release at the neuromuscular junction, likely through the inhibition of calcium influx into nerve endings. Patients who develop paralysis as a result of hypermagnesemia should be treated with intravenous calcium gluconate.

> Araki K, et al. Hypermagnesemia in a 20-month-old healthy girl caused by the use of a laxative: A case report. *J Med Case Rep*. 2021;15:129.

22.5. Answer: D. Acute pyridoxine neuropathy is caused by massive doses of pyridoxine, which disrupt the cellular metabolism of the dorsal root ganglion. The clinical picture is one of development of widespread sensory loss. Because the pathologic process involves only the dorsal root ganglion, motor function is unimpaired. Appendicular ataxia is marked and is a consequence of sensory ataxia rather than involvement of the cerebellum. There is some autonomic instability in the acute form of the overdose, but it does not appear to be attributable to abnormalities at the neuromuscular junction.

Albin RL, et al. Acute sensory neuropathy-neuronopathy from pyridoxine overdose. *Neurology* 1987;37:1729-1732.

22.6. Answer: E. Parkinson disease is characterized by tremor, rigidity, akinesia, and postural instability. Drug-induced parkinsonism is caused by xenobiotics that either destroy cells in the substantia nigra (eg, 1-methyl-4-phenyl-1,2,3,6-tetrahydropyridine [MPTP]) or, much more commonly, antagonize the effects of dopamine, either pre- or postsynaptically in the nigrostiatal pathway. The use of antipsychotics is the most common reversible cause of parkinsonism. MPTP-induced parkinsonism was reported almost exclusively in individuals using a synthetic opioid that contained MPTP. The syndrome differs from that of idiopathic Parkinson disease in its rapidity of onset. In most patients, the effects appear to be permanent.

Fukuda T. Neurotoxicity of MPTP. *Neuropathology*. 2001;21:323-332.

22.7. Answer: D. The eosinophilia-myalgia syndrome was associated with ingestion of the amino acid L-tryptophan. The clinical picture was that of sudden-onset severe myalgias, cutaneous involvement, and a peripheral eosinophilia. Pathologically, an eosinophilic myositis and fasciitis were found.

Hertzman PA, et al. Association of the eosinophilia-myalgia syndrome with the ingestion of tryptophan. *N Engl J Med.* 1990;322:869-873.

22.8. Answer: D. Tetanus infection results in the formation of a neurotoxin that affects the neuromuscular junction, the sympathetic pathways, the spinal cord, and the brain. Tetanospasmin, the clinically important exotoxin of *Clostridium tetani*, travels from the point of entry, largely via the axon, to the CNS. There, it blocks release of inhibitory neurotransmitters, thus producing disinhibition with associated widespread muscular spasm and autonomic instability.

Weinstein LW. Tetanus. *N Engl J Med.* 1973;289:1293-1296.

22.9. Answer: A. This patient is presenting with epidemic spastic paraparesis, also known as konzo, which occurs as a result of improperly prepared *Manihot esculenta* (cassava), which contains the cyanogenic glycoside linamarin. The exact mechanism for this disease is not fully elucidated, and there is still no known definitive treatment.

Banea-Mayambu JP, et al. Geographical and seasonal association between linamarin and cyanide exposure from cassava and the upper motor neuron disease konzo in former Zaire. *Trop Med Int Health.* 1997;2:1143-1151.

22.10. Answer: E. This patient is presenting with cocaine washout, which occurs after depletion of exicitatory amino acids (EAA) and dopamine. Patients present sleepy but rousable and oriented. Patients are often mildly bradycardic. There is no therapy; recovery occurs over time as the patient's own neurotransmitters regenerate. The time course of cocaine washout is sometimes as long as 24 hours.

Roberts JR, Greenberg MI. Cocaine washout syndrome. *Ann Intern Med* 2000;132:679-680.

Oncologic Principles

QUESTIONS

23.1. Which organ system is most commonly affected in patients who are hospitalized as a result of an adverse effect of a chemotherapeutic?
A. Cardiac
B. Pulmonary
C. Hematologic
D. Gastrointestinal
E. Dermatologic

23.2. Deoxyribonucleic acid (DNA) replication occurs during which phase of the cell cycle?
A. G_0
B. G_1
C. G_2
D. S
E. M

23.3. Cells deficient in interstrand cross-link repair mechanisms are susceptible to inhibition of replication caused by which of the following chemotherapeutics?
A. Topotecan
B. 6-Mercaptopurine
C. Methotrexate
D. Vincristine
E. Mechlorethamine

23.4. A 24-year-old man is started on a chemotherapy regimen for the treatment of acute T-cell lymphoblastic leukemia. Two weeks later, he is involved in a motor vehicle collision. A complete blood count demonstrates myelosuppression. Which of the following chemotherapeutics is most likely to be responsible for this finding?
A. Vincristine
B. Mechlorethamine
C. Cisplatin
D. Carmustine
E. Cyclophosphamide

23.5. What is the general order of differentiation by cell type in a cell lineage?
A. Specialized cell, progenitor cell, stem cell
B. Specialized cell, stem cell, progenitor cell
C. Progenitor cell, stem cell, specialized cell
D. Stem cell, specialized cell, progenitor cell
E. Stem cell, progenitor cell, specialized cell

23.6. Which of the following statements is true about stem cell niches?
A. Niches degenerate once stem cells are depleted
B. Cellular components are exclusively responsible for maintaining the niche
C. Disruption of the niche plays a role in neoplastic transformation
D. Stem cells in niches are protected from injury by radiation
E. Niches only respond to endocrine hormones

23.7. Vinblastine disrupts cell replication by which of the following mechanisms?
A. Inhibiting CDK activity in G_1 phase
B. Inhibition of cyclin D binding to CDK 4 and 6
C. Activation of transcription factor E2F
D. Spindle alignment complex inhibition of the anaphase-promoting complex
E. Production of INK4 proteins

23.8. Which of these protein complexes activates p53, triggering a cascade of processes that halts cell replication?
A. Spindle alignment complex (SAC)
B. Ataxia-telangiectasia mutated kinase (ATM) and Rad3-related complex (ATR)
C. Cyclin D-CDK4
D. p16-retinoblastoma protein (pRB)
E. Transcription factor E2F

23.9. A 23-year-old woman with Hodgkin lymphoma is started on a chemotherapeutic regimen that includes bleomycin. After 2 weeks on this regimen, she develops a nonproductive cough. On examination, she has bibasilar crackles, and a chest radiograph demonstrates basilar infiltrates. The mechanism of toxicity of bleomycin is most like which of the following xenobiotics?

A. Paraquat
B. Cyclosporine
C. Oxaliplatin
D. Colchicine
E. Bevacizumab

23.10. A 45-year-old man is being treated for stage III colon cancer. Which of the following chemotherapeutics would cause both intrastrand and interstrand cross-linking of DNA in this patient?
A. Folinic acid
B. Cisplatin
C. Oxaliplatin
D. Irinotecan
E. 5-Fluorouracil

ANSWERS

23.1. Answer: D. Gastrointestinal complications are the leading cause for chemotherapy-related hospitalizations, followed by infectious, hematologic, and cardiac. This is because cells with rates of high turnover are sensitive to most chemotherapeutics.

Hassett MJ, et al. Chemotherapy-related hospitalization among community cancer center patients. *Oncologist.* 2011;16:378-387.

23.2. Answer: D. The phases of the cell cycle are G_0 (resting phase), G_1 (gap 1), S (synthesis), G_2 (gap 2), and M (mitosis). Replication of DNA occurs during S phase. In the S phase, DNA unwinds using the CMG helicase complex, elongates, and undergoes synthesis. The replisome accomplishes these steps during DNA replication, which includes assembly of supporting proteins, unwinding, polymerization, synthesis of RNA primers, and coordination of the polymerization between the leading and lagging strands of DNA.

Heijink AM, et al. The DNA damage response during mitosis. *Mutat Res.* 2013;750:45-55.

23.3. Answer: E. Alkylating agents cause interstrand cross-linking of deoxyribonucleic acid (DNA), which is significant as these mutations are not easily repaired. Detection of these errors by the DNA damage response initiates a cascade leading to apoptosis.

Huang Y, Li L. DNA crosslinking damage and cancer—a tale of friend and foe. *Transl Cancer Res.* 2013;2:144-154.

23.4. Answer: A. This patient is likely receiving vincristine as part of his chemotherapeutic regimen. Cell cycle phase-specific chemotherapeutics cause early onset of myelosuppression, whereas nonspecific chemotherapeutics cause late and prolonged myelosuppression.

Hoagland HC. Hematologic complications of cancer chemotherapy. *Semin Oncol.* 1982;9:95-102.

23.5. Answer: E. Differentiation of cells progresses from stem cells, which exist in the G_0 phase; progenitor cells, which are continuously active in the cell cycle; and specialized or mature cells.

Fukushima N, Ohkawa H. Hematopoietic stem cells and microenvironment: The proliferation and differentiation of stromal cells. *Crit Rev Oncol Hematol.* 1995;20:255-270.

23.6. Answer: C. The niche is a microenvironment that protects and provides support to stem cells. A niche consists of support cells, extracellular matrix proteins, blood vessels that supply nutrients and carry hormonal signals to stem cells, and neuronal inputs. A niche retains its function even if the stem cells are depleted by radiation or chemotherapy, allowing for recruitment of stem cells from other niches or induction of more pluripotent stem cells from other organ systems. Disruption of the niche plays a role in neoplastic transformation.

Boulais PE, Frenette PS. Making sense of hematopoietic stem cell niches. *Blood.* 2015;125:2621-2629.

23.7. Answer: D. Vinca alkaloids prevent the assembly of kinetochore microtubules, activating the spindle alignment complex (SAC), which in turn blocks activation of the anaphase-promoting complex (APC).

Yamada HY, Gorbsky GJ. Spindle checkpoint function and cellular sensitivity to antimitotic drugs. *Mol Cancer Ther*. 2006;5:2963-2969.

23.8. Answer: B. Activation of the ATR complex leads to phosphorylation of p53, ultimately leading to cell senescence.

Heijink AM, et al. The DNA damage response during mitosis. *Mutat Res*. 2013;750:45-55.

23.9. Answer: A. Both paraquat and bleomycin cause pulmonary toxicity through free radical cycling, which is enhanced with oxygen therapy. Cyclosporine is a calcineurin inhibitor used for immune suppression. Oxaliplatin is believed to crosslink DNA and is associated with peripheral neuropathy and nephrotoxicity. Colchicine is a microtubule inhibitor associated with alopecia after acute overdose. Bevacizumab is a VEGF inhibitor that inhibits angiogenesis, associated with hypertension, proteinuria, and poor wound healing.

Borges EL, et al. Effect of Lung fibrosis on glycogen content in different extrapulmonary tissues. *Lung*. 2014;192;125-131.

23.10. Answer: C. Platinum coordination complexes form both interstrand and intrastrand cross-linkages. Of these agents, oxaliplatin is used in the treatment of colorectal cancer as part of the FOLFOX (folinic acid, fluorouracil, and oxaliplatin) regimen. Folinic acid is used in the treatment of colorectal cancer to enhance the cytotoxicity of capecitabine and 5-fluorouracil (5-FU). Cisplatin is a platinum coordination complex used in the treatment of testicular, ovarian, bladder, esophageal, gastric, lung, head and neck, anal, and breast cancers, but not rectal or colon cancer. Irinotecan inhibits topoisomerase I and is used in the treatment of colorectal cancers. 5-FU is used in the treatment of colorectal cancer and inhibits thymidylate synthase.

Pang SK, et al. East-west fusion-necrosis and apoptosis acting in concert by demethylcantharidin-integrated platinum complexes. *Anticancer Agents Med Chem*. 2014;14:756-761.

Ophthalmic Principles

QUESTIONS

24.1. Which of the following options is true of ocular irrigation after chemical exposures?
  A. Use of a scleral shell irrigating device (e.g., Morgan lens) should be avoided
  B. Outcome is worse if water is used instead of commercially available solutions
  C. Regardless of the exposure, irrigation should be continued for 2 hours
  D. Measurement of conjunctival pH is an unreliable indicator of adequate irrigation
  E. Prolonged irrigation is important after severe alkali burns, but not severe acid burns

24.2. A 32-year-old woman presents to the emergency department with her eye closed shut. She relates that she was using cyanoacrylate glue to fix a broken piece of pottery and she unintentionally touched her eyelid. She has no pain but cannot open her eye. Which therapy is best indicated?
  A. Apply acetone to dissolve the glue
  B. Trim the eyelashes and gently pull apart the lids
  C. Consult ophthalmology for surgical repair
  D. Irrigate with sterile mineral oil
  E. Apply antibiotic ointment and cover the eye

24.3. Which of the following is true regarding irrigation of a patient with an ocular exposure to hydrofluoric acid (HF)?
  A. Emergency needle paracentesis of the anterior chamber is indicated
  B. A 10% calcium gluconate solution should be used if available
  C. Commercial amphoteric solutions are proven to be superior to 0.9% saline

  D. Only a single liter of irrigation solution is recommended for each eye
  E. Magnesium sulfate should be added to irrigation solutions

24.4. Which of the following treatments is recommended for a phenol exposure to the eye?
  A. Irrigation with a low-molecular-weight polyethylene glycol (PEG), such as PEG-400
  B. Irrigation with PEG electrolyte lavage solution
  C. Irrigation with a dilute copper sulfate solution
  D. Irrigation with an amphoteric lavage solution
  E. No therapy as this is a benign event

24.5. Which of the following is true of the ocular toxicity of methanol?
  A. Funduscopic abnormalities consistently precede visual changes
  B. The primary site of toxicity is the retina
  C. Toxicity is due to the metabolite formaldehyde
  D. Visual changes are consistently completely reversible
  E. Folate or folinic acid is not indicated once acidosis is evident

24.6. Which of the following options is true of the ocular toxicity of quinine?
  A. It only occurs after a massive, acute overdose
  B. It is caused by retinal vasoconstriction
  C. Full recovery of vision is expected, even after complete blindness
  D. It is well correlated to blood quinine concentration
  E. Funduscopic abnormalities consistently precede visual changes

24.7. Which of the following options contributes to the risk of systemic absorption and toxicity from eye drops?

A. Greater dose-to-body weight ratio in children

B. Preexisting conditions in the elderly

C. Lack of first-pass metabolism of drugs absorbed from the conjunctiva

D. Lack of familiarity with potential adverse effects

E. All of the above

24.8. Which of the following xenobiotics causes optic neuritis?

A. Amiodarone

B. Corticosteroids

C. Chloroquine

D. Ethambutol

E. Quinine

24.9. Which of the following xenobiotics characteristically causes vertical nystagmus?

A. Carbamazepine

B. Phenytoin

C. Phencyclidine

D. Ethanol

E. Diazepam

24.10. Occupational exposure to which of the following xenobiotics causes color blindness?

A. Lead

B. Carbon monoxide

C. Ultraviolet light

D. Thallium

E. Styrene

ANSWERS

24.1. Answer: D. Irrigating lenses do not increase injury and improve the consistency of irrigation. Water is less comfortable, but there is no evidence that it is less effective. Severe acid and alkali burns should be irrigated for two or more hours, but most other exposures require only brief irrigation. Limitations of paper strips, contamination by irrigation solutions, and failure of conjunctival pH to reflect anterior chamber pH are among the reasons that normal pH should be a necessary but not sufficient endpoint.

Herr RD, et al. Clinical comparison of ocular irrigation fluids following chemical injury. *Am J Emerg Med.* 1991;9:228-231.

Pfister RR. Chemical injuries of the eye. *Ophthalmology* 1983;90:1246-1253.

24.2. Answer: E. Cyanoacrylate exposures to the eye are generally benign. Although acetone is used in other areas to dissolve the glue, the risk of acetone to the eye outweighs the potential benefit. Similarly, aggressive mechanical attempts rip tissues and result in disfigurement. In general, the eye will open once the skin sheds, but the addition of an ointment will hasten the recovery. Once the eye is open, a complete examination is recommended.

Kimbrough RL, et al. Conservative management of cyanoacrylate ankyloblepharon: A case report. *Ophthalmic Surg.* 1986;17:176-177.

24.3. Answer: D. Ocular exposure to HF causes severe burns but requires specialized management. Although systemic calcium and magnesium are often needed for patients with systemic toxicity, both salts are irritating to the eye and

unproven to improve outcome. Anterior chamber paracentesis is rarely necessary in patients with alkaline injuries. In an animal model, prolonged irrigation is associated with a worse outcome. While this is not demonstrated in humans, prolonged irrigation is usually unnecessary.

McCulley JP. Ocular hydrofluoric acid burns: Animal model, mechanism of injury and therapy. *Trans Am Ophthalmol Soc.* 1990;88:649-684.

24.4. Answer: A. Phenol tends to form an adherent mass when exposed to water. Low-molecular-weight polyethylene glycol (PEG-400) is the dermal irrigating solution of choice, and its use in the eye has some literature support. Higher molecular weight polyethylene glycol solutions, such as those used for bowel irrigation, have no role. Copper sulfate is used for dermal phosphorus exposures. There is little support for amphoteric solutions for any exposure. If, however, PEG-400 is not immediately available, then irrigation with 0.9% sodium chloride, lactated Ringer solution, or a balanced salt solution should proceed immediately.

Lang K. Treatment of phenol burns of the eye with polyethyleneglycol-400. *Z Arztl Fortbild.* 1969;63:705-708.

24.5. Answer: B. Formate produced by methanol metabolism is the cause of ocular toxicity, which primarily affects the retina. Funduscopic examination is most often normal when visual symptoms first appear. Treatment with folate or folinic acid speeds the degradation of formate and prevents retinal folate depletion. The presence of acidosis indicates the need for folate or folinic acid therapy. Patients with severe methanol toxicity often progress to develop complete blindness. Some patients develop a delayed loss of vision, despite an initial improvement in their vision.

Benton CD, Calhoun FP. The ocular effects of methyl alcohol poisoning: Report of a catastrophe involving 320 persons. *Am J Ophthalmol.* 1953;36:1677-1685.

Garner CD, et al. Role of retinal metabolism in methanol-induced retinal toxicity. *J Toxicol Environ Health.* 1995;44:43-56.

24.6. Answer: D. Serum concentrations of quinine above 20 mcg/mL within 10 hours of overdose consistently predict visual defects. Early funduscopic examination is often normal in the face of significant visual loss. The exact cause is unknown, but vasoconstriction is excluded. Partial recovery is common after serious visual deficits. Less severe visual loss occurs after quinine exposure in settings other than acute overdose.

Boland ME, et al. Complications of quinine poisoning. *Lancet.* 1985; 1:384-385.

24.7. Answer: E. All answers choices contribute to the risk of systemic absorption and toxicity from eye drops.

Adverse systemic effects from ophthalmic drugs. *Med Lett Drugs Ther.* 1982;24:53-54.

Hugues FC, Le Jeune C. Systemic and local tolerability of ophthalmic drug formulations. An update. *Drug Safety.* 1993;8:365-380.

24.8. Answer: D. Ethambutol is one of the toxicologic causes of optic neuritis. Amiodarone and chloroquine cause corneal deposits; steroids cause cataracts; quinine causes retinal abnormalities.

Chan RY, Kwok AK. Ocular toxicity of ethambutol. *Hong Kong Med J.* 2006;12:56-60.

24.9. Answer: C. Vertical nystagmus is usually suggestive of severe central nervous system disease but also occurs commonly with phencyclidine use. Horizontal nystagmus is a common finding in medical disorders, as an adverse drug effect (phenytoin, carbamazepine), and as a complication of many common overdoses, including ethanol and other sedative-hypnotics.

McCarron MM, et al. Acute phencyclidine toxicity: Incidence of clinical findings in 1,000 cases. *Ann Emerg Med.* 1981;10:237-242.

24.10. Answer: E. Styrene causes loss of color discrimination that is one of the earliest manifestations of neurotoxicity following exposure. Lead is associated with optic nerve injury. Carbon monoxide causes cortical blindness. Exposure to ultraviolet light causes a severe keratitis. Thallium is associated with cranial nerve abnormalities and optic neuritis.

Choi AR, et al. Occupational styrene exposure and acquired dyschromatopsia: A systematic review and meta-analysis. *Am J Ind Med.* 2017;60:930-946.

Otolaryngologic Principles

QUESTIONS

25.1. The odor of violets on a patient's urine is associated with an exposure to which of the following xenobiotics?
A. Cyanide
B. Methyl salicylate
C. Turpentine
D. Ethchlorvynol
E. Nitrobenzene

25.2. Which of the following xenobiotics is most likely to cause reversible hearing loss?
A. Cisplatin
B. Bromates
C. Arsenic
D. Quinine
E. Neomycin

25.3. In addition to stimulating the olfactory nerve, ammonia, acetone, and menthol also stimulate which other cranial nerve?
A. Facial
B. Trigeminal
C. Vagal
D. Hypoglossal
E. Glossopharyngeal

25.4. Which of the following options best describes the major function of the stria vascularis?
A. Regenerates hair cells of the cochlea
B. Maintains the electrochemical gradient between the endolymph and the perilymph
C. Conducts neural transmission to the cochlear nucleus and the inferior colliculus

D. Secretes G proteins for the hair cells
E. Provides negative feedback for hair cell transmissions

25.5. Which of the following xenobiotics demonstrates rapid olfactory fatigue at concentrations exceeding 100-150 ppm?
A. Carbon monoxide
B. Phosgene
C. Cyanide
D. Hydrogen sulfide
E. Hydrofluoric acid

25.6. Angiotensin-converting enzyme (ACE) inhibitors cause taste distortion by which of the following mechanisms?
A. Inhibit adenylate cyclase at the stria vascularis
B. Antagonize calcium conduction
C. Decrease angiotensin II, an important protein for cochlear function
D. Cause angioedema
E. Chelate zinc at the taste receptors and the salivary proteins

25.7. A 62-year-old man presents to the emergency department with shortness of breath. He is diagnosed with acute congestive heart failure. In the intensive care unit, he develops hearing loss. Which of the following sites is affected by loop diuretics, leading to his presentation?
A. Stria vascularis
B. Outer hair cells
C. Basilar membrane
D. Reisner membrane
E. Spiral ganglion

25.8. A 23-year-old woman presents to the emergency department because she is concerned that she has lost her ability to smell. A COVID test is negative. Exposure to which of the following xenobiotics explains her symptoms?
   A. Corticosteroids
   B. Morphine
   C. Amphetamines
   D. Methanol
   E. Oral contraceptives

25.9. A 32-year-old man presents to the emergency department because he noticed that every time he drinks a carbonated beverage it tastes terrible. He said that these symptoms only began after he was started on a new medication. Which of the following xenobiotics is the most likely cause of his presentation?

   A. Colchicine
   B. Ibuprofen
   C. Acetazolamide
   D. Lisinopril
   E. Furosemide

25.10. Noise-induced hearing impairment is most likely demonstrated by testing at which of the following ranges?
   A. Testing at 3-6 kHz range
   B. Testing at 10-15 kHz range
   C. Testing at 15-20 kHz range
   D. Testing at greater than 20 kHz range
   E. Testing at any range

ANSWERS

25.1. Answer: C. An odor of violets is associated with an overdose of turpentine because of metabolites that are excreted in the urine. Cyanide is associated with a bitter almond smell. Methyl salicylate is associated with a wintergreen odor. Ethchlorvynol is associated with a plastic or vinyl smell. An odor of shoe polish is suggestive of nitrobenzene exposure.

Goldfrank LR, et al. Teaching the recognition of odors. *Ann Emerg Med.* 1982;11:684-686.

25.2. Answer: D. The primary mechanism of quinine-induced ototoxicity is related to prostaglandin inhibition. Quinine inhibits phospholipase A_2, which converts phospholipids to arachidonic acid. Quinine also inhibits calcium channels that interact with prostaglandins. These effects tend to be reversible. All the other xenobiotics cause loss of hair cells of the cochlea, causing mostly irreversible hearing loss.

Jung TTK, et al. Ototoxicity of salicylate, nonsteroidal anti-inflammatory drugs, and quinine. *Otolaryngol Clin North Am.* 1993;26:791-810.

Schacht J. Molecular mechanisms of drug-induced hearing loss. *Hearing Res.* 1986;22:297-304.

25.3. Answer: B. Primary odor detection is a function of the olfactory (I) nerve. For some irritant odors, such as ammonia and acetone, neurotransmission is also conducted through the trigeminal (V) nerve.

Doty RL. A review of olfactory dysfunction in man. *Am J Otolaryngol.* 1979;1:57-79.

Schneider BA. Anosmia: Verification and etiologies. *Ann Otol.* 1972;81:272-277.

25.4. Answer: B. The production of the cochlear fluids and the maintenance of the electrochemical gradient between the endolymph and the perilymph are functions of the stria vascularis. The stria vascularis contains a high concentration of oxidative enzymes, Na^+-K^+-ATPase, adenylate cyclase, and carbonic anhydrase, which are susceptible to toxins. The cochlear fluids are critical to conduct sound waves to the hair cells, to provide nutrients and waste removal for the cells lining the cochlear duct, to control pressure distribution in the cochlea, and to maintain an electrochemical gradient for the function of the hair cells.

Huang MY, Shacht J. Drug-induced ototoxicity: Pathogenesis and prevention. *Med Toxicol.* 1989;4:452-467.

25.5. Answer: D. Olfactory fatigue is the process of olfactory adaptation after exposure to a stimulus for a variable period of time, leading to temporal diminution of the smell. For example, hydrogen sulfide, a toxin that binds to cytochrome oxidase, is readily detectable as a distinct and offensive substance at the very low concentration of 0.025 ppm. At the higher and potentially toxic concentration of 50 ppm, the odor is less offensive, and recognition disappears after 2-15 minutes of exposure. At even higher concentrations, when toxicity is likely, the onset of olfactory fatigue is more rapid.

Audeau FM, et al. Hydrogen sulfide poisoning: Associated with pelt processing. *NZ Med J.* 1985;98:145-147.

Stine R, et al. Hydrogen sulfide intoxication. *Ann Intern Med.* 1976;85:756-758.

25.6. Answer: E. Angiotensin-converting enzyme (ACE) inhibitors such as captopril, enalapril, and lisinopril are among the most common medications that cause gustatory impairment, usually hypogeusia and dysgeusia. Since ACE inhibitors work by inhibiting zinc-dependent ACE, they also inhibit taste receptors resulting in distorted taste.

Henkin RI. Drug-induced taste and smell disorders. Incidence, mechanisms and management related primarily to treatment of sensory receptor dysfunction. *Drug Safety.* 1994;11:318-377.

25.7. Answer: A. Furosemide and other loop diuretics, such as bumetanide and ethacrynic acid, cause physiologic dysfunction and edema at the stria vascularis, which leads to reversible hearing loss. This is due to the inhibition of potassium pumps and G proteins that are associated with adenylate cyclase. The permanent hearing loss is due to direct inference with oxidative metabolism in the outer hair cells.

Verdel BM, et al. Drug-related nephrotoxic and ototoxic reactions—a link through a predictive mechanistic commonality. *Drug Saf.* 2008;31:877-884.

Matz GJ. The ototoxic effects of ethacrynic acid in man and animals. *Laryngoscope.* 1976;86:1065-1086.

25.8. Answer: A. Anosmia, or the loss or inability to smell, is most commonly caused by viral infections, trauma, tumors and congenital disorders. However, many xenobiotics also lead to anosmia. The anosmia from inhaled corticosteroids is caused by the local effects on the epithelium as well as direct effects on both G proteins and adenylate cyclase.

Henkin RI. Drug-induced taste and smell disorders. Incidence, mechanisms and management related primarily to treatment of sensory receptor dysfunction. *Drug Saf.* 1994;11:318-377.

25.9. Answer: C. Acetazolamide is associated with cacogeusia, or a foul taste, when carbonated beverages are consumed. While the exact mechanism is not fully known, it is believed to be a result of the inhibition of carbonic anhydrase causing carbon dioxide accumulation and an increased tissue bicarbonate.

Joyce PW. Taste disturbance with acetazolamide. *Lancet.* 1990; 336:1446.

25.10. Answer: A. The section of the cochlea most at risk from loud noises is at the 9-13 mm region (the total length is 32 mm). This region is responsible for hearing at the 3-6 kHz range, corresponding to the typical noise-induced hearing-loss pattern. Even though human speech is composed of mostly low-frequency sounds, the ability to perceive higher frequency sounds is extremely important in speech recognition. Because of this, the major impairment in patients with noise-induced hearing loss is an inability to discriminate speech, particularly from background noise.

McGill TJ, Schuknecht HF. Human cochlear changes in noise induced hearing loss. *Laryngoscope.* 1976;86:1293-1302.

Alberti PW. Noise-induced hearing loss. *BMJ.* 1992;304:522.

Psychiatric Principles

26.1. Which of the following factors is associated with a protective effect against suicide?
A. Caucasian race
B. Elderly age
C. Male gender
D. Pregnancy
E. Impulsivity

26.2. What percentage of persons who completed suicide gave some warning of their intent?
A. None
B. 10%
C. 25-33%
D. 50-70%
E. >90%

26.3. Major mental illness is a factor in what percentage of adult suicides?
A. 5-10%
B. 33%
C. 50%
D. 75%
E. >90%

26.4. Which of the following scenarios demonstrates an instance in which patient-doctor confidentiality is allowed to be breached?
A. The patient's employer needs to know a date of return to work
B. The patient's family threatens to sue if information is not released

C. The disclosure is in the interest of protecting the patient or other third party from further harm or decline
D. The patient is a prominent person and law enforcement is making an inquiry
E. The patient's case history is unique enough to warrant a published case report

26.5. Which of the following statements fits *Diagnostic and Statistical Manual of Mental Disorders*, Fifth Edition (DSM-5) criteria for alcohol use disorder?
A. Alcohol is often taken in smaller amounts over a longer period than was intended
B. There is no desire to cut down alcohol use
C. Minimal time is spent in activities necessary to obtain alcohol
D. There is a markedly diminished effect with continued use of the same amount of alcohol
E. Attendance at occupational activities is increased

26.6. Men complete suicide at more than three times the rate of women. Which of the following methods is the most common way that men commit suicide?
A. Hanging
B. Drowning
C. Carbon monoxide inhalation
D. Ingestion
E. Firearm

26.7. The general legal standard for capacity requires assessment and documentation of a few basic skills. Which of the following statements is necessary to state that a person has capacity?
A. Unable to communicate a choice
B. Unable to speak English
C. Understands the relevant information
D. Has no appreciation for the situation and the consequences
E. Is unable to explain the reasons behind the treatment options

26.8. Which of the following options suggest a medical cause of new-onset psychiatric symptoms?
A. Age greater than 40
B. Normal vital signs
C. Normal cognition
D. Normal physical examination
E. Gradual onset of symptoms

26.9. A 27-year-old man is being evaluated in the emergency department for medical clearance prior to transfer to the psychiatric emergency department. A blood ethanol concentration greater than which of the following concentrations would mandate the patient be kept in the emergency department and not be medically cleared?
A. 50 mg/dL (10.9 mmol/L)
B. 80 mg/dL (17.4 mmol/L)
C. 100 mg/dL (21.7 mmol/L)
D. 200 mg/dL (43.4 mmol/L)
E. There is no mandated concentration

26.10. Which of the following statements regarding the assessment of the suicidal patient is true?
A. No individual observation is necessary
B. Acute intoxication does not interfere with the identification of underlying psychiatric illness
C. Direct questions about suicidal ideation will not cause the patient to become more impulsive and self-injurious
D. Patients rarely require involuntary hospitalization
E. Alcoholism does not increase the risk of suicide

ANSWERS

26.1. Answer: D. Patients need to be assessed for modifiable risk factors providing opportunities for intervention. There are certain protective factors that mitigate the risk for suicide. These include pregnancy; children in the home; effective clinical care for mental, physical, and substance use disorders; family and community support positive social support; religious beliefs and cultural practices; and skills in problem solving and conflict resolution.

McClatchey K, et al. Protective factors of suicide and suicidal behavior relevant to emergency healthcare settings: A systematic review and narrative synthesis of post-2007 reviews. *Arch Suicide Res.* 2019;23: 411-427.

26.2. Answer: D. Psychological autopsy studies examined clinical and demographic variables of persons who had completed suicide, including the communication of suicidal intent. Intent was viewed as a direct statement about ending one's life or an indirect remark about "no longer being here" or being "better off dead." A review of 100 cases of suicide found that 55% of people who completed suicides gave some warning of their intention. Another study of 134 cases of suicide found that 69% of people who completed suicides gave a warning.

Barraclough B, et al. A hundred cases of suicide: Clinical aspects. *Br J Psychiatry.* 1974;125:355-373.

Robins E, et al. Some clinical considerations in the prevention of suicide based on a study of 134 successful suicides. *Am J Public Health.* 1959;49:888-889.

26.3. Answer: E. Suicide risk for individuals with severe mental illness is approximately 20-40 times higher than the risk for the general population. Psychological autopsy studies consistently reveal major psychiatric illness to be present in 93% of adult suicides. The increased rate of psychiatric illness is also true for those who have serious suicide attempts.

Inskip HM, et al. Lifetime risk of suicide for affective disorder, alcoholism and schizophrenia. *Br J Psychiatry.* 1998;172:35-37.

Kochanek KD, et al. Deaths: Final data for 2002. *Natl Vital Stat Rep.* 2004;53:1-115.

26.4. Answer: C. Confidentiality is a vital part of the physician-patient relationship. A patient's request for confidentiality should be honored unless the patient is a danger to self or others. Reasons for breaching confidentiality should be recorded in the patient's chart. In clinical situations when a patient is threatening to harm a person, the physician has a duty to warn the potential victim. This duty arose from the *Tarsoff* ruling of 1973 in the United States.

Simon RI. *Clinical Psychiatry and the Law*. 2nd ed. Washington, DC: American Psychiatric Press; 1992:268-269, 319-320.

26.5. Answer: D. There are many diagnostic criteria that are used to diagnose alcohol use disorder, these include the following: alcohol is often taken in larger amounts or over a longer period than was intended; there is a persistent or unsuccessful desire to cut down on alcohol use; a great deal of time is spent in activities necessary to obtain alcohol; important social, occupational, or recreational activities are given up because of alcohol use; and patients exhibit tolerance, such that they have a markedly diminished effect with continued use of the same amount.

American Psychiatric Association. *Diagnostic and Statistical Manual of Mental Disorders*. 5th ed. Arlington, VA: American Psychiatric Association; 2013.

26.6. Answer: E. While women attempt suicide at a higher rate than men, men account for approximately 77% of completed suicides in the United States. The majority of the completed suicides are by use of firearms (55.6% of male suicides), followed by suffocation (26.9%), and then self-poisoning (10%). Women's most common method of completed suicide is self-poisoning (33.4%), followed by firearms (30.5%) and then suffocation (26.7%).

Karch DL, et al. Surveillance for violent deaths—National Violent Death Reporting System, 16 states, 2009. *MMWR Surveill Summ*. 2012;61:1-43.

26.7. Answer: C. Assessing for capacity is a fluid process, and a patient's capacity fluctuates depending on multiple factors, including their medical condition, the time of day, or the amount of pain that they are in. To accurately assess a patient's capacity, the conversation needs to be performed in the patient's native language. The physician performing the capacity assessment needs to keep in mind the patient's health literacy. The patient needs to communicate a choice. The patient needs to understand the relevant information. The patient also needs to appreciate the situation and its consequences. The patient must be able to appreciate treatment options.

Grisso T, et al. The MacCAT-T: A clinical tool to assess patients' capacities to make treatment decisions. *Psychiatr Serv*. 1997;48:1415-1419.

26.8. Answer: A. There are certain signs that are concerning that the etiology of a patient's presentation is medical and not psychiatric. That includes new-onset symptoms in a patient older than 40, abnormal vital signs or physical examination, recent memory loss, or clouded sensorium. Patients who are elderly or very young; patients with substance use, abnormal movements, or abrupt onset of symptoms; and patients with no prior psychiatric history have a high risk of medical instability.

Gregory RJ, et al. Medical screening in the emergency department for psychiatric admissions: A procedural analysis. *Gen Hosp Psychiatry*. 2004;26:405-410.

26.9. Answer: E. There is no evidence-based data to support that patients regain decision-making capacity at a particular blood ethanol concentration. Depending on tolerance, cognition varies widely, and certain patients will, in fact, begin to withdraw at significantly elevated blood ethanol concentrations. The decision to medically clear someone should be based on a patient's clinical sobriety as a particular ethanol concentration is not necessarily reflective of a patient's degree of intoxication.

Dhossche D, Rubinstein J. Drug detection in a suburban psychiatric emergency room. *Ann Clin Psychiatry*. 1996;8:59-69.

Lukens TW, et al. Clinical policy: Critical issues in the diagnosis and management of the adult psychiatric patient in the emergency department. *Ann Emerg Med*. 2006;47:79-99.

26.10. Answer: C. Patients will not be "provoked" into suicidal crisis by a discussion of their suicidal ideation and thoughts about death. Many patients will be relieved that the physician is willing to speak openly with them about their distress. Patients who are being evaluated for suicidality should be supervised continuously by a health professional to prevent further self-injurious behavior. Acute intoxication interferes with the identification of underlying psychiatric illness. Patients will frequently require involuntary hospitalization. The presence of alcoholism increases the risk of suicide.

Fawcett J, et al. Assessing and treating the patient at risk for suicide. *Psychiatr Ann* 1993;23:244-255.

Renal Principles

27.1. Which of the following choices is associated with nontraumatic myoglobinuric acute kidney failure?
A. Phencyclidine
B. *Tricholoma equestre*
C. Amphetamine
D. Cisplatin
E. *Cortinarius orellanus*

27.2. A 40-year-old man develops acute kidney injury following an intentional acetaminophen overdose. Which of the following findings would be most supportive of a diagnosis of hepatorenal syndrome as opposed to acute tubular necrosis?
A. The urinary sediment has dirty brown casts
B. The serum creatinine concentration is rapidly rising
C. The fractional extraction of urea is >50%
D. The fractional extraction of sodium is <1%
E. The patient has isosthenuria

27.3. A 27-year-old man presents to the emergency department with metabolic acidosis and kidney failure after ingesting a liquid found in his garage. Later, he develops acute renal cortical necrosis. Which of the following xenobiotics did he most likely drink?
A. Ethylene glycol
B. Diethylene glycol
C. Propylene glycol
D. Ethylene glycol monobutyl ether
E. Methanol

27.4. A 56-year-old man develops nephrotic syndrome. Which of the following exposures is most likely causative?
A. Bismuth
B. Arsenic
C. Gold
D. Lithium
E. Lead

27.5. A 57-year-old man eats a meal that consists of grass carp gallbladder. Two weeks later, he presents to the hospital with nausea, fatigue, and generalized weakness. Which pathophysiologic lesion do you expect to find?
A. Focal glomerulosclerosis
B. Acute interstitial nephritis
C. Obstructive uropathy
D. Acute tubular necrosis
E. Prerenal acute kidney injury

27.6. Crystaluria is an important complication of which of the following xenobiotics?
A. Ethylene glycol
B. Acyclovir
C. Methotrexate
D. Melamine
E. All of the above

27.7. Prerenal acute kidney injury commonly results from salt and water depletion. Which xenobiotic causes prerenal acute kidney injury by another mechanism?
A. Ketoprofen
B. Ergotamine
C. Ethylene glycol
D. Amphetamines
E. Cisplatin

27.8. A 33-year-old woman presents to the hospital complaining of bilateral flank pain and is found to have hydronephrosis with an acute kidney injury. Imaging confirms retroperitoneal fibrosis. Which of the following xenobiotics was most likely responsible?
A. Gentamicin
B. Ethylene glycol
C. Iodinated radiocontrast agents
D. Bromocriptine
E. Mercuric chloride

27.9. A 52-year-old man with chronic back pain who regularly takes simultaneous maximal doses of salicylates, acetaminophen, and another analgesic he bought while traveling abroad develops kidney disease. Which of the following findings is most suggestive of analgesic nephropathy?
A. Eosinophiluria
B. Papillary necrosis
C. Focal glomerulosclerosis
D. Membranous glomerulonephritis
E. Acute tubular necrosis

27.10. A 47-year-old woman has been taking a new herbal remedy for one week because of progressive weakness and fatigue. She presents to the hospital and is found to have kidney failure. Which of the following options best suggests that her kidney disease predates her new herbal medication use?
A. Normal-sized kidneys on ultrasound
B. A normal hemoglobin
C. A low serum calcium
D. Hyperkalemia
E. Acidemia

ANSWERS

27.1. Answer: B. All of the choices listed cause either severe muscle injury and myoglobinuric acute kidney injury (choices A and C) or acute kidney injury without muscle damage (choices D and E), but only the mushroom *Tricholoma equestre* causes nontraumatic rhabdomyolysis and acute kidney injury. Other causes of nontraumatic muscle injury include the HMG-CoA reductase inhibitors (statins), doxylamine, carbon monoxide, and rarely cocaine.

Bedry R, et al. Wild-mushroom intoxication as a cause of rhabdomyolys. *N Engl J Med.* 2001;345:798-802.

27.2. Answer: D. The hepatorenal syndrome resembles prerenal acute kidney injury and results from hormonally mediated renal vasoconstriction. It is characterized by a benign urinary sediment, a low fractional excretion of sodium, a low fractional excretion of urea, and usually only recovers if liver function is restored. While the blood urea nitrogen: creatinine ratio tends to be higher in prerenal acute kidney injury, both concentrations climb. Choices A, C, and E are suggestive of acute tubular necrosis.

Salerno F, et al. Diagnosis, treatment and survival of patients with hepatorenal syndrome: A survey on daily medical practice. *J Hepatol.* 2011;55:1241-1248.

27.3. Answer: B. Diethylene glycol causes metabolic acidosis, acute kidney injury, and neurologic toxicity. Renal cortical necrosis is also described. Ethylene glycol causes acidosis, acute kidney injury, and rarely neurologic toxicity, but the pathophysiology of the kidney injury is acute tubular necrosis. While most ingestions of ethylene glycol monobutyl ether are benign, large ingestions are rarely associated with acidosis and hemolysis, but not kidney injury.

Marraffa JM, et al. Diethylene glycol: Widely used solvent presents serious poisoning potential. *J Emerg Med.* 2008;35:401-406.

27.4. Answer: C. Nephrotic syndrome is characterized by proteinuria and edema, usually without hypertension. While many xenobiotics are associated with nephrotic syndrome, of the ones listed, gold is most likely.

Hall CL. Gold nephropathy. *Nephron.* 1988;50:265-272.

27.5. Answer: D. The grass carp gallbladder contains 5 alpha-cyprinol sulphate, a xenobiotic that produces both liver and kidney injury. Patients often present with mild gastroenteritis that develop elevated hepatic aminotransferases and acute tubular necrosis. Some patients will require hemodialysis.

Kung SW, et al. Acute renal failure and hepatitis following ingestion of carp gallbladder. *Clin Toxicol (Phila).* 2008;46:753-757.

27.6. Answer: E. All of the choices produce crystalluria, which contributes to kidney injury. Other xenobiotics implicated in crystalluria include vitamin C, fluorinated anesthetics, sulfonamides, fluoroquinolone antibiotics, and certain antiretrovirals.

Daudon M, Frochot V. Crystalluria. *Clin Chem Lab Med*. 2015;53(suppl 20): s1479-1487.

Osborne CA, et al. Melamine and cyanuric acid-induced crystalluria, uroliths, and nephrotoxicity in dogs and cats. *Vet Clin North Am Small Anim Pract*. 2009;39:1-14.

27.7. Answer: A. Nonsteroidal antiinflammatory drugs (NSAIDs) inhibit cyclooxygenase, which prevents the conversion of arachidonic acid to vasodilatory prostaglandins. The net reduction in renal perfusion mimics salt and water depletion and is essentially indistinguishable from other causes of prerenal acute kidney injury. Adverse drug reactions occur commonly when NSAIDs are prescribed to patients who take medicines that are normally very dependent on renal perfusion, such as lithium. The other choices all produce acute kidney injury by other mechanisms.

Nobre G, et al. Pathophysiological aspects of nephropathy caused by non-steroidal anti-inflammatory drugs. *J Bras Nefrol*. 2019;41:124-130.

27.8. Answer: D. All of the listed choices are associated with kidney injury, but only bromocriptine is associated with post renal acute kidney injury from retroperitoneal fibrosis. This is an uncommon injury pattern, and other implicated xenobiotics include *Aristolochia* spp, hydralazine, methysergide, gadolinium, and methyldopa.

Alberti C. Drug-induced retroperitoneal fibrosis: Short aetiopathogenetic note, from the past times of ergot-derivatives large use to currently applied bio-pharmacology. *G Chir*. 2015;36:187-191.

27.9. Answer: B. Papillary necrosis follows the chronic interstitial inflammation of analgesic nephropathy. Eosinophiluria characterizes hypersensitivity reactions. Choices C, D, and E represent other forms of kidney injury.

Shelley JH. Pharmacologic mechanisms of analgesic neuropathy. *Kidney Int*. 1978;13:15-26.

27.10. Answer: C. Chronic kidney disease is associated with small shrunken kidneys, anemia (from loss of erythropoietin), and hypocalcemia (from loss of vitamin D activation). Both acute kidney injury and chronic kidney disease cause acidemia and hyperkalemia.

Allgrove J, Shaw NJ. A practical approach to vitamin D deficiency and rickets. *Endocr Dev*. 2015;28:119-133.

Respiratory Principles

QUESTIONS

28.1. A 26-year-old man presents to the emergency department unresponsive after an opioid overdose. He is difficult to ventilate because of chest wall rigidity. Which xenobiotic is most likely responsible?
A. Morphine
B. Fentanyl
C. Diacetylmorphine
D. Codeine
E. Hydromorphone

28.2. A 23-year-old man is brought into the emergency department after a reported overdose. A chest radiograph demonstrates pneumomediastinum. Which of the following xenobiotics most likely contributed to this finding?
A. Acetaminophen
B. Salicylate
C. Caffeine
D. Intravenous heroin
E. Crack cocaine

28.3. Which of the following mechanisms best explains the generation of opioid-induced acute respiratory distress syndrome (ARDS)?
A. Hypoxia
B. Aspiration during a period of unconsciousness
C. Elevation of catecholamines produced by hypercapnia
D. Direct opioid-induced alterations in pulmonary capillary integrity
E. Acute myocardial dysfunction from high concentrations of opioid

28.4. A 62-year-old woman presents to the emergency department with shortness of breath and is diagnosed with hypersensitivity pneumonitis. Chronic use of which of the following medications led to this diagnosis?
A. Nitrofurantoin
B. Acetaminophen
C. Albuterol
D. Clonidine
E. Enalapril

28.5. A 23-year-old man is pulled out of his apartment unresponsive after a suicide attempt. He has complete resolution of his symptoms following removal from his apartment and administration of oxygen. Which of the following gases best explain his presentation?
A. Helium
B. Hydrogen sulfide
C. Cyanide
D. Phosphine
E. Phosgene

28.6. A 31-year-old woman with a history of heavy menstrual bleeding presents to the emergency department with shortness of breath. She has a hemoglobin of 7.5 g/dL. Her oxygen saturation is 95%. What is the expected oxygen content of this patient's blood?
A. 4.3 mL O_2/dL
B. 10.2 mL O_2/dL
C. 20.1 mL O_2/dL
D. 25.4 mL O_2/dL
E. 51.8 mL O_2/dL

28.7. Nebulized 2-4% sodium bicarbonate is a reasonable treatment option for which of the following pulmonary irritants?
A. Nitrogen dioxide
B. Chloroacetophenone
C. Chlorine
D. Ammonia
E. Ozone

28.8. In 1986, an earthquake in Lake Nyos, Cameroon, caused a release of a gas from a volcanic lake that led to the death of 1,700 people. Most survivors recovered without complications. Which of the following gases was responsible for this disaster?
A. Phosgene
B. Hydrogen sulfide
C. Carbon monoxide
D. Carbon dioxide
E. Ozone

28.9. A 22-year-old man is placed on end-tidal CO_2 monitoring after an intentional overdose. The patient's end-tidal CO_2 is 65 mmHg. Which of the following is a reasonable intervention to attempt?
A. Sodium bicarbonate
B. Midazolam
C. 100% oxygen through a face mask
D. Methylene blue
E. Naloxone

28.10. A 31-year-old man presents after an intentional ingestion of a large amount of liquid nicotine in a suicide attempt. Which of the following markers is most helpful in deciding whether to intubate this patient?
A. Pulse oximeter
B. Chest radiograph
C. Auscultation
D. Butylcholinesterase concentration
E. Negative inspiratory force

ANSWERS

28.1. Answer: B. Fentanyl is unique among the opioids in that it produces severe chest wall rigidity of a degree that compromises ventilation. Although the exact mechanism for this effect is unknown, it is relieved by both naloxone and neuromuscular blockers.

> Caspi J, et al. Delayed respiratory depression following fentanyl anesthesia for cardiac surgery. *Crit Care Med.* 1988;16:238-240.

> Christian CM, et al. Postoperative rigidity following fentanyl anesthesia. *Anesthesiology.* 1983;58:275-277.

28.2. Answer: E. Pneumomediastinum is associated with insufflating drugs such as marijuana and crack cocaine. This is likely due to barotrauma secondary to insufflation followed by a prolonged Valsalva maneuver to maximize drug effect, which leads to rupture of an alveolar bleb.

> Shesser R, et al. Pneumomediastinum and pneumothorax after inhaling alkaloidal cocaine. *Ann Emerg Med.* 1981;10:213-215.

28.3. Answer: C. Experimental evidence in animals demonstrates that there is a profound increase in catecholamine concentrations associated with opioid-induced hypercapnia. This results in ARDS following opioid overdose, especially when the opioid is reversed prior to correction of the hypercapnia. Hypoxia alone is insufficient to give the same effect. Although other models are important, this study helps link "opioid-induced noncardiogenic pulmonary edema" to other causes of ARDS (such as neurogenic edema).

> Mill CA, et al. Cardiovascular effects of fentanyl reversed by naloxone at varying arterial carbon dioxide tensions in dogs. *Anesth Analg.* 1988;67:730-736.

28.4. Answer: A. Hypersensitivity pneumonitis is also known as extrinsic allergic alveolitis. It is both drug induced and non–drug induced. Common causes of medication-induced hypersensitivity pneumonitis include nitrofurantoin, amiodarone, and minocycline.

> Watts MM, Grammer LC. Hypersensitivity pneumonitis. *Allergy Asthma Proc.* 2019;40:425-428.

28.5. Answer: A. Simple asphyxiants have little or no toxicity except for their ability to displace oxygen. Simply removing the patient from the enclosed space and providing oxygen supplementation are curative if the patient has not suffered permanent damage because of hypoxia. Examples of simple asphyxiants include argon, helium, ethane, methane, and propane.

> Borron SW, Bebarta VS. Asphyxiants. *Emerg Med Clin North Am.* 2015;33:89-115.

28.6. **Answer: B.** Oxygen content is equal to the hemoglobin (Hb) bound to oxygen added to the dissolved oxygen. Assuming a PO_2 of 100 mmHg, this patient would have an oxygen content of 10.2 mL O_2/dL.

$$
\begin{aligned}
O_2 \text{ content} = {} & (Hb)(O_2 \text{ sat})(1.39 \text{ mL } O_2/g\%) \\
& + (0.003 \text{ mL } O_2/dL/mmHg)(PO_2) \\
= {} & (7.5 \text{ g/dL})(95\%)(1.39 \text{ mL } O_2/g\%) \\
& + (0.003 \text{ mL } O_2/dL/mmHg)(100 \text{ mmHg}) \\
= {} & 10.2 \text{ mL } O_2/dL
\end{aligned}
$$

If this patient had a hemoglobin of 15 g/dL, her oxygen content would be 20.1 mL/O_2.

Treacher DF, Leach RM. Oxygen transport-1. Basic principles. *BMJ.* 1998;317:1302-1306.

28.7. **Answer: C.** An inhaled solution of dilute (2-4%) sodium bicarbonate provides relief from pain and cough in patients exposed to chlorine gas. This probably results from neutralization of hydrochloric acid that forms when chlorine gas dissolves in lung water.

Chisholm CD, et al. Inhaled sodium bicarbonate therapy for chlorine inhalational injuries. *Ann Emerg Med.* 1989;18;466.

28.8. **Answer: D.** A volcanic lake in Lake Nyos, Cameroon, released a cloud of carbon dioxide of approximately one-quarter million tons. The cloud flowed into low-lying valleys and killed approximately 1,700 people. Countless other people were also affected because of hypoxia. Patients who did not have permanent effects of hypoxia recovered with no complications.

Freeth SJ. Lake Nyos disaster. *BMJ.* 1989;299:513.

28.9. **Answer: E.** End-tidal CO_2 is the maximum partial pressure of CO_2 at the end of respiration. An elevated end-tidal CO_2 reading corresponds with an elevated $PaCO_2$; however, low values are frequently spurious. This patient's elevated end-tidal CO_2 reading corresponds with respiratory depression, and given the history of an overdose, a dose of naloxone is reasonable. Unfortunately, the sensitivity and specificity of end-tidal CO_2 in predicting complications of hypoventilation in patients who present to the emergency department following an overdose are 46 and 86%, respectively.

Viglino D, et al. Noninvasive end tidal CO_2 is unhelpful in the prediction of complications in deliberate drug poisoning. *Ann Emerg Med.* 2016;68:62-70.

28.10. **Answer: E.** Negative inspiratory force (NIF), also known as maximum inspiratory pressure, identifies subclinical diaphragmatic weakness. A NIF that is worse (closer to zero) than negative 30 cmH$_2$O is predictive of respiratory failure. Patients who present with toxicity from xenobiotics such as nicotine, botulism, and elapid envenomation should have a NIF performed every 2-4 hours after the initial presentation to identify changes in a patient's condition and to anticipate the need for intubation.

Lawn ND, et al. Anticipating mechanical ventilation in Guillain-Barré Syndrome. *Arch Neurol.* 2001;58:893-898.

Thermoregulatory Principles

QUESTIONS

29.1. The thermosensitive neurons are predominantly located in what area of the central nervous system?
A. Posterior hypothalamus
B. Substantia nigra
C. Locus ceruleus
D. Anterior hypothalamus
E. Thalamus

29.2. Which of the following neurotransmitters causes stimulation of sweat glands?
A. Norepinephrine
B. Serotonin
C. Acetylcholine
D. Antidiuretic hormone
E. Glycine

29.3. Which of the following processes is the main thermoregulatory response to cold in adult humans?
A. Vasoconstriction
B. Shivering
C. Gluconeogenesis
D. Mobilization of brown fat
E. Piloerection

29.4. Which of the following options best describes the classic electrocardiographic change associated with hypothermia?
A. PR segment prolongation
B. QT interval shortening
C. Peaked T waves
D. U waves
E. J-point deflection

29.5. Heatstroke is characterized by which of the following physical examination findings?
A. Excessive sweating
B. Temperature >104 °F (40.0 °C)
C. Altered mental status
D. Hypotension
E. Bradycardia

29.6. A 25-year-old man presents to the emergency department after he was found sleeping on the sidewalk in the winter. His vital signs are: blood pressure, 100/80 mmHg; heart rate, 55 beats/min; respiratory rate, 14 breaths/min; core temperature, 89 °F (31.7 °C); and oxygen saturation, 100%. Which of the following rewarming techniques is indicated?
A. Removing wet clothes and covering the patient with a blanket
B. Active external rewarming, with a goal of reaching 98.6 °F (37 °C) within 20 minutes
C. Peritoneal lavage with warmed dialysate
D. Extracorporeal venovenous rewarming
E. Bilateral chest tube insertion with thoracic lavage

29.7. Dantrolene is the initial treatment of choice in which of the following conditions?
A. Exertional heatstroke
B. Neuroleptic malignant syndrome
C. Malignant hyperthermia
D. Classic heatstroke
E. Strychnine poisoning

29.8. Hyperthermia occurs in which of the following conditions?
A. Thiamine deficiency
B. Phenobarbital poisoning
C. Hypoglycemia
D. Carbon monoxide poisoning
E. Salicylate poisoning

29.9. Which of the following options is of greatest prognostic significance in hypothermia?
A. Temperature 70–80 °F (21–27 °C)
B. K^+ >10 mEq/L

C. Frostbite
D. Unconsciousness
E. Ethanol intoxication

29.10. Which of the following statements is correct regarding drug metabolism in hypothermia?
A. Hepatic metabolism increases
B. Renal clearance increases
C. Glomerular filtration rate increases
D. Volume of distribution increases
E. Neuromuscular blockade is prolonged

ANSWERS

29.1. Answer: D. Thermosensitive neurons are located predominantly in the preoptic area of the anterior hypothalamus, although some are found in the posterior hypothalamus. Heating or cooling of the hypothalamus in conscious animals results in appropriate thermoregulatory responses.

Boulant JA. Hypothalamic neurons. Mechanisms of sensitivity to temperature. *Ann N Y Acad Sci.* 1998;856:108-115.

29.2. Answer: C. Sweat glands are controlled by sympathetic postganglionic nerve fibers that are cholinergic. Large amounts of acetylcholinesterase and a number of peptides are involved in neural transmission. Anticholinergic xenobiotics impair sweat gland function and predispose individuals to heat illness.

Hensel H. Neural processes in thermoregulation. *Physiol Rev.* 1973;53:948-1007.

29.3. Answer: B. Shivering is the main thermoregulatory response to cold in humans, except in neonates, where nonshivering thermogenesis prevails. Shivering is initiated in the posterior hypothalamus. Efferent stimuli from the posterior hypothalamus travel through the midbrain, pons, and lateral medullary reticular formation to the motor pathways of the tectospinal and rubrospinal tract, resulting in shivering. Heat produced without muscle contraction is nonshivering thermogenesis. Brown fat, the most important site of nonshivering thermogenesis, is found primarily in neonates.

Birzis L, Hemingway A. Descending brain stem connections controlling shivering in cat. *J Neurophysiol.* 1956;19:37-43.

Bruck K. Non-shivering thermogenesis and brown adipose tissue in relation to age, and their integration in the thermoregulatory system. In: Lindberg O, ed. *Brown Adipose Tissue.* Amsterdam: Elsevier/North-Holland; 1970:117-154.

29.4. Answer: E. A deflection occurring at the junction of the QRS and ST segment, known as the Osborn wave, was first described in 1938. This J-point deflection is invariably found in hypothermic patients with temperatures <90 °F (32.2 °C) when multiple electrocardiographic leads are obtained.

Vassallo SU, et al. A prospective evaluation of the electrocardiographic manifestations of hypothermia. *Acad Emerg Med.* 1999;6:1121-1126.

29.5. Answer: C. Heatstroke is defined as a temperature >106 °F (41.1 °C) in the setting of mental status alteration. The altered mental status is very common, but not universal; some young patients present with lethargy and others with seizures. Although absence of sweating was once thought to comprise part of the definition of heatstroke, many patients with heatstroke maintain the ability to sweat. Hypotension is exceptionally common, but not sufficient for diagnosing heatstroke.

Malamud N, et al. Heatstroke: A clinico-pathologic study of 125 fatal cases. *Milit Surg.* 1946;99:397-444.

Bouchama A, Knochel JP. Heat stroke. *N Engl J Med.* 2002;346: 1978-1988.

29.6. Answer: A. Passive external rewarming by removing wet clothes and covering the patient with a blanket is the appropriate therapy for this patient. As opposed to hyperthermia, in which patients need to be cooled rapidly, patients who are hypothermic are able to be safely rewarmed more slowly. Rewarming rates are usually about 1.80 °F (1.0 °C) an hour. Patients who rewarm at a slower rate than that need to be evaluated for an underlying infection or alternative source of hypothermia. Options C-D are not indicated for this degree of hypothermia. Extracorpeal methods of active internal rewarming should be reserved for patients with a temperature <80 °F (<27 °C) or those with unstable cardiac rhythms attributed to hypothermia.

> White JD. Hypothermia: The Bellevue Experience. *Ann Emerg Med.* 1982;11:417-424.

> Delaney KA, et al. Rewarming rates in urban patients with hypothermia: Prediction of underlying infection. *Acad Emerg Med.* 2006;13:913-921.

> Althaus U, et al. Management of profound accidental hypothermia with cardiorespiratory arrest. *Ann Surg.* 1982;195:492-495.

29.7. Answer: C. Dantrolene is the preferred drug in the treatment of malignant hyperthermia. Dantrolene acts on the ryanodine receptor of skeletal muscles and either inhibits the release of calcium or increases calcium uptake in the sarcoplasmic reticulum. Dantrolene does not improve outcome from heatstroke.

> Bouchama A, et al. Ineffectiveness of dantrolene sodium in the treatment of heatstroke. *Crit Care Med.* 1991;19:176-180.

> Gronert GA. Controversies in malignant hyperthermia. *Anesthesiology.* 1983;59:273-274.

> Amsterdam JT, et al. Dantrolene sodium for treatment of heatstroke victims: Lack of efficacy in a canine model. *Am J Emerg Med.* 1986;4:399-405.

29.8. Answer: E. Thiamine deficiency, sepsis, hypoglycemia, and carbon monoxide poisoning predispose to hypothermia.

Salicylates cause uncoupling of oxidative phosphorylation and predispose to hyperthermia.

> Maickel RP. Interaction of drugs with autonomic nervous function and thermoregulation. *Fed Proc.* 1970;29:1973-1979.

29.9. Answer: B. Prolonged cardiorespiratory arrest and absolute temperature do not predict poor outcome. Profound hyperkalemia is associated with the inability to successfully resuscitate severely hypothermic patients.

> Althaus U, et al. Management of profound accidental hypothermia with cardiorespiratory arrest. *Ann Surg.* 1982;195:492-495.

> Hauty MG, et al. Prognostic factors in severe accidental hypothermia: Experiences from the Mt. Hood tragedy. *J Trauma.* 1987;27:1107-1112.

> Mair P, et al. Prognostic markers in patients with severe accidental hypothermia and cardiocirculatory arrest. *Resuscitation.* 1994;27:47-54.

29.10. Answer: E. Neuromuscular blockade is prolonged in hypothermic patients. Hepatic metabolism decreases, renal clearance decreases, glomerular filtratation rates decrease, and volume of distribution decreases.

> Wislicki L. Effects of hypothermia and hyperthermia on the action of neuromuscular blocking agents. I. Suxamethonium. *Arch Int Pharmacodyn Ther.* 1960;126:68–78.

> Ham J, et al. Pharmacokinetics and pharmacodynamics of D-tubocurarine during hypothermia in the cat. *Anesthesiology.* 1978;49:324–329.

Reproductive and Perinatal Principles

QUESTIONS

30.1. Which of the following signs and symptoms is associated with neonatal opioid abstinence syndrome (NAS)?
A. Sleepiness
B. Increased feeding
C. Acidosis
D. Hypotonia
E. Myoclonic jerking

30.2. A 31-year-old woman presents to the emergency department at 28 weeks of gestation with abdominal pain and vomiting after self-medicating for dental pain. Her laboratory analysis demonstrates an aspartate aminotransferase of 1462 U/L, an international normalized ratio (INR) of 2.3, and an acetaminophen concentration of 63 mg/L (417.1 micromol/L). Which of the following statements is most correct?
A. *N*-acetylcysteine (NAC) administration will reduce the likelihood of adverse fetal outcome
B. Exchange transfusion is first-line therapy for fetal acetaminophen poisoning
C. Fetal hepatotoxicity is unlikely to occur because fetal tissues do not express CYP2E1
D. NAC is unlikely to cross human placenta
E. The fetus should be urgently delivered

30.3. A 25-year-old woman presents to the emergency department after an intentional overdose of iron tablets. She is pregnant at 22 weeks of gestation. Her vital signs are: blood pressure, 95/60 mmHg; heart rate, 118 beats/min; respiratory rate, 20 breaths/min; and temperature, 98.4 °F (36.9 °C). She has six episodes of emesis. Her laboratory studies are significant for acidemia and an elevated anion gap. Her abdominal radiograph demonstrates iron tablets in the stomach. Which of the following options is the best treatment strategy for this patient?
A. Deferoxamine and whole bowel irrigation should both be avoided
B. Deferoxamine should be avoided, but whole bowel irrigation should be administered
C. Deferoxamine should be administered, but whole bowel irrigation should be avoided
D. Deferoxamine and whole bowel irrigation should both be administered
E. No data exists to make an informed recommendation on deferoxamine or whole bowel irrigation in pregnant women

30.4. Which of the following pharmacokinetic properties facilitates xenobiotic transfer to breast milk?
A. Large molecular weight
B. Weak base
C. Low lipid solubility
D. Highly protein bound
E. Ionized in plasma

30.5. Which of the following antidotes is associated with known human teratogenicity?
A. Hyperbaric oxygen
B. Fomepizole
C. Deferoxamine
D. Penicillamine
E. Pralidoxime

30.6. Which of the following statements regarding fetal alcohol syndrome is correct?
  A. After the first trimester, alcohol is no longer teratogenic
  B. At least 60 mL/day of 100% alcohol is usually necessary to cause fetal alcohol syndrome
  C. Alcohol is second only to nicotine as the leading cause of birth defects
  D. Neonatal alcohol withdrawal should be treated with tincture of opium
  E. Children with fetal alcohol syndrome are generally large for gestational age

30.7. Which of the following medications is most commonly ingested in overdose during pregnancy in the United States?
  A. Acetaminophen
  B. Diazepam
  C. Ferrous sulfate
  D. Ampicillin
  E. Salicylates

30.8. Which of the following statements about carbon monoxide poisoning in human pregnancy is true?
  A. Peak maternal carboxyhemoglobin exceeds peak fetal carboxyhemoglobin
  B. Lower fetal PO_2 diminishes the adverse effects of fetal carboxyhemoglobin
  C. Therapy with 100% oxygen should be discontinued when the maternal carboxyhemoglobin returns to a normal level

  D. Hyperbaric oxygen therapy should be administered for a period of time equal to twice the standard length of treatment
  E. Fetal toxicity is generally greater than maternal toxicity

30.9. A 27-year-old woman presents to the emergency department with severe abdominal pain and vaginal bleeding. She is pregnant at 32 weeks of gestation. She is diagnosed with abruptio placentae and is emergently taken to the operating room. Which of the following xenobiotics most likely contributed to her presentation?
  A. Heroin
  B. Cocaine
  C. Ethanol
  D. Ibuprofen
  E. Carbon monoxide

30.10. A 16-year-old girl takes a xenobiotic in an attempt to induce abortion. She is unsuccessful and the child is born with hypoplasia of the eighth nerve and deafness. Which of the following teratogens was the child exposed to in utero?
  A. Quinine
  B. Tetracycline
  C. Polychlorinated biphenyls
  D. Diazepam
  E. Amiodarone

ANSWERS

30.1. Answer: E. Neonatal opioid abstinence syndrome (NAS) occurs following chronic maternal exposure to opioids. The onset of symptoms depends on the type of opioid to which the mother was exposed. Heroin withdrawal occurs within 24 hours of delivery, while withdrawal from methadone and buprenorphine usually occurs within 2-3 days of delivery. Patients present with feeding difficulty, irritability, respiratory distress, yawning, sneezing, and fevers. Babies with NAS are very jittery with myoclonic jerking.

Doberczak TM, et al. Relationship between maternal methadone methadone dosage, maternal-neonatal methadone levels, and neonatal withdrawal. *Obstet Gynecol.* 1993;81:936-940.

30.2. Answer: A. Pregnant women with acetaminophen toxicity should be treated with *N*-acetylcysteine (NAC). While NAC does not cross sheep placenta, it was found in the cord blood of recently delivered infants who were treated in utero. Fetal tissues express CYP2E1 as early as 16 weeks of gestation, but at reduced concentrations than adults. While exchange transfusion is used in the setting of fetal toxicity with elevated cord acetaminophen concentrations, it is a high-risk procedure with little data to support its use. Urgent delivery is only indicated if fetal instability occurs. The outcome of pregnancy seems to best corelate with maternal outcome.

Miller MS, et al. Drug metabolic enzymes in developmental toxicology. *Fundam Appl Toxicol.* 1996;34:165-175.

Horowitz RS, et al. Placental transfer of *N*-acetylcysteine following human maternal acetaminophen toxicity. *J Toxicol Clin Toxicol.* 1997;35:447-451.

30.3 Answer: D. This patient has significant iron toxicity and requires treatment for her overdose. The risk of maternal distress to the fetus is greater than the potential teratogenicity of deferoxamine; therefore, deferoxamine should be administered when signs and symptoms indicate severe poisoning. Whole bowel irrigation (WBI) is also safe in pregnant women. Iron overdose is one of the few specific indications for WBI.

Singer ST, Vichinsky EP. Deferoxamine treatment during pregnancy: Is it harmful? *Am J Hematol.* 1999;60:24-26.

Van Ameyde KJ, Tenenbein M. Whole bowel irrigation during pregnancy. *Am J Obstet Gynecol.* 1989;160:646-647.

30.4. Answer: B. Xenobiotics that are weak bases are largely nonionized in plasma and easily diffuse into the breast milk. Xenobiotics with a large molecular weight, defined as 500-600 D and greater are unlikely to cross into the breast milk of lactating mothers. Lipid solubility is important for both the diffusion and accumulation of the xenobiotic in the breast milk as breast milk is rich in fat. Only free xenobiotics transverse the mammary alveolar body.

Sachs HC. Committee on Drugs. The transfer of drugs and therapeutics into human breast milk: An update on selected topics. *Pediatrics.* 2013;132:e796-e809.

30.5. Answer: D. Penicillamine use during pregnancy is associated with the development of cutis laxa and hyperflexibility of joints, although the risk is probably low. The other antidotes are used clinically for acute poisoning during pregnancy. Hyperbaric oxygen and deferoxamine are associated with teratogenic effects in some animal models.

Shepard TH, Lemire RJ. *Catalog of Teratogenic Agents.* 13th ed. Baltimore, MD: Johns Hopkins University Press; 2010.

Bosque MA, et al. Assessment of the developmental toxicity of deferoxamine in mice. *Arch Toxicol.* 1995;69:467-471.

30.6. Answer: B. Fetal alcohol syndrome (FAS) is characterized by (1) intrauterine or postnatal growth retardation; (2) facial dysmorphogenesis, particularly microcephaly, short palpebral fissures, epicanthal folds, maxillary hypoplasia, cleft palate, hypoplastic philtrum, and micrognathia; and (3) developmental delay or behavioral abnormalities. These effects occur after consumption of the equivalent of 2-3 ounces of absolute ethanol (4-6 drinks of distilled spirits) per day throughout pregnancy. The craniofacial effects probably represent early teratogenic effects on the embryo, whereas the central nervous system abnormalities result from adverse effects later in gestation. Benzodiazepines are the recommended therapy for neonatal alcohol withdrawal. The leading cause of birth defects is unknown, but FAS is one of the leading preventable causes of developmental delay.

Sokol RJ, et al. Fetal alcohol spectrum disorder. *JAMA.* 2003;290:2996-2999.

30.7. Answer: A. Analgesics are the most commonly ingested xenobiotics during pregnancy, and acetaminophen is the most commonly ingested analgesic. At therapeutic doses, acetaminophen is considered safe in pregnancy. However, in overdose, there is an increased incidence of spontaneous abortions, particularly in the setting of delayed *N*-acetylcysteine administration. Most pregnant women survive an acetaminophen overdose with appropriate NAC therapy and recover without adverse effects to either themselves or their babies.

Li DK, et al. Exposure to non-steroidal anti-inflammatory drugs during pregnancy and risk of miscarriage: Population based cohort study. *BMJ.* 2003;327:368.

Rayburn W, et al. Drug overdose during pregnancy: An overview from a metropolitan poison control center. *Obstet Gynecol.* 1984;64:611-614.

Riggs BS, et al. Acute acetaminophen overdose during pregnancy. *Obstet Gynecol.* 1989;74:247-253.

30.8. Answer: E. The fetus is at greater risk of toxicity from carbon monoxide than the mother. Peak fetal carboxyhemoglobin generally exceeds maternal levels and occurs at a later time. For this reason, it is recommended that oxygen therapy be continued for a period of time five times as long as it takes to lower the maternal level to normal. Lower fetal PO$_2$ exacerbates the effects of fetal carboxyhemoglobin.

Hyperbaric therapy is appropriate for cases of carbon monoxide poisoning in pregnancy. Therapy should follow standard treatment protocols for time and pressure.

Elkharrat D, et al. Acute carbon monoxide intoxication and hyperbaric oxygen in pregnancy. *Intensive Care Med.* 1991;17:289-292.

van Hoesen KB, et al. Should hyperbaric oxygen be used to treat the pregnant patient for acute carbon monoxide poisoning? A case report and literature review. *JAMA.* 1989;261:1039-1043.

30.9. Answer: B. Cocaine use during pregnancy increases the risk of developing abruptio placentae. Cocaine use is also associated with perinatal seizures, strokes, and intraventricular hemorrhages in the newborn. Toxicity is likely secondary to vascular mechanisms, including increased uterine vascular resistance and decreased uterine blood flow.

Chiriboga CA. Neurological correlates of fetal cocaine exposure. *Ann N Y Acad Sci.*1998;846:109-125.

Shiono PH, et al. The impact of cocaine and marijuana use on low birth weight and preterm birth: A multicenter study. *Am J Obstet Gynecol.* 1995;172:19-27.

Flowers D, et al. Cocaine intoxication associated with abruptio placentae. *J Natl Med Assoc.* 1991;83:230-232.

30.10. Answer: A. Fetal exposure to quinine, especially at higher doses, is associated with hypoplasia of the eighth nerve and deafness. Tetracycline leads to yellow or brown discoloration of the teeth. Polychlorinated biphenyls lead to hyperpigmentation of the skin. Diazepam potentially leads to cleft palate formation, although this is controversial. Amiodarone leads to transient neonatal hypothyroidism and hyperthyroidism.

Shepard TH, Lemire RJ. *Catalog of Teratogenic Agents.* 13th ed. Baltimore, MD: Johns Hopkins University Press; 2010.

Pediatric Principles

QUESTIONS

31.1. Which of following statements is true regarding child-resistant containers?
A. Child-resistant containers prevent all children from opening them
B. Child-resistant containers are mandatory for the dispensing of all pharmaceuticals
C. Child-resistant containers are responsible for a significant decline in morbidity related to childhood poisoning
D. Children generally ingest medications contained in child-resistant containers
E. Child-resistant containers are designed to function even when pill dust or liquid residue sticks to the cap or screw top

31.2. Which of the following scenarios is suspicious of child abuse in the setting of a childhood ingestion?
A. An 18-month-old girl was observed to ingest two acetaminophen tablets from her mother's bedside table
B. A 30-month-old boy is found comatose on the living room floor after their parent's 10th anniversary party
C. A 16-month-old boy ingests 10 iron sulfate pills that resemble candy
D. A 12-month-old boy swallows a small button battery that he found on the floor of the living room
E. A 6-month-old girl ingests five aspirin tablets that she found in her mother's purse

31.3. In addition to the sedative-hypnotic effects of acute ethanol ingestion, ethanol is associated with which of the following toxicities in young children?
A. Hypoglycemia
B. Hyperthermia
C. Constipation
D. Methemoglobinemia
E. Thiamine deficiency

31.4. A 4-year-old girl presents to the emergency department unresponsive after an unintentional ingestion of her grandfather's glimepiride. She is hypoglycemic in triage, and 25 g of 50% dextrose is administered. The patient regains consciousness; however, she immediately begins screaming in pain and points to the infusion site. Which of the following is true regarding complications of 50% dextrose extravasation?
A. It is benign
B. It is safely treated with local infiltration of insulin
C. Warm compresses are usually sufficient as treatment
D. It needs surgical consult for potential debridement
E. It should be treated with dimethylsulfoxide (DMSO)

31.5. A 2-year-old girl presents to the emergency department unresponsive after ingesting one of her mother's hydrocodone/acetaminophen tablets. Which of the following gastric decontamination techniques would be appropriate?
A. Induced emesis
B. Orogastric lavage
C. Activated charcoal through a nasogastric tube
D. Whole bowel irrigation
E. No gastric decontamination

31.6. A 4-month-old boy presents to the emergency department with vomiting, tachypnea, hyperpnea, and lethargy following a salicylate ingestion. He deteriorates further and requires intubation. He has already received large amounts of sodium bicarbonate, potassium supplementation, multiple doses of activated charcoal, and whole bowel irrigation. Nephrology is unable to perform hemodialysis given his small size. Which of the following therapies could be attempted?
    A. High-dose insulin euglycemia therapy
    B. Methylene blue
    C. Fomepizole
    D. Exchange transfusion
    E. No further therapies are possible

31.7. A 3-month-old boy develops abdominal distension, vomiting, metabolic acidosis, and worsening pallid cyanosis while he is being treated for a *Haemophilus influenzae* infection. Which of the following xenobiotics led to his presentation?
    A. Chloramphenicol
    B. Benzyl alcohol
    C. Aniline dye
    D. Melamine
    E. Propofol

31.8. Which of the following gastrointestinal decontamination techniques causes the *least* fluid and electrolyte abnormalities in pediatric patients?
    A. Magnesium sulfate
    B. Magnesium citrate
    C. Sorbitol
    D. Sodium phosphate
    E. Polyethylene glycol ELS

31.9. A 4-year-old girl presents to the emergency department after a witnessed ingestion of six atropine-diphenoxylate pills 2 hours ago. She is currently asymptomatic with normal vital signs. What is the next best step in management?
    A. Observe the patient in the emergency department for 2 hours and then discharge home
    B. Discharge immediately with outpatient follow-up in 1 week
    C. Order a urine drug screen, and if negative, discharge home
    D. Administer physostigmine
    E. Admit the patient to the hospital for 24 hours of observation

31.10. What is the best way to prevent unsupervised ingestions in the home?
    A. Ensure medication is up and away, out of a children's reach and sight
    B. Store medication in the dashboard of the car
    C. If medication comes in child-resistant containers, unsupervised ingestions never occur
    D. Ensure properly functioning child-resistant containers for supplies and store them in a cabinet under the sink in the bathroom
    E. Remove all materials that could potentially be toxic from the home

ANSWERS

31.1. Answer: C. Child-resistant packaging means that packaging must be effective at preventing 85% of children from opening the packaging, and yet allow 90% of adults to open the container. Child-resistant containers (CRCs) are believed to be responsible for the almost 90% decline in mortality from childhood poisonings over the past 30 years. CRCs are not 100% effective. Not all medications are required to be dispensed in them. Children sometimes open them. CRCs will not function properly if there is pill or liquid residue around the closure. Children often find pills outside of the CRC from which they were originally dispensed.

Walton WW. An evaluation of the Poison Prevention Packaging Act. *Pediatrics*. 1982;69:363-370.

Wiseman HM, et al. Accidental poisoning in childhood: A multicenter survey. 2. The role of packaging in accidents involving medications. *Hum Toxicol*. 1987;6:303-314.

31.2. Answer: E. A 6-month-old child does not have the developmental skills to get to the mother's purse, open it, and remove pills. When the history of the ingestion conflicts with the child's developmental abilities, child abuse must be suspected. Choices A and D are typical ingestion scenarios in toddlers. Choice B illustrates a common problem when a child wakes up early on the morning after a party and discovers leftover ethanol that has not yet been cleaned up. Choice C illustrates the problem of poison look-alikes, substances that resemble other tasty nontoxic substances with which the child is familiar.

Dine MS, McGovern ME. Intentional poisoning of children—an overlooked category of child abuse: Report of seven cases and review of the literature. *Pediatrics*. 1982;70:32-35.

31.3. Answer: A. In children, ethanol is associated with sedative-hypnotic effects as well as ethanol-induced hypoglycemia. This results in an increased risk for seizures and the exacerbation of central nervous system toxicity from ethanol. Children are at particular risk for hypoglycemia because of their reduced hepatic glycogen stores.

Cummins LH. Hypoglycemia and convulsions in children following alcohol ingestion. *J Pediatr.* 1961;58:23-26.

31.4. Answer: D. Children should not receive 50% dextrose as part of the management of hypoglycemia. The more appropriate concentration of dextrose in infants and young children is 10%. The osmolarity of 50% dextrose is 2,525 mOsm/L and is associated with thrombophlebitis, limb necrosis and amputation after soft tissue extravasation. Large boluses of 50% dextrose in children are associated with seizures, brain hemorrhage, and hyperosmolar coma.

Arad I, Benady S. Letter: Gangrene following intraumbilical injection of hypertonic glucose. *J Pediatr.* 1976;89:327-328.

DeLorenzo RA, Vista JP. Another hazard of hypertonic dextrose. *Am J Emerg Med.* 1994;12:262-263.

31.5. Answer: E. While historically syrup of ipecac was used to induce emesis in pediatric patients who present after an overdose, it is no longer recommended given its limited benefit and the risk of adverse effects. Small children are unlikely to tolerate a large orogastric tube for lavage, and realistically, a small tube is not effective in removing pills; therefore, orogastric lavage is limited to adolescents and adults. Regardless, this ingestion is not one that would warrant orogastric lavage anyway. There are very rare, if any, occasions in which a nasogastric tube should be inserted in a child for the sole purpose of administering activated charcoal as there is a significant risk of aspiration. Had this child been awake and able to safely drink, then activated charcoal would be reasonable. However, in this case, the possible risks of activated charcoal far outweigh the benefits. There is no reason to perform whole bowel irrigation. No gastric decontamination is indicated in this patient.

Osterhoudt KC, et al. Risk factors for emesis after therapeutic use of activated charcoal in acutely poisoned children. *Pediatrics.* 2004;113:806-810.

31.6. Answer: D. Certain centers are unable to perform hemodialysis on very small infants, and peritoneal dialysis does not effectively remove toxins. Some xenobiotics, such as salicylate, are amenable to enhanced elimination through exchange transfusion. In this patient, an exchange transfusion was performed, and his salicylate concentration went from 70.1 mg/dL (5.1 mmol/L) to 34.4 mg/dL (2.5 mmol/L). He eventually had a complete recovery and was discharged home.

Manikian A, et al. Exchange transfusion in severe infant salicylism. *Vet Hum Toxicol.* 2002;44:224-227.

31.7. Answer: A. This patient is presenting with gray baby syndrome because of high-dose chloramphenicol administration. Gray baby syndrome consists of abdominal distension, vomiting, metabolic acidosis, progressive pallid cyanosis, irregular respirations, hypothermia, hypotension, and vasomotor collapse.

Holt D, et al. Chloramphenicol toxicity. *Adverse Drug React Toxicol Rev.* 1993;12:83-95.

31.8. Answer: E. Cathartics, such as magnesium sulfate, magnesium citrate, and those containing phosphate, are frequently associated with fluid and electrolyte abnormalities. Sorbitol has fewer problems when a single dose is used but is associated with similar complications after multiple-dose use. Polyethylene glycol electrolyte lavage solution (ELS) is a whole bowel irrigating solution that was originally developed as a preparation for bowel surgery. It was subsequently incorporated into poison management strategies, particularly for xenobiotics such as iron, which are not adsorbed to activated charcoal.

Tenenbein M. Whole bowel irrigation in iron poisoning. *J Pediatr.* 1987;111:142-145.

Tuggle DW, et al. The safety and cost effectiveness of polyethylene glycol electrolyte solution bowel preparation in infants and children. *J Pediatr Surg.* 1987;22:513-515.

31.9. Answer: E. Atropine-diphenoxylate (Lomotil) is associated with serious morbidity and mortality, especially in children. Symptoms following ingestion are occasionally delayed for as long as 24 hours. Patients who ingest atropine-diphenoxylate should be admitted to the hospital for 24 hours of observation, even if they are initially asymptomatic.

Cutler EA, et al. Delayed cardiopulmonary arrest after Lomotil ingestion. *Pediatrics.* 1980;65:157-158.

McCarron MM, et al. Diphenoxylate-atropine (Lomotil) overdose in children: An update (report of eight cases and review of the literature). *Pediatrics.* 1991;87:694-700.

31.10. Answer: A. Unsupervised ingestions is the term preferred by certain epidemiologists to describe unintentional poisoning in children. The Centers for Disease Control and Prevention (CDC) estimates that approximately 50,000 children present to the emergency department because of an unsupervised ingestion. The CDC currently supports an "Up and Away" campaign that highlights the importance of safe medication storage. Medication should be stored up and away from children's reach and sight any time a medication is taken. While child-resistant packaging decreases the likelihood of a child opening a container, at least 15% of children are still able to open containers. Other important aspects of the campaign include teaching children about what medicine is and why an adult needs to supervise the ingestion and ensuring that children are never told that medicine is candy. It is impossible to remove all toxic materials from the home.

https://www.cdc.gov/medicationsafety/protect/campaign.html. Accessed May 28, 2021.

Geriatric Principles

QUESTIONS

32.1. The Beers Criteria, developed by Dr Mark H. Beers in 1991, were created to address which of the following?
A. A steep rise in intentional overdoses
B. Adverse drug reactions that occur in the geriatric population
C. Risk stratification to determine need for admission after toxicologic exposure
D. Identification of substance use disorders in the geriatric population
E. Differentiation of adverse drug reactions from common geriatric syndromes

32.2. Which of the following medications will exhibit an age-related increase in the volume of distribution that will prolong the elimination half-life?
A. Salicylate
B. Acetaminophen
C. Lithium
D. Flurazepam
E. Ibuprofen

32.3. Which of the following antidotes should be used with caution in geriatric patients?
A. *N*-acetylcysteine
B. Succimer
C. Deferoxamine
D. Polyvalent crotalid antivenom
E. Sodium bicarbonate

32.4. Adverse drug events in the geriatric population are typically identified during which phase of clinical trials?
A. Phase I
B. Phase II
C. Phase III
D. Phase IV
E. Phase V

32.5. What is a possible explanation for the enhanced central nervous system (CNS) effects of xenobiotics in the geriatric population?
A. Decreased concentrations of cyclic adenosine monophosphate (cAMP) leading to decreased calcium efflux into neurons and increased impedance in the neuron
B. Degradation of the extracellular portion of 7-transmembrane receptors, with resultant decreased activity of G protein-coupled receptor activity
C. Increased potassium efflux from neurons in the CNS by way of passive diffusion, resulting in decreased signal propagation
D. Age-related denaturing of synaptobrevin, resulting in decreased release of acetylcholine
E. Decreased P-glycoprotein activity, resulting in decreased efflux of substrate from the brain

32.6. Which of the following options is most commonly found in the urine toxicology analysis of geriatric trauma patients?
A. Amphetamines
B. Opioids
C. Tricyclic antidepressants
D. Cannabinoids
E. Cocaine

32.7. Which of the following options is true for people over the age of 65 as compared to younger adults?
A. They account for a disproportionately high number of poisonings
B. They have a higher mortality rate following poisoning
C. They have a lower suicide rate
D. They have a lower rate of critical care admissions from emergency departments
E. They take fewer medications than people 40–50 years of age

32.8. A 72-year-old man presents to the emergency department in alcohol withdrawal. He is tremulous, diaphoretic, and delirious. Escalating doses of diazepam are administered to treat his symptoms. He remains comatose for several days, with eventual improvement of his symptoms. What pharmacodynamic property best explains his prolonged sedation?

A. Genetically inherited deficiency of CYP2C19 with a resultant prolonged half-life
B. Slowed gastrointestinal motility, leading to prolonged absorption of diazepam
C. Decreased hepatic oxidation, resulting in a prolonged half-life
D. Decreased enterohepatic circulation, leading to a prolonged half-life
E. Synergistic effects of ethanol and benzodiazepines on gamma-aminobutyric acid (GABA) receptors

32.9. Highly protein bound basic drugs will be most affected by an age-related increase in which of the following options?
A. Alpha$_1$-acid glycoprotein synthesis
B. Hepatic perfusion
C. Renal clearance
D. Albumin synthesis
E. Calcium

32.10. Compared to younger adults, which of the following characteristics of alcohol metabolism contributes to toxicity in geriatric patients?
A. Peak effect of alcohol occurs more slowly
B. Peak effect of alcohol is diminished
C. Gastric alcohol dehydrogenase decreases
D. The half-life of alcohol is prolonged
E. There is a larger volume of distribution

ANSWERS

32.1. Answer: B. The Beers Criteria or Beers List is a set of guidelines developed in 1991 to encourage better prescribing practices in the geriatric population. It defines a list of potentially inappropriate medications (PIM) that should be avoided in older adults. It undergoes constant revision.

American Geriatrics Society 2015 Beers Criteria Update Expert Panel. American Geriatrics Society 2015 Beers Criteria for potentially inappropriate medications use in older adults. *J Am Geriatr Soc.* 2015;63:2227-2246.

By the 2019 American Geriatrics Society Beers Criteria® Update Expert Panel. American Geriatrics Society 2019 Updated AGS Beers Criteria® for Potentially Inappropriate Medication Use in Older Adults. *J Am Geriatr Soc.* 2019;67:674-694.

Croke L. Beers Criteria for Inappropriate Medication Use in Older Patients: An update from the AGS. *Am Fam Physician.* 2020;101:56-57.

32.2. Answer: D. The fat-to-lean ratio increases with advancing age. Highly lipid-soluble drugs have an increased volume of distribution. As a result, there is a delay prior to achieving steady state; therefore, peak effect and toxicity are delayed. This mechanism is part of the reason drugs such as diazepam and flurazepam have a prolonged half-life in otherwise healthy geriatric patients.

Novak LP. Aging, total body potassium, fat-free mass, and cell mass in males and females between ages 18 and 85 years. *J Gerontol.* 1972;27:428-443.

32.3. Answer: E. All the listed antidotes are used to treat geriatric patients with overdoses appropriate for these drug therapies. Sodium bicarbonate predisposes patients with underlying cardiovascular disease to congestive heart failure, pulmonary edema, and hypertension, and should be used with caution when indicated.

Puczynski MS, et al. Sodium intoxication caused by baking soda as a home remedy. *Can Med Assoc J.* 1983;128:821-822.

Maher D, et al. Alterations in drug disposition in older adults: A focus on geriatric syndromes. *Expert Opin Drug Metab Toxicol.* 2021;17:41-52.

32.4. Answer: D. Very few people over the age of 75 are subjects in clinical trials of new drugs in the United States, but this is probably due to problems recruiting appropriate, disease-free geriatric subjects, as there are no government regulations that would hinder their participation. Enhanced effects of many, but not all, substances increase the risk of serious adverse drug events among geriatric patients. Likewise, geriatric patients take more prescription and nonprescription drugs than do other age groups, increasing exposure to potentially harmful drugs as well as increasing the risk of clinically important drug–drug interactions. Pharmacokinetic changes increase the risk; delayed elimination of active substances delays peak action, so toxicity is delayed, sometimes for days, when long-acting agents are ingested. Adverse drug events are most commonly discovered after US Food and Drug Administration (FDA) approval. This takes place during phase IV of clinical trials. Phase V does not exist and phases I, II, and III typically do not include a large enough sample size or time span to study drug effects on geriatric patients, especially those on multiple medications. In 2019, the National Institutes of Health (NIH) proposed a new policy called "Inclusion Across the Lifespan," which requires participants of all ages to be included in clinical trials unless a specific ethical or scientific exclusion reason is stated.

Bugeja G, et al. Exclusion of elderly people from clinical research: A descriptive study of published reports. *Br Med J.* 1997;315:1059.

Lee PY, et al. Representation of elderly persons and women in published randomized trials of acute coronary syndromes. *JAMA.* 2001;286:708-713.

Shenoy P, Harugeri A. Elderly patients' participation in clinical trials. *Perspect Clin Res.* 2015;6:184-189.

32.5. Answer: E. Decreased P-glycoprotein activity is implicated in the accumulation of specific xenobiotics in brain tissue. This leads to an increased volume of distribution and enhanced or prolonged effects of a particular xenobiotic. None of the other answer choices are demonstrated to specifically enhance CNS effects of xenobiotics in geriatric patients.

Van Assema DM, et al. Blood-brain barrier P-glycoprotein function in Alzheimer's disease. *Brain.* 2012;135:181-189.

Finch A, Pillans P. P-glycoprotein and its role in drug-drug interactions. *Aust Prescr.* 2014;37:137-139.

32.6. Answer: B. Opioids are the most common xenobiotics found in urine toxicology analysis of geriatric trauma patients. It is important, however, to address one limitation of this finding; the study was unable to exclude iatrogenic administration of opioids during transport.

Ekeh AP, et al. The prevalence of positive drug and alcohol screens in elderly trauma patients. *Subst Abus.* 2014;35:51-55.

32.7. Answer: B. Although patients over 65 account for only 5% of poisoning exposures, nearly 19% of deaths from poisoning occur among geriatric patients. This is likely due to the presence of disease or physiologic changes in various organ systems. Physiologic vulnerability leading to life-threatening complications from poisonings, and serious nontoxicologic illness account for the high rate of critical care admissions of geriatric patients. The rate of completed suicides increases with age, particularly among white men, although most suicides among men are associated with firearms rather than drug overdose.

Tadros G, Salib E. Age and methods of fatal self harm (FSH). Is there a link? *Int J Geriatr Psychiatry.* 2000;15:848-852.

Meehan PJ, et al. Suicides among older United States residents: Epidemiologic characteristics and trends. *Am J Public Health.* 1991;81:1198-1200.

32.8. Answer: C. Diazepam, which is metabolized by hepatic oxidation, is eliminated more slowly with age. An increased percentage of body fat in geriatric patients further prolongs the half-life of diazepam, primarily through an increased volume of distribution. The increased percentage of body fat is especially significant in lipid-soluble drugs, such as diazepam.

Greenblatt DJ, et al. Slow accumulation and elimination of diazepam and its active metabolite with extended treatment in the elderly. *J Clin Pharmacol.* 2021;61:193-203.

32.9. Answer: A. Basic drugs bind primarily to alpha$_1$-acid glycoprotein. Alpha$_1$-acid glycoprotein is an acute-phase reactant that increases rather than decreases with age. It is unclear if this increase is related to certain disease states or to age. The significance is that it increases the ratio of bound to unbound medication.

Abernethy DR, Kerzner L. Age effects on alpha-1-acid glycoprotein concentration and imipramine plasma protein binding. *J Am Geriatr Soc.* 1984;32:705-708.

Svensson CK, et al. Free drug concentration monitoring in clinical practice. Rationale and current status. *Clin Pharmacokinet.* 1986;11:450-469.

32.10. Answer: C. Gastric alcohol dehydrogenase declines with age, possibly due to atrophy of the gastric mucosa. The resulting decrease of "gastric first pass" metabolism leads to a higher blood ethanol concentration and an enhanced effect of alcohol. Many studies report no alteration in the metabolism of ethanol in older adults.

Pozzato G, et al. Ethanol metabolism and aging: The role of "first pass metabolism" and gastric alcohol dehydrogenase activity. *J Gerontol.* 1995;50:B135-B141.

Meier P, Seitz HK. Age, alcohol metabolism and liver disease. *Curr Opin Clin Nutr Metab Care*. 2008;11:21-26.

Acetaminophen

33

QUESTIONS

33.1. Which of the following statements is true of the toxic acetaminophen metabolite *N*-acetyl-*p*-benzoquinoneimine (NAPQI)?
A. It reacts readily with available electrophiles
B. It is formed only in the liver
C. In the liver, it is mostly formed in zone III
D. It is formed after acetaminophen overdose but not after recommended dosing
E. Glutathione stores must remain near normal to prevent toxicity

33.2. A 27-year-old woman presents to the emergency department (ED) with right upper quadrant pain. She had an intentional overdose of acetaminophen approximately 36 hours prior to arrival in the ED. Which of the following laboratory abnormalities is a poor prognostic marker?
A. An international normalized ratio (INR) of 1.8
B. A serum creatinine of 3.7 mg/dL (327 micromol/L)
C. A serum bilirubin of 6.2 mg/dL (106.02 micromol/L)
D. An aspartate aminotransferase of >10,000 IU/L
E. An alanine aminotransferase of >5,000 IU/L

33.3. A 19-year-old woman develops fulminant hepatic failure after an intentional acetaminophen overdose. She is treated in the intensive care unit and survives. A biopsy of her liver performed 1 year after the overdose will most likely reveal which of the following findings?

A. Significant fibrosis
B. Nonalcohol fatty liver disease
C. Cirrhotic liver
D. Persistent inflammatory changes
E. Normal liver

33.4. Which of the following statements is true of *N*-acetylcysteine (NAC)?
A. It is a glutathione substitute but does not lead to increased glutathione supply
B. It is a glutathione substitute and prevents the formation *N*-acetyl-*p*-benzoquinoneimine (NAPQI)
C. It decreases the capacity for sulfation of acetaminophen
D. If administered within 8 hours of an acute acetaminophen ingestion it prevents liver failure
E. It interferes with the acetaminophen assay

33.5. Which of the following is true of acetaminophen overdose in pregnancy?
A. *N*-Acetylcysteine (NAC) does not cross the human placenta
B. The fetus is incapable of producing *N*-acetyl-*p*-benzoquinoneimine (NAPQI) until late in the third trimester
C. NAC directly protects the fetus from serious toxicity
D. The fetus should be urgently delivered if at a viable gestational age
E. In nearly all cases, both maternal and fetal outcome is good if NAC is used in a timely manner

33.6. A 27-year-old man presents to the emergency department after a massive ingestion of acetaminophen. His blood pressure is 60/30 mmHg and heart rate is 145 beats/min. He has altered mental status and is intubated for airway protection. His acetaminophen concentration is 1,000 mcg/mL (6,615 micromol/L). He is immediately started on *N*-acetylcysteine therapy. Which of the following therapies is also indicated?
   A. Hemodialysis
   B. Methylene blue
   C. Immediate liver transplantation
   D. Hydroxocobalamin
   E. Intravenous lipid emulsion

33.7. Which of the following statements is true of acetaminophen exposure in patients younger than 5 years old?
   A. They have increased capacity for sulfation, providing them with protection from acetaminophen-induced hepatic injury
   B. They are less likely than adults to suffer toxicity related to repeated excessive dosing
   C. Acute febrile illness decreases the risk of acetaminophen-induced liver injury
   D. The lower incidence of liver injury after acute acetaminophen exposure in these patients is related to the amount of exposure, time to treatment, or decreased susceptibility
   E. The acetaminophen nomogram does not apply to children

33.8. Which of the following statements regarding acute kidney injury after acetaminophen exposure is correct?
   A. Hepatorenal syndrome is the only cause of acetaminophen-induced kidney injury
   B. The incidence of kidney injury is the same regardless of the degree of liver injury
   C. Renal CYP2E1 metabolism of acetaminophen leads to the formation of *N*-acetyl-*p*-benzoquinoneimine (NAPQI)

   D. Pancreatic injury is more common than kidney injury
   E. Kidney injury does not occur in the absence of liver injury

33.9. Which of the following statements regarding the administration of activated charcoal after acetaminophen ingestion is correct?
   A. Activated charcoal does not interfere with the absorption of oral *N*-acetylcysteine (NAC)
   B. Activated charcoal does not decrease acetaminophen absorption
   C. Interference with absorption of oral NAC is rarely a clinical concern
   D. If a patient has a depressed mental status, a nasogastric tube should be inserted for the administration of charcoal
   E. Activated charcoal increases the absorption of acetaminophen

33.10. For which of the following cases is the acetaminophen nomogram **not** applicable?
   A. A patient who is comatose with a serum acetaminophen concentration of 20 mcg/mL (132 micromol/L) and no history regarding the time of ingestion
   B. A patient who presents with a history of single acute acetaminophen ingestion with a serum acetaminophen concentration of 20 mcg/mL (132 micromol/L) 28 hours after his ingestion
   C. A patient who is taking 10 g of acetaminophen per day for 3 days and has a serum acetaminophen concentration of 50 mcg/mL (330.8 micromol/L) 4 hours after his last dose
   D. A patient who gives a history of acute acetaminophen ingestion in a self-harm attempt who has right upper quadrant tenderness with a serum acetaminophen concentration of 30 mcg/mL (198.5 micromol/L) and an aspartate aminotransferase (AST) of 450 IU/L 12 hours after his ingestion
   E. All of the above

ANSWERS

33.1. Answer: C. NAPQI is itself an electrophile, formed primarily in centrilobular (zone III) regions of liver, in which most oxidative drug metabolism occurs. It is also formed in the kidney and other sites. It is always formed during acetaminophen metabolism, but results in toxicity only when glutathione depletion is extensive.

Mitchell JR, et al. Acetaminophen-induced hepatic necrosis. IV. Protective role of glutathione. *J Pharmacol Exp Ther.* 1973;187:211-217.

33.2. Answer: B. The King's College Criteria are used to help prognosticate outcomes of patients who are poisoned by acetaminophen and help to guide transfer to a liver transplant center. These criteria include an arterial pH <7.3 or a lactate concentration >3.0 mmol/L after fluid resuscitaton, a creatinine >3.3 mg/dL (291.8 micromol/L), a prothrombin time > 100 sec (or an international normalized ratio of >6.5), or grade III or IV encephalopathy. Survival rates have continued to improve, and now the survival of patients who meet King's College Criteria who are not transplated is 25-40%.

Grady JG, et al. Early indicators of prognosis in fulminant hepatic failure. *Gastroenterology.* 1989;97:439-445.

Larson AM, et al. Acetaminophen-induced acute liver failure: Results of a United States multicenter, prospective study. *Hepatology.* 2005;42:1364-1372.

33.3. Answer: E. Patients typically die of their fulminant liver failure within 3-5 days of an acetaminophen overdose. Patients who survive beyond that time enter a recovery phase. Survivors have complete hepatic regeneration, and their liver biopsies are expected to be normal.

Portmann B, et al. Histopathological changes in the liver following a paracetamol overdose: Correlation with clinical and biochemical parameters. *J Pathol.* 1975;117:169-181.

Lesna M, et al. Evaluation of paracetamol-induced damage in liver biopsies. *Virchows Arch Pathol.* 1976;370:333-344.

33.4. Answer: D. There is no loss of efficacy if *N*-acetylcysteine (NAC) is given within 8 hours of acetaminophen ingestion. NAC acts as a glutathione substitute and also increases glutathione supply. NAC detoxifies *N*-acetyl-*p*-benzoquinoneimine (NAPQI) but does not block its formation. NAC increases the sulfation of acetaminophen.

Lauterburg BH, et al. Mechanism of action of N-acetylcysteine in the protection against hepatotoxicity of acetaminophen in rats in vivo. *J Clin Invest.* 1983;71:980-991.

Smilkstein MJ, et al. Efficacy of oral N-acetylcysteine in the treatment of acetaminophen overdose: Analysis of the national multicenter study (1976–1985). *N Engl J Med.* 1988;319:1557-1562.

33.5. Answer: E. The fetus is able to form NAPQI during most of pregnancy and is at risk for toxicity. Although NAC treatment leads to a good outcome in nearly all cases, it is unclear whether NAC is effective in directly treating the fetus. Even though NAC fails to cross the placenta in experimental animals, it does cross the human placenta. Good maternal outcome, is the best way to ensure good fetal outcome.

Horowitz RS, et al. Placental transfer of N-acetylcysteine following human maternal acetaminophen toxicity. *J Toxicol Clin Toxicol.* 1997;35:447-451.

Riggs BS, et al. Acute acetaminophen overdose during pregnancy. *Obstet Gynecol.* 1989;74:247-253.

33.6. Answer: A. Hemodialysis (HD) increases elimination of acetaminophen. HD is recommended in patients who have a serum acetaminophen concentration >700 mcg/mL (4,630 micromol/L) with altered mental status, an elevated lactate concentration, and metabolic acidosis. Hemodialysis is also reccomended for patients with a concentration >1,000 mcg/mL (6,615 micromol/L) regardless of other therapies performed. It is important to remember that *N*-acetylcysteine (NAC) is also removed during dialysis; therefore, it is reasonable to double the dose of NAC during hemodialysis to compensate. Volume resuscitation is indicated before attempting HD as patients with low blood pressures are unlikely to tolerate the procedure. Of note, fomepizole is currently being studied as an adjunct therapy in the treatment of massive acetaminophen overdoses.

Gosselin S, et al. Extracorporeal treatment for acetaminophen poisoning: Recommendations from the EXTRIP workgroup. *Clin Toxicol (Phila).* 2014;52:856-867.

Hernandez SH, et al. The pharmacokinetics and extracorporeal removal of *N*-acetylcysteine during renal replacement therapies. *Clin Toxicol.* 2015;53:941-949.

Shah KR, et al Fomepizole as an adjunctive treatment in severe acetaminophen ingestions: A case series. *Clin Toxicol.* 2021;59:71-72.

33.7. Answer: D. When all cases with initial acetaminophen concentrations above the Rumack-Matthew treatment line are reviewed, the incidence of hepatotoxicity is lower in children under 5 years of age than in adults. However, these cases were not stratified by both serum concentration of acetaminophen and time to treatment with *N*-acetylcysteine (NAC). This makes amount of exposure, delay to treatment, and decreased susceptibility all possible explanations for the lower incidence of liver injury. Although the fraction of acetaminophen metabolized by sulfation is increased in children, this does not necessarily confer decreased risk of NAPQI formation. The relative risk of chronic excessive dosing for children is not known, but children with acute febrile illnesses comprise one of the few groups in which toxicity after repeated excessive dosing is described.

Day A, Abbott GD. Chronic paracetamol poisoning in children: A warning to health professionals. *N Z Med J.* 1994;107:201.

Rumack BH. Acetaminophen overdose in young children: Treatment and effects of alcohol and other additional ingestants in 417 cases. *Am J Dis Child.* 1984;138:428-433.

Tenenbein M. Why young children are resistant to acetaminophen poisoning. *J Pediatr.* 2000;137:891-892.

33.8. Answer: C. Kidney injury after acute acetaminophen overdose is typically due to acute tubular necrosis, which is likely caused by local production of NAPQI by renal CYP2E1 enzymes. NAPQI formation through the renal COX-2 and prostaglandin-mediated renal medullary ischemia are one of the mechanisms of the chronic analgesic nephropathy caused by acetaminophen. Kidney injury occurs in as many as 25% of cases with significant hepatotoxicity and in more than 50% of those with hepatic failure. Pancreatic injury is rarely reported.

Hart SG, et al. Acetaminophen nephrotoxicity in CD-1 mice. I. Evidence of a role for in situ activation in selective covalent binding and toxicity. *Toxicol Appl Pharmacol.* 1994;126:267-275.

Prescott LF, et al. Paracetamol-induced acute renal failure in the absence of fulminant liver damage. *Br Med J.* 1982;284:421-422.

Wilkinson SP, et al. Frequency of renal impairment in paracetamol overdose compared with other causes of acute liver damage. *J Clin Pharmacol.* 1977;30:220-224.

33.9. Answer: C. Activated charcoal decreases acetaminophen absorption. It also adsorbs NAC. Because NAC is effective if given within 8 hours and activated charcoal is most effective if given early after ingestion, it is very rare that the administration of charcoal and oral NAC could not be separated by at least 2 hours. In any case, currently, NAC is almost always administered intravenously. It is always important to weigh the risks and the benefits of any intervention; in the setting of acetaminophen overdose, the risks of the placement of a nasogastric tube for activated charcoal administration in a sedated patient far outweigh the benefits. Therefore, we recommend activated charcoal administation to patients with an acetaminophen overdose only in patients who are awake and are safely able to drink the activated charcoal, or in patients who are already intubated for another reason.

Buckley NA, et al. Activated charcoal reduces the need for N-acetylcysteine treatment after acetaminophen (paracetamol) overdose. *J Toxicol Clin Toxicol.* 1999;37:753-757.

Ekins B, et al. The effect of activated charcoal on N-acetylcysteine absorption in normal subjects. *Am J Emerg Med.* 1987;5:483-487.

33.10. Answer: E. The Rumack Matthew Nomogram applies to a single acute ingestion. In order to apply the nomogram, the time of the ingestion must be known, and an acetaminophen concentration must be obtained between 4 and 24 hours after ingestion. The nomogram cannot be used to exclude the risk of liver injury after repeat excessive dosing. In the circumstance when a patient has an acetaminophen concentration below the treatment line but has evidence of liver injury by physical and laboratory examination, reevaluation and treatment are indicated.

Rumack BH, et al. Acetaminophen overdose. 662 cases with evaluation of oral acetylcysteine treatment. *Arch Intern Med.* 1981;141:380-385.

Smilkstein MJ, et al. Acetaminophen poisoning and liver function. *N Engl J Med.* 1994;330:1310-1311.

Colchicine, Podophyllin, and the Vinca Alkaloids

QUESTIONS

34.1. Which of the following options best represents the primary pathophysiology of colchicine toxicity?
A. Inhibition of neutrophil and synovial cell release of glycoproteins
B. Inhibition of microtubule polymerization
C. Reduction in expression of adhesion molecules on white blood cells (WBCs)
D. Increased antagonism at $GABA_A$ receptors
E. Pancytopenia

34.2. A 62-year-old woman presents to the emergency department with cellulitis. She is already prescribed colchicine for her gout. Which antibiotic should be avoided because it would increase the risk of colchicine toxicity?
A. Doxycycline
B. Amoxicillin
C. Levofloxacin
D. Clarithromycin
E. Azithromycin

34.3. Which of the following potential complications of a colchicine overdose typically occurs weeks after the event?
A. Seizures
B. Leukocytosis
C. Alopecia
D. Anemia
E. Pancreatitis

34.4. A 10-year-old boy receives a vincristine overdose as the result of a medication dosing error. What life-threatening complication is he at risk for developing?
A. Congestive heart failure
B. Anaphylaxis
C. Seizures
D. Delirium
E. Stevens-Johnson syndrome

34.5. A 34-year-old woman presents to the emergency department with several episodes of vomiting and diarrhea. On review of her history, she reveals that she ate a plant in her garden 8 hours ago. Her complete blood count is remarkable for a white blood cell count of 30,000/mm³. She is admitted to the intensive care unit for observation and, 24 hours later, has a sudden cardiac arrest. The patient has return of spontaneous circulation; however, she is now pancytopenic, has oliguria, and hepatotoxicity. Which of the following plants did she ingest?
A. *Gloriosa superba*
B. *Datura stramonium*
C. *Convallaria majalis*
D. *Aconitum napellus*
E. *Catha edulis*

34.6. A 13-year-old boy is admitted to the intensive care unit after an intentional overdose of colchicine 4 hours prior to presentation. Which of the following therapies should be performed to decrease the amount of colchicine in his body?
A. Activated charcoal
B. Urinary alkalinization
C. Hemodialysis
D. Hemoperfusion
E. Colchicine-specific antibodies

34.7. A 62-year-old man presents to the emergency department obtunded 12 hours after an intentional overdose of a topical medication he was prescribed for warts. His initial laboratory analysis reveals a leukocytosis. Forty-eight hours later, he progresses to pancytopenia. If this patient survives this overdose, which of the following long-term complications is he at greatest risk of developing?
A. Bone marrow dysfunction
B. Peripheral sensorimotor axonopathy
C. Limb necrosis
D. Chloracne
E. Nephrocalcinosis

34.8. A 22-year-old man is transferred to the intensive care unit following an unintentional vincristine overdose. Which of the following therapies will lead to a significant decrease in vincristine concentrations?
A. Methotrexate
B. Vinca-specific antibodies
C. Leucovorin
D. Plasmapheresis
E. Hemodialysis

34.9. While vinca alkaloids and colchicine share much in common, which of the following toxicities occurs only with the vinca alkaloids?
A. Delirium
B. Seizures
C. Gastrointestinal effects
D. Syndrome of inappropriate antidiuretic hormone secretion
E. Multisystem organ dysfunction

34.10. A 3-year-old girl presents to the emergency department with bilateral ptosis and is diagnosed with bilateral cranial nerve III palsies. Which of the following medications caused this finding?
A. Vincristine
B. Lithium
C. Aspirin
D. Gabapentin
E. Digoxin

ANSWERS

34.1. Answer: B. Colchicine causes toxicity primarily through inhibition of microtubule polymerization, which eventually produces multiorgan disfunction.

> Finkelstein Y, et al. Colchicine poisoning: The dark side of an ancient drug. *Clin Toxicol (Phila)*. 2010;48:407-414.

34.2. Answer: D. Clarithromycin is a strong inhibitor of both CYP3A4 and P-glycoprotein, both of which metabolize and eliminate colchicine. Coadministration of clarithromycin and colchicine leads to supratherapeutic concentrations of colchicine.

> Villa Zapata L, et al. Evidence of clinically meaningful drug-drug interaction with concomitant use of colchicine and clarithromycin. *Drug Saf*. 2020;43:661-668.

34.3. Answer: C. Alopecia is delayed up to 2-3 weeks following exposure to a toxic dosage of colchicine.

> Putterman C, et al. Colchicine intoxication: Clinical pharmacology, risk factors, features, and management. *Semin Arthritis Rheum*. 1991;21:143-155.

34.4. Answer: C. Seizures are the most common complication among pediatric cancer patients who develop vincristine toxicity.

> Hurwitz RL, et al. Reversible encephalopathy and seizures as a result of conventional vincristine administration. *Med Pediatr Oncol*. 1988;16:216-219.

34.5. Answer: A. Colchicine is derived from two plants, *Colchicum autumnale* (autumn crocus) and *Gloriosa superba* (glory lily). There is a case report of a patient who mistook the tubers of a glory lily for sweet potatoes.

> Putterman C, et al. Colchicine intoxication: Clinical pharmacology, risk factors, features, and management. *Semin Arthritis Rheum*. 1991;21:143-155.

34.6. Answer: A. Activated charcoal adsorbs colchicine and is recommended as part of the management of colchicine toxicity. A single case report describes the use of colchicine-specific antibodies in a patient who had colchicine toxicity. The company no longer manufactures this product, and therefore, it is not available for use. Colchicine has a very large volume of distribution, and therefore, hemodialysis and hemoperfusion will not remove a significant amount of toxin. Because of enterohepatic circulation and the lack of effective antidotes, it would be reasonable to give activated charcoal even several hours after ingestion.

Bismuth C. Biological valuation of extra-corporeal techniques in acute poisoning. *Acta Clin Belg Suppl.* 1990;13:20-28.

34.7. Answer: B. This patient ingested podophyllin in a suicide attempt. Patients who survive an overdose of podophyllin are at greatest risk of developing a peripheral sensorimotor axonopathy. Weeks to months are needed to fully recover.

Chang MH, et al. Acute ataxic sensory neuronopathy resulting from podophyllin intoxication. *Muscle Nerve.* 1992;15:513-514.

34.8. Answer: D. Plasmapheresis was performed on a patient who had a vincristine overdose, and his serum concentrations dropped by 23%. Vincristine is highly protein bound, and therefore, hemodialysis will not be as effective. Leucovorin is thought to shorten the duration of the peripheral neuropathy; however, there are insufficient data to routinely recommend its use for that indication. Vinca-specific alkaloid antibodies are not available at this time.

Pierga JY, et al. Favourable outcome after plasmapheresis for vincristine overdose. *Lancet.* 1992;340:185.

34.9. Answer: D. Overdose on vinca alkaloids is associated with the development of syndrome of inappropriate antidiuretic hormone secretion (SIADH). This occurs as a result of the vinca alkaloids directly stimulating the hypothalamus. Serum electrolytes need to be monitored for 10 days following an overdose.

Rosenthal S, Kaufman S. Vincristine neurotoxicity. *Ann Intern Med.* 1974;80:733-737.

34.10. Answer: A. Vincristine, a vinca alkaloid, is associated with several different types of peripheral neuropathies. The neuropathies typically present 2 weeks following an overdose. Patients present with parasthesias, wrist drop, foot drop, and cranial nerve defects. There were several reported cases of patients with vincristine toxicity presenting with bilateral cranial nerve III palsies and resultant ptosis.

Hatzipantelis E, et al. Bilateral eyelid ptosis, attributed to vincristine, treated successfully with pyridoxine and thiamine in a child with acute lymphoblastic leukemia. *Toxicol Int.* 2015;22:162-164.

Nonsteroidal Antiinflammatory Drugs

35.1. A 33-year-old woman with collagen vascular disease presents to the emergency department with a temperature of 101.4 °F (38.6 °C), headache, and nuchal rigidity. Which nonsteroidal antiinflammatory drug (NSAID) is most likely to have caused these symptoms?
A. Naproxen
B. Sulindac
C. Ibuprofen
D. Indomethacin
E. Ketorolac

35.2. Aplastic anemia is most commonly associated with use of which of the following nonsteroidal antiinflammatory drugs (NSAIDs)?
A. Sulindac
B. Phenylbutazone
C. Naproxen
D. Ketorolac
E. Ibuprofen

35.3. Which of the following statements about ibuprofen is true?
A. It is poorly dialyzable in most overdoses due to a high volume of distribution
B. It is poorly dialyzable in most overdoses due to high protein binding
C. It is poorly dialyzable in most overdoses due to its high molecular weight
D. It is well dialyzed in most overdoses due to its low molecular weight
E. It is well dialyzed in most overdoses due to its low protein binding

35.4. A 67-year-old man presents to the emergency department for evaluation of chronic knee pain. On history, he endorses frequent nonsteroidal antiinflammatory drug (NSAID) use for his pain. Which of the following deleterious effects would be expected from his chronic NSAID use?
A. Hyponatremia
B. Hypokalemia
C. Narrow anion gap
D. Edema
E. Hypochloremia

35.5. A 37-year-old woman presents to the emergency department following an intentional overdose of a nonsteroidal antiinflammatory drug (NSAID) prescribed to treat her severe menstrual cramps. The ingestion occurred approximately 5 hours prior to presentation. While being evaluated, the patient develops a generalized tonic-clonic seizure. Which of the following NSAIDs did she ingest?
A. Mefenamic acid
B. Indomethacin
C. Meloxicam
D. Diclofenac
E. Celecoxib

35.6. Which of the following options is the most common adverse effect from chronic nonsteroidal antiinflammatory drug (NSAID) use?
A. Hyperkalemia
B. Gastrointestinal irritation
C. Chronic kidney disease
D. Hemolytic anemia
E. Lower and upper intestinal tract bleeding

35.7. Selective COX-2 inhibitors lead to increased cardiovascular events via which of the following mechanisms?
  A. Greater inhibition of thromboxane synthesis than prostacyclin synthesis
  B. Greater inhibition of prostacyclin synthesis than thromboxane synthesis
  C. Greater inhibition of prostaglandin synthesis than thromboxane synthesis
  D. Greater inhibition of thromboxane synthesis than prostaglandin synthesis
  E. Greater inhibition of prostaglandin synthesis than prostacyclin synthesis

35.8. Which of the following medications caused significant cardiovascular risk and was removed from the United States (US) market?
  A. Celecoxib
  B. Rofecoxib
  C. Indomethacin
  D. Mefenamic acid
  E. Diclofenac

35.9. Which of the following options is true of concurrent use of nonsteroidal antiinflammatory drugs (NSAIDs) with anticoagulants?

  A. These medications can be safely prescribed together
  B. Elderly patients on both drugs have a twofold increased risk of gastrointestinal bleeding
  C. The two drugs compete for protein binding and both affect hemostasis
  D. NSAIDs promote gastrointestinal bleeding by mechanical and antiprostaglandin effects that are augmented by the procoagulant effects on factors II, VII, IX, and X
  E. Pediatric patients are at particular risk for adverse drug interactions with this combination of drugs

35.10. An 80-year-old woman with a past medical history of atrial fibrillation presents to the emergency department following a loss of consciousness. Her electrocardiogram demonstrates slow atrial fibrillation at a rate of 32 beats/min. She is having frequent premature ventricular contractions on the monitor. Which of the following medications did she recently start taking?
  A. Ibuprofen
  B. Acetaminophen
  C. Olanzapine
  D. Diphenhydramine
  E. Glyburide

ANSWERS

35.1. Answer: C. This patient has aseptic meningitis. Analysis of cerebrospinal fluid in patients with aseptic meningitis demonstrates pleocytosis with a neutrophil predominance, elevated protein, normal or low glucose, and negative cultures. While naproxen and sulindac are reported to cause aseptic meningitis, ibuprofen is most commonly implicated, likely due to its widespread use. While the incidence is low, aseptic meningitis occurs with frequent use of these NSAIDs. An immunologic mechanism is also suggested because aseptic meningitis occurs more often in patients with systemic lupus erythematosus. Indomethacin and ketorolac are not implicated.

Auriel E, et al. Non steroidal anti-inflammatory drugs exposure and the central nervous system. *Hand Clin Neurol.* 2014;119;577-584.

35.2. Answer: B. Aplastic anemia occurs with therapeutic dosing of phenylbutazone. Although sale of this drug is now restricted in the United States, it is still available as a veterinary medication. Aplastic anemia is also rarely reported in patients using indomethacin and etodolac.

Court H, Volans G. Poisoning after overdose with nonsteroidal antiinflammatory drugs. *Adv Drug Reaction Acc Poison.* 1984;3:1-21.

35.3. Answer B. Ibuprofen has a low molecular weight, a volume of distribution of 0.1-0.2 L/kg, and is a highly albumin-bound nonsteroidal antiinflammatory drug (NSAID) both at therapeutic and most supratherapeutic concentrations. Due to its high protein binding, it is poorly dialyzable in most overdoses. In massive overdoses, however, albumin-binding sites are saturated, and the increased free fraction is more readily dialyzed.

Le HT. Ibuprofen overdose complicated by renal failure, adult respiratory distress syndrome and metabolic acidosis. *J Toxicol Clin Toxicol.* 1994;32:315-320.

35.4. Answer: D. NSAIDs can have many deleterious effects on the kidney. The most common is an acute tubulointerstitial nephritis (ATIN), which occurs with short-term use and usually improves within 2 weeks of discontinuation. Patients develop sodium retention, hyperkalemia, and edema, with both chronic and acute NSAID use. Acute overdoses lead to an elevated anion gap metabolic acidosis. Hypochloremia is not typically associated with NSAID use.

Whelton A. Nephrotoxicity of nonsteroidal anti-inflammatory drugs: Physiologic foundations and clinical implications. *Am J Med.* 1999;106: 13S-24S.

35.5. Answer: A. An overdose of mefenamic acid leads to muscle twitching as well as generalized tonic-clonic seizures. The seizures typically occur within 7 hours of ingestion. Seizures also occur following ibuprofen overdoses. The mechanism of the seizures is unknown at this time.

Balali-Mood M, et al. Mefenamic acid overdosage. *Lancet Lond Engl.* 1981;1:1354-1356.

35.6. Answer: B. While all of the listed choices occur with varying frequency in patients taking NSAIDs, gastrointestinal irritation is the most common adverse effect from chronic use.

Brooks PM, Day RO. Nonsteroidal antiinflammatory drugs: Differences and similarities. *N Engl J Med.* 1991;324:1716-1725.

35.7. Answer: B. PGI_2, a prostacyclin, blocks platelet activation and causes vasodilation. TXA_2, a thromboxane, is a platelet stimulator and vasoconstrictor. COX-2 inhibitors block the synthesis of both TXA_2 and PGI_2 but affect TXA_2 less, leading to a more prothrombotic environment.

Mukherjee D, et al. Risk of cardiovascular events associated with selective COX-2 inhibitors. *JAMA.* 2001;266:954-959.

35.8. Answer: B. Rofecoxib and valdecoxib were removed from the US market due to increased cardiovascular risk. Celecoxib is currently still labelled with a black box warning. Diclofenac, meloxicam, indomethacin, and ibuprofen show a trend toward increased cardiovascular risk.

Bresalier RS, et al. Cardiovascular events associated with rofecoxib in a colorectal adenoma chemo prevention trial. *N Engl J Med.* 2005;352:1092-1102.

35.9. Answer: C. These medications should not be prescribed together. The risk for gastrointestinal bleeding is an order of magnitude larger than if only one is given: one study reports a 13-fold increase in relative risk with this drug combination. It is safer to find another analgesic if a patient requires anticoagulation. Elderly patients are at particular risk for adverse drug interactions with this combination of drugs. NSAIDs promote gastrointestinal bleeding by mechanical and antiprostaglandin effects that are augmented by anticoagulant effects on factors II, VII, IX, and X.

Shorr RO, et al. Concurrent use of nonsteroidal antiinflammatory drugs and oral anticoagulants places elderly persons at high risk for hemorrhagic peptic ulcer disease. *Arch Intern Med.* 1993;153:1665-1670.

35.10. Answer: A. Nonsteroidal anti-inflammatory drugs (NSAIDs) interact with many medications that are used in the treatment of patients with cardiovascular disease, and they should be used with extreme caution. Patients who are chronically taking digoxin are at risk of developing an elevation in their serum digoxin concentrations when an NSAID is newly initiated.

Stöllberger C, Finsterer J. Nonsteroidal anti-inflammatory drugs in patients with cardio- or cerebrovascular disorders. *Z Kardiol.* 2003;92: 721-729.

Opioids

36

QUESTIONS

36.1. Which of the following opioid receptor subtypes contributes the most to the development of respiratory depression?
A. Mu$_1$
B. Mu$_2$
C. Delta
D. Kappa
E. Omega

36.2. A 56-year-old man presents to the emergency department extremely lethargic and unresponsive to external stimuli. During his evaluation, the patient has a generalized tonic-clonic seizure. Which of the following xenobiotics best explains his presentation?
A. Morphine
B. Fentanyl
C. Tramadol
D. Oxycodone
E. Diacetylmorphine

36.3. A 25-year-old woman presents to the emergency department unresponsive. On examination, she has pinpoint pupils and a respiratory rate of 4 breaths/min. Naloxone is administered intravenously, and the patient's respiratory rate improves to 15 breaths/min. Opioids are not detected on the standard urine drug. Which of the following xenobiotics best explains her presentation?
A. Diacetylmorphine
B. Morphine
C. Fentanyl
D. Codeine
E. Hydromorphone

36.4. Which of the following patients is at an increased risk of developing an adverse reaction to naloxone administration?
A. 32-year-old marathon runner
B. 2-year-old following an ingestion of her mother's methadone
C. 61-year-old with a spinal cord injury
D. 53-year-old opioid-naïve patient with hepatic encephalopathy
E. 23-year-old who is unresponsive following a gamma-hydroxybutyrate overdose

36.5. A 26-year-old woman with a history of opioid use disorder presents to the emergency department with nausea, vomiting, abdominal cramping, yawning, and piloerection. Exposure to which of the following xenobiotics best explains her presentation?
A. Flumazenil
B. Clonidine
C. Diacetylmorphine
D. Buprenorphine
E. Methadone

36.6. A 26-year-old man presents to the emergency department with nausea, chest pain, palpitations, and tremor following intravenous heroin use. On examination, he is tachycardic. His laboratory studies are notable for hyperglycemia, hypokalemia, and an elevated lactate concentration. Which of the following xenobiotics best explains this patient's presentation?
A. Diphenhydramine
B. Scopolamine
C. Quinine
D. Strychnine
E. Clenbuterol

36.7. A 37-year-old man with a long-standing history of opioid use disorder presents to the emergency department with pinpoint pupils and a respiratory rate of 4 breaths/min. Which of the following doses of intravenous naloxone is the best starting dose?
A. 0.04 mg
B. 0.4 mg
C. 2 mg
D. 4 mg
E. 10 mg

36.8. Which of the following xenobiotics produces psychotomimesis by acting on the kappa opioid receptor?
A. Hydromorphone
B. Salvinorin A
C. Dextromethorphan
D. Tramadol
E. Dermorphin

36.9. A 22-year-old woman with a past medical history of depression develops an elevated temperature, lower extremity rigidity, and sustained ankle clonus while

in the hospital. The symptoms occurred after which of the following opioids was administered?
A. Hydromorphone
B. Morphine
C. Codeine
D. Oxycodone
E. Meperidine

36.10. A 22-year-old man is brought to the emergency department directly from an international airport due to concern for internal drug concealment. Which of the following statements regarding "body packers" is correct?
A. Body packers ingest illicit substances prior to arrest to avoid discovery of their drugs by police
B. It is usually impossible to differentiate cocaine body packers from heroin body packers without toxicology analysis
C. Patients are often asymptomatic for hours or days before developing toxicity
D. Opioid toxicity is an absolute indication for surgical removal of the packets
E. Asymptomatic patients should receive cascara or other potent irritant cathartics

ANSWERS

36.1. Answer: B. Opioids not only depress ventilatory response to hypoxia, but also reduce the sensitivity of medullary chemoreceptors to hypercapnea, resulting in a decreased stimulus to breathe. Mu$_2$ receptors, specifically, are consistently implicated in the respiratory depressant effects of opioids.

Sarton E, et al. Naloxone reversal of opioid-induced respiratory depression with special emphasis on the partial agonist/antagonist buprenorphine. *Adv Exp Med Biol.* 2008;605:486-491.

Shook JE, et al. Differential roles of opioid receptors in respiration, respiratory disease, and opiate induced respiratory depression. *Am Rev Respir Dis.* 1990;142:895-909.

36.2. Answer: C. Tramadol is a synthetic analgesic that has both opioid and nonopioid mechanisms. Case reports and case series describe tramadol-associated seizures both at therapeutic doses and in overdose. Although tramadol-related seizures do not respond to naloxone, they are treated successfully with benzodiazepines.

Ryan NM, Isbister GK. Tramadol overdose causes seizures and respiratory depression but serotonin toxicity appears unlikely. *Clin Toxicol.* 2015;53:545-550.

36.3. Answer: C. This patient presented with symptoms that are characteristic of an opioid overdose, and her respiratory rate improved with naloxone. The standard urine drug screen detects metabolites of diacetylmorphine (heroin), codeine, and morphine. As fentanyl is a synthetic opioid and does not contain any metabolites, it is not detected on routine drug screens. The ability to detect hydromorphone is variable.

Moeller KE, et al. Clinical interpretation of urine drug tests: What clinicians need to know about urine drug screens. *Mayo Clin Proc.* 2017;92:774-796.

36.4. Answer: A. In general, naloxone produces almost no side effects in patients who are opioid naïve, even those who present after an acute opioid overdose. In fact, spinal cord injury patients who received massive doses of naloxone as part of a research study had no adverse clinical effects. Athletes, however, develop a sense of well-being and euporhia known as "runner's high" mediated by endogenous opioid peptides, which is reversed by naloxone and leads to dysphoria. Naloxone will not produce withdrawal in patients who are opioid naïve and solely overdosed on gamma-hydroxybutyrate. While flumazenil is used more commonly than naloxone for hepatic encephalopathy, there are case reports of naloxone being used as part of the management of hepatic encephalopathy.

Sgherza AL, et al. Effect of naloxone on perceived exertion and exercise capacity during maximal cycle ergometry. *J Appl Physiol.* 2002;93:2023-2028.

Janal MN, et al. Pain sensitivity, mood and plasma endocrine levels in man following long-distance running: Effects of naloxone. *Pain.* 1984;19:13-25.

Bracken MB, et al. A randomized, controlled trial of methylprednisolone or naloxone in the treatment of acute spinal-cord injury. Results of the Second National Acute Spinal Cord Injury Study. *N Engl J Med.* 1990;322:1405-1411.

36.5. Answer: D. Buprenorphine, a partial mu opioid receptor agonist, has a very high affinity for and slow rate of dissociation from the mu receptor, which prevents other opioids from binding to the receptor. Though buprenorphine is used as part of the management in patients with opioid use disorder, in patients who are opioid dependent, it behaves as an opioid antagonist when most other opioids are present.

Pasternak GW. Multiple opiate receptors: Déjà vu all over again. *Neuropharmacology.* 2004;47(suppl 1):312-323.

36.6. Answer: E. While all the xenobiotics listed are adulterants of heroin, this patient's presentation is most consistent with clenbuterol. Clenbuterol, a $beta_2$ adrenergic receptor agonist, has a rapid onset and a long duration of action. Patients develop tachycardia and hypotension. Characteristic laboratory abnormalities include hyperglycemia, hypokalemia, and an elevated lactate concentration. Treatment includes beta adrenergic receptor antagonism, with a medication such as esmolol, and potassium supplementation.

Hoffman RS, et al. A descriptive study of an outbreak of clenbuterol-containing heroin. *Ann Emerg Med.* 2008;52:548-553.

Wingert WE, et al. Detection of clenbuterol in heroin users in twelve postmortem cases at the Philadelphia medical examiner's office. *J Anal Toxicol.* 2008;32:522-528.

36.7. Answer: A. The goal of naloxone therapy is to restore respiration; however, large doses increase the risk of precipitated opioid withdrawal. To minimize this risk, 0.04 mg of intravenous naloxone is a reasonable initial dose. If patients do not respond to an initial 0.04 mg, this dose can be repeated and increased followed by a continuous infusion if necessary.

Kim HK, Nelson LS. Reversal of opioid-induced ventilatory depression using low-dose naloxone (0.04 mg): A case series. *J Med Toxicol.* 2016;12:107-110.

36.8. Answer: B. Stimulation of the kappa opioid receptor by salvinorin A, an active compound found in the salvia plant, leads to psychotomimesis as compared to the euphoria that occurs with mu opioid receptor agonists.

Sheffler DJ, et al. The magic mint hallucinogen finds a molecular target in the kappa opioid receptor. *Trends Pharmacol Sci.* 2003;24:107-109.

36.9. Answer: E. In addition to its opioid effects, meperidine blocks presynaptic serotonin reuptake. Meperidine is associated with the development of serotonin toxicity, particularly in patients who are taking monoamine oxidase inhibitors. Normeperidine, a metabolite of meperidine, causes excitatory neurotoxicity and leads to delirium, tremor, myoclonus, and seizures. Given the significant side effect profile of meperidine and the availably of other opioids, it is now very rarely used.

Sinclair JG, Lo GH. The blockade of serotonin uptake and the meperidine monoamine oxidase inhibitor interaction. *Proc West Pharmacol Soc.* 1977;20:373-374.

36.10. Answer: C. Body packers are patients who ingest large numbers of multiply wrapped packages of concentrated cocaine or heroin to transport illicit drugs from one country to another. Body stuffers hurriedly ingest unprotected drug to avoid police detection. Although generally asymptomatic, body packers are at risk for delayed and prolonged toxicity from packet leakage or rupture. Unlike patients body packing cocaine, in whom surgery is mandatory upon the development of symptoms, those with heroin packets are often managed nonoperatively with continuous-infusion naloxone, activated charcoal, and whole-bowel irrigation. Irritant cathartics should be avoided due to the potential for bag rupture. Observation, however, must be performed by trained personnel and airway support or naloxone must be rapidly available. Although rapid urine testing for drugs of abuse occasionally assists in determining the packet content, often people who are selected to be body packers have no history of drug use and, if the packets have not ruptured, they often have a negative urine drug screen. The number of packages and the type of drug contained are usually obtained more quickly and reliably by asking the patient, determining the country of origin, or identifying toxidromes.

Utecht MJ, et al. Heroin body packers. *J Emerg Med.* 1993;11:33-40.

Salicylates

37

QUESTIONS

37.1. A 19-year-old man presents to the hospital 6 hours following an intentional ingestion of aspirin. Which of the following acid–base abnormalities would be expected in this patient?
A. Respiratory alkalosis, alkalemia
B. Respiratory acidosis, acidemia
C. Respiratory alkalosis, metabolic acidosis, alkalemia
D. Respiratory alkalosis, metabolic acidosis, acidemia
E. Respiratory acidosis, metabolic acidosis, acidemia

37.2. A 22-year-old woman is brought into the emergency department by her roommate following an intentional overdose of aspirin. On examination, she is very confused. A point-of-care glucose is 100 mg/dL (7.24 mmol/L). Which of the following statements best describes the effects of salicylate poisoning on glucose metabolism?
A. Most patients are hyperglycemic
B. Most patients are hypoglycemic
C. The cerebrospinal fluid (CSF) glucose concentration is consistent with the blood glucose concentration
D. The rate of CSF glucose utilization exceeds the rate of supply even in the presence of a normal serum glucose
E. The CSF glucose concentrations are consistently high, even when serum glucose is normal and low

37.3. A 29-year-old man is admitted to the hospital for the management of alcoholic pancreatitis. This diagnosis was established because of an elevated serum lipase concentration. He is awake, alert, and participatory with the examination. At the time of consultation, the patient has no abdominal pain. His vital signs on arrival are: blood pressure, 120/80 mmHg; heart rate, 86 beats/min; respiratory rate, 12 breaths/min; and oxygen saturation, 100% on room air. A salicylate concentration is obtained as part of his admission profile and returns at >100 mg/dL (7.24 mmol/L). His anion gap is 11 mEq/L with a serum bicarbonate of 23 mEq/L. The patient's serum creatinine and urine output are within normal limits. What would be the best next step in the management of this patient?
A. Begin serum and urine alkalinization, with a goal serum pH of 7.55 and a urine pH of 8
B. Consult nephrology for immediate hemodialysis
C. Check serum triglycerides and initiate insulin therapy
D. Administer intravenous lipid emulsion therapy
E. Administer activated charcoal orally

37.4. A 10-kg toddler ingests 10 mL of pure oil of wintergreen. Assuming oil of wintergreen has a density of 1 g/mL, a volume of distribution of 0.1 L/kg, 100% bioavailability, and instantaneous absorption, approximately what is the expected peak serum salicylate concentration?
A. 1 mg/dL (0.07 mmol/L)
B. 10 mg/dL (0.72 mmol/L)
C. 100 mg/dL (7.24 mmol/L)
D. 1,000 mg/dL (72.41 mmol/L)
E. 10,000 mg/dL (724.11 mmol/L)

37.5. Which of the following signs and symptoms of salicylate poisoning is most indicative of severe life-threatening toxicity?

A. Tinnitus
B. Vertigo
C. Lethargy
D. Hyperthermia
E. Agitation

37.6. A 19-year-old-woman presents to the emergency department after an intentional overdose of aspirin. Her initial serum salicylate concentration is 78 mg/dL (5.65 mmol/L). A bolus followed by an infusion of sodium bicarbonate is administered. Two hours following the initiation of this therapy, the patient's serum pH is 7.55 and her urine pH is 4.2. What intervention is likely necessary to achieve appropriate urine alkalinization?

A. Administration of acetazolamide
B. Increase the rate of the sodium bicarbonate infusion
C. Potassium supplementation
D. Emergent hemodialysis utilizing a high-bicarbonate bath
E. Immediate intubation and hyperventilation

37.7. Which of the following groups of patients is **least** likely to manifest tinnitus from salicylate toxicity?

A. Elderly
B. Males
C. Those with concomitant use of quinine
D. Children
E. Pregnant women

37.8. Which of the following statements regarding salicylate-induced acute respiratory distress syndrome (ARDS) is true?

A. It occurs more commonly in nonsmokers
B. It is more likely to occur after an acute salicylate ingestion

C. It reflects underlying cardiac disease, particularly congestive heart failure
D. It has never been identified in children
E. It almost always occurs in adults over 30 years of age

37.9. An 89-year-old man is admitted to the hospital for altered mental status and a presumed diagnosis of urosepsis. The nursing notes document that the patient is hearing impaired. Two days into the hospital course, the patient is still delirious with minimal improvement despite intravenous antibiotics and fluids. The patient is tachypneic, with a respiratory rate of 28 breaths/min. A radiograph of the chest demonstrates bilateral fluffy infiltrates consistent with acute respiratory distress syndrome (ARDS). A salicylate concentration is ordered and returns at 58 mg/dL (4.2 mmol/L). What are the next management steps?

A. Immediate intubation and ventilation
B. Addition of intravenous acyclovir
C. Administration of a sodium bicarbonate bolus and infusion
D. Nephrology consultation for immediate hemodialysis
E. Administration of a sodium bicarbonate bolus and infusion in addition to nephrology consultation for immediate hemodialysis

37.10. A patient presents following a witnessed salicylate overdose. On examination, he is tachypneic and hyperpneic. His laboratory analysis reveals an anion gap of 12 mEq/L. What is the likely cause of his normal anion gap?

A. A negative salicylate concentration
B. A falsely elevated chloride concentration
C. A renal tubular alkalosis
D. A serum bilirubin greater than 20 mg/dL (342 micromol/L)
E. Elevated triglycerides in the serum

ANSWERS

37.1. Answer: C. Salicylates act directly on the respiratory center in the brainstem, causing hyperventilation and respiratory alkalosis. At the same time, salicylates, which are weak acids, interfere with the Krebs cycle, limit ATP production, generate lactate, and cause a ketoacidosis. Although the metabolic acidosis begins with the earliest stages of salicylate toxicity, the respiratory alkalosis predominates initially, leaving the patient with a respiratory alkalosis, metabolic acidosis, and alkalemia. An adult presenting early after a salicylate overdose with respiratory acidosis almost certainly ingested a concomitant CNS depressant or has an aspiration pneumonitis. The combination of acute respiratory alkalosis, metabolic acidosis, and acidemia is an ominous finding indicating an immediately life-threatening salicylate overdose. Although it takes some time after ingestion for this pattern to develop in adults, children present with these findings at an earlier stage. Until arterial blood gas (ABG) determinations became commonly available and the precise combinations of pH and PCO_2 values for each of the primary disturbances were established, "respiratory alkalosis" was said to be the typical adult response in the early phase of salicylate poisoning. Even when metabolic acidosis predominates, the respiratory alkalosis is not merely compensatory.

Gabow PA, et al. Acid-base disturbances in the salicylate-intoxicated adult. *Arch Intern Med.* 1978;138:1481-1484.

Temple AR. Acute and chronic effects of aspirin toxicity and their treatment. *Arch Intern Med.* 1981;141:364-369.

Tenney SM, Miller RM. The respiratory and circulatory action of salicylate. *Am J Med.* 1955;19:498-508.

37.2. Answer: D. Despite a normal plasma glucose, cerebrospinal fluid (CSF) glucose fell by a third in salicylate-poisoned mice, indicating an excessive utilization of glucose in the central nervous system (CNS). There are also case reports of patients with salicylate toxicity and a normal serum glucose whose mental status improved with an intravenous dextrose bolus. For this reason, glucose supplementation is an important component in treating salicylate-poisoned patients, even when serum salicylate concentrations are normal. Serum glucose concentrations are low, normal, or high, but do not correlate well with CSF glucose concentrations. As noted above, the CSF concentrations are typically lower than the plasma concentrations.

Thurston JH, et al. Reduced brain glucose with normal plasma glucose in salicylate poisoning. *Clin Invest.* 1970;49:2139-2145.

Kuzak N, et al. Reversal of salicylate-induced euglycemic delirium with dextrose. *Clin Toxicol.* 2007;45:526-529.

37.3. Answer: C. This patient's normal vital signs, normal serum bicarbonate, and normal anion gap are inconsistent with a significant salicylate overdose. Furthermore, this patient has an elevated serum lipase with no abdominal pain. All these factors point toward the possibility of a laboratory error. Elevated triglycerides lead to erroneously elevated salicylate and lipase concentrations. A "strawberry milkshake" color to the blood assists in making this diagnosis. In the setting of an elevated salicylate concentration, it is important to ensure that the presentation is consistent with the reported concentration and not due to a laboratory error.

Biary R, et al. Falsely elevated salicylate concentration in a patient with hypertriglyceridemia. *Toxicol Commun.* 2018; 2:1-2.

37.4. Answer: D. Assuming complete absorption and no elimination, this child could have a concentration as high as 1,000 mg/dL (72.4 mmol/L). This is calculated because concentration is equal to dose / (volume of distribution × weight in kilograms). Pure oil of wintergreen contains 98% methyl salicylate, which is hydrolyzed in the liver to form salicylate. Ingesting a very small amount is associated with consequential salicylate concentrations. One teaspoon (5 mL) is approximately equivalent to a 7-g ingestion of salicylate. Oil of wintergreen has a pleasant, minty taste and, as a result, poses a significant hazard to children.

Stevenson CS. Oil of wintergreen (methyl salicylate) poisoning report of three cases, one with autopsy, and a review of the literature. *Am J Med Sci.* 1937;193:772-788.

Done AK, Otterness LJ. Exchange transfusion in the treatment of oil of wintergreen (methyl salicylate) poisoning. *Pediatrics.* 1956;18:80-85.

37.5. Answer: D. Markedly elevated temperatures due to salicylate poisoning are the result of the uncoupling of oxidative phosphorylation and, in this circumstance, almost always represents a preterminal event. Deafness, with or without antecedent tinnitus, vertigo, lethargy, and other altered states of consciousness, except for coma and hyperventilation, are all associated with salicylism or salicylate poisoning at various stages following an acute ingestion and at various salicylate concentrations obtained after chronic ingestions. Coma is rare and generally occurs following massive ingestions (serum salicylate concentrations greater than 100 mg/dL [7.24 mmol/L]). Tragically, many of the signs and symptoms of salicylate poisoning are mistaken for signs and symptoms of the condition for which the salicylate was taken in the first place, prompting additional self-medication with disastrous consequences.

Miyahara JT, Karler R. Effect of salicylate on oxidative phosphorylation and respiration of mitochondrial fragments. *Biochem J.* 1965;97: 194-198.

37.6. Answer: C. If the urine pH is 4.2 despite appropriate serum alkalinization, a likely cause is that the patient is hypokalemic. The patient's potassium must be addressed to ensure urine alkalinization and appropriate excretion of salicylate. As the patient's serum pH is 7.55, there is no need to increase the rate of the sodium bicarbonate infusion. Although acetazolamide alkalinizes the urine, it causes acidemia and is associated with worse outcomes in salicylate poisoning. Acetazolamide is therefore contraindicated in the treatment of salicylate toxicity. There is no indication to intubate this patient currently, as she is protecting her airway and the risks of intubation and hyperventilation far outweigh the benefits.

Heller I, et al. Significant metabolic acidosis induced by acetazolamide: Not a rare complication. *Arch Intern Med.* 1985;145:1815-1817.

Vree TB, et al. Effect of urinary pH on the pharmacokinetics of salicylate acid, with its glycine and glucuronide conjugates in human. *Int J Clin Pharm Ther.* 1994;32:550-558.

37.7. Answer: A. Tinnitus associated with salicylates usually begins at the high therapeutic or low toxic concentration (approximately 20-40 mg/dL or 1.4-2.9 mmol/L). However, tinnitus is not as evident in elderly patients with hearing impairment despite significantly elevated salicylate concentrations.

Mongan E, et al. Tinnitus as an indication of therapeutic serum salicylate levels. *JAMA.* 1973;226:142-145.

37.8. Answer: E. Among the risks for developing salicylate-induced acute respiratory distress syndrome (ARDS) (previously called noncardiogenic pulmonary edema [NCPE]) are salicylate concentrations >30 mg/dL (2.17 mmol/L), age >30 years, cigarette smoking, chronic salicylate ingestion, and the presence of neurologic symptoms on admission. Although in one study the average salicylate concentration for those patients who developed salicylate-induced "pulmonary edema" was about 57 mg/dL (4.13 mmol/L), this was also the average concentration for patients in the study who did not develop salicylate-induced ARDS. Salicylate-induced ARDS does not reflect underlying cardiac disease. Treatment includes ventilation, oxygenation, and hemodialysis, but not diuresis. While uncommon, ARDS is reported in children.

Fisher CJ, et al. Salicylate induced pulmonary edema. Clinical characteristics in children. *Am J Emerg Med.* 1985;3:33-37.

Walters JS, et al. Salicylate induced pulmonary edema. *Radiology.* 1983;146:289-293.

37.9. Answer: E. Chronic salicylate toxicity is more common in elderly patients. There is typically a significant delay to diagnosis, as long as 72 hours, and often patients are misdiagnosed as having sepsis, delirium, or dementia. Patients with chronic salicylate toxicity demonstrate signs of more severe toxicity with lower serum concentrations. The mortality associated with chronic salicylate toxicity is as high as 25%. Given this patient's altered mental status and ARDS, immediate initiation of serum alkalinization and concurrent nephrology consultation are indicated.

Anderson RJ, et al. Unrecognized adult salicylate intoxication. *Ann Intern Med.* 1976;85:745-748.

Juurlink DN, et al. Extracorporeal treatment for salicylate poisoning: Systematic review and recommendations from the EXTRIP Workgroup. *Ann Emerg Med.* 2015;66:165-181.

37.10. Answer: B. The patient had a witnessed salicylate overdose and his respiratory rate is consistent with the reported ingestion. It is important not to rely on a normal anion gap as a sole marker of the degree of toxicity as severe salicylate toxicity sometimes causes a falsely elevated chloride and thus a narrow anion gap. Salicylates also lead to a metabolic acidosis with a normal anion gap because of renal tubular acidosis. Elevated bilirubin concentrations lead to a falsely elevated acetaminophen concentration. Elevated triglycerides cause a falsely elevated serum salicylate concentration.

Kaul V, et al. Negative anion gap metabolic acidosis in salicylate overdose—a zebra! *Am J Emerg Med.* 2013;31:1536 e3-4.

Botulism

38.1. Which of the following monitoring parameters is the most reliable determinant of the need for intubation in patients who present with botulism?
A. Peak inspiratory flow rate
B. Pulse oximetry
C. The presence of a gag reflex
D. End-tidal CO_2
E. Negative inspiratory force

38.2. The prompt management of wound botulism is vital to prevent further progression of toxicity; therefore, in combination with thorough wound debridement, which of the following antibiotics is also recommended?
A. Clindamycin
B. Azithromycin
C. Meropenem
D. Penicillin G
E. Amoxicillin

38.3. A 34-year-old man presents to the emergency department with a descending paralysis. His family noted that his weakness was preceded by fatigue, dysphagia, and diplopia. What is the mechanism of action of the toxin that is causing these symptoms?
A. Inhibition of presynaptic release of acetylcholine
B. Impaired metabolism of acetylcholine
C. Inhibition at the presynaptic glycine receptor
D. Inhibition at the postsynaptic glycine receptor
E. Obstruction of voltage-gated sodium channels

38.4. Which of the following diagnostic tests is the gold standard for the diagnosis of botulism?
A. Stool anaerobic culture
B. Enzyme-linked immunosorbent assay (ELISA)
C. Endopeptidase assay
D. Immuno-polymerase chain reaction (immuno-PCR)
E. Bioassay

38.5. Which of the following findings is found in patients with wound botulism but not foodborne botulism?
A. Respiratory paralysis
B. Fever
C. Dysphagia
D. Dysphonia
E. Gastrointestinal symptoms

38.6. A 5-month-old boy is found lethargic and limp at home. He has no past medical history and was developmentally normal. The patient was constipated for the past several days and has been feeding poorly since yesterday. The patient is breastfed. His father is employed as a construction worker. On physical examination, the child has dilated pupils, hypotonia, poor anal sphincter tone, and a feeble cry. He is afebrile. What is the next best step in management of this patient?
A. Electrophysiologic testing
B. Antibiotic therapy following results of blood cultures
C. Edrophonium testing
D. Administer human botulism immune globulin
E. Administer equine botulism antitoxin

38.7. What are the first cranial nerves that are affected in a patient who has foodborne botulism?
A. II, III, IV, VI, IX
B. III, VI, IX, X, XI
C. III, IV, V, VI, IX, X
D. II, III, IV, VI, IX
E. II, IV, IX, X, XI

38.8. Which of the following statements about infant botulism is correct?
A. It is associated with the ingestion of nonpasteurized milk in children <3 years of age
B. It usually affects immunocompromised children
C. Tremor and myoclonus are commonly observed
D. The mechanism involves the germination of *Clostridium botulinum* spores in the gut with a slow elaboration of toxin
E. Spores and toxin are found in the infant's urine for many weeks after recovery

38.9. Which of the following statements about botulism is correct?
A. Botulinum toxin is lethal to humans at 1 pg/kg
B. The toxin binds reversibly to the peripheral neuromuscular junction
C. Cholinesterase inhibitors will restore neuromuscular activity in patients with botulism
D. Botulinum toxin is heat stable
E. Outbreaks of foodborne botulism generally involve more than two victims

38.10. Which of the following diagnoses is most likely to be a botulism mimic?
A. Mercury poisoning
B. Lead poisoning
C. *Shigella* food poisoning
D. Guillain-Barré syndrome
E. Clonidine toxicity

ANSWERS

38.1. Answer: E. Respiratory compromise is the most common cause of death in patients with botulism. It is important to look for early signs of impending respiratory failure as a marker for the need for intubation. While all the answer choices listed are used to monitor a patient's respiratory status, it is the negative inspiratory force (NIF) that is the most reliable test that is used to determine the correct time to intubate a patient. A vital capacity that is <20 mL/kg or an NIF that is poorer than −30 cmH$_2$O is an indication for intubation.

Schmidt-Nowara WW, et al. Early and late pulmonary complications of botulism. *Arch Intern Med*. 1983;143:451-456.

Lawn ND, et al. Anticipating mechanical ventilation in Guillain-Barré syndrome. *Arch Neurol*. 2001;58:893-898.

38.2. Answer: D. In patients with wound botulism, penicillin G has excellent antimicrobial efficacy against *C. botulinum* and is therefore recommended as part of the management. It is important to note that there is no role for antibiotics in patients who present with either adult (foodborne) botulism or infant botulism, as antibiotics do not treat preformed toxin and do not prevent gut spores from germinating. Aminoglycosides, fluoroquinolones and clindamycin interfere with neuromuscular transmission, so they should be used with caution in patients who present with botulism.

Swenson JM, et al. Susceptibility of *Clostridium botulinum* to thirteen antimicrobial agents. *Antimicrob Agents Chemother*. 1980;18:13-19.

Santos JI, et al. Potentiation of *Clostridium botulinum* toxin aminoglycoside antibiotics: Clinical and laboratory observations. *Pediatrics*. 1981;68:50-54.

38.3. Answer: A. The patient in this scenario is presenting with a descending paralysis concerning for botulism. Botulinum toxin travels to peripheral cholinergic terminals, binds irreversibly the cell membrane, and impairs presynaptic release of acetylcholine.

Lamanna C, Carr CJ. The botulinal, tetanal, and enterostaphylococcal toxins: A review. *Clin Pharmacol Ther*. 1967;8:286.

38.4. Answer: E. Mouse lethal bioassays remain the gold standard for the diagnosis of botulism, with a detection limit of 0.01 ng/mL. A sample (serum, stool, or food) is injected intraperitoneally into mice; the mice are then observed for the development of signs and symptoms of botulism. A medication list should be included with samples sent for bioassay due to possible drug inferences or independent toxicity to the mice.

Lindstrom M, Korkeala H. Laboratory diagnostics of botulism. *Clin Microbiol Rev*. 2006;19:298-314.

38.5. Answer: B. Because patients have an infected wound in wound botulism, a fever often develops. A fever is distinctly unusual with foodborne botulism. Respiratory paralysis, dysphagia, and dysphonia are described with all forms of botulism. Gastrointestinal symptoms are found in many patients with foodborne botulism but are not found in patients with wound botulism.

> Merson MH, Dowell VR. Epidemiologic, clinical and laboratory aspects of wound botulism. *N Engl J Med.* 1973;289:1005-1010.

38.6. Answer: D. Treatment of botulism should not be delayed for diagnostic testing. Infant botulism is treated with human-derived botulism antitoxin antibodies as botulism immune globulin (BabyBIG). Sensory nerve action potentials in botulism are expected to be normal; motor potentials in affected muscles will have lower amplitudes but normal velocity. However, there are no pathognomonic findings for botulism and electrophysiologic testing is most useful for excluding alternative diagnoses. Routine blood cultures are not useful in confirming a diagnosis of botulism. Edrophonium testing is used to diagnose myasthenia gravis. Equine-derived botulism antitoxin is used in the treatment of botulism in adults.

> Arnon SS, et al. Human botulism immune globulin for the treatment of infant botulism. *N Engl J Med.* 2006;354:462-471.

38.7. Answer: B. Patients who have foodborne botulism present initially with diplopia, ptosis, blurred vision, and a lateral rectus palsy. The first cranial nerves that are affected are III, VI, IX, X, and XI.

> Terranova W, et al. Ocular findings in botulism type B. *JAMA.* 1979;241:475-477.

38.8. Answer: D. The infant's gastrointestinal tract lacks bile acids and gastric acid, both of which inhibit clostridial growth in older children and adults. Pasteurization would not be capable of destroying either spores or toxin. Infant botulism does not require an immunocompromised infant. Decreased muscle tone and a "floppy baby" develop, not tremor and myoclonus. Spores and toxin are isolated from the stool, not the urine or blood.

> Schreiner MS, et al. Infant botulism: A review of 12 years experience at Children's Hospital of Philadelphia. *Pediatrics.* 1991;87:159-165.

38.9. Answer: A. Botulinum toxin is the most powerful toxin known to man. It will cause respiratory depression at a dose of 1 pg/kg. The toxin binds irreversibly to the presynaptic nerve ending, inhibiting calcium-dependent exocytosis of acetylcholine. Cholinesterase inhibitors will cause only a minimal improvement in muscle contractility. This enables botulism to be differentiated from myasthenia gravis, in which a dramatic improvement will occur. Botulinum toxin is destroyed by heating to 212 °F (100 °C) for 10 minutes at sea level. More than 60% of botulism outbreaks involve only one victim.

> Dowell UR Jr, et al. Coproexamination for botulinal toxin and *Clostridium botulinum. JAMA.* 1977;238:1829-1832.

38.10. Answer: D. The Miller Fisher variant of Guillain-Barré syndrome is commonly confused with the diagnosis of botulism. Both cause a descending paralysis. The distinction between the two is often made when protein is found in the cerebrospinal fluid of the patient with Guillain-Barré. None of the other choices would be expected to cause a descending paralysis. The gastrointestinal symptoms with both mercury and *Shigella* food poisoning are likely to be far more severe than with botulism. Metallic material is occasionally visible in the gastrointestinal tract with either lead or mercury poisoning. Clonidine causes respiratory depression in children; however, the children commonly start breathing after stimulation. Clonidine also causes miosis, bradycardia, and hypotension, which is unusual with botulism.

> McKhann GM, et al. Acute motor axonal neuropathy: A frequent cause of flaccid paralysis in China. *Ann Neurol.* 1993;33:333-336.

Food Poisoning

QUESTIONS

39.1. A 16-year-old girl presents to an emergency department in Washington State, USA with perioral and extremity numbness. She later develops dysphagia and dysarthria. On history, she endorses eating shellfish approximately 30 minutes prior to the onset of her symptoms. Which toxin caused her illness?
A. Brevetoxin
B. Saxitoxin
C. Domoic acid
D. Tetrodotoxin
E. Ciguatoxin

39.2. A 57-year-old man presents with 2 weeks of painful paresthesias to his hands. He states that when he washes his hands, the cold water that comes out of the tap feels hot. What medication will most likely help his symptoms?
A. Amitriptyline
B. Midazolam
C. Calcium gluconate
D. Hypertonic saline
E. Mannitol

39.3. A 62-year-old woman presents to the emergency department with anuria and abdominal pain 4 days after attending a barbeque. The patient also has persistent bloody diarrhea. Which of the following options should be the first priority?
A. Fluid and supportive care
B. Treatment with ciprofloxacin or vancomycin
C. Treatment with ampicillin and aminoglycosides
D. Immediate stool Gram stain
E. Observation in isolation

39.4. A 26-year-old man presents to the emergency department with nausea, vomiting, abdominal pain, and rectal burning. He also has reversal of hot and cold temperatures. His symptoms began 14 hours after eating shellfish. What is the mechanism of action of this toxin?
A. Histamine release and anaphylaxis
B. Obstruction of voltage-sensitive sodium channels
C. Action as an analog of the neurotransmitter glutamic acid
D. Stimulation of sodium flux through voltage-gated sodium channels
E. Binding glycolipid receptors, ribosomal inactivation, and cell death

39.5. A 24-year-old woman presents to the emergency department shortly after eating dinner. She describes a burning sensation to her chest, headache, and flushing. On physical examination, she has diffuse expiratory wheezing. What toxin best explains her symptoms?
A. Ciguatoxin
B. Tetrodotoxin
C. Brevetoxin
D. Saxitoxin
E. Monosodium glutamate

39.6. A 48-year-old woman presents to an emergency department in Nova Scotia Canada with memory loss approximately 5 hours after ingesting mussels. On examination, she has purposeless chewing and grimacing. What is the mechanism of action of the suspected toxin?
A. Histamine and anaphylaxis
B. Obstruction of voltage-sensitive sodium channels
C. Analog of the neurotransmitter glutamic acid
D. Stimulation of sodium flux through voltage-gated sodium channels
E. Binding glycolipid receptors, ribosomal inactivation, and cell death

39.7. A 31-year-old man presents to the emergency department with diffuse erythema of the face, neck, and upper torso. He does not have shortness of breath or difficulty swallowing. He ate tuna at a restaurant 45 minutes prior to presentation. What is the mechanism of action of the suspected toxin?
A. Histamine ingestion
B. Obstruction of voltage-sensitive sodium channels
C. Analog of the neurotransmitter glutamic acid
D. Stimulation of sodium flux through voltage-gated sodium channels
E. Binding glycolipid receptors, ribosomal inactivation, and cell death

39.8. A 28-year-old woman presents to the emergency department with nausea and vomiting. Upon examination, the patient has severe upper abdominal pain associated with rebound and guarding. She states that the pain began 6 hours after ingesting sushi at a Japanese restaurant. What is the most probable cause for her symptoms?
A. *Amanita phalloides*
B. *Diphyllobothrium* spp
C. *Eustrongylides anisakis*
D. *Pseudoterranova decipiens*
E. Tetrodotoxin poisoning

39.9. In 2002 in China, patrons of a snack bar developed seizures that did not respond to benzodiazepines and other antiepileptics. Forty-two people died. What xenobiotic was responsible for this outbreak?
A. 4-Aminopyridine
B. Isoniazid
C. *Gyromitra* mushrooms
D. Tetramine
E. Strychnine

39.10. In 2008 in China, 50,000 children were hospitalized as a result of nephrolithiasis and secondary complications, including acute kidney injury. All of these children had been given the same powdered infant formula. What xenobiotic was found in this formula?
A. Melamine
B. Tetramine
C. Strychnine
D. Cadmium
E. Chromium

ANSWERS

39.1. Answer: B. Saxitoxin is produced by the dinoflagellate *Protogonyaulax tamarensis*, which causes paralytic shellfish poisoning (PSP). The mechanism of toxicity is through sodium channel blockade. Shellfish implicated are clams, oysters, mussels, and scallops. Neurologic symptoms predominate and include paresthesias and numbness of the mouth and extremities, a sensation of floating, headache, ataxia, vertigo, muscle weakness, paralysis, and cranial nerve dysfunction manifested by dysphagia, dysarthria, dysphonia, and transient blindness. Gastrointestinal symptoms are less common and include nausea, vomiting, abdominal pain, and diarrhea. Fatalities occur due to respiratory failure, usually within the first 12 hours after symptom onset.

Levin R. Paralytic shellfish toxins: Their origin, characteristics and methods of detection: A review. *J Food Biochem.* 1991;15:405-407.

39.2. Answer: A. This patient has symptoms that are consistent with ciguatera poisoning. Ciguatoxin causes sodium channel opening, with resultant paresthesias and temperature reversal. Amitriptyline, a sodium channel blocker, is used to treat the paresthesias. Intravenous mannitol is potentially beneficial to alleviate severe neurologic symptoms if administered early, but this patient is now 2 weeks into his course.

Bowman PB. Amitriptyline and ciguatera. *Med J Aust.* 1984;140:802.

Palafox NA, et al. Successful treatment of ciguatera fish poisoning with intravenous mannitol. *JAMA.* 1988;259:2740-2742.

39.3. Answer: A. The patient is currently suffering from hemolytic uremic syndrome given that her symptoms of anuria and bloody stool are consistent with the epidemiology of *Escherichia coli (E. coli)* O157:H7. Treatment with antibiotics is not recommended at this time as a definitive pathogen has not yet been identified. Therefore, only fluid and supportive care are indicated.

Fakhouri F, et al. Haemolytic uraemic syndrome *Lancet*. 2017;390: 681-696.

39.4. Answer: D. This patient developed neurotoxic shellfish poisoning, which is caused by brevetoxin. This toxin is produced by *Ptychodiscus brevis* and is a lipid-soluble, heat-stable polyether ladder toxin. It stimulates sodium in flux through the sodium channel of both nerve and muscle. Neurotoxic shellfish toxicity resembles the toxicity caused by ciguatoxin. Neurotoxic shellfish poisoning is not fatal, and the treatment is largely supportive.

Asai S, et al. The site of action of *Ptychodiscus brevis* toxin within the parasympathetic axonal sodium channel H gate in airway smooth muscle. *J Allergy Clin Immunol*. 1984;73:824-828.

Levin R. Paralytic shellfish toxins: Their origin, characteristics and methods of detection: A review. *J Food Biochem*. 1991;15:405-407.

39.5. Answer: E. This patient is presenting with symptoms consistent with exposure to monosodium glutamate (MSG). MSG is added to food as a flavor enhancer. Symptoms typically resolve within 1 hour of ingestion and are usually benign, although MSG is rarely associated with life-threatening bronchospasm. Interestingly, in young children, a seizurelike syndrome, or "shudder attacks," are described.

Schaumburg HH, et al. Monosodium L-glutamate: Its pharmacology and role in the Chinese restaurant syndrome. *Science*. 1969;163:826-828.

39.6. Answer: C. The etiologic agent of amnestic shellfish poisoning (ASP) is domoic acid, which is produced by the diatom *Nitzschia pungens* and is a structural analog of glutamic and kanaic acids. ASP is characterized by nausea, vomiting, abdominal cramps, diarrhea, memory loss, and, less frequently, coma, seizures, hemiparesis, ophthalmoplegia, purposeless chewing, and grimacing. The mortality rate is 2%, with death most frequently occurring in older patients who suffer more severe neurologic symptoms. Ten percent of victims suffer long-term anterograde memory deficits as well as motor and sensory neuropathy.

Teitelbaum JS, et al. Neurologic sequelae of domoic acid intoxication due to ingestion of contaminated mussels. *N Engl J Med*. 1990;322:1781-1787.

Perl TM, et al. An outbreak of toxic encephalopathy caused by eating mussels contaminated with domoic acid. *N Engl J Med*. 1990;322:1775-1780.

39.7. Answer: A. This patient is presenting with symptoms consistent with scombroid poisoning. Certain fish, such as tuna, have high concentrations of histidine in their dark meat. Bacteria present on the surface of the fish contain histadine decarboxylase and convert histadine to histamine. The treatment is supportive, and patients usually improve with antihistamine therapy alone.

Kim R. Flushing syndrome due to mahimahi (scombroid fish) poisoning. *Arch Dermatol*. 1979;115:963.

39.8. Answer: C. *Eustrongylides anisakis*, an intestinal parasitic infection, is associated with abdominal cramping, nausea, and vomiting with rebound and guarding. Symptoms occur within 1 to 12 hours of ingestion as opposed to that of *Diphyllobothrium* spp, which has an incubation period of 1 to 2 weeks after ingestion.

Kristmundsson A, Helgason S. Parasite communities of eels Anguilla anguilla in freshwater and marine habitats in Iceland in comparison with other parasite communities of eels in Europe. *Folia Parasitol (Praha)*. 2007;54:141-153.

39.9. Answer: D. Tetramine is a rodenticide that causes status epilepticus. It causes seizures due to its noncompetitive, irreversible binding to the chloride channel on the gamma-aminobutyric acid receptor complex. The seizures are not effectively treated with benzodiazepines. As a result of the inability to control the seizures, tetramine leads to grave neurologic injury. In this case, tetramine was used as a deliberate form of mass poisoning.

Croddy E, Croddy E. Rat poison and food security in the People's Republic of China: Focus on tetramethylene disulfotetramine (tetramine). *Arch Toxicol*. 2004;78:1-6.

39.10. Answer: A. Melamine, which is used in the production of plastic, has a high nitrogen content. The Kjeldahl method is used to measure nitrogen content, which was used by criminals to assure high nitrogen contents in contaminated foods. Watered-down milk would have been recognized because of the low nitrogen content, so melamine was added to disguise the quality and protein concentration of milk sold. Melamine leads to the development of nephrolithiasis and secondary obstructive nephropathy.

Ingelfinger JR. Melamine and the global implications of food contamination. *N Engl J Med*. 2008;359:2745-2748.

Dieting Xenobiotics and Regimens

40.1. The diet drug rimonabant, an endocannabinoid receptor inverse agonist, was withdrawn from the market in Europe due to which significant side effect?
A. Small bowel obstruction
B. Hemorrhagic strokes
C. Cardiac dysrhythmias
D. Hyperthermia
E. Dysphoria

40.2. Which of the following options accounts for the potential mechanism of dinitrophenol as a weight loss agent?
A. Blockade of amylase and thus starch breakdown
B. Prevention of glucagon release
C. Uncoupling of oxidative phosphorylation
D. Increasing insulin release
E. Development of dysgeusia

40.3. How does liraglutide lead to weight loss?
A. Impairing absorption of fatty acids
B. Directly acting on hypothalamus to suppress appetite
C. Uncoupling oxidative phosphorylation
D. Increasing energy expenditure
E. Direct expansion in the stomach leading to a sensation of fullness

40.4. Ma huang is an "herbal" supplement used to increase energy and lose weight. This product is structurally and pharmacologically similar to which of the following xenobiotics?
A. Caffeine
B. Cocaine
C. Amphetamine
D. Nicotine
E. Digoxin

40.5. Cal-Ban 300 was a guar gum mixture that worked by absorbing water in the stomach and expanding, thus giving the sensation of a full stomach. This caused weight loss by producing early satiety. Which of the following options was the most consequential toxicity associated with this xenobiotic?
A. Dehydration
B. Constipation
C. Esophageal and intestinal obstruction
D. Hyperthermia
E. Nausea and bloating

40.6. A 29-year-old woman presents to the hospital with headache and blurry vision after ingesting an old medication she found under the sink in her mother's bathroom. Her vital signs are: blood pressure of 180/110 mmHg; heart rate of 58 beats/min; temperature of 99.3 °F (37.4 °C); and respiratory rate of 20 breaths/min. What weight loss xenobiotic did she take?
A. Dinitrophenol
B. Phenylpropanolamine
C. Liraglutide
D. Syrup of ipecac
E. Orlistat

40.7. A 43-year-old woman had a colonoscopy performed that demonstrated melanosis coli. What medication has this patient been taking chronically?
  A. Aspirin
  B. Acetaminophen
  C. Liraglutide
  D. Senna
  E. Phenylpropanolamine

40.8. A 55-year-old woman presents to the emergency department with shortness of breath and is diagnosed with a cardiomyopathy. She had a 15-year history of an eating disorder. What xenobiotic could have contributed to her cardiomyopathy?
  A. Dinitrophenol
  B. Syrup of ipecac
  C. Senna
  D. Orlistat
  E. Liraglutide

40.9. A 29-year-old woman presents to the emergency department with confusion and ataxia. She has a recent history of bariatric surgery. What treatment is most indicated?
  A. Thiamine
  B. Pyridoxine
  C. Folate
  D. Levetiracetam
  E. Alteplase

40.10. Fenfluramine is a weight loss agent that was removed from the US market due to which significant side effect?
  A. Depression
  B. Cardiac valvulopathy
  C. Hypoglycemia
  D. Hyponatremia
  E. Migraine headaches

ANSWERS

40.1. Answer: E. Rimonabant is an endocannabinoid receptor inverse agonist that was proposed as a weight loss xenobiotic. Its effects on central cannabinoid receptor type 1 (CB1) receptors has a negative effect on the reward pathway and also decreases appetite via the hypothalamus. Preliminary studies demonstrated significant weight loss. This drug never reached the US market and was withdrawn from the European market due to its association with serious dysphoria.

> Ruilope LM, et al. Effect of rimonabant on blood pressure in overweight/obese patients with/without co-morbidities: Analysis of pooled RIO study results. *J Hypertens.* 2008;26:357-367.

40.2. Answer: C. Dinitrophenol uncouples oxidative phosphorylation and thus prevents formation of ATP (calorie yield) from ingested foods. This extra energy is then lost as heat, which results in hyperthermia and precludes any safe use of this xenobiotic as a diet aid.

> Cutting WC, et al. Action and uses of dinitrophenol. *JAMA.* 1933;101:193-195.

> Tainter ML, et al. Febrile, respiratory and some other actions of dinitrophenol. *J Pharmacol Exp Ther.* 1933;48:410-429.

40.3. Answer: B. Glucagon-like peptide-1 (GLP-1) xenobiotics, such as liraglutide, lead to weight loss by acting directly on the hypothalamus and suppressing appetite. Liraglutide also stimulates insulin release and decreases glucagon secretion. There are reports of hypoglycemia secondary to the use of this weight loss supplement.

> Burcelin R, Gourdy P. Harnessing glucagon-like peptide-1 receptor agonists for the pharmacological treatment of overweight and obesity. *Obes Rev.* 2017;18:86-98.

40.4. Answer: C. Ma huang and Chinese ephedra are synonymous with ephedrine, the sympathomimetic amine with properties like *d*-amphetamine. It was sold over the counter as an unregulated "herbal" supplement and was abused as a stimulant and anorexiant. Many adverse events are reported, with toxicity resulting from its amphetaminelike properties.

> Perotta DM, et al. Adverse events associated with ephedrine containing products - Texas, December 1993-September 1995. *MMWR.* 1996;45:689-693.

40.5. Answer: C. Multiple reports of esophageal obstruction caused by Cal-Ban 300 led to the removal of the product from the US pharmaceutical market.

> Lewis JH. Esophageal and small bowel obstruction from guar-gum containing diet pills: Analysis of 26 cases reported to the Food and Drug Administration. *Am J Gastroenterol.* 1992;87:1424-1428.

40.6.   Answer: B. Phenylpropanolamine is a sympathomimetic and was a common weight loss xenobiotic. It causes hypertension that is associated with intracranial hemorrhages, seizures, and death. The hypertension is mediated by alpha adrenergic agonism and leads to a concomitant reflex bradycardia. This xenobiotic is no longer approved in the United States (US) for weight loss.

Lake CR, et al. Adverse drug effects attributed to phenylpropanolamine: A review of 142 case reports. *Am J Med.* 1990;89:195-208.

40.7.   Answer: D. Patients who abuse anthraquinone laxatives, such as senna, develop characteristic findings on their colonoscopy. Melanosis coli is benign a dark staining of colonic mucosa and is pathognomonic for senna use.

Müller-Lissner SA. Adverse effects of laxatives: Fact and fiction. *Pharmacology.* 1993;47(suppl 1):138-145.

40.8.   Answer: B. Syrup of ipecac was available over the counter and was commonly abused by patients with eating disorders. In addition to electrolyte abnormalities caused by induced vomiting, patients were also at risk of developing a cardiomyopathy after chronic use. Emetine is the alkaloid in syrup of ipecac that is responsible for the development of this adverse effect. In 2003 the US FDA recommended against the use of ipecac is now rare to see patients who have toxicity from ipecac.

Palmer EP, et al. Reversible myopathy secondary to abuse of ipecac in patients with major eating disorders. *N Engl J Med.* 1985;313:1457-1459.

40.9.   Answer: A. Weight loss surgery, such as gastric bypass surgery, is associated with significant, sustained weight loss. With weight loss, patients often have resolution of their diabetes and hypertension. Bariatric surgery, however, leads to thiamine deficiency and is a risk factor for the development of Wernicke encephalopathy. Thiamine therapy should be prescribed to all patients who have a history of bariatric surgery. In this case, high-dose intravenous thiamine hydrochloride therapy should be given immediately.

Aasheim ET. Wernicke encephalopathy after bariatric surgery: A systematic review. *Ann Surg.* 2008;248:714-720.

40.10.   Answer: B. Fenfluramine is a serotonin agonist that was used for weight loss until it was removed from the US market due to significant cardiac toxicity, specifically valvulopathies. The cardiac valvulopathies occurred as a result of the action of fenfluramine on the 5-HT$_{2B}$ receptor. Other notable toxicities from this xenobiotic included hallucinations, pulmonary hypertension, and serotonin toxicity.

Brenot F, et al. Primary pulmonary hypertension and fenfluramine use. *Br Heart J.*1993;70:537-541.

Halford JCG, et al. Serotonergic anti-obesity agents: Past experience and future prospects. *Drugs.* 2011;71:2247-2255.

41

Athletic Performance Enhancers

QUESTIONS

41.1. A 27-year-old man presents to the hospital with confusion, a plethoric appearance, blackened toes, and decreased pulses. His hematocrit is 72%. The patient states that he is currently training for a marathon. Which of the following performance-enhancing medications explains his presentation?
A. Human growth hormone
B. Testosterone
C. Human chorionic gonadotropin
D. Erythropoietin
E. Meldonium

41.2. Human chorionic gonadotropin (HCG) is used by male athletes for which of the following reasons?
A. Prevent testicular atrophy
B. Increase muscle mass
C. Burn fat
D. Increase exercise capacity
E. Increase fertility

41.3. A 32-year-old man presents to the emergency department with abdominal pain. His laboratory investigations are notable for an aspartate aminotransferase (AST) 163 IU/L, alanine aminotransferase (ALT) 241 IU/L, and mildly elevated total bilirubin and gamma-glutamyltransferase (GGT). A computed tomography (CT) scan of his abdomen demonstrates blood-filled sinuses in the liver. He says that he is using a prescription athletic performance enhancer. Which of the following complications does this drug put him at greatest risk of developing?
A. Red cell aplasia
B. Polycythemia

C. Thrombocytosis
D. Thrombocytopenia
E. Leukemia

41.4. A 27-year-old man presents to the hospital with complaints of breast enlargement. He has been using anabolic steroids, although he does not know which ones. He also says that he was supposed to take "some other pill" but could not afford it. Which of the following is the xenobiotic that he was unable to afford?
A. Dehydroepiandrosterone
B. Estradiol
C. Human chorionic gonadotropin
D. Aminoglutethimide
E. Meldonium

41.5. Which of the following adverse effects of anabolic steroid use is fully reversible in women athletes?
A. Baldness
B. Deepening of the voice
C. Increased facial hair
D. Clitoral hypertrophy
E. Amenorrhea

41.6. Which of the following athletic performance enhancers has a similar mechanism of action as valproic acid?
A. Erythropoietin
B. Insulinlike growth factor-1
C. Meldonium
D. Dehydroepiandrosterone
E. Anastrozole

41.7. A 22-year-old man presents to the emergency department following an episode of loss of consciousness while exercising. His vital signs are notable for a heart rate of 142 beats/min and a blood pressure of 60/30 mmHg. His laboratory analysis demonstrates a potassium of 6.2 mEq/L and a creatinine of 2.5 mg/dL (221 micromol/L). Which of the following athletic performance enhancers best explain this patient's presentation?
A. Spironolactone
B. Clenbuterol
C. Erythropoietin
D. Insulinlike growth factor-1
E. Testosterone

41.8. Which of the following laboratory techniques is the current gold standard for the detection of anabolic-androgenic steroids?
A. Atomic absorption
B. Gas chromatography
C. Thin-layer chromatography
D. Gas chromatography + mass spectrometry
E. Immunoassay

41.9. Why do some bodybuilders consume gamma hydroxybutyrate (GHB)?
A. Stimulation of insulin production
B. Increase in total testosterone concentrations
C. Decrease in androgenic side effects of steroids
D. Increase in growth hormone associated with onset of sleep
E. Maintain a normal sleep pattern

41.10. A 20-year-old-man is accused of using testosterone as an athletic performance-enhancer. Which of the following tests should be ordered to evaluate this allegation?
A. Gas chromatography + mass spectrometry
B. Liquid chromatography + mass spectrometry
C. Testosterone-to-epitestosterone ratio
D. Monoclonal antibody test
E. C-peptide

ANSWERS

41.1. Answer: D. Erythropoietin (EPO) is a hormone that induces erythropoiesis. EPO increases exercise capacity and hemoglobin production. Patients develop very elevated hematocrits, which increase the risk of thromboembolic events. The treatment involves discontinuing the EPO, intravenous hydration, and in certain circumstances, phlebotomy.

Zelman G, et al. Erythropoietin overdose treated with emergency erythropheresis. *J Toxicol Clin Toxicol.* 999;37:602-603.

41.2. Answer: A. Human chorionic gonadotropin (HCG) is used by male athletes to prevent testicular atrophy, both during and after androgen administration. HCG causes an increase in both testosterone and epitestosterone production.

Kicman AT, et al. Human chorionic gonadotrophin and sport. *Br J Sports Med.* 1991;25:73-80.

41.3. Answer: B. This patient has peliosis hepatis, which are blood-filled sinuses in the liver that are at risk of rupture. This condition develops because of the use of alkylated androgens. Testosterone and other androgens are also associated with polycythemia. They increase red blood cell counts by stimulating erythropoietin expression. Other common complications of extreme testosterone supplementation include peripheral edema, cardiac and hepatic dysfunction, and gonadal atrophy.

The other answers listed are rarely associated with androgen supplementation, if at all.

Bagheri SA, Boyer JL. Peliosis hepatis associated with androgenic-anabolic steroid therapy. A severe form of hepatic injury. *Ann Intern Med.* 1974;81:610-618.

41.4. Answer: D. Aminoglutethimide is an aromatase inhibitor that is taken in conjunction with exogenous testosterone to prevent feminization.

Mareck U, et al. Identification of the aromatase inhibitor aminoglutethimide in urine by gas chromatography/mass spectrometry. *Rapid Commun Mass Spectrom.* 2002;16:2209-2214.

41.5. Answer: E. All the listed answer choices are adverse effects of anabolic steroid use. Amenorrhea and acne are usually completely reversible with the cessation of use of anabolic steroids. All the other effects are often irreversible.

Hickson RC, et al. Adverse effects of anabolic steroids. *Med Toxicol Adverse Drug Exp.* 1989;4:254-271.

41.6. Answer: C. Meldonium inhibits the carnitine transporter type 2, reducing L-carnitine biosynthesis and transport in a manner that resembles valproic acid. Erythropoietin stimulates erythropoiesis. Insulinlike growth factor-1 release is stimulated by human growth hormone and increases glucose utilization, amino acid uptake, and protein synthesis. Dehydroepiandrosterone is a testosterone precursor that is converted to androstenedione after ingestion. Anastrozole is an aromatase inhibitor that prevents conversion of androstenedione and testosterone into estrogen.

> Dambrova M, et al. Pharmacological effects of meldonium: Biochemical mechanisms and biomarkers of cardiometabolic activity. *Pharmacol Res.* 2016;113:771-780.

41.7. Answer: A. Diuretic abuse is common among bodybuilders as it gives physique definition. Certain other athletes, such as jockeys, abuse diuretics to achieve a certain weight. Patients will present with symptoms consistent with volume depletion, such as tachycardia, hypotension, and acute kidney injury. Potassium-sparing diuretics, such as spironolactone, also cause hyperkalemia.

> al-Zaki T, Taibot-Stern J. A bodybuilder with diuretic abuse presenting with symptomatic hypotension and hyperkalemia. *Am J Emerg Med.* 1996;14:96-98.

41.8. Answer: D. While gas chromatography detects approximately 95% of all doping positive results, mass spectrometry is added for the detection of further substances. The current standard for detection of anabolic-androgenic steroids is gas chromatography and mass spectrometry.

> Catlin DH, et al. Testing urine for drugs. *Ann Biol Clin (Paris).* 1992;50:359-366.

41.9. Answer: D. An epidemic of GHB abuse was first reported in body builders, who believed that GHB had some properties to increase muscle bulk. This was due to an increase in growth hormone associated with onset of sleep. However, the euphoric effects of GHB were discovered at the same time, and GHB instead gained favor as a drug that was used recreationally. Due to the concern for drug-facilitated sexual assault, the Food and Drug Administration (FDA) banned nonprescription GHB use.

> Dyer JE, et al. Multistate outbreak of poisonings associated with illicit use of gamma hydroxybutyrate. *MMWR.* 1990;39:861-863.

> Van Cauter E, et al. Simultaneous stimulation of slow-wave sleep and growth hormone secretion by gamma-hydroxybutyrate in normal young men. *J Clin Invest.* 1997;100:745-753.

41.10. Answer: C. A testosterone-to-epitestosterone ratio is the best way to ascertain if a patient is using exogenous testosterone. A ratio of greater than 4:1 is considered evidence that a patient is using exogenous testosterone. Gas chromatography + mass spectrometry is unable to distinguish endogenous testosterone from exogenous testosterone. Erythropoietin is detected using a monoclonal erythropoietin antibody test. Liquid chromatography-mass spectrometry is used for further testing when there is a concern for a xenobiotic added to the urine as a masking agent. C-peptide concentrations are used to evaluate for exogenous insulin administration.

> Catlin DH, et al. Issues in detecting abuse of xenobiotic anabolic steroids and testosterone by analysis of athletes' urine. *Clin Chem.* 1997;43:1280-1288.

Essential Oils

QUESTIONS

42.1. The primary toxin in wormwood has a similar mechanism of action as which of the following toxins?
A. Picrotoxin
B. Batrachotoxin
C. Saxitoxin
D. Brevetoxin
E. Ciguatoxin

42.2. An 11-year-old boy is brought to the pediatrician by his mother for a routine visit. The pediatrician notes that the patient is developing undesired breast tissue. Which of the following essential oils is the most likely culprit?
A. Peppermint oil
B. Clove oil
C. Eucalyptus oil
D. Lavender oil
E. Oil of sycamore

42.3. A 41-year-old woman presents to the emergency department with abdominal pain. Her vital signs are: blood pressure, 111/73 mmHg; heart rate, 111 beats/min; respiratory rate, 18 breaths/min; temperature, 98.7 °F (37.1 °C), and oxygen saturation, 100%. On examination, she has scleral icterus and jaundice. The patient reports that she took an alternative medicine to induce an abortion. Which of the following essential oils did this patient most likely ingest?
A. Oil of wintergreen
B. Pine oil
C. Eucalyptus oil
D. Peppermint oil
E. Pennyroyal oil

42.4. Which of the following statements regarding tea tree oil is correct?
A. Is a commonly used and generally safe acne treatment
B. Neuropathy is the most common effect following topical exposure
C. Tea tree oil is an antioxidant
D. There are many reported deaths caused by tea tree oil
E. Typical symptoms following ingestion include vomiting and hyperreflexia

42.5. A 25-year-old man presents to the emergency department with altered mental status. His vital signs are: blood pressure, 150/90 mmHg; heart rate, 105 beats/min; respiratory rate, 15 breaths/min; temperature, 98.7 °F (37.1 °C), and oxygen saturation, 99%. Prior to presentation, he drank an essential oil and was initially very giddy but now is hallucinating and complaining of a sense of impending doom. Which essential oil ingestion best explains this patient's symptoms?
A. Clove oil
B. Oil of wintergreen
C. Nutmeg oil
D. Pennyroyal oil
E. Pine oil

42.6. A 2-year-old girl presents to the emergency department with altered mental status, fever to 101.3 °F (38.5 °C), and tachypnea to 30 breaths/min. Which of the following statements is true regarding oil of wintergreen?
A. Methyl salicylate is not dermally absorbed in significant amounts
B. Children are at a greater risk for toxicity given their lower surface area-to-weight ratio
C. Methyl salicylate undergoes hydrolysis in the liver to form salicylic acid
D. Cold increases dermal absorption of methyl salicylate
E. A mouthful of oil of wintergreen in a pediatric patient has a low risk of serious toxicity

42.7. Which of the following statements best describes the characteristics of eugenol?
A. It is both renally metabolized and eliminated
B. It is structurally similar to cantharidin
C. It forms a reactive intermediate that requires glutathione for elimination
D. It is used to treat otitis media and otitis externa
E. It upregulates prostaglandin synthetase

42.8. A 16-year-old boy presents to the emergency department after he ingested oil of wormwood. Which of the following findings would be expected on his urinalysis?
A. Myoglobinuria
B. Blue urine
C. Elevated urine pH

D. Pyuria
E. Nitrite positivity

42.9. A 16-year-old boy presents 7 hours following an intentional ingestion of camphor in a suicide attempt. He is currently asymptomatic. An acetaminophen concentration is undetectable, and his liver function tests are within normal limits. Which of the following options is the best next step in his management?
A. Administer 1 g/kg of activated charcoal
B. Load with phenobarbital
C. Administer lorazepam empirically to prevent status epilepticus
D. Admit to the intensive care unit for 24 hours of observation
E. Discharge to psychiatry

42.10. An 18-year-old woman presents to the emergency department with respiratory distress following intravenous self-administration of an essential oil in a suicide attempt. A computed tomography (CT) scan of her chest is performed and is consitent with acute respiratory distress syndrome (ARDS). Which of the following essential oils most likely caused her presentation?
A. Camphor
B. Thujone
C. Pulegone
D. Mysristicin
E. Pine oil

ANSWERS

42.1. Answer: A. The primary toxin in wormwood, alpha thujone, is a noncompetitive GABA$_A$ receptor antagonist. Picrotoxin, found in Indian fish berries, is also a GABA$_A$ receptor antagonist. Batrachatoxin comes from the poison dart frog and is a sodium channel opener. Saxitoxin causes paralytic shellfish poisoning and blocks sodium channels. Brevetoxin causes neurotoxic shellfish poisoning and is a sodium channel opener. Ciguatoxin causes ciguatera fish poisoning and is also a sodium channel opener.

Hold KM, et al. Alpha-thujone (the active component of absinthe): Gamma-aminobutyric acid type A receptor modulation and metabolic detoxification. *Proc Natl Acad Sci USA*. 2000;97:3826-3831.

42.2. Answer: D. There are several case reports that describe the development of gynecomastia in prepubertal boys using lavender oil. Like estradiol, lavender oil elicits a dose-dependent increase in estrogen responsivity and antiandrogenic activity in breast cancer cell cultures. The gynecomastia resolves when the oil is discontinued. Clove, eucalyptus, and peppermint oil are not associated with gynecomastia. Oil of sycamore is not an essential oil.

Block SL. The possible link between gynecomastia, topical lavender, and tea tree oil. *Pediatr Ann*. 2012;41:56-58.

Diaz A, et al. Prepubertal gynecomastia and chronic lavender exposure: Report of three cases. *J Pediatr Endocrinol Metab*. 2016;29:103-107.

Kemper KJ, et al. Prepubertal gynecomastia linked to lavender and tea tree oils. *N Engl J Med*. 2007;356:2541-2542.

42.3. Answer: E. Pennyroyal oil has been used for centuries as an abortifacient. Most cases of severe toxicity involve women ingesting large amounts to induce an abortion. The active ingredient in pennyroyal oil is pulegone, which is responsible for the hepatotoxicity. Oil of wintergreen, pine oil, eucalyptus oil, and peppermint oil are not traditionally used as abortifacients.

Gordon WP, et al. The metabolism of the abortifacient terpene, (r)-(+)-pulegone, to a proximate toxin, menthofuran. *Drug Metab Dispos.* 1987;15:589-594.

42.4. Answer: A. Tea tree oil is composed of terpene hydrocarbons, with 1,8-cineole implicated as the main irritating component. Tea tree oil is used as a topical antiseptic. Skin irritation and allergic reactions are the most common adverse effects following topical exposures. Tea tree oil also has antiinflammatory, not antioxidant, properties. There are no reported cases of deaths from pediatric or adult oral tea tree oil poisoning. Typical symptoms following ingestion include drowsiness and slurred speech.

Carson CF, et al. Melaleuca alternifolia (tea tree) oil: A review of antimicrobial and other medicinal properties. *Clin Microbiol Rev.* 2006;19:50.

42.5. Answer: C. Following nutmeg oil ingestion, symptoms such as gastrointestinal distress and tachycardia are common. The central nervous system effects, caused by the active ingredient myristicin, range from giddiness to hallucinations, delusions, and a sense of impending doom. Oil of wintergreen, clove oil, pennyroyal oil, and pine oil do not typically cause hallucinations or giddiness.

Akesson HO, Walinder J. Nutmeg intoxication. *Lancet.* 1965;1:1271-1272.

Anonymous. Nutmeg poisoning. *Br Med J.* 1959;2:1466-1467.

42.6. Answer: C. Methyl salicylate undergoes hydrolysis in the liver to form salicylic acid. Methyl salicylate is absorbed from both the gastrointestinal (GI) tract and the skin in significant amounts, and either route of exposure causes toxicity. Children are at a higher risk of toxicity given a higher surface area-to-weight ratio and more permeable skin. Heat or broken skin increases absorption of methyl salicylate, as does prolonged use of occlusive dressings. Because a single teaspoon of oil of wintergreen contains over 7 g of salicylate, a mouthful of oil of wintergreen is potentially lethal in children.

Davison C, et al. Metabolism and toxicity of methyl salicylate. *J Pharmacol Exp Ther.* 1961;132:207.

42.7. Answer: C. Eugenol, the active component of clove oil, undergoes sulfonation and glucuronidation in the liver. There is a minor pathway that involves CYP enzymes where a reactive intermediate is formed and requires glutathione for elimination. Eugenol is structurally similar to capsaicin and inhibits prostaglandin synthetase. It is used to treat dental pain, and is just as effective as topical benzocaine for analgesia.

Thompson DC, et al. Metabolism and cytotoxicity of eugenol in isolated rat hepatocytes. *Chem Biol Interact.* 1991;77:137-147.

Hume WR. The pharmacological and toxicological properties of zinc oxide-eugenol. *J Am Dent Assoc.* 1986;113:789-791.

42.8. Answer: A. Although the etiology is unclear, rhabdomyolysis with subsequent myoglobinuria and acute kidney injury occur after ingestion of oil of wormwood.

Weisbord SD, et al. Poison on line—acute renal failure caused by oil of wormwood purchased through the Internet. *N Engl J Med.* 1997;337:825-827.

42.9. Answer: E. Camphor leads to gastrointestinal irritation followed by central nervous system toxicity. Patients develop confusion, agitation, delirium, and hallucinations. Seizures occur within minutes to a few hours of exposure. There is a very low likelihood of developing seizures if patients are asymptomatic more than 6 hours after ingestion, and therefore, it is appropriate to transfer this patient to psychiatry for further management.

Manoguerra AS, et al. Camphor poisoning: An evidence-based practice guideline for out-of-hospital management. *Clin Toxicol.* 2006;44: 357-370.

42.10. Answer: E. Pine oil is used as a household cleaner, varnish, and polish. Aspiration pneumonitis occurs commonly following ingestion or inhalation. Intravenous injection leads to acute respiratory distress syndrome (ARDS). While the exact mechanism of intravenous pine oil leading to ARDS is unknown, this toxicity is reproduced in animal models.

Sperling F, et al. Acute effects of turpentine vapor on rats and mice. *Toxicol Appl Pharmacol.* 1967;10:8-20.

Plant- and Animal-Derived Dietary Supplements

43

QUESTIONS

43.1. A 52-year-old woman with a history of lupus nephritis and a stable kidney allograft presents to the emergency department with progressive fatigue, oliguria, and abdominal pain. Her serum creatinine is 4.2 mg/dL (371 micromol/L), which is increased from her baseline creatinine of 1.1 mg/dL (97 micromol/L). She is compliant with her medications, which include cyclosporine, mycophenolate mofetil (MMF), and hydroxychloroquine. She also started taking an herbal supplement 1 month prior to presentation to help with depressed mood. Which of the following interactions most likely contributed to her presentation?
A. CYP3A4 inhibition leading to supratherapeutic cyclosporine concentrations
B. P-glycoprotein inhibition leading to subtherapeutic MMF concentrations
C. Monoamine oxidase (MAO) reuptake inhibition leading to supratherapeutic cyclosporine concentrations
D. CYP3A4 induction leading to subtherapeutic cyclosporine concentrations
E. P-glycoprotein upregulation leading to supratherapeutic cyclosporine concentrations

43.2. A 22-year-old woman is brought into the emergency department 5 hours after an intentional ingestion of the dietary supplement vitamin B_{17}. Shortly after presentation, she has a generalized tonic-clonic seizure and becomes hypotensive to 50/20 mmHg. Which of the following antidotes should be administered immediately?
A. Physostigmine
B. Fomepizole

C. Naloxone
D. Methylene blue
E. Hydroxocobalamin

43.3. A 14-year-old boy presents to the hospital with generalized fatigue and hypertension after repeatedly consuming a candy over the last 2 weeks. He purchased the candy while on vacation in Europe last month. Which electrolyte abnormalities would you expect?
A. Hypokalemia and sodium retention
B. Hyperkalemia and sodium loss
C. Hypermagnesemia and potassium loss
D. Hypernatremia and hyperchloremia
E. Hyponatremia and hypomagnesemia

43.4. Which statement concerning the US Food and Drug Administration (FDA) regulations of herbal preparations is true?
A. The FDA approves marketing of preparations that are proven safe and efficacious
B. The FDA regulates marketing of herbal preparations to prevent misidentification, mislabeling, and misleading claims
C. Herbal preparations are considered to be medications by the FDA
D. Herbal preparations are considered to be dietary supplements by the FDA
E. The FDA ensures that herbal preparations are manufactured according to federal standards of quality control

43.5. A 42-year-old woman presents to the emergency department 2 hours after ingesting the herbal supplement chuan wu. She has paresthesias of her oral mucosa, nausea, vomiting, and diarrhea. During her admission, she develops progressive skeletal muscle weakness and a tachydysrhythmia. Which of the following therapies would you give?
A. Sodium bicarbonate
B. Phenytoin
C. Esmolol
D. Procainamide
E. Digoxin-specific Fab

43.6. Which of the following options is an appropriate therapy for ch'an su induced tachydysrhythmias?
A. Sodium bicarbonate
B. Phenytoin
C. Lidocaine
D. Procainamide
E. Digoxin-specific Fab

43.7. Betel (*Areca catechu*) is used recreationally by more than 200 million people. Which of the following listed plants contains an active ingredient that most closely resembles the active ingredient in betel?
A. Blue cohosh
B. Wormwood
C. Monkshood
D. Green plum seeds
E. Cassava

43.8. A 38-year-old woman presents to the emergency department with colicky abdominal pain. On physical examination, she has significant pallor and a pronounced foot drop. She recently started taking a *rasa shastra* Ayurvedic medication. Which of the following xenobiotics best explains her presentation?
A. Wormwood
B. Aconite
C. Lead
D. Arsenic
E. Aristolochic acid

43.9. A 32-year-old man presents to the emergency department after his outpatient bloodwork revealed agranulocytosis. The patient takes no prescription medication. He is, however, taking the herbal preparation marketed as Chui Fong Tou Ku Wan. Which of the following xenobiotics is the likely cause for this patient's agranulocytosis?
A. Garlic
B. Ginseng
C. Pyrrolizidine alkaloid
D. Phenylbutazone
E. Aristolochic acid

43.10. Which of the following xenobiotics is found in the herbal preparation maqianzi?
A. Aconite
B. Strychnine
C. Lead
D. Wormwood
E. Bufadienolides

ANSWERS

43.1. Answer: D. This patient is presenting with acute allograft rejection. St. John's Wort (*Hypericum perforatum*) is an herbal supplement that acts as a monoamine oxidase (MAO) reuptake inhibitor. It also induces CYP3A4, upregulates P-glycoprotein, and is associated with reduced serum cyclosporine concentrations and increased risk of rejection. Mycophenolate mofetil (MMF) is predominantly inactivated by glucuronidation and undergoes renal elimination, so alteration in CYP3A4 activity is unlikely to directly affect its metabolism or elimination.

Izzo AA, Ernst E. Interactions between herbal medicines and prescribed drugs: An updated systematic review. *Drugs*. 2009;69:1777-1798.

43.2. Answer: E. Vitamin B_{17} is sold in many health food stores and is touted as being a cure for cancer. Vitamin B_{17} is, in fact, not a vitamin; it is instead the name under which amygdalin, a cyanogenic glycoside, is sold. Patients who overdose on this xenobiotic are at risk of developing cyanide toxicity and should be treated with hydroxocobalamin.

Shively RM, et al. Rebound metabolic acidosis following intentional amygdalin supplement overdose. *Clin Toxicol*. 2020;58:290-293.

43.3. Answer A. The patient ate licorice, which is derived from the licorice root, *Glycyrrhiza glabra*. It is widely used in candies, herbal preparations, and as a root to chew. Glycyrrhizin inhibits the conversion of cortisol to cortisone by inhibiting 11-beta-hydroxysteroid dehydrogenase, increasing mineralocorticoid activity. The syndrome mimics hyperaldosteronism and leads to hypokalemia, sodium and water retention, peripheral edema, hypertension, and weakness.

Walker BR, Edwards CR. Licorice-induced hypertension and syndromes of apparent mineralocorticoid excess. *Endocrinol Metab Clin North Am*. 1994;23:359-377.

43.4. Answer: D. In 1994, the US Congress passed the Dietary Supplement and Health Education Act, which reduced the Food and Drug Administration's (FDA) oversight of products categorized as dietary supplements. This includes vitamins, minerals, herbals, amino acids, and any product that is sold as a "supplement" before October 15, 1994. Herbal products are marketed without any testing for efficacy or safety. The FDA must prove an herbal product is unsafe before it can be challenged. These products are manufactured without any federal standards of quality control. Although packaging claims to cure or prevent a specific disease are not permitted, claims detailing how a product affects the "body's structure or function" are acceptable. No FDA approval is required with regard to packaging or marketing.

Food and Drug Administration. Federal register. Part II 21 CFR Part 101. Food labeling; Final Rule and Proposed Rules. December 28, 1995.

43.5. Answer: D. This patient is presenting with aconite toxicity following the ingestion of chuan wu. Aconite toxicity is due to aconite alkaloids, including aconitine, mesaconitine, and hypoaconitine, which increase sodium influx through the sodium channel, delaying the final repolarization phase of the action potential and initiating premature excitation. There is no specific antidote to aconite toxicity. Case reports of aconite toxicity demonstrate a benefit from sodium channel blockers such as procainamide or flecainide. One case of aconite-induced refractory tachydysrhythmias was successfully managed with a ventricular assist device.

Tai YT, et al. Cardiotoxicity after accidental herb-induced aconite poisoning. *Lancet.* 1992;340:1254-1256.

43.6. Answer: E. Ch'an su is a traditional herbal remedy derived from the secretions of the parotid and sebaceous glands of the toads, *Bufo bufo gargarizans* or *Bufo melanosticus.* It is used as a topical anesthetic and cardiac medication. In New York City, it is also marketed as an aphrodisiac and is sold under names such as "Stone," "Love Stone," "Black Stone," and "Rock Hard." Ch'an su contains two cardioactive steroids of the bufadienolide class, and bufotenine. Digoxin-specific Fab is used to treat ch'an su toxicity and should be empirically administered for any suspected case of ch'an su cardiotoxicity. Digoxin-specific Fab should also be empirically administered to other herbal cardiac glycoside toxins, including oleander (*Nerium oleander*), squill (*Urginea maritima*), lily of the valley (*Convallaria majalis*), and yellow oleander (*Thevetia peruviana*).

Brubacher JR, et al. Treatment of toad venom poisoning with digoxin-specific Fab fragments. *Chest.* 1996;110:1282-1288.

43.7. Answer: A. The active ingredient in betel is arecoline, which is a direct-acting nicotinic agonist. Other plants with nicotinic constituents include blue cohosh, nicotine, horse chestnut, and lobelia. The active substance in wormwood is thujone; in monkshood, it is aconite; green plum seeds contain amygdalin; and cassava contains linamarin.

Norton SA. Betel: Consumption and consequences. *J Am Acad Dermatol.* 1998;38:81-88.

43.8. Answer: C. *Rasa shastra* is a form of Ayurvedic remedy that is based on ancient traditional healing in India. It deliberately combines metals such as lead, gold, zinc, and copper in the products. Patients present with toxicity consistent with the metal that is in the product. It is important to counsel patients regarding the use Ayurvedic medication. It is also important to keep a high clinical suspicion for metal toxicity in patients who present with vague complaints and are taking Ayurvedic medication.

Centers for Disease Control and Prevention (CDC). Lead poisoning associated with ayurvedic medications—five states, 2000-2003. *MMWR Morb Mortal Wkly Rep.* 2004;53:582-584.

43.9. Answer: D. Many plant- and animal-derived dietary supplements actually contain unlisted and potentially harmful ingredients. Herbalists will also sometimes combine pharmaceutical medication into herbal medication. These pharmaceutical medications are not listed on the packaging. Chui Fong Tou Ku Wan contained phenylbutazone and aminopyrine, both of which lead to agranulocytosis.

Ridker PM. Toxic effects of herbal teas. *Arch Environ Health.* 1987;42:133-136.

43.10. Answer: B. Maqianzi is derived from the dried seeds of the plant *Strychnos nux vomica.* It is used in traditional Chinese medicine to treat rheumatism and musculoskeletal complaints. Patients develop signs of mild toxicity, even at the standard dosing regimen.

Chan TYK. Herbal medicine causing likely strychnine poisoning. *Hum Exp Toxicol.* 2002;21:467-468.

Kong H-Y, et al. Safety of individual medication of Ma Qian Zi (semen strychni) based upon assessment of therapeutic effects of Guo's therapy against moderate fluorosis of bone. *J Tradit Chin Med Chung Tsa Chih Ying Wen Pan.* 2011;31:297-302.

44

Vitamins

QUESTIONS

44.1. A 55-year-old man starts a new therapy for elevated triglycerides. Four days later, he calls his doctor to report flushing, itching, and tingling, which he finds intolerable. His doctor recommends he take another medication to lessen these effects. How does the new medication improve his symptoms?
A. Cyclooxygenase inhibition
B. Prostaglandin D_2 production
C. Glutamic acid decarboxylase (GAD) production
D. Regeneration of tocopherol
E. Promotion of osteoblastic activity

44.2. A 35-year-old woman presents to the emergency department with 3 months of worsening tingling and weakness to her lower extremities. On examination, she has severe distal impairment of proprioception and a pronounced ataxia. Her speech and cognition are entirely normal. Excess of which of the following vitamins could explain her symptoms?
A. Vitamin A
B. Vitamin B_6
C. Vitamin C
D. Vitamin D
E. Niacin

44.3. Which of the following formulations of vitamin A is a teratogen?
A. Retinoid
B. 11-*cis*-Retinal
C. Topical tretinoin
D. Isotretinoin
E. Prenatal vitamin A

44.4. A 52-year-old man is admitted to the hospital due to a new finding of hepatotoxicity. Which of the following findings would be consistent with vitamin A as the etiology of his liver dysfunction?
A. Centrilobular necrosis
B. Periportal necrosis
C. Cirrhosis
D. Kupffer cell–mediated inflammation
E. Proliferation of bile ducts

44.5. A 35-year-old woman presents to the emergency department with bilateral flank pain, diarrhea, and epigastric burning. She states that she goes to a wellness clinic for a "preventative" regimen of dietary supplements including oral and intravenous (IV) preparations. Which vitamin is most likely to be causing her symptoms?
A. Vitamin A
B. Vitamin B_{17}
C. Vitamin C
D. Vitamin D
E. Vitamin E

44.6. A 26-year-old woman is diagnosed with a pulmonary embolism. Due to insurance issues, she is only able to be prescribed warfarin therapy. Which of the following vitamins interferes with her current anticoagulation regimen?
A. Vitamin B_6
B. Vitamin B_{12}
C. Vitamin C
D. Vitamin D
E. Vitamin E

44.7. A 6-week-old boy is brought into the emergency department due to concern for poor weight gain and lethargy. He has an ultrasound of his abdomen performed that demonstrates bilateral medullary nephrocalcinosis. Administration of which of the following vitamins by his parents explains his presentation?
A. Vitamin B_6
B. Vitamin B_{12}
C. Vitamin C
D. Vitamin D
E. Vitamin E

44.8. A 24-year-old woman with cystic acne presents to the emergency department with a severe headache. As part of her evaluation, she has a lumbar puncture performed that only demonstrates elevated opening pressures. Which of the following medications should she be prescribed?
A. Isoretinoin
B. Nicardapine
C. Carbamazepine
D. Acetazolamide
E. Metoclopramide

44.9. A 57-year-old man presents to the emergency department with a fever, a pericardial effusion, pulmonary infiltrates, and new kidney failure. Further history reveals that he has a history of acute promyelocytic leukemia. Which of the following medications explains his new symptoms?
A. Retinoid
B. 11-*cis*-Retinal
C. Tretinoin
D. Isotretinoin
E. Prenatal vitamin A

44.10. Patients with niacin-induced hepatic toxicity also have which of the following characteristics?
A. Are likely to develop the niacin flush syndrome
B. Have a liver biopsy demonstrating centrilobular necrosis
C. Are taking sustained-release niacin preparations
D. Are allergic to aspirin
E. Have an alcohol use disorder

ANSWERS

44.1. Answer: A. This patient initially began niacin as a therapy for his elevated triglycerides. It should be noted that niacin is no longer considered an indicated therapy for dyslipidemias. Niacin commonly causes vasodilatory cutaneous flushing secondary to the production of prostaglandin D_2 and E_2 in capillaries. A dose of aspirin of 325 mg, ideally 30 minutes prior to niacin, diminishes this flushing by decreasing production of prostaglandins via cyclooxygenase inhibition. Prostaglandin production is the mechanism of flushing, not the mechanism for relief. Pyridoxine assists in glutamic acid decarboxylase (GAD) production. Vitamin E promotes regeneration of tocopherol. Vitamin D promotes osteoblastic activity.

Whelan A, et al. The effect of aspirin on niacin-induced cutaneous reactions. *J Fam Pract.* 1992;34:165-168.

Kamanna VS, et al. The mechanism and mitigation of niacin-induced flushing. *Int J Clin Pract.* 2009;63:1369-1377.

44.2. Answer: B. Pyridoxine, or vitamin B_6, leads to toxicity in both excess and deficiency. Chronic overdoses of pyridoxine, in which patients ingested 2-6 g/day for between 2 and 40 months, led to severe ataxia and dysfunction of the distal peripheral nerves. Chronic doses as low as 200 mg/day,

however, are also reported to cause this presentation. On biopsy, patients had nonspecific axonal degeneration. When pyridoxine is discontinued, patients have gradual improvement in their neuropathy. Acute neurotoxicity also occurs following a single massive overdose of pyridoxine. Large overdoses of pyridoxine lead to ataxia, seizures, and death.

Schaumburg H, et al. Sensory neuropathy from pyridoxone abuse: A new megavitamin syndrome. *N Engl J Med.* 1983;309:445-448.

Parry GJ, Bredesen DE. Sensory neuropathy with low-dose pyridoxine. *Neurology.* 1985;35:1466-1468.

44.3. Answer: D. Isotretinoin (13-*cis*-retinal) is a synthetic vitamin A derivative used to treat severe cystic acne. Its use is contraindicated in pregnant women (US FDA pregnancy category X) because of interference with fetal skeletal differentiation and growth. Other congenital defects include craniofacial, cardiovascular, neurologic, and thymic abnormalities. Women of childbearing age are enrolled under the iPLEDGE program, a mandatory US FDA risk evaluation and mitigation strategy (REMS) program that tracks and educates health professionals of its risk of use. Tretinoin is a synthetic vitamin A derivative that is minimally absorbed when applied topically and is not a teratogen. However, if tretinoin is used systemically as a chemotherapeutic agent to treat promyelocytic leukemia, it is listed as US FDA pregnancy category D agent and should be avoided in the first trimester.

Binkley N, Krueger D. Hypervitaminosis A and bone. *Nutr Rev.* 2000; 58:138-144.

iPLEDGE. https://www.ipledgeprogram.com. Accessed March 30, 2017.

Lammer EJ, et al. Retinoic acid embryopathy. *N Engl J Med.* 1985; 313:837-841.

44.4. Answer: C. Vitamin A hepatotoxicity is histologically defined as cirrhosis. This is secondary to the proliferative effect vitamin A has on hepatic stellate (Ito) cells. These cells deposit excessive amounts of collagen and result in scarring.

Kowalski T, et al. Vitamin A hepatotoxicity. A cautionary note regarding 25,000 IU supplements. *Am J Med.* 1994;97:523-528.

44.5. Answer: C. Oral vitamin C ingestions are associated with osmotic diarrhea and esophagitis. Ascorbic acid is metabolized to oxalate, but there is not a clear risk of nephrolithiasis in patients taking oral vitamin C supplements except in those with a prior history of nephrolithiasis. Several case reports describe nephrolithiasis in patients receiving IV vitamin C supplements. Amygdalin is often wrongly referred to as vitamin B_{17} and leads to cyanide toxicity.

Hoyt C. Diarrhea from vitamin C. *JAMA.* 1980;244:1674.

McAllister C. Renal failure secondary to massive infusion of vitamin C. *JAMA.*1984;252:1684.

44.6. Answer: E. Absorption of vitamin K is impaired by large doses of vitamin E in animal studies. This, coupled with the inhibitory effect vitamin E has on the epoxidation of vitamin K to its active form, means that excessive vitamin E supplementation prolongs prothrombin times in patients taking warfarin.

Anonymous. Vitamin K, vitamin E and the coumarin drugs. *Nutr Rev.* 1982;40:180-181.

Roberts H. Perspective of vitamin E as therapy. *JAMA.* 1981;246:129-131.

44.7. Answer: D. Excess vitamin D supplementation leads to severe hypercalcemia. Vitamin D promotes calcium absorption from the gut and mobilization of calcium from the bones. The symptoms of vitamin D overdose correspond to the degree of hypercalcemia and include weakness, fatigue, irritability, and, in rare cases, nephrocalcinosis. The treatment includes immediate discontinuation of vitamin D and any calcium supplementation, and intravenous fluid hydration. Depending on the severity of the hypercalcemia, calcitonin and bisphosphonates are also used.

Lee K, et al. Iatrogenic vitamin D intoxication. Report of a case and review of vitamin D physiology. *Connecticut Med.* 1999;63:399-403.

44.8. Answer: D. This patient is presenting with idiopathic intracranial hypertension (IIH), formerly known as pseudotumor cerebri, likely because of the isoretinoin therapy she is prescribed for her acne. It is postulated that oral retinoids create imbalances in cerebrospinal fluid (CSF) and are directly toxic to arachnoid villi function. Acetazolamide is the most commonly used medication in the treatment of IIH. Acetazolamide leads to a reduction in CSF production. If acetazolamide is not successful or is not tolerated, furosemide is added as a second-line treatment.

Randhawa S, Van Stavern G. Idiopathic intracranial hypertension (pseudotumor cerebri). *Curr Opin Ophthalmol.* 2008;19:445-453.

Tintle SJ, et al. Safe use of therapeutic-dose oral isotretinoin in patients with a history of pseudotumor cerebri. *JAMA Dermatol.* 2016; 152:582-584.

44.9. Answer: C. All-*trans*-retinoic acid (ATRA), or tretinoin, is a chemotherapeutic that is used to treat acute promyelocytic leukemia. It is associated with the development of acute promyelocytic leukemia differentiation syndrome (DS), which was formerly known as ATRA syndrome. This syndrome includes at least three of the following symptoms: fever, dyspnea, weight gain, pleural or pericardial effusions, pulmonary infiltrates, and kidney failure.

Patatanian E, Thompson D. Retinoic acid syndrome: A review. *J Clin Pharm Ther.* 2008;33:331-338.

44.10. Answer: C. Niacin-induced hepatitis appears to be more frequent and more severe among those with hyperlipidemias treated with high doses of sustained-release preparations compared to patients receiving crystalline or immediate-release niacin. Hepatotoxicity is consistent with hepatocellular necrosis and rarely cholestasis. These manifestations are dose related and not a hypersensitivity response.

Rader JI, et al. Hepatic toxicity of unmodified and time release preparations of niacin. *Am J Med.* 1992;92:77-81.

Iron

QUESTIONS

45.1. Which of the following formulations of iron contains the highest percentage of elemental iron?
A. Ferrous chloride
B. Ferrous fumarate
C. Ferrous gluconate
D. Ferrous sulfate
E. All contain the same amount of elemental iron

45.2. A 17-year-old girl is admitted to the hospital after an acute iron overdose. Three days into her hospital stay, she develops a fever, abdominal pain, and blood in her stool. Which of the following choices best explains this patient's current symptoms?
A. Unresolved iron toxicity
B. *Yersinia* infection
C. *Pseudomonas* infection
D. *Enterococcus* infection
E. *Vibrio* infection

45.3. Which adverse effect is the main reason to limit the use of the use of deferoxamine to 24 hours?
A. Hypotension
B. Nephrotoxicity
C. Pulmonary toxicity
D. Hepatotoxicity
E. Neurotoxicity

45.4. A 20-month-old girl is brought to the emergency department 3 hours after possibly ingesting 100 mg/kg of elemental iron. She has already vomited four times. An abdominal radiograph reveals multiple radiopaque iron fragments in the stomach. Which of the following decontamination techniques would be the best to perform in this patient?
A. 1 g/kg of activated charcoal
B. Administer oral magnesium citrate
C. Orogastric lavage with deferoxamine
D. Orogastric lavage with normal saline
E. Whole-bowel irrigation with polyethylene glycol electrolyte lavage solution

45.5. Significant toxicity following an iron overdose is **unlikely** to occur in patients who have which of the following findings?
A. A white blood cell count (WBC) <15,000/mm^3
B. A serum glucose <150 mg/dL (8.32 mmol/L)
C. A total iron binding capacity (TIBC) that is greater than the serum iron concentration
D. Have been asymptomatic for 6 hours in the emergency department (ED)
E. A normal serum potassium

45.6. Deferoxamine therapy should be discontinued when which of the following findings occurs?
A. The urine turns brownish red
B. The total iron binding capacity (TIBC) exceeds the serum iron concentration
C. The white blood cell count (WBC) and glucose return to normal
D. The anion gap acidosis resolves and the patient appears well
E. Vomiting and diarrhea resolve

45.7. A 50-year-old woman presents to the emergency department after she received a five-fold over-dose of intravenous iron. One hour following the infusion, her iron concentration is 1,301 mcg/dL (232.9 micromol/L). She has no vomiting; her vital signs and anion gap are normal. Which of the following interventions should be performed next on this patient?
A. Intravenous fluid bolus
B. Hemodialysis
C. Deferoxamine infusion
D. Oral deferasirox
E. No therapy at this time

45.8. Which of the following statements about iron poisoning in pregnancy is true?
A. Iron crosses the placenta by passive diffusion
B. Maternal toxicity from iron exceeds direct fetal toxicity from iron
C. The use of deferoxamine is contraindicated in pregnancy
D. Iron is the most commonly ingested pharmaceutical substance during pregnancy
E. The maternal serum iron concentration directly correlates with fetal toxicity

45.9. A reported dose of elemental iron that is greater than which of the following amounts warrants a child be referred to the hospital for further evaluation?
A. 5 mg/kg
B. 10 mg/kg
C. 20 mg/kg
D. 35 mg/kg
E. 50 mg/kg

49.10. Which of the following statements best explains the mechanism of the acidosis that occurs following an iron overdose?
A. Iron ions disrupt mitochondrial oxidative phosphorylation
B. Iron leads to a decrease in the build up of unused hydrogen ions
C. Absorption of iron from the gastrointestinal tract leads to conversion of ferric iron to ferrous iron
D. Ferrous iron exceeds the binding capacity of plasma leading to the formation of ferric hydroxide
E. Iron mediates its effects as a reducing agent

ANSWERS

45.1. Answer: B. Ferrous fumarate contains the highest amount of elemental iron at 33%. Ferrous chloride contains 28% elemental iron, ferrous sulfate contains 20% elemental iron, and ferrous gluconate contains 12% elemental iron. These are all oral ionic formulations of iron.

Melamed N, et al. Iron supplementation in pregnancy—does the preparation matter? *Arch Gynecol Obstet.* 2007;276:601-604.

45.2. Answer: B. Patients who have acute iron toxicity develop *Yersinia* infections as a complication of both the iron overdose and the deferoxamine treatment. Iron-rich environments provide a growth factor for bacterial overgrowth, which enhances the virulence of *Yersinia entercolitica*. *Yersinia* should be suspected in patients who develop abdominal pain, fever, or bloody diarrhea following an iron overdose. Deferoxamine therapy is also associated with the development of *Klebsiella* spp, *Vibrio* spp, *Aeromonas hydrophila, and Mucorales* spp infections.

Melby K, et al. Septicaemia due to *Yersinia enterocolitica* after oral overdoses of iron. *Br Med J (Clin Res Ed).* 1982;285:467-468.

45.3. Answer: C. The duration of deferoxamine therapy is limited to 24 hours to minimize the risk of pulmonary toxicity. Prolonged use is associated with the development of acute respiratory distress syndrome (ARDS). Hypotension is a rate-related factor with regard to deferoxamine administration.

Tenenbein M, et al. Pulmonary toxic effects of continuous administration in acute iron poisoning. *Lancet.* 1992;339:699-701.

45.4. Answer: E. This patient is actively vomiting; furthermore, she is only 20 months old and a large orogastric tube should not be placed. Therefore, orogastric lavage is not the appropriate gastrointestinal decontamination method in this patient. Orogastric lavage with deferoxamine increases toxicity due to increased concentrations of ferrioxamine. Activated charcoal does adsorb iron. The use of whole-bowel irrigation (WBI) in iron overdose is supported by case reports and one case series. Given that there are multiple radiopaque iron fragments on this patient's radiograph, it is reasonable to perform WBI.

Tenenbein M. Whole bowel irrigation in iron poisoning. *J Pediatr.* 1987;111:142-145.

45.5. Answer: D. Iron poisoning is a clinical diagnosis. Patients who appear well with normal vital signs and no symptoms after 6 hours in the ED are unlikely to become ill. A WBC >15,000/mm^3 and a serum glucose >150 mg/dL (8.8 mmol/L) were associated with an iron concentration >300 mcg/dL (53.7 micromol/L) in pediatric patients, although other patients with WBC <15,000/mm^3 and with glucose <150 mg/dL (8.3 mmol/L) also had iron concentrations >300 mcg/dL (53.7 micromol/L). Clinical iron toxicity was thought not to occur if the serum iron concentration was less than the TIBC because insufficient circulating non–transferrin-bound iron was present to cause tissue damage. The error in interpretation results from the limitations of measuring TIBC values. The in vitro value of TIBC factitiously increases because of iron poisoning and thus tends to apparently increase above a concurrently measured serum iron concentration. The TIBC as currently determined has limited, if any, value in the assessment of iron-poisoned patients.

Burkhart KK, et al. The rise in the total iron binding capacity after iron overdose. *Ann Emerg Med.* 1991;20:532-535.

Lacouture PG, et al. Emergency assessment of severity in iron overdose by clinical and laboratory methods. *J Pediatr.* 1981;99:89-91.

45.6. Answer: D. Although much debate has centered on criteria for discontinuation of deferoxamine therapy in the iron-poisoned patient, most authors agree that when the patient looks well and the anion gap acidosis resolves, it is reasonable to discontinue deferoxamine. In the uncommon event that symptoms persist beyond 24 hours post ingestion, the risks and benefits of continued deferoxamine therapy are best evaluated with a toxicology consultant.

Mills KC, Curry SC. Acute iron poisoning. *Emerg Med Clin North Am.* 1994;12:397-413.

45.7. Answer: E. Intravenous iron is complexed to carbohydrates, which lead to serum concentrations that do not correlate with severity of symptoms. The decision to perform further therapy should depend on the patient's clinical status. This patient is asymptomatic with a normal anion gap; therefore, no further therapy is indicated at this time.

Biary R, et al. Intravenous iron overdose: Treat the patient not the number. *Toxicol Commun.* 2019;3:37-39.

45.8. Answer: B. Maternal iron toxicity exceeds fetal toxicity; fetal toxicity is related to maternal hemodynamic and physiologic status, not fetal iron poisoning. Since iron crosses biologic membranes by a process of receptor-mediated endocytosis, little iron reaches the fetus. Concern about deferoxamine is related to references to teratogenic effects in animal models; however, deferoxamine is used successfully in human poisonings. Acetaminophen is the most ingested pharmaceutical substance during pregnancy.

Curry S, et al. An ovine model of maternal iron poisoning in pregnancy. *Ann Emerg Med.* 1990;19:632-638.

Olenmark M, et al. Fatal iron intoxication in late pregnancy. *J Toxicol Clin Toxicol.* 1987;25:347-359.

45.9. Answer: C. Children who appear well with unintentional ingestions <20 mg/kg of elemental iron and only an isolated episode of vomiting are managed at home with close consultation with a poison control center. There are certain guidelines that exist that use a 40 mg/kg dose as the limit to send patients into healthcare; however, we recommend a more conservative approach and would prefer children who ingest >20 mg/kg be evaluated in the hospital.

Manoguerra AS, et al. Iron ingestion: An evidence-based consensus guideline for out-of-hospital management. *Clin Toxicol (Phila).* 2005;43: 553-570.

45.10. Answer: A. Iron leads to a metabolic acidosis through several different mechanisms. Iron induces oxidative stress. The initial oxidative damage to the gastrointestinal epithelium permits iron ions to enter systemic circulation. Iron ions disrupt mitochondrial oxidative phosphorylation, which then lead to a build up of unused hydrogen ions. Iron from the gastrointestinal tract leads to the conversion of ferrous iron (Fe^{2+}) to ferric iron (Fe^{3+}). It is the ferric iron that exceeds the binding capacity of plasma, leading to the formation of ferric hydroxide and subsequent release of three protons. Patients also develop decreased cardiac output and shock, which further exacerbates the acidosis.

Reissmann KR, Coleman TJ. Acute intestinal iron intoxication II. Metabolic, respiratory and circulatory effects of absorbed iron salts. *Blood.* 1955;10:46-51.

Tenenbein M. Toxicokinetics and toxicodynamics of iron poisoning. *Toxicol Lett.* 1998;102-103:653-656.

Pharmaceutical Additives

46

QUESTIONS

46.1. A 21-year-old man presents to the emergency department in status epilepticus. He is intubated, placed on a high-dose lorazepam infusion, and admitted to the neurologic intensive care unit (ICU). On the third day of his ICU stay, he remains on a continuous infusion of lorazepam and develops progressive tachypnea and hemodynamic instability. What do you expect his laboratory investigations to now show?
A. Decreased pH, increased anion gap, normal lactate
B. Normal pH, increased anion gap, increased lactate
C. Decreased pH, normal anion gap, normal lactate
D. Normal pH, decreased anion gap, normal lactate
E. Decreased pH, increased anion gap, increased lactate

46.2. The "gasping" syndrome described in neonates resulted from which of the following options?
A. A decreased ability to metabolize benzyl alcohol
B. A decreased ability to metabolize benzoic acid
C. A glucose-6-phosphate dehydrogenase (G6PD) deficiency
D. Sterile water for injection
E. Methanol

46.3. Exposure to benzyl alcohol is associated with which of the following sequelae?
A. Guillain-Barré syndrome
B. Selective mutism
C. Autism spectrum disorder
D. Neuromyelitis optica
E. Cerebral palsy

46.4. In 1983, a new parental medication was introduced that resulted in a fatal syndrome that included thrombocytopenia, acute kidney injury, cholestasis, hepatomegaly, and ascites. It was never approved by the US Food and Drug Administration (FDA) but was marketed as a nutritional supplement and was used intravenously (IV) in neonates. This product was recalled from the market 4 months after release. What medication was this?
A. Benzyl alcohol
B. E-Ferol
C. Phenformin
D. Thalidomide
E. Isoretinoin

46.5. A 28-year-old woman presents to the emergency department due to severe pain to her right eye with associated decreased vision. Her corneal examination reveals superficial, punctate erosions of the epithelium. On medication reconciliation, she reveals that she unintentionally used drops that were intended for her ear in her eye. What led to her ocular toxicity?
A. Benzalkonium chloride
B. Benzyl alcohol
C. Methylparaben
D. Polyethylene glycol
E. Propylene glycol

46.6. A 38-year-old man presents to the emergency department with central nervous system depression. He was found next to an old bottle of Seducaps. Chlorobutanol is listed on the ingredient list. Which of the following compounds has a similar chemical structure?
   A. Trichloroethanol
   B. Perchloroethylene
   C. Vinyl chloride
   D. Clorpromazine
   E. Polyvinyl chloride

46.7. A 33-year-old woman is brought into to the emergency department after she developed ventricular tachycardia in a clinic. While there, she had lost consciousness as she was undergoing a regimen to treat acne scars. Which of the following is responsible for her dysrhythmia?
   A. Benzyl alcohol
   B. Polyethylene glycol
   C. Phenol
   D. Sorbitol
   E. Chlorobutanol

46.8. A 48-year-old man presents to the emergency department after an intentional ingestion of polyethylene glycol (PEG)-200. What toxicity might be expected?
   A. Profuse diarrhea
   B. Renal tubular necrosis
   C. Bradycardia and QRS widening
   D. Cerebral intravascular hemorrhage
   E. Breakdown of the corneal epithelium

46.9. A 22-year-old woman presents to the emergency department after an intentional oral overdose of a medication that contains sorbitol. What toxicity might be expected?
   A. Profuse diarrhea
   B. Renal tubular necrosis
   C. Bradycardia and QRS widening
   D. Cerebral intravascular hemorrhage
   E. Breakdown of the corneal epithelium

46.10. Between 1995 and 1996, in Haiti, at least 86 children developed acute anuric kidney failure after ingesting acetaminophen syrup. Which of the following xenobiotics led to the kidney toxicity?
   A. 5-Oxoproline
   B. Glutathione
   C. *N*-Acetyl-*p*-benzoquinone
   D. Diethylene glycol
   E. Propylene glycol

ANSWERS

46.1. Answer: E. Propylene glycol is the typical diluent for lorazepam and causes hemodynamic instability, both as a rate-related event and in the setting of progressive lactic acidosis as it is metabolized. Propylene glycol causes hyperosmolarity, an elevated anion gap metabolic acidosis, and an increased lactate concentration. Propylene glycol also causes nephrotoxicity due to renal tubular necrosis.

Arroliga AC, et al. Relationship of continuous infusion lorazepam to serum propylene glycol concentration in critically ill adults. *Crit Care Med*. 2004;32:1709-1714.

Horinek EL, et al. Propylene glycol accumulation in critically ill patients receiving continuous intravenous lorazepam infusions. *Ann Pharmacother*. 2009;43:1964-1971.

Wilson KC, et al. Propylene glycol toxicity: A severe iatrogenic illness in ICU patients receiving IV benzodiazepines: A case series and prospective, observational pilot study. *Chest*. 2005;3:1674-1681.

46.2. Answer: B. Though the "gasping" syndrome was originally attributed to the immature metabolic capabilities of neonates, it was later found that neonates actually have an increased ability to metabolize benzyl alcohol to benzoic acid. Neonates have a glycine deficiency and therefore cannot further metabolize benzoic acid to hippuric acid. These neonates were exposed to benzyl alcohol through medications reconstituted with bacteriostatic (not sterile water for injection) water preserved with benzyl alcohol.

Brown WJ, et al. Fatal benzyl alcohol poisoning in an neonatal intensive care unit. *Lancet*. 1982;1:1250.

Gershanik J, et al. The gasping syndrome and benzyl alcohol poisoning. *N Engl J Med*. 1982;307:1384-1388.

46.3. Answer: E. In very low birth weight infants, in addition to "gasping" syndrome benzyl alcohol is also associated with increased rates of intracerebral hemorrhage, developmental delay, and cerebral palsy.

Benda GI, et al. Benzyl alcohol toxicity. Impact on neurologic handicaps among surviving very-low-birth-weight infants. *Pediatrics*. 1986; 77:507-512.

46.4. Answer: B. E-Ferol was a parenteral formulation of vitamin E that led to at least 38 deaths. It contained 25 units/mL of alpha-tocopherol acetate, 90% polysorbate 80, 1% polysorbate 20, and water. The toxicity was due to the polysorbate emulsifiers.

Alade SL, et al. Polysorbate 80 and E-Ferol toxicity. *Pediatrics.* 1986;77:593-597.

46.5. Answer: A. Benzalkonium chloride (BAC) is a commonly used preservative in ophthalmic, otic, and nasal formulations. When it is used as an ophthalmic preservative, the concentration ranges from 0.004-0.01%. Higher concentrations are associated with increased ocular toxicity. BAC leads to intracellular matrix dissolution and loss of epithelial superficial layers. Patients report intractable pain and photophobia.

Lemp MA, Zimmerman LE. Toxic endothelial degeneration in ocular surface disease treated with topical medications containing benzalkonium chloride. *Am J Ophthamol.* 1988;105:670-673.

46.6. Answer: A. Chlorobutanol is closely related to trichloroethanol, the active metabolite of chloral hydrate. Chlorobutanol causes central nervous system depression following acute poisonings. Because chlorobutanol, is a chlorinated hydrocarbon, it also sensitizes the myocardium to catecholamines.

Borody T, et al. Chlorobutanol toxicity and dependence. *Med J Aust.* 1979;1:288.

DeChristoforro R, et al. High dose morphine complicated by chlorobutanol-somnolence. *Ann Intern Med.* 1983;98:335-336.

Nordt SP. Chlorobutanol toxicity. *Ann Pharmacother.* 1996;30:1179-1180.

46.7. Answer: C. Systemic toxicity from topical phenol occurs when high concentrations are used as a chemical peel solution. There are case reports of patients who developed dysrhythmias, including ventricular tachycardia, who improved with local irrigation of the skin and intravenous lidocaine.

Unlu RE, et al. Phenol intoxication in a child. *J Craniofac Surg.* 2004;15:1010-1013.

46.8. Answer: B. Patients who ingest low-molecular-weight PEG (200 and 300) (not to be confused with high-molecular-weight PEG that is used for whole bowel irrigation) develop acute tubular necrosis, oliguria, and an anion gap metabolic acidosis. The metabolic acidosis is due to the metabolism of lower weight PEG by alcohol dehydrogenase to hydroxyacid and diacid metabolites.

Erickson TB, et al. Acute renal toxicity after ingestion of lava light liquid. *Ann Emerg Med.* 1996;27:781-784.

Sturgill BC, et al. Renal tubular necrosis in burn patients treated with topical polyethylene glycol. *Lab Invest.* 1982;46:81A.

Herold DA, et al. Oxidation of polyethylene glycols by alcohol dehydrogenase. *Biochem Pharmacol.* 1989;38:73-76.

46.9. Answer: A. Sorbitol leads to fluid shifts within the gastrointestinal tract and, in large ingested doses, produces abdominal cramping, flatulence, vomiting, and profuse diarrhea with ensuing electrolyte disturbances. Since sorbitol is metabolized to fructose in the liver, people with hereditary fructose deficiency are also at risk of developing hypoglycemia and death.

Hill DB, et al. Osmotic diarrhea by sugar-free theophylline solution in critically ill patients. *J Parenter Enteral Nutr.* 1991;15:332-336.

46.10. Answer: D. Many outbreaks were reported in the last century in which diethylene glycol was used as a solvent for liquid medication. These events occurred in the United States, Haiti, South Africa, Bangladesh, Nigeria, and Panama and were usually discovered when multiple cases of anuric kidney failure occurred simultaneously. In addition to kidney failure, these patients developed a metabolic acidosis followed by neurologic findings that, included a bilateral cranial nerve VII palsy, peripheral neuropathy, and encephalopathy.

Centers for Disease Control and Prevention. Fatalities associated with ingestion of diethylene glycol-contaminated glycerin used to manufacture acetaminophen syrup—Haiti, November 1995–June 1996. *MMWR Morb Mortal Wkly Rep.* 1996;45:649-650.

Antidiabetics and Hypoglycemics/Antiglycemics

47

QUESTIONS

47.1. Which of the following laboratory findings is diagnostic of an exogenous insulin overdose in a hypoglycemic patient with a high insulin concentration?
- A. A persistent blood glucose concentration <50 mg/dL (3.3 mmol/L)
- B. An alpha-acid glycoprotein concentration >3 mg/mL (0.75 µmol/L)
- C. A low C-peptide concentration
- D. The elevated insulin concentration alone is sufficient
- E. A low glucagon concentration

47.2. A 4-year-old malnourished girl is brought into an emergency department in India after she was found seizing in an orchard. Her point-of-care blood glucose is 39 mg/dL (2.16 mmol/L). She was found next to a pile of fruits. What toxin is responsible for the patient's presentation?
- A. Methylenecyclopropylglycine
- B. Pyrinuron
- C. Oleandrin
- D. Alloxan hydrate
- E. Chlorpyrifos

47.3. Which of the following options is the most appropriate therapy for patients with recurrent hypoglycemia following a sulfonylurea overdose?
- A. Dextrose then octreotide
- B. Dextrose then diazoxide
- C. Octreotide then streptozotocin
- D. Dextrose then fructose
- E. Octreotide is the first-line therapy

47.4. Which of the following drugs was withdrawn from the US market due to significant hepatic toxicity associated with therapeutic dosing?
- A. Repaglinide
- B. Troglitazone
- C. Rosiglitazone
- D. Pioglitazone
- E. Acarbose

47.5. A 22-year-old woman presents to the hospital following an intentional ingestion of her friend's quinidine. Her point-of-care blood glucose is 25 mg/dL (1.4 mmol/L). Despite receiving intravenous dextrose, she has recurrent episodes of hypoglycemia. What antidote is indicated at this time?
- A. Octreotide
- B. Glucagon
- C. Calcium gluconate
- D. Liraglutide
- E. Diazoxide

47.6. A 37-year-old man presents to the emergency department approximately 5 hours following an oral overdose of a long-acting insulin. His vital signs and blood glucose are within normal limits, as are the remainder of his laboratory values. He has an undetectable acetaminophen concentration. What are the next steps in management for this patient?
- A. Oral activated charcoal
- B. Initiation of a 10% dextrose infusion
- C. Admission for 24-hour observation with blood glucose checks every 2 hours
- D. Empiric administration of N-acetylcysteine
- E. Transfer to psychiatry

47.7. A 45-year-old woman develops an altered mental status following an overdose of aspirin. She is being treated with a sodium bicarbonate infusion. Her pH is 7.52 with an associated anion gap metabolic acidosis. Her salicylate concentration returns at 75 mg/dL (5.4 mmol/L). Her point-of-care blood glucose is 80 mg/dL (4.4 mmol/L). What is the next step in management?

A. Intubation
B. Administration of 25 g of dextrose intravenously
C. Immediate hemodialysis
D. Increase the rate of her sodium bicarbonate to three times maintenance
E. Administration of intravenous lipid emulsion therapy

47.8. A 67-year-old man presents to the emergency department after going out to a bar with friends. He feels very flushed, nauseated, and has vomited several times. He is visiting from another country, and his only medical history is diabetes, for which he takes an oral medication. What medication likely contributed to his presentation?

A. Glyburide
B. Metformin
C. Acarbose
D. Glimipiride
E. Chlorpropamide

47.9. A 52-year-old-man presents to the emergency department with abdominal cramping. He has a known history of diabetes and was recently started on a new medication. His point-of-care blood glucose in the emergency department is 100 mg/dL (5.55 mmol/L). His blood work reveals a pH of 7.25, a lactate of 1.0 mmol/L, and an anion gap of 18 mEq/L. A urinalysis is performed, and it shows negative nitrites, negative leukocytes, and moderate ketones. What medication is this patient taking for his diabetes?

A. Glyburide
B. Metformin
C. Canagliflozin
D. Acarbose
E. Chlorpropamide

47.10. A 27-year-old woman presents to the emergency department after an intentional ingestion of her grandmother's medication. Her blood work demonstrates a pH of 6.89, a lactate concentration of >25 mmol/L, an undetectably low serum bicarbonate and an anion gap of 38 mEq/L. Her serum glucose is 105 mg/dL (5.83 mmol/L). Which medication did this patient overdose on?

A. Glyburide
B. Metformin
C. Canagliflozin
D. Acarbose
E. Chlorpropamide

ANSWERS

47.1. Answer: C. A C-peptide concentration of <0.2 nmol/L is diagnostic of an exogenous insulin exposure in a hypoglycemic patient with an elevated insulin concentration. Endogenous insulin increases both insulin and C-peptide concentrations as does administration of a sulfonylurea. All the commercially available insulins do not contain C-peptide. Proinsulin is present with endogenous insulin and sulfonylureas but would be absent with exogenous insulin. Urinary concentrations of sulfonylurea metabolites would distinguish between a sulfonylurea and an insulinoma as the cause of hypoglycemia.

Bauman WA, Yalow RS. Hyperinsulinemic hypoglycemia: Differential diagnosis by determination of the species of circulatory insulin. *JAMA.* 1984;252:2730-2734.

47.2. Answer: A. In the Muzaffarpur district of Bihar state in India, there are outbreaks of acute neurologic illness among children, typically starting in June and lasting several weeks. Patients with worse outcomes are more likely to have

a serum blood glucose of <70 mg/dL (3.89 mmol/L). This seasonal epidemic is linked to methylenecyclopropylglycine, a toxin found in lychee, as well as hypoglycin A, which is also found in unripe ackee fruit. Susceptibility is generally related to the patient's underlying nutritional status. Alloxan is a glucose analogue that destroys pancreatic beta cells. Pyrinuron (PNU), which was sold under the brand name Vacor, leads to beta islet cell destruction and resultant hyperglycemia and drug-induced type 1 diabetes mellitus (DM). Chlorpyrifos is an organophosphate compound, and toxicity would include muscarinic findings; it does not typically cause hypoglycemia. Oleandrin is a cardioactive steroid found in the oleander plant and leads to cardiac toxicity that resembles digoxin toxicity.

Shrivastava A, et al; Centers for Disease Control and Prevention (CDC). Outbreaks of unexplained neurologic illness - Muzaffarpur, India, 2013-2014. *MMWR Morb Mortal Wkly Rep.* 2015;64:49-53.

47.3. Answer: A. Following resolution of the hypoglycemia, octreotide is the drug of choice and is indicated in the management of sulfonylurea-related hypoglycemia that is refractory to or recurrent following dextrose administration. Diazoxide, like octreotide, inhibits sulfonylurea-induced insulin release from beta islet cells. However, hypotension occurs as a side effect, and the treatment is not readily available. Streptozotocin, a medication that destroys pancreatic islet cells, is used to treat patients with insulinomas; however, it takes hours to days to increase glucose concentrations and occasionally results in permanent diabetes. Fructose will have no effect on increasing the blood glucose.

Boyle PJ, et al. Octreotide reverses hyperinsulinemia and prevents hypoglycemia induced sulfonylurea overdoses. *J Clin Endrocrinol Metab.* 1993;76:752-756.

McLaughlin SA, et al. Octreotide: An antidote for sulfonylurea-induced hypoglycemia. *Ann Emerg Med.* 2000;36:133-138.

Palatnick W, et al. Clinical spectrum of sulfonylurea overdose and experience with diazoxide therapy. *Arch Intern Med.* 1991;151:1859-1862.

47.4. Answer: B. Troglitazone was withdrawn from the US pharmaceutical market in 2000 because of liver toxicity which developed in patients on therapeutic doses. Some cases were severe, requiring liver transplantation. A defect in metabolism of a unique side chain that produces a highly reactive metabolite is thought to be the cause, and likely why rosiglitazone and pioglitazone are rarely implicated in causing liver toxicity. Elevated aminotransferase concentrations occur in some patients receiving acarbose, but most patients are asymptomatic, and resolution occurs after medication discontinuation.

Gitlin N, et al. Two cases of severe clinical and histologic hepatotoxicity associated with troglitazone. *Ann Intern Med.* 1998;129:36-38.

Hollander P. Safety of acarbose, an alpha-glucosidase inhibitor. *Drugs.* 1992;21:20-24.

Neuschwander-Tetri BA, et al. Troglitazone-induced hepatic failure leading to liver transplantation. A case report. *Ann Intern Med.* 1998;129:38-41.

47.5. Answer: A. Quinidine and quinine cause hypoglycemia in overdose. They act on the ligand-gated potassium channels and prevent the efflux of potassium, which then causes a secondary rise in intracellular calcium concentrations and eventually increased insulin release. This mechanism of action is similar to that of the sulfonylureas.

Octreotide inhibits calcium entry through the calcium channel and inhibits insulin release. Historically, diazoxide was used to treat sulfonylurea-induced hypoglycemia, but it is no longer used for that indication due to its significant side effect profile.

Phillips RE, et al. Effectiveness of SMS 201–995, a synthetic long-acting somatostatin analogue in treatment of quinine-induced hyperinsulinaemia. *Lancet.* 1986;1:713-716.

47.6. Answer: E. Intramuscular and subcutaneous insulin overdoses are associated with hypoglycemia. Following overdoses of long-acting insulin, 24-hour admission for frequent blood glucose monitoring is indicated. However, *oral* insulin is degraded by gut enzymes, does not have significant systemic absorption, and is, therefore, benign. While there is a case report of hypoglycemia following an oral overdose of 3,000 units of insulin, this is incredibly unusual. Unless there is another concerning ingestion, there is no indication for oral activated charcoal or admission to the hospital. Given that this patient has a negative acetaminophen concentration and normal laboratory studies, it is safe to medically clear and transfer to the psychiatric service for further management.

Svingos RS, et al. Life-threatening hypoglycemia associated with intentional insulin ingestion. *Pharmacotherapy.* 2013;33:e28-e33.

47.7. Answer: B. Aspirin toxicity is associated with neuroglycopenia. Patients develop an altered mental status despite a normal serum blood glucose. In patients who develop an altered mental status, the initial management should be empiric administration of intravenous dextrose, even if the point-of-care dextrose is normal. If a patient's mental status does not improve following administration of dextrose, then the patient should receive emergent hemodialysis. There is no indication for intubation in this patient, and empiric intubation should be avoided as acidemia is associated with a significant risk of mortality. The patient's pH is 7.52, so there is no indication to increase the rate of the bicarbonate infusion. Intravenous lipid emulsion therapy is not indicated following overdose of aspirin.

Kuzak N, et al. Reversal of salicylate-induced euglycemic delirium with dextrose. *Clin Toxicology.* 2007;45:526-529.

47.8. Answer: E. Chlorpropamide, a very-long-acting first-generation sulfonylurea, is no longer used as a treatment for diabetes in the US. It causes a disulfiram-like reaction by blocking the metabolism of acetaldehyde, the first by-product of ethanol metabolism. It also causes the syndrome of inappropriate antidiuretic hormone secretion (SIADH).

These two side effects are uncommon with the newer generation sulfonylureas.

Podgainy H, Bressler R. Biochemical basis of the sulfonylurea-induced Antabuse syndrome. *Diabetes*. 1968;17:679-683.

47.9. Answer: C. Canagliflozin is a sodium-glucose cotransporter-2 (SGLT2) inhibitor and causes euglycemic diabetic ketoacidosis, even in therapeutic doses. As patients taking this medication have a normal serum glucose, diabetic ketoacidosis is easily overlooked. It is very important to pay attention to the serum bicarbonate concentration and check for urinary ketones in patients who are on an SGLT2 inhibitor.

Taylor SI, et al. SGLT2 inhibitors may predispose to ketoacidosis. *J Clin Endocrinol Metab*. 2015;100:2849-2852.

47.10. Answer: B. Metformin is a biguanide that leads to a metabolic acidosis with an elevated lactate concentration (MALA). The mechanism leading to an elevated lactate is complex; however, the biguanides interfere with cellular aerobic metabolism and lead to mitochondrial dysfunction. MALA occurs more frequently in patients who have underlying renal dysfunction. It is important to note that the Cochrane review that states that metformin is not associated with MALA is erroneous, as their review did not assess patients who had an intentional overdose or who had underlying kidney dysfunction.

Calello DP, et al. Extracorporeal treatment for metformin poisoning: Systemic review and recommendations from the extracorporeal treatments in poisoning workgroup. *Crit Care Med*. 2015;43:1716-1730.

Antiepileptics

48

QUESTIONS

48.1. A 45-year-old woman with a past medical history of a mood disorder presents to the emergency department after an intentional ingestion of her own medication. On physical examination, she is drowsy and mildly tachypneic. Her initial venous blood gas shows: pH, 7.35; PCO_2, 32 mmHg; bicarbonate, 17 mmol/L; and lactate, 1.5 mmol/L. Her serum electrolytes are: sodium, 139 mmol/L; potassium, 4.2 mmol/L, chloride, 112 mmol/L; bicarbonate, 17 mmol/L; blood urea nitrogen, 12 mg/dL (4.3 mmol/L); and creatinine, 0.8 mg/dL (70.7 micromol/L). What did she most likely overdose on?
A. Lamotrigine
B. Topiramate
C. Lithium
D. Valproate
E. Carbamazepine

48.2. A 27-year-old woman presents to the emergency department with 1 day of fevers, a rash, facial edema, and elevated hepatic aminotransferases. Six weeks earlier, her neurologist added carbamazepine to her treatment regimen. Of the following alternative antiepileptics, which is safe for her to take once she recovers from her current presentation?
A. Valproic acid
B. Phenytoin
C. Lamotrigine
D. Levetiracetam
E. Phenobarbital

48.3. A 42-year-old man presents to the hospital after ingesting a handful of his seizure medication. He now has difficulty walking, lethargy, and nystagmus. His symptoms persist for nearly 5 days. Serum antiepileptic concentrations are persistently elevated, dropping only 50% after 3 days. What mechanism would most likely explain the persistent symptoms and elevated serum concentration?
A. Pharmacobezoar
B. Continued ingestion while hospitalized
C. Saturation of hydroxylation reaction
D. Redistribution of drug from adipose tissue
E. Increased circulating unbound drug

48.4. Children who overdose on carbamazepine develop which of the following findings that does not typically occur in adults?
A. Ileus
B. Hypoglycemia
C. Electrocardiographic abnormalities
D. Choreoathetosis
E. Hyponatremia

48.5. Which of the following anticonvulsants has a metabolite that is almost as active as the parent compound?
A. Phenytoin
B. Carbamazepine
C. Gabapentin
D. Vigabatrin
E. Lamotrigine

48.6. A 44-year-old man with a history of epilepsy and acid reflux presents to the emergency department with ataxia and sedation. His phenytoin concentration is 50 mcg/mL (198 micromol/L). The therapeutic range of phenytoin is 10-20 mcg/mL (39.6-79.3 micromol/L). Which xenobiotics is most likely responsible for his presentation?

A. Ranitidine
B. Cimetidine
C. Famotidine
D. Cyproheptadine
E. Diphenhydramine

48.7. Which of the following anticonvulsants causes a prolonged QRS complex duration after an acute ingestion?

A. Gabapentin
B. Felbamate
C. Lamotrigine
D. Vigabatrin
E. Tiagabine

48.8. A 52-year-old man presents to the emergency department comatose after an intentional overdose of valproic acid. A serum valproic acid concentration returns at 1,000 mg/L (6,934 micromol/L). The therapeutic concentration for valproic acid is 50-100 mg/L (347-693 micromol/L). Which of the following therapies is recommended?

A. Oral L-carnitine
B. Fomepizole
C. *N*-Acetylcysteine
D. Exchange transfusion
E. Hemodialysis

48.9. A 54-year-old man with a long-standing history of gabapentin use presents to the emergency department with agitation, confusion, and tachycardia. His wife notes that he abruptly discontinued his gabapentin. Which of the following medications is most reasonable to treat his withdrawal?

A. Gabapentin
B. Clonidine
C. Lorazepam
D. Chlordiazepoxide
E. Phenobarbital

48.10. A 27-year-old man develops edema and a purple discoloration to his right hand 7 hours after receiving an intravenous antiepileptic medication. The discoloration progresses to the point of necrosis, and he requires an amputation. Which of the following antiepileptics led to this patient's presentation?

A. Levetiracetam
B. Valproic acid
C. Phenytoin
D. Topiramate
E. Phenobarbital

ANSWERS

48.1. Answer: B. The patient has hyperchloremia and a primary non-anion gap metabolic acidosis with respiratory compensation, most consistent with topiramate overdose. Topiramate is a weak carbonic anhydrase II inhibitor that causes a renal tubular acidosis (RTA) through its action at the proximal tubule. Lithium is associated with a normal or reduced anion gap in overdose. The other choices are not associated with a specific primary acid–base abnormality.

Fakhoury T, et al. Topiramate overdose: Clinical and laboratory features. *Epilepsy Behav.* 2002;3:185-189.

Traub SJ, et al. Acute topiramate toxicity. *J Toxicol Clin Toxicol.* 2003;41:987-990.

48.2. Answer: A. This patient has drug-induced hypersensitivity syndrome (DIHS), formally known as drug reaction with eosinophilia and systemic symptoms (DRESS). Treatment begins with discontinuing the offending drug and starting a corticosteroid. In one study, 90% of patients showed an in vitro cross-reactivity to other aromatic antiepileptics, so they should be avoided. Acceptable alternatives include valproic acid, benzodiazepines, gabapentin, topiramate, and tiagabine.

Knowles S, et al. Anticonvulsant hypersensitivity syndrome: An update. *Expert Opin Drug Saf.* 2012;11:767-778.

48.3. Answer: C. This patient overdosed on phenytoin based on his clinical findings and the demonstration of a prolonged apparent half-life after ingestion. Phenytoin typically exhibits first-order kinetics in therapeutic ranges. However, at increased concentrations, it begins to demonstrate metabolism closer to zero-order due to saturation of hydroxylation, which results in an apparent half-life of 20-105 hours. This type of kinetics is known as Michaelis-Menten kinetics.

Craig S. Phenytoin poisoning. *Neurocrit Care.* 2005;3:161-170.

48.4. Answer: D. There is a higher incidence of dystonic reactions, seizures, and choreoathetosis in children who overdose on carbamazepine. Hyponatremia is associated with chronic carbamazepine toxicity in adults. The other electrolyte abnormalities do not typically occur following carbamazepine overdoses. Pediatric carbamazepine overdoses are not associated with ileus, although carbamazepine has mild anticholinergic activity.

Gandelman MS. Review of carbamazepine-induced hyponatremia. *Prog Neuro-Psychopharmacol Biol Psychiatry*. 1994;18:211-233.

Stremski ES, et al. Pediatric carbamazepine intoxication. *Ann Emerg Med*. 1995;25:624-630.

48.5. Answer: B. Gabapentin, felbamate, lamotrigine, and phenytoin have no active metabolites. Carbamazepine-10,11-epoxide is a carbamazepine metabolite that is almost as active as the parent compound. Therapeutic serum concentrations of carbamazepine are 4-12 mg/L (169-508 micromol/L). Carbamazepine-10,11-epoxide concentrations are 1-10 mg/L and exceed 10 mg/L when lamotrigine or valproic acid is co-ingested due to epoxide hydrolase inhibition. Because of this active metabolite, patients are at risk of developing toxicity following the addition of lamotrigine or valproic acid.

Dichter MA, Brodie MJ. New antiepileptic drugs. *N Engl J Med*. 1996;334:1583-1590.

48.6. Answer: B. Cimetidine is responsible for numerous drug-drug interactions because it inhibits several cytochrome P450 enzymes, including CYP2C19. Phenytoin is metabolized by CYP2C19, so inhibitors will increase phenytoin concentrations. Ranitidine and famotidine are H_2 antihistamines but do not have the same hepatic metabolism. Cyproheptadine and diphenhydramine are H_1 antihistamines that do not affect CYP metabolism.

Bartle WR, et al. Dose-dependent effect of cimetidine on phenytoin kinetics. *Clin Pharmacol Ther*. 1983;33:649-655.

48.7. Answer: C. Patients who overdose on lamotrigine frequently present with a prolonged QRS complex duration, Brugadalike electrocardiographic abnormalities, and third-degree heart block. The prolonged QRS complex duration is likely due to sodium channel blockade.

Strimel WJ, et al. Brugada-like electrocardiographic pattern induced by lamotrigine toxicity. *Clin Neuropharmacol*. 2010;33:265-267.

Nogar JN, et al. Severe sodium channel blockade and cardiovascular collapse due to massive lamotrigine overdose. *J Toxicol Clin Toxicol*. 2011;49:854-857.

48.8. Answer: E. While valproic acid is tightly bound to protein, following a massive overdose protein saturation occurs and a greater proportion of free valproic acid is present. Hemodialysis is recommended in patients who have valproic acid concentrations that are >900 mg/L (6,241 micromol/L), patients who are comatose, have respiratory depression, or have a pH <7.10. While L-carnitine is added on to the treatment regimen of patients who are poisoned with valproic acid, intravenous L-carnitine is recommended for patients who are symptomatic. Currently, there is no role for fomepizole, *N*-acetylcysteine, or exchange transfusion in the management of valproic acid toxicity.

Ghannoum M, et al. The extracorporeal treatment of valproic acid poisoning: Systematic review and recommendations from the EXTRIP workgroup. *Clin Toxicol*. 2015;53:454-465.

48.9. Answer: A. While gabapentin is structurally like gamma-aminobutyric acid (GABA), it does not mimic GABA when it is applied to GABA neurons. Patients who withdraw from gabapentin develop agitation, confusion, tachycardia, and seizures. Unfortunately, gabapentin withdrawal does not respond well to benzodiazepines; therefore, patients who present with gabapentin withdrawal should be treated with tapering doses of gabapentin.

Mersfelder TL, Nichols WH. Gabapentin: Abuse, dependence, and withdrawal. *Ann Pharmacother*. 2016;50:229-233.

48.10. Answer: C. This patient developed purple glove syndrome as a complication of intravenous phenytoin administration. The exact pathophysiology is unclear; however, it is hypothesized to occur as a result of micro-extravasations. Symptoms typically occur between 2 and 12 hours following the intravenous drug infusion. The symptoms begin as edema and discoloration distal to the site of administration. Severe cases progress to necrosis and occasionally need amputation. Purple glove syndrome also occurs with fosphenytoin; however, the risk is lower than with phenytoin.

Burneo JG, et al. A prospective study of the incidence of the purple glove syndrome. *Epilepsia*. 2001;42:1156-1159.

Garbovski LA, et al. Purple glove syndrome after phenytoin or fosphenytoin administration: Review of reported cases and recommendations for prevention. *J Med Toxicol*. 2015;11:445-459.

Antihistamines and Decongestants

QUESTIONS

49.1. Terfenadine and astemizole inhibit which of the following sites?
A. The slow calcium channel
B. The H_2 receptor
C. Efferent chloride currents
D. The delayed rectifier potassium channel
E. Efferent calcium fluxes at the sarcoplasmic reticulum

49.2. Which of the following decongestants is most likely to cause hypertension and bradycardia?
A. Phenylpropanolamine
B. Pseudoephedrine
C. Terbutaline
D. Ephedrine
E. Isoephedrine

49.3. A 27-year-old woman presents to the emergency department with a severe headache and left-sided weakness after ingesting a decongestant that she found in her parent's attic. A computed tomography (CT) scan of her brain demonstrates an intracranial hemorrhage. Which of the following decongestants most likely caused her presentation?
A. Phenylpropanolamine
B. Pseudoephedrine

C. Terbutaline
D. Ephedrine
E. Isoephedrine

49.4. A 22-year-old man presents to the emergency department after an intentional overdose of an antihistamine. His laboratory analysis reveals a creatine phosphokinase that is higher than the laboratory upper limit of reporting, consistent with rhabdomyolysis. Which of the following antihistamines best explains this finding?
A. Loratadine
B. Brompheniramine
C. Doxylamine
D. Pyrilamine
E. Astemizole

49.5. A 24-year-old woman presents to the emergency department following an intentional overdose of an antihistamine. She has a generalized tonic-clonic seizure that resolves following a dose of lorazepam. An electrocardiogram is performed and demonstrates a QRS interval of 140 msec. Which of the following antihistamines best explains her presentation?
A. Loratadine
B. Cetirizine
C. Doxylamine
D. Ranitidine
E. Diphenhydramine

49.6. An 18-year-old man presents to the emergency department after having a generalized tonic-clonic seizure at home. His vital signs are: blood pressure, 168/90 mmHg; heart rate, 154 beats/min; respiratory rate, 15 breaths/min; and temperature 100.8 °F (38.2 °C). On examination, he has dilated pupils that react only minimally, dry mucous membranes, garbled speech, and a very distended bladder. He has active hallucinations and appears to be picking at things. An electrocardiogram is performed, which demonstrates a QRS interval of 89 msec. Which of the following interventions would be the best next step to perform on this patient?
A. Computed tomography (CT) scan of the patient brain
B. Lumbar puncture
C. Administer lorazepam
D. Administer ceftriaxone, vancomycin, and acyclovir
E. Administer physostigmine

49.7. A 5-year-old boy presents to the emergency department following an ingestion of oxymetazoline nasal spray. Which of the following signs or symptoms is likely to occur initially following this ingestion?
A. Hypertension
B. Tachycardia
C. Agitation

D. Tachypnea
E. Hypertonia

49.8. Which of the following imidazolines also acts as a histamine H_2 agonist?
A. Xylometazoline
B. Naphazoline
C. Oxymetazoline
D. Tetrahydrozoline
E. Neumotazoline

49.9. Which of the following therapies is reasonable in a 3-year-old boy who presents following an ingestion of naphazoline?
A. Naloxone
B. Lorazepam
C. Flumazenil
D. Clonidine
E. Physostigmine

49.10. *Citrus aurantium*, also known as bitter orange, contains which of the following active ingredients?
A. Ephedra
B. Ephedrine
C. Pseudoephedrine
D. *p*-Synephrine
E. Tetrahydrozoline

ANSWERS

49.1. Answer: D. Terfenadine and astemizole are antihistamines that are no longer approved for use in the United States. Terfenadine inhibits the outward potassium current of the delayed rectifier potassium channel, leading to prolongation of the QT interval and an increased risk of torsade de pointes. The cardiac toxicity occurred because of accumulation of the parent drug (terfenadine) due to inhibition of drug elimination by other xenobiotics, such as astemizole.

Yang T, et al. Mechanism of block of a human cardiac potassium channel by terfenadine racemate and enantiomers. *J Pharmacol.* 1995;115:267-274.

49.2. Answer: A. Phenylpropanolamine (PPA) is a pure alpha adrenergic agonist. It commonly causes a reflex bradycardia. The other medications have beta adrenergic activity and cause tachycardia.

Woo OF, et al. Atrioventricular conduction block caused by phenylpropanolamine. *JAMA.* 1985;253:2646-2647.

49.3. Answer: A. As described in Question 49.2, phenylpropanolamine (PPA) is an alpha adrenergic agonist. There were at least 22 cases of hemorrhagic strokes reported to the US Food and Drug Administration (FDA) between 1991 and 2000 and >30 cases reported in the literature. A statistical analysis demonstrated that PPA was an independent risk factor for the development of hemorrhagic stroke in women. This led to the FDA recommending the removal of PPA from the United States market in 2000.

Kernan WN, et al. Phenylpropanolamine and the risk of hemorrhagic stroke. *N Engl J Med.* 2000;343:1826-1832.

Cantu C, et al. Stroke associated with sympathomimetics contained in over-the-counter cough and cold drugs. *Stroke.* 2003;34:1667-1672.

49.4. Answer: C. Doxylamine is unique among the antihistamines in that in overdose it causes rhabdomyolysis. This is a nontraumatic rhabdomyolysis and occurs in the absence of seizures or prolonged coma.

Mendoza FS, et al. Rhabdomyolysis complicating doxylamine overdose. *Clin Pediatr.* 1987;26:595-597.

49.5. Answer: E. Diphenhydramine is associated with seizures when adults ingest a dose >1.5 g. Diphenhydramine also causes sodium channel blockade, and in overdose, leads to QRS prolongation with findings on the electrocardiogram that are similar in appearance to the electrocardiogram of patients who overdose on tricyclic antidepressants. Hypertonic sodium bicarbonate reverses the QRS prolongation that occurs with diphenhydramine overdose.

Radovanovic D, et al. Dose-dependent toxicity of diphenhydramine overdose. *Hum Exp Toxicol.* 2000;19:489-495.

Jang DH, et al. Status epilepticus and wide-complex tachycardia secondary to diphenhydramine overdose. *Clin Toxicol (Phila).* 2010;48:945-948.

Sharma AN, et al. Diphenhydramine-induced wide complex dysrhythmia responds to treatment with sodium bicarbonate. *Am J Emerg Med.* 2003;21:212-215.

49.6. Answer: E. In most circumstances, patients who have an elevated temperature, altered mental status, and a seizure should be treated empirically for encephalitis; they should also have a head CT and a lumbar puncture performed. As this patient has a narrow QRS interval and an examination consistent with antimuscarinic toxicity, we recommend starting by treating with physostigmine. Physostigmine is both therapeutic and diagnostic. Physostigmine also leads to less interventions (such as a lumbar puncture), less imaging, and a shorter hospital stay. Physostigmine is also safer than benzodiazepines in the treatment of antimuscarinic poisoning.

Burns MJ, et al. A comparison of physostigmine and benzodiazepines for the treatment of anticholinergic poisoning. *Ann Emerg Med.* 2000;35:374-381.

49.7. Answer: A. When ingested, oxymetazoline is a pure central and peripheral alpha$_2$ adrenergic receptor agonist. Toxicity resembles that of clonidine. Patients present acutely with hypertension, which eventually progresses to hypotension. They also have bradycardia, hypoventilation, and central nervous system depression.

Higgins G, et al. Pediatric poisoning from over-the-counter imidazoline-containing products. *Ann Emerg Med.* 1991;20:655-658.

49.8. Answer: D. Tetrahydrozoline, which is available without prescription in the US as an ophthalmic preparation to decrease conjunctival injection, is also a histamine H$_2$ agonist in addition to an alpha adrenergic agonist. Stimulation of H$_2$ increases the production of acid in the stomach. Neumotazoline is not a decongestant.

Higgins GL, et al. Pediatric poisoning from over-the-counter imidazoline-containing products. *Ann Emerg Med.* 1991;20:655-658.

49.9. Answer: A. Naphazoline, which is an imidazoline, causes toxicity that resembles clonidine when ingested. There are case reports of children with respiratory depression following an imidazoline overdose who responded to naloxone. While the data are sparse, naloxone is well tolerated in opioid-naïve children, and therefore, it is a reasonable intervention.

Katar S, et al. Naloxone use in a newborn with apnea due to tetrahydrozoline intoxication. *Pediatr Int.* 2010;52:488-489.

49.10. Answer: D. The US Food and Drug Administration (FDA) banned the sale of dietary supplements that contain ephedra in 2004 as there was a high incidence of cardiovascular events associated with their abuse. Since then, manufactures have substituted *Citrus aurantium* and have marketed their products as "ephedra free." The main ingredient in *Citrus aurantium* is *p*-synephrine. There are reports of "ephedra-free" dietary supplements leading to ischemic strokes.

Retamero C, et al. "Ephedra-free" diet pill-induced psychosis. *Psychosomatics.* 2011;52:579-582.

Bouchard NC, et al. Ischemic stroke associated with use of an ephedra-free dietary supplement containing synephrine. *Mayo Clin Proc.* 2005;80:541-545.

Chemotherapeutics

50

QUESTIONS

50.1. A 57-year-old man was unintentionally administered three times the intended amount of cisplatin intravenously. The possible side effects of this chemotherapeutic include nephrotoxicity, myelosuppression, seizures, retinal toxicity, and a sensory neuropathy. Which antidote is most appropriate to prevent the nephrotoxicity?

A. Amifostine

B. Dexrazoxane

C. Mesna

D. Glucarpidase

E. Uridine triacetate

50.2. A 28-year-old man is undergoing treatment for Hodgkin lymphoma. He is inadvertently prescribed a 10-fold overdose of one of his chemotherapeutics. He is found to have pancytopenia. All his medications are stopped, and he is started on granulocyte colony-stimulating factor (G-CSF). However, after 5 weeks of treatment, his cell lines have not yet recovered. Which of the following chemotherapeutics best explains this patient's prolonged pancytopenia?

A. Amygdalin

B. Doxorubicin

C. Brentuximab

D. Vinblastine

E. Lomustine

50.3. A 21-year-old man with recurrent stage IIIB seminoma presents to the emergency department for fever, hematuria, and dysuria. He is currently undergoing his third of four etoposide-ifosfamide-cisplatin (VIP) treatment cycles. Which of the following statements is most accurate?

A. Methylene blue should be administered

B. Most cases of hemorrhagic cystitis are prevented with medication pretreatment

C. Bladder irrigation with thiosulfate solution is indicated

D. A chest radiograph is indicated to exclude drug-induced lung injury

E. A localizing Rinne and Weber test suggests cisplatin ototoxicity

50.4. A 45-year-old man is on the FOLFIRI regimen, which includes 5-fluorouracil, leucovorin, and irinotecan, as a treatment for colon cancer. He is also taking ondansetron for occasional nausea and acetaminophen for pain. Shortly after the infusion is complete, he begins to feel dizzy and weak and has difficulty breathing. He has abdominal cramping and diarrhea. His vitals after the episode demonstrated a heart rate of 35 beats/min. He is very diaphoretic and has diffuse expiratory wheezing. An adverse effect of which therapy best explains his symptoms?

A. 5-Fluorouracil

B. Leucovorin

C. Irinotecan

D. Ondansetron

E. Acetaminophen

50.5. Which of the following cardiac manifestations is a dose-dependent response to doxorubicin?
A. Dysrhythmias
B. QT interval prolongation
C. Pericarditis
D. Myocarditis
E. Cardiomyopathy

50.6. Which of the following antidotes helps to minimize the dose-dependent cardiac toxicity that occurs with doxorubicin?
A. Mesna
B. Methylene blue
C. Glucarpidase
D. Uridine triacetate
E. Dexrazoxane

50.7. Syndrome of inappropriate secretion of antidiuretic hormone (SIADH) is an adverse effect of which of the following chemotherapeutics?
A. Methotrexate
B. Cisplatin
C. Vincristine
D. Daunorubicin
E. Mitoxantrone

50.8. Which of the following chemotherapeutics has mono-amine oxidase inhibitor (MAO-I) activity?
A. Doxorubicin
B. Procarbazine
C. Carboplatin
D. Vinblastine
E. Chlorambucil

50.9. A 67-year-old man presents to the emergency department for further evaluation of abdominal pain. An upright chest radiograph is performed that demonstrates free air under the diaphragm. Which of the following chemotherapeutics best explains this patient's presentation?
A. Paclitaxel
B. Cytarabine
C. Bleomycin
D. Procarbazine
E. Doxorubicin

50.10. Which of the following xenobiotics is responsible for cyclophosphamide-induced hemorrhagic cystitis?
A. Pulegone
B. Acrolein
C. 1,2-Dibromo-3-chloropropane
D. Cantharidin
E. Trichosanthin

ANSWERS

50.1. Answer: A. Cisplatin, a platinum-based chemotherapeutic, causes acute kidney injury, sensory neuropathy, seizures, encephalopathy, ototoxicity, retinal toxicity, and myelosuppression. Both amifostine and thiosulfate are used to treat cisplatin-induced toxicity. Amifostine, which is a precursor to a thiol free radical scavenger, prevents cisplatin-induced nephrotoxicity. Dexrazoxane treats anthracycline overdoses. Mesna treats nitrogen mustard overdoses. Glucarpidase treats methotrexate overdoses. Uridine triacetate treats 5-fluorouracil overdoses.

Santini V, Giles FJ. The potential of amifostine: From cytoprotective to therapeutic agent. *Hematologia*. 1999;84:1035-1042.

50.2. Answer: E. Lomustine, an alkylating agent, is primarily used to treat central nervous system (CNS) tumors but is also used as a second-line agent for Hodgkin lymphoma. As it is directly toxic to progenitor cells, it leads to prolonged pancytopenia, significantly greater than the 2 weeks expected for other myelosuppressive chemotherapeutics.

Trent KC, et al. Multiorgan failure associated with lomustine overdose. *Ann Pharmacother*. 1995;29:384-386.

50.3. Answer: B. VIP is used to treat refractory germ cell cancer when there is a contraindication to bleomycin. When given prophylactically along with ifosfamide, mesna prevents most cases of cystitis. Methylene blue (intravenous or oral) improve ifosfamide-associated encephalopathy through an ill-defined mechanism. Other potential treatments for ifosfamide encephalopathy include diazepam, thiamine, albumin, and hemodialysis. Thiosulfate is given subcutaneously for certain chemotherapeutic extravasations. None of this patient's active chemotherapeutics are classically associated with lung injury. Cisplatin ototoxicity in VIP is common and is typically a bilateral sensorineural type.

Andriole GL, et al. The efficacy of mesna (2-mercaptoethane sodium sulfonate) as a uroprotectant in patients with hemorrhagic cystitis receiving further oxazaphosphorine chemotherapy. *J Clin Oncol*. 1987;5:799-803.

50.4. Answer: C. The patient in this case has symptoms that are consistent with a cholinergic toxidrome. Irinotecan, a topoisomerase I inhibitor, is used in the treatment of patients who have metastatic colon cancer. Irinotecan is associated with cholinergic toxicity.

Blandizzi C, et al. Cholinergic toxic syndrome by the anticancer drug irinotecan: Acetylcholinesterase does not play a major role. *Clin Pharmacol Ther*. 2002;71:263-271.

50.5. Answer: E. The incidence of developing congestive cardiomyopathy in patients receiving doxorubicin is between 1 and 10% when the cumulative dose is <450 mg/m^2 and becomes greater than 20% when >550 mg/m^2 is administered.

von Hoff DD, et al. Risk factors for doxorubicin induced congestive heart failure. *Ann Intern Med*. 1979;91:710-717.

50.6. Answer: E. Dexrazoxane helps to minimize the cardiomyopathy caused by anthracyclines, such as doxorubicin. The mechanism is postulated to be due to dexrazoxane's ability to chelate iron and therefore suppress superoxide radical formation. Mesna is used to treat the hemorrhagic cysititis caused by cyclophosphamide and ifosfamide. Methylene blue is used to treat the encephalopathy caused by ifosfamide. Glucarpidase is used to treat methotrexate overdoses. Uridine triacetate is used in the treatment of 5-fluorouracil overdoses.

Liesse K, et al. Dexrazoxane significantly reduces anthracycline-induced cardiotoxicity in pediatric solid tumor patients: A systematic review. *J Pediatr Hematol Oncol*. 2018;40:417-425.

50.7. Answer: C. Vincristine stimulation of the hypothalamus is responsible for the fevers and SIADH associated with vincristine administration. Serum electrolytes need to be monitored for 10 days following therapy.

Rosenthal S, Kaufman S. Vincristine neurotoxicity. *Ann Intern Med*. 1974;80:733-737.

50.8. Answer: B. Procarbazine, an alkylating agent, has both disulfiramlike and MAO-I activity. Patients should be counseled to avoid ethanol as well as foods with a high tyramine content. Drug interactions also need to be checked every time a new medication is initiated.

Livingston MG, Livingston HM. Monoamine oxidase inhibitors. *Drug Safety*. 1996;14:219-227.

50.9. Answer: A. This patient is presenting with gastrointestinal perforation that was caused by paclitaxel. Taxane-based chemotherapeutics lead to colitis, with >40% of patients requiring hospitalization. Rarely, taxane-induced colitis also progresses to colonic perforation.

Chen E, et al. Clinical characteristics of colitis induced by taxane-based chemotherapy. *Ann Gastroenterol*. 2020;33:59-67.

50.10. Answer: B. Up to 46% of patients receiving cyclophosphamide develop hemorrhagic cystitis. Acrolein is the metabolite that damages the urothelium and leads to this finding. The hemorrhagic cystitis that occurs following ifosfamide also occurs because of acrolein.

Droller MJ, et al. Prevention of cyclophosphamide-induced hemorrhagic cystitis. *Urology*. 1982;20:256-258.

Methotrexate, 5-Fluorouracil, and Capecitabine

QUESTIONS

51.1. Methotrexate is an analogue of which of the following options?
A. Citrate
B. Folate
C. Pyruvate
D. Succinate
E. Thymidylate

51.2. Which of the following mechanisms best explains the kidney injury caused by methotrexate?
A. Acute glomerulonephritis
B. Acute ischemic cortical necrosis
C. Acute interstitial nephritis
D. Acute tubular necrosis
E. Acute renal vein thrombosis

51.3. Glucarpidase (carboxypeptidase G_2, $CPDG_2$) cleaves methotrexate to produce 2,4-diamino-N(10)-methylpteroic acid (DAMPA) and which of the following metabolites?
A. Asparagine
B. Aspartate
C. Cysteine
D. Glutamate
E. Tryptophan

51.4. Which of the following intravenous pharmaceuticals is protective against methotrexate-associated kidney injury?
A. Cisplatin
B. Gentamicin
C. Ketorolac
D. Piperacillin
E. Sodium bicarbonate

51.5. Following intravenous administration of glucarpidase (carboxypeptidase G_2, $CPDG_2$), methotrexate concentrations should be determined using which of the following laboratory techniques?
A. Atomic absorption spectroscopy (AAS)
B. Chemiluminescent microparticle immunoassay (CMIA)
C. Enzyme multiplied immunoassay (EMIT)
D. Fluorescence polarization immunoassay (FPIA)
E. High-performance liquid chromatography (HPLC)

51.6. Following intravenous administration, which of the following locations would achieve the highest concentration of glucarpidase (carboxypeptidase G_2, $CPDG_2$)?
A. Blood
B. Central nervous system
C. Gastrointestinal lumen
D. Intracellular compartment
E. Urinary collecting system

51.7. Which of the following xenobiotics is an antidotal therapy for 5-fluorouracil (5-FU) toxicity?
A. Dexrazoxane
B. Glucarpidase
C. Leucovorin (folinic acid)
D. Mercaptoethane sulfonate
E. Uridine triacetate

51.8. Dihydropyrimidine dehydrogenase (DPD) deficiency is a risk factor for developing toxicity from which of the following xenobiotics?
   A. Capecitabine
   B. Cisplatin
   C. Doxorubicin
   D. Irinotecan
   E. Methotrexate

51.9. Uridine triacetate supports synthesis of which of the following options?
   A. Deoxyribonucleic acid
   B. Glycine

   C. Methionine
   D. Ribonucleic acid
   E. Tetrahydrofolate

51.10. Capecitabine toxicity is worsened by high activity rates of which of the following options?
   A. Cytidine deaminase
   B. Dihydrofolate reductase
   C. Dihydropyrimidine dehydrogenase
   D. Glomerular filtration
   E. Pepsin

ANSWERS

51.1. Answer: B. Methotrexate (MTX) is a structural analogue of folate. It inhibits dihydrofolate reductase (DHFR). MTX and its metabolites inhibit 5-aminoimidazole-4-carboxamide ribonucleotide (AICAR) transformylase, phosphoribosylpyrophosphate amidotransferase (PPAT), and thymidylate synthase (TYMS).

> Jackson RC, Grindley GB. The biochemical basis for methotrexate cytotoxicity. In: Sirotnak FM, et al, eds. *Folate Antagonists as Therapeutic Agents*. New York, NY: Academic Press; 1984:289-315.

51.2. Answer: D. Methotrexate and the relatively insoluble drug metabolites 7-hydroxy methotrexate (7-OH-MTX) and 2,4-diamino-N(10)-methylpteroic acid (DAMPA) accumulate and precipitate in the renal tubules, causing reversible acute tubular necrosis. Prerenal azotemia (dehydration) is a risk factor in developing methotrexate nephrotoxicity.

> Abelson HT, et al. Methotrexate-induced renal impairment: Clinical studies and rescue from systemic toxicity with high-dose leucovorin and thymidine. *J Clin Oncol*. 1983;1:208-216.

51.3. Answer: D. Glucarpidase cleaves methotrexate to DAMPA and glutamate. The other amino acids are incorrect. Intracellular methotrexate polyglutamate derivatives are responsible for persistent cytotoxic effects.

> Voraxaze. (glucaripdase) [package insert]. West Conshohocken, PA: BTG International Inc; 2012. https://www.accessdata.fda.gov/drugsatfda_docs/label/2012/125327lbl.pdf. Accessed July 6, 2021.

51.4. Answer: E. Methotrexate (MTX) is excreted by glomerular filtration and active tubular secretion. The solubility of MTX in the urine is pH dependent and is low in acidic urine. 7-Hydroxy methotrexate (7-OH-MTX) and 2,4-diamino-N(10)-methylpteroic acid (DAMPA) are even less soluble in urine than methotrexate. Patients who are at

increased risk include the elderly and those with a glomerular filtration rate (GFR) of <60 mL/min. Other risk factures include coingestion of medications that decrease blood flow, such as nonsteroidal antiinflammatory drugs (NSAIDs), nephrotoxic drugs, such as aminoglycosides; or drugs that inhibit renal secretion, such as the weak organic acids salicylates and piperacillin.

> Christensen ML, et al. Effect of hydration on methotrexate plasma concentrations in children with acute lymphocytic leukemia. *J Clin Oncol*. 1988;6:797-801.

51.5. Answer: E. Following administration of glucarpidase, high-performance liquid chromatography must be used to accurately determine methotrexate concentrations. The 2,4-diamino-N(10)-methylpteroic acid (DAMPA) metabolite created by glucarpidase interferes with immunoassay-based tests.

> Brandsteterova E, et al. HPLC determination of methotrexate and its metabolite in serum. *Neoplasma*. 1990;37:395-403.

51.6. Answer: A. When given intravenously, the large protein size (83-kDa) of glucarpidase does not permit it to cross the blood–brain barrier, to cross the cell membranes to act intracellularly, cross the gut lumen or urinary collecting system, or to treat methotrexate extravasation. Therefore, when administered intravenously, the highest concentration of glucarpidase is in the blood. Glucarpidase is safe to be administered directly into the intrathecal space when needed.

> DeAngelis LM, et al. Carboxypeptidase G2 rescue after high-dose methotrexate. *J Clin Oncol*. 1996;14:2145-2149.

51.7. Answer: E. Early administration of uridine triacetate reduces mortality in patients who develop 5-fluorouracil (5-FU) and capecitabine toxicity. Leucovorin (folinic acid) worsens 5-FU toxicity. Dexrazoxane is an antidote for anthracycline toxicity. Glucarpidase (carboxypeptidase G_2) is an antidote for methotrexate toxicity. Mercaptoethane sulfonate (mesna) is an antidote for nitrogen mustards.

> Ma WW, et al. Emergency use of uridine triacetate for the prevention and treatment of life-threatening 5-fluorouracil and capecitabine toxicity. *Cancer.* 2017;123:345-356.

51.8. Answer: A. Common risk factors for toxicity from 5-fluorouracil (5-FU) and its prodrug capecitabine, include genetic polymorphisms such as dihydropyrimidine dehydrogenase (DPD) deficiency, which impairs metabolism. Other risk factors for developing 5-FU toxicity include underlying liver, kidney, and coronary artery diseases.

> Mercier C, Ciccolini J. Severe or lethal toxicities upon capecitabine intake: Is DPYD genetic polymorphism the ideal culprit? *Trends Pharmacol Sci.* 2007;28:597-598.

51.9. Answer: D. Uridine triacetate is deacetylated by nonspecific esterases to uridine. Uridine is activated to uridine triphosphate (UTP), which is utilized for RNA synthesis. It does not support DNA synthesis, as there is no uridine in DNA. Methionine is synthesized from homocysteine and 5-methyl-tetrahydrofolate, and glycine is synthesized from serine as part of folate cycling, which leucovorin administration would support. Tetrahydrofolate is an active folate central to folate cycling, which is sustained by leucovorin.

> Ma WW, et al. Emergency use of uridine triacetate for the prevention and treatment of life-threatening 5-fluorouracil and capecitabine toxicity. *Cancer.* 2017;123:345-356.

51.10. Answer: A. Capecitabine is an oral chemotherapeutic prodrug that is metabolized by carboxylesterase and cytidine deaminase, and then thymidine phosphorylase to 5-fluorouracil (5-FU). Cytidine deaminase "rapid metabolizers" form higher than expected concentrations of 5-FU from capecitabine and experience early gastrointestinal and hematopoietic toxicity. A deficiency of dihydropyrimidine dehydrogenase (DPD), the enzyme that inactivates approximately 80% of 5-FU, increases 5-FU or capecitabine toxicity. Low glomerular filtration rates (GFR) (<30 mL/min) are a contraindication to administration because capecitabine is predominately excreted by the kidneys. Dihydrofolate reductase is inhibited by methotrexate.

> Mercier C, et al. Early severe toxicities after capecitabine intake: Possible implication of a cytidine deaminase extensive metabolizer profile. *Cancer Chemother Pharmacol.* 2009;63:1177-1180.

Antimigraine Medications

52.1. A 26-year-old woman with a history of migraines takes six doses of subcutaneous sumatriptan in one day. Later that evening, she develops pain and tinging in both of her hands. Which of the following interventions is an appropriate treatment in this patient?
A. Intravenous hydration and analgesia
B. Activated charcoal
C. Tissue plasminogen activator (TPA)
D. Aspirin, heparin, and nitroglycerin
E. Methylprednisolone

52.2. A 58-year-old woman presents with vomiting after taking several extra doses of her migraine medication because her headache was not improving. She reports a burning sensation to her extremities. Her blood pressure is 190/95 mmHg, and her left foot is pale with absent pulses. Which of the following therapies is an appropriate next step?
A. Consult interventional radiology for angiogram
B. Administer tissue plasminogen activator
C. Perform a transmetatarsal amputation
D. Administer sodium nitroprusside
E. Provide reassurance

52.3. Which of the following foods has an increased risk of contamination with an ergot-containing substance?
A. Pokeweed
B. Rye bread
C. Cassava
D. Rhubarb
E. Lychee

52.4. Which of the following findings is associated with chronic ergotamine use?
A. Neutropenia
B. Aortic valve regurgitation
C. Vasculitis
D. Pulmonary fibrosis
E. Alopecia

52.5. Which of the following options is the most concerning adverse effect that occurs with triptan use?
A. Chest pressure
B. Esophageal spasm
C. Flushing
D. Paresthesias
E. Vomiting

52.6. A 25-year-old woman presents to the emergency department with mild to moderate pain and blanching of the toes in her left foot. The symptoms began after using an ergot product to treat her migraine. Which of the following treatments would be reasonable in this patient?
A. Warm water soaks
B. Immediate-release nifedipine
C. High-dose aspirin
D. Topical nitroglycerin
E. Intravenous heparin

52.7. Which of the following statements regarding the pharmacokinetics of ergotamine is correct?
A. Ergots are well absorbed by the oral route
B. Ergots are eliminated unmetabolized in the urine
C. The volume of distribution of the ergot alkaloids is 0.2 L/kg
D. The elimination half-life of the ergots is >24 hours
E. Rectal bioavailability is 20 times greater than oral

52.8. Which of the following ergot medications is most likely to cause retroperitoneal fibrosis?
A. Ergotamine
B. Ergonovine
C. Bromocriptine
D. Dihydroergotamine
E. Methysergide

52.9. Which of the following cardiac dysrhythmias is most likely to occur in a patient with ergot toxicity?
A. Sinus tachycardia
B. Sinus bradycardia
C. Atrioventricular block
D. Premature ventricular contractions
E. Ventricular tachycardia

52.10. Which of the following ergotamine preparations is used in obstetric care to stimulate contraction of the uterus?
A. Ergonovine
B. Ergotamine
C. Ergocristine
D. Dihydroergotamine
E. Ergometrine

ANSWERS

52.1. Answer: A. Excessive triptan use is associated with vasoconstriction and tachyphylaxis. Patients respond to simple hydration and analgesia. Activated charcoal is not useful in most sumatriptan overdoses because sumatriptan is administered subcutaneously, although it is reasonable in oral triptan overdoses. TPA is not required because the neurologic symptoms are secondary to vasoconstriction not clotting. Aspirin, heparin, and nitroglycerin are used to treat triptan-associated myocardial ischemia. Methylprednisolone is a poorly supported treatment for ergotamine-induced lower extremity arterial vasospasm.

Fulton JA, et al. Renal infarction during the use of rizatriptan and zolmitriptan: Two case reports. *Clin Toxicol (Phila)*. 2006;44:177-180.

52.2. Answer: D. This patient is presenting with severe peripheral artery vasospasm following triptan use. When triptan-induced vasoconstriction produces ischemic changes that include angina, myocardial infarction, cerebral ischemia, intermittent claudication, and internal organ ischemia, reasonable therapies include phentolamine, sodium nitroprusside, and intravenous calcium channel blockers titrated until resolution of vasoconstriction.

Carliner N, et al. Sodium nitroprusside treatment of ergotamine-induced peripheral ischemia. *JAMA*. 1974;227:308-309.

52.3. Answer: B. Ergot is the product of *Claviceps purpurea*, a fungus that contaminates rye and other grains. The spores of the fungus are windborne and transported by insects to young rye. Pokeweed produces profound gastrointestinal distress and significant leukocytosis. Cassava contains linamarin, a cyanogenic glycoside. The leafy part of rhubarb contains calcium oxalate and leads to oropharyngeal edema and pain. Lychee is associated with outbreaks of hypoglycemia from hypoglycin A, as occurs with unripe ackee fruit.

Belser-Ehrlich S et al. Human and cattle ergotism since 1900: Symptoms, outbreaks, and regulations. *Toxicol Ind Health*. 2013;29:307-316.

52.4. Answer: B. Ergots, including ergotamine, dihydroergotamine, pergolide, and cabergoline, cause mitral and aortic valve leaflet thickening and immobility resulting in valvular regurgitation. The mitral and aortic valves and pulmonary arteries have high concentrations of 5-HT$_{2B}$ receptors. The ergot-derived medications are potent 5-HT$_{2B}$ receptor agonists, and stimulation activates cellular kinases leading to fibroblast proliferation and collagen synthesis.

Redfield MM, et al. Valve disease associated with ergot alkaloid use: Echocardiographic and pathologic correlations. *Ann Intern Med*. 1992;117:50-52.

Flaherty KR, Bates JR. Mitral regurgitation caused by chronic ergotamine use. *Am Heart J*. 1996;131:603-606.

52.5. Answer: A. While all the listed options are common adverse effects that occur following triptan use, the most consequential adverse effects are chest pressure and vasoconstriction. Chest pressure is reported in up to 15% of sumatriptan users.

Ottervanger JP, et al. Postmarketing study of cardiovascular adverse reactions associated with sumatriptan. *BMJ*. 1993;307:1185.

52.6. Answer: B. This patient is presenting with mild symptoms of vasospasm following ergot exposure. Immediate-release oral nifedipine is a reasonable therapy for patients with mild symptoms of vasospasm, such as dysesthesias and minimal ischemic pain of the digits.

Dagher FJ, et al. Severe unilateral ischemia of the lower extremity caused by ergotamine: Treatment with nifedipine. *Surgery.* 1985;97:369-373.

52.7. Answer: E. Rectal bioavailability is 20 times greater than oral. The ergots are poorly absorbed by the oral route because they undergo extensive first-pass metabolism. The volume of distribution is 2 L/kg, and the half-life ranges from 90 to 360 minutes.

Ibraheem JJ, et al. Kinetics of ergotamine after intravenous and intramuscular administration of migraine sufferers. *Eur J Clin Pharmacol.* 1982;23:235-240.

Orton DA, Richardson RJ. Ergotamine absorption and toxicity. *Postgrad Med J.* 1982;58:6-11.

52.8. Answer: E. Methysergide causes retroperitoneal fibrosis as well as pleuropericardial, endocardial, and endovascular fibrosis. The exact mechanism is not entirely clear; however, it is hypothesized to occur because of the serotonin antagonist effects, which lead to increased endogenous serotonin and, consequently, fibrosis.

Bucci JA, Manoharan A. Methysergide-induced retroperitoneal fibrosis: Successful outcome and two new laboratory features. *Mayo Clin Proc.* 1997;72:1148-1150.

Cai FZ, et al. Methysergide-induced retroperitoneal fibrosis and pericardial effusion. *Intern Med J.* 2004;34:297-298.

52.9. Answer: B. The bradycardia that occurs in patients with ergot toxicity is caused by a reflex baroreceptor-mediated phenomenon associated with vasoconstriction. A reduction in sympathetic tone, direct myocardial depression, and increased vagal activity are also factors in causing the bradycardia.

Sanders-Bush E, Mayer SE. 5-Hydroxytryptamine (serotonin) receptor agonists and antagonists. In: Brunton LL, et al, eds. *Goodman and Gilman's The Pharmacological Basis of Therapeutics.* 11th ed. New York, NY: McGraw-Hill; 1992:297-315.

52.10. Answer: A. Ergonovine is used in obstetric practice because it stimulates uterine smooth muscle contraction. Ergonovine was also formerly used in cardiac stress tests.

Rall TW, Schleifer LS. Oxytocin, prostaglandins, ergot alkaloids and other tocolytic agents. In: Gilman AG, et al, eds. *Goodman & Gilman's The Pharmacological Basis of Therapeutics.* 8th ed. New York, NY: Macmillan; 1990:933-953.

Thyroid and Antithyroid Medications

53.1. Which of the following medications produces hypo-thyroidism as an adverse effect in approximately 25% of patients?
- A. Amiodarone
- B. Lithium
- C. Prednisone
- D. Sucralfate
- E. Aminoglutethimide

53.2. Which of the following options is associated with carcinoma of the thyroid?
- A. Arsenic
- B. Ionizing radiation
- C. Vincristine
- D. Hexavalent chromium
- E. Ricin

53.3. Which of the following statements best describes the effect of thyroid hormones on the cardiovascular system?
- A. Upregulation of beta adrenergic receptors
- B. Downregulation of alpha adrenergic receptors
- C. Enhanced activity of L-type voltage-gated calcium channels
- D. Enhanced activity of protein kinase A
- E. All of the above

53.4. Which of the following statements best describes the Wolff-Chaikoff effect?
- A. Iodine administration prevents the peripheral conversion of tetraiodothyronine (T_4) to triiodo-thyronine (T_3)
- B. Iodine, which is essential for the formation of thyroid hormone, prevents iodination of thyroglobulin
- C. Iodine administration suppresses thyroid-stimulating hormone
- D. Iodine, which is essential for the formation of thyroid hormone, inhibits thyroid hormone release
- E. Iodine administration to patients with hypothyroid goiter produces thyrotoxicosis

53.5. The majority of circulating thyroid hormones are bound to thyroid-binding globulin. Which of the following statements is true of the remainder of thyroid hormones in the circulation?
- A. They are primarily bound to albumin
- B. They are primarily bound to alpha-1-acid glycoprotein
- C. Tetraiodothyronine is bound to albumin and triiodothyronine is bound to alpha-1-acid glycoprotein
- D. Tetraiodothyronine is bound to alpha-1-acid glycoprotein, and triiodothyronine is bound to albumin
- E. They are free in circulation

53.6. A 24-year-old woman presents with tremor, tachycardia, hypertension, fever, and diarrhea and is clinically diagnosed with thyrotoxicosis. In addition to controlling her heart rate and blood pressure, which of the following is another desirable effect of propranolol use?
   A. It prevents the conversion of tetraiodothyronine (T_4) to triiodothyronine (T_3) in the thyroid gland
   B. It prevents the peripheral conversion of T_4 to T_3
   C. It prevents iodination of thyroglobulin
   D. It prevents the release of T_4 and T_3 from the thyroid gland
   E. It suppresses thyroid-stimulating hormone (TSH)

53.7. The two major thioamides used to treat hyperthyroidism are methimazole and propylthiouracil. What is a major reason to use one drug over the other in certain high-risk patients?
   A. Propylthiouracil is preferred in pregnancy because of concerns of methimazole embryopathy
   B. Propylthiouracil is easier to dose in patients with chronic kidney disease
   C. Methimazole does not need dose adjustment in patients with liver disease
   D. Low doses of propylthiouracil are less likely to cause agranulocytosis
   E. Cardiotoxicity is less common in patients treated with methimazole

53.8. A 5-year-old boy presents to the hospital 1 hour after ingesting seven (125 mcg each) of his mother's prescription levothyroxine (T_4) medication. He is given a dose of activated charcoal, and you are contacted regarding further management strategies. Which of the following options is the best approach?

   A. Admit to the pediatric intensive care unit for inevitable thyrotoxicosis
   B. Check concentrations of thyroid-stimulating hormone (TSH) and tetraiodothyronine (T_4) and base management on the results
   C. Begin oral metoprolol and discharge
   D. Observe for 4-6 hours for symptoms and treat accordingly
   E. Discharge with strict return precautions

53.9. A 4-year-old girl presents to the hospital 1 hour after ingesting seven (50 mcg each) of her mother's prescription liothyronine (T_3) medication. She is given a dose of activated charcoal, and you are contacted regarding further management strategies. Which of the following is the best approach?
   A. Admit to the pediatric intensive care unit for inevitable thyrotoxicosis
   B. Check concentrations of thyroid-stimulating hormone (TSH) and tetraiodothyronine (T_4) and base management on the results
   C. Begin oral metoprolol and discharge
   D. Observe for 4-6 hours for symptoms and treat accordingly
   E. Discharge with strict return precautions

53.10. Addition of which of the following medications is likely to result in clinical hyperthyroidism in a patient who is already taking supplemental levothyroxine (T_4) therapeutically?
   A. Rifampin
   B. Cholestyramine
   C. Salicylates
   D. Carbamazepine
   E. Antacids

ANSWERS

53.1. Answer: A. All the choices reduce circulating concentrations of thyroid hormone by various mechanisms, and some, such as lithium, are common causes of drug-induced hypothyroidism. None affect thyroid function as commonly as amiodarone, which also causes thyrotoxicosis in patients with iodine deficiency.

Harjai KJ, Licata AA. Effects of amiodarone on thyroid function. *Ann Intern Med*. 1997;126:63-73.

53.2. Answer: B. The effects of large doses of ionizing radiation are best described in the survivors of the nuclear detonations at Hiroshima and Nagasaki. In exposed survivors,

multiple types of thyroid cancer have been reported, likely as a direct result of the uptake of radioactive iodine into the thyroid gland. Similar results are emerging following the release at Chernobyl.

Ermak G, et al. Genetic aberrations in Chernobyl-related thyroid cancers: Implications for possible future nuclear accidents or nuclear attacks. *IUBMB Life*. 2003;55:637-41.

Suzuki K, et al. Radiation-induced thyroid cancers: Overview of molecular signatures. *Cancers (Basel)*. 2019;11:1290.

53.3. Answer: E. While the exact mechanism of action of thyroid hormones on the cardiovascular system is complex and incompletely understood, all of these effects are supported by some evidence. Interestingly, the effects on alpha adrenergic receptors explain why beta adrenergic antagonism is used safely in patients with hyperthyroidism without producing paradoxical hypertension from unopposed alpha adrenergic agonism as occurs with cocaine or pheochromocytoma.

Bachman ES, et al. The metabolic and cardiovascular effects of hyperthyroidism are largely independent of beta-adrenergic stimulation. *Endocrinology.* 2004;145:2767-2774.

Danzi S, Klein I. Thyroid hormone and the cardiovascular system. *Med Clin North Am.* 2012;96:257-268.

Kahaly GJ, Dillmann WH. Thyroid hormone action in the heart. *Endocr Rev.* 2005;26:704-728.

53.4. Answer: D. In the Wolff-Chaikoff effect, high intrathyroidal iodide concentrations inhibit the release of thyroid hormone into circulation. Thus, iodine and similarly negatively charged anions, such as thiocyanate, are used to treat hyperthyroidism. The effect is transient and serves as a temporizing therapy until other modalities become effective.

Markou K, et al. Iodine-Induced hypothyroidism. *Thyroid.* 2001;11: 501-510.

53.5. Answer: A. Because a large percentage of thyroid hormones in circulation are bound to albumin, xenobiotics that are highly albumin bound have the potential to displace thyroid hormones and exacerbate hyperthyroidism.

Schussler GC. The thyroxine-binding proteins. *Thyroid.* 2000;10:141-149.

53.6. Answer: B. Propranolol and other beta adrenergic antagonists are used to treat many of the cardiovascular and neurologic manifestations of hyperthyroidism. One additional benefit of propranolol, atenolol, and possibly other members of the class is that they reduce the conversion of circulating T_4 to T_3. T_4 has far less physiologic activity than to T_3.

Wiersinga WM. Propranolol and thyroid hormone metabolism. *Thyroid.* 1991;1:273-277.

53.7. Answer: A. Both thioamides are effective in hyperthyroidism, but the overall safety profile favors the use of methimazole. However, propylthiouracil is favored in pregnancy because methimazole has a slightly greater risk of teratogenicity. Both drugs cause agranulocytosis, especially as total daily dosing increases.

Bartalena L, et al. Adverse effects of thyroid hormone preparations and antithyroid drugs. *Drug Saf.* 1996;15:53-63.

Inoue M, et al. Hyperthyroidism during pregnancy. *Can Fam Physician.* 2009;55:701-703.

53.8. Answer: E. Most unwitnessed ingestions of levothyroxine (T_4) in children produce no or minimal symptoms because the T_4 is metabolized and eliminated before it is converted to T_3. These children are typically managed entirely as outpatients since symptoms rarely occur. If symptoms do occur, there is a 5-7 day delay to symptom onset. Parents should be instructed to watch for irritability or tremor and be taught how to check the child's pulse. For large ingestions (greater than about 3 mg in a child), activated charcoal is reasonable if the child presents to health care. While much greater ingestions produce toxicity, these are exceptionally uncommon, especially in children. We discourage obtaining blood concentrations of thyroid hormones as they will typically result as extreme panic values and have no bearing on treatment or prognosis.

Golightly LK, et al. Clinical effects of accidental levothyroxine ingestion in children. *Am J Dis Child.* 1987;141:1025-1027.

53.9. Answer: D. Since liothyronine (T_3) is biologically active, patients who ingest liothyronine are expected to display symptoms fairly rapidly. Should symptoms occur, most are easily treated with a beta adrenergic antagonist alone as they are generally mild and transient in children. Anti-thyroid medications are not indicated as the thyroid gland itself is normal.

He ZH, et al. Thyrotoxicosis after massive triiodothyronine (LT3) overdose: A coast-to-coast case series and review. *Drugs Context.* 2020; 15;9:2019-8-4.

Dahlberg PA, et al. Triiodothyronine intoxication. *Lancet.* 1979;29;2:700.

53.10. Answer: C. Because salicylates are highly albumin bound, they have the potential to displace thyroid hormone and exacerbate toxicity. All the other choices decrease circulating thyroid hormones either by preventing absorption (B, E) or enhancing metabolism (A, D).

Surks MI, Sievert R. Drugs and thyroid function. *N Engl J Med.* 1995;333:1688-1694.

Antibacterials, Antifungals, and Antivirals

54

QUESTIONS

54.1. A 67-year-old woman is prescribed trimethoprim-sulfamethoxazole (TMP-SMX) to treat a urinary tract infection. Her initial serum creatinine is 1.5 mg/dL (133 micromol/L). She returns for a follow-up visit 1 week later. She is feeling much better and has no symptoms. Her creatinine has increased to 2.0 mg/dL (177 micromol/L). What is the most likely etiology of this rise in creatinine?
- A. Destruction of phospholipids on the brush border membranes in the proximal renal tubule
- B. Distal renal tubule damage causing renal artery vasoconstriction
- C. Precipitation of crystals within the renal tubules
- D. Inhibition of renal tubular secretion of creatinine
- E. Prostaglandin-mediated renal medullary ischemia

54.2. A 34-year-old man with pulmonary aspergillosis is administered intravenous amphotericin B. Less than an hour after the infusion is started, he develops a fever, headache, and rigors. What is the most appropriate initial method of treating these adverse effects?
- A. Discontinuing amphotericin B and starting ketoconazole
- B. Switching to liposomal amphotericin B
- C. Increasing the infusion rate
- D. Administering hydrocortisone and acetaminophen
- E. Performing an exchange transfusion

54.3. After an anaphylactic (IgE-mediated) reaction to penicillin, which of the following options describes the risk for anaphylaxis to a third-generation cephalosporin?
- A. Twice the general population risk (0.04%)
- B. Ten times the general population risk (1%)
- C. Fifty times the general population risk (10%)
- D. One thousand times the population risk (20%)
- E. Negligible increased risk

54.4. A 26-year-old woman is referred to the emergency department after her outpatient laboratory analysis revealed cholestatic hepatitis. Her only medication is an antibiotic she began taking 8 days prior to presentation. Which of the following antibiotics best explains her abnormal liver function tests?
- A. Levofloxacin
- B. Metronidazole
- C. Trimethoprim-sulfamethoxazole
- D. Amoxicillin-clavulanic acid
- E. Nitrofurantoin

54.5. A 6-month-old boy who is prescribed chronic antibiotic therapy to treat osteomyelitis presents to the emergency department with blood in his stool. The nurse notes that he has prolonged bleeding at the site of an intravenous catheter. His international normalized ratio (INR) is 6. Which of the following antibiotics best explains his presentation?
- A. Ampicillin
- B. Cefazolin
- C. Trimethoprim-sulfamethoxazole
- D. Amoxicillin-clavulanic acid
- E. Chloramphenicol

54.6. A 3-month-old boy develops vomiting, abdominal distention, green stools, lethargy, and an ashen color in the pediatric intensive care unit. His laboratory analysis is notable for a metabolic acidosis. Which of the following antibiotics best explains his presentation?
   A. Ampicillin
   B. Cefazolin
   C. Gentamicin
   D. Chloramphenicol
   E. Amoxicillin-clavulanic acid

54.7. A 62-year-old woman with a past medical history of myasthenia gravis is admitted to the hospital for treatment of an infection with intravenous antibiotics. She then develops sweating, vomiting, profuse diarrhea, and shortness of breath. On examination, she has notable wheezing to both lung fields. Which of the following antibiotics best explains her presentation?
   A. Telithromycin
   B. Clindamycin
   C. Vancomycin
   D. Doxycycline
   E. Erythromycin

54.8. A 26-year-old woman with a past medical history of depression presents to the emergency department with a urinary tract infection. She is admitted and is treated with antibiotics. While in the hospital, she becomes hyperthermic to 106.5 °F (41.4 °C). She has lower extremity rigidity with clonus and a marked tremor in her hands. Which of the following antibiotics led to her presentation?

   A. Vancomycin
   B. Piperacillin-tazobactam
   C. Aztreonam
   D. Imipenem
   E. Linezolid

54.9. A 54-year-old man with a past medical history of myasthenia gravis develops paralysis as he is being administered an intravenous antibiotic. He requires intubation and mechanical ventilation. Which of the following antibiotics best explains his presentation?
   A. Piperacillin-tazobactam
   B. Ceftriaxone
   C. Gentamicin
   D. Chloramphenicol
   E. Vancomycin

54.10. A 27-year-old man develops extreme apprehension and auditory hallucinations while being treated for an infection in the emergency department. His heart rate is 135 beats/min and his blood pressure is 168/95 mmHg. He has no history of psychiatric illness and no recent substance use. Which of the following antimicrobials explains this patient's symptoms?
   A. Ganciclovir
   B. Nitrofurantoin
   C. Penicillin G
   D. Ceftriaxone
   E. Azithromycin

ANSWERS

54.1. Answer: D. While TMP-SMX causes an increase in serum creatinine concentration of 13-35%, this is independent of glomerular filtration rate (GFR) and resolves when the TMP-SMX is discontinued. Choice A is the mechanism of aminoglycoside-associated kidney injury. Choice B is the mechanism of amphotericin B–associated kidney injury. Choice C is the mechanism of acyclovir-related kidney injury. Choice E is one of the mechanisms of acetaminophen-associated kidney injury.

Delanaye P, et al. Trimethoprim, creatinine and creatinine-based equations. *Nephron Clin Pract.* 2011;119:c187-c193.

54.2. Answer: D. Infusion of amphotericin B results in fever, headache, and rigors. Slowing the infusion rate and pretreating patients with diphenhydramine decreases the incidence of this reaction. Patients who do develop these symptoms

should be treated with acetaminophen and hydrocortisone. Liposomal amphotericin B is preferred as it is associated with a lower incidence of infusion-related fevers, headaches, rigors, and nephrotoxicity. Liposomal amphotericin B is also associated with fewer breakthrough fungal infections.

Tynes BS, et al. Reducing amphotericin B reactions. A double-blind study. *Am Rev Respir Dis.* 1963;87:264-268.

54.3. Answer: E. The general population risk of anaphylaxis is 0.02%. The cross-reactivity between penicillin and a first- or second-generation cephalosporin is approximately 1%. Third-, fourth-, and fifth-generation cephalosporins, however, have a dissimilar antigenic side chain; therefore, the cross-reaction between cephalosporins and penicillin is negligible.

Campagna JD, et al. The use of cephalosporins in penicillin-allergic patients: A literature review. *J Emerg Med.* 2012;42:612-620.

54.4. Answer: D. The liver injury in this patient is caused by the amoxicillin, which is a second-generation penicillin. Liver injury induced by penicillins is usually a cholestatic hepatitis. Penicillin-induced liver injury is the most common cause of drug-induced liver injury in the United States. The mechanism of hepatotoxicity is not fully elucidated. Most patients have clinical resolution with just supportive care and discontinuation of the drug.

Björnsson ES. Drug-induced liver injury: An overview over the most critical compounds. *Arch Toxicol*. 2015;89:327-334.

Chawla A, et al. Rapidly progressive cholestasis: An unusual reaction to amoxicillin/clavulanic acid therapy in a child. *J Pediatr*. 2000;136:121-123.

54.5. Answer: B. Cefazolin is a cephalosporin that contains an *N*-methylthiotetrazole (nMTT) side chain. This side chain is associated with a disulfiram reaction. Less commonly, however, the nMTT side chain also leads to depletion of vitamin K–dependent clotting factors through the inhibition of vitamin K epoxide reductase. Patients who present with bleeding should be treated with clotting factor replacement and vitamin K administration.

Bhat RV, Deshmukh CT. A study of Vitamin K status in children on prolonged antibiotic therapy. *Indian Pediatr*. 2003;40:36-40.

54.6. Answer: D. This patient is presenting with "gray baby syndrome" following chronic chloramphenicol administration. In addition to this patient's presenting symptoms, some patients progress to hypotension and cardiovascular collapse. Infants are at a higher risk of developing this syndrome because they have a limited capacity to form a glucuronide conjugate of chloramphenicol as well as a limited ability to excrete the chloramphenicol in the urine.

Mulhall A, et al. Chloramphenicol toxicity in neonates: Its incidence and prevention. *Br Med J (Clin Res Ed)*. 1983;287:1424-1427.

Weisberger AS, et al. Mechanisms of action of chloramphenicol. *JAMA*. 1969;209:97-103.

54.7. Answer: A. Telithromycin is a ketolide with similar pharmacology to macrolides. Telithromycin contains a carbamate side chain that interferes with normal function of neuronal cholinesterase. Patients with myasthenia gravis, especially those taking pyridostigmine, are at a much higher risk of developing a cholinergic crisis.

Perrot X, et al. Myasthenia gravis exacerbation or unmasking associated with telithromycin treatment. *Neurology*. 2006;67:2256-2258.

54.8. Answer: E. Linezolid has monoamine oxide inhibition activity and leads to a vasopressor response to tyramine. It also leads to serotonin toxicity when it is administered to patients who are already taking a selective serotonin reuptake inhibitor.

Huang V, Gortney JS. Risk of serotonin syndrome with concomitant administration of linezolid and serotonin agonists. *Pharmacotherapy*. 2006;26:1784-1793.

54.9. Answer: C. Aminoglycosides, such as gentamicin, exacerbate concomitant neuromuscular blockade. They do this by inhibiting presynaptic calcium channels, which inhibits the release of acetylcholine from presynaptic nerve terminals. Patients with a history of myasthenia gravis are at a particularly high risk of developing this toxicity.

Paradelis AG. Aminoglycoside antibiotics and neuromuscular blockade. *J Antimicrob Chemother*. 1979;5:737-738.

54.10. Answer: C. This patient is presenting with Hoigne syndrome, which occurs after large doses of procaine penicillin G. Procaine rather than penicillin implicated as the etiology in this syndrome. Patients develop extreme apprehension, hallucinations, tachycardia, and hypertension. Occasionally patients also develop seizures. The symptoms occur within minutes following the administration of the penicillin G.

Utley PM, et al. Acute psychotic reactions to aqueous procaine penicillin. *South Med J*. 1966;59:1271-1274.

Ilechukwu ST. Acute psychotic reactions and stress response syndromes following intramuscular aqueous procaine penicillin. *Br J Psychiatry J Ment Sci*. 1990;156:554-559.

Antimalarials

QUESTIONS

55.1. Which of the following statements about the pharmacokinetics of quinine is correct?
- A. Quinine is slowly and incompletely absorbed by the oral route
- B. Peak plasma concentrations occur within 3 hours
- C. Fifty percent of quinine is plasma protein bound
- D. Most of quinine is excreted unchanged in the urine
- E. The volume of distribution of quinine is 5 L/kg

55.2. Quinine has pharmacologic effects similar to which of the following classes of xenobiotics?
- A. Sulfonylureas
- B. Thiazide diuretics
- C. Beta adrenergic antagonists
- D. Calcium channel blockers
- E. Phenothiazines

55.3. Malaria protects patients from quinine toxicity because it increases which of the following processes or substances?
- A. Hepatic clearance
- B. Renal clearance
- C. Alpha-1-acid glycoprotein
- D. The volume of distribution
- E. The number of sickle cells

55.4. Which of the following symptoms most commonly develops in patients with cinchonism?
- A. Diplopia
- B. Mydriasis
- C. Scotomata
- D. Blurred vision
- E. Tinnitus

55.5. Which of the following medications would be the best option to treat the cardiac toxicity from the cinchona alkaloids?
- A. Propranolol
- B. Disopyramide
- C. Procainamide
- D. Sodium bicarbonate
- E. Bretylium

55.6. A 19-year-old woman presents to the emergency department after an intentional ingestion of chloroquine. Which of the following therapies would best treat her chloroquine toxicity?
- A. Atropine and sodium bicarbonate
- B. Pilocarpine and diphenhydramine
- C. Corticosteroids
- D. Diazepam and epinephrine
- E. Sodium bicarbonate and quinidine

55.7. Which of the following electrolyte abnormalities is most likely to occur in patients who overdose on chloroquine?
- A. Hypokalemia
- B. Hypernatremia
- C. Hyponatremia
- D. Hypochloremia
- E. Hyperglycemia

55.8. A 22-year-old woman presents to the emergency department for further evaluation of insomnia and very vivid dreams. Which of the following antimalarials best explains her presentation?
A. Chloroquine
B. Hydroxychloroquine
C. Mefloquine
D. Halofantrine
E. Primaquine

55.9. A 35-year-old man presents to the emergency department after an unintentional overdose of his antimalarial medication. He is cyanotic and has a pulse oximeter reading of 87%. He is diagnosed with methemoglobinemia and treated with methylene blue. Which of the following antimalarial medications best explains his presentation?

A. Chloroquine
B. Hydroxychloroquine
C. Mefloquine
D. Halofantrine
E. Primaquine

55.10. A 54-year-old man presents to the hospital for further evaluation of a rash. On examination, the rash is most consistent with purpura. His laboratory analysis reveals thrombocytopenia. Which of the following antimalarials best explains his presentation?
A. Hydroxychloroquine
B. Halofantrine
C. Lumefantrine
D. Piperaquine
E. Quinine

ANSWERS

55.1. Answer: B. Peak plasma concentrations occur within 3 hours. Quinine is rapidly and almost completely absorbed following oral administration. Approximately 85% is protein bound. The volume of distribution is 1.8 L/kg. Approximately 80% of quinine is metabolized with only 20% excreted unchanged in the urine.

Bateman DN, et al. Pharmacokinetics and clinical toxicity of quinine overdosage: Lack of efficacy of techniques intended to enhance elimination. *Q J Med.* 1985;54:125-131.

55.2. Answer: A. Quinine causes inhibition of the adenosine triphosphate (ATP)-sensitive potassium channels of pancreatic beta cells, which leads to a release of insulin in the same way that sulfonylureas do. The risk of developing hypoglycemia is highest in patients receiving high-dose intravenous quinine, intentional overdoses, and patients with other metabolic stresses. Patients who overdose on quinine and develop hypoglycemia are treated with octreotide for the same reasons and at the same dose that is used to treat sulfonylurea overdoses (1 mcg/kg with a maximum dose of 50 mcg subcutaneously every 6 hours).

Davis TM. Antimalarial drugs and glucose metabolism. *Br J Clin Pharmacol.* 1997;44:1-7.

Taylor WR, White NJ. Antimalarial drug toxicity: A review. *Drug Saf.* 2004;27:25-61.

55.3. Answer: C. Patients who are severely ill with malaria do not demonstrate signs of cinchonism at concentrations of quinine that typically lead to toxicity. This is due to an increase in plasma alpha-1-acid glycoprotein that occurs with malaria, which reduces the free fraction of quinine present.

Silamut K, et al. Alpha 1-acid glycoprotein (orosomucoid) and plasma protein binding of quinine in falciparum malaria. *Br J Clin Pharmacol.* 1991;32:311-315.

55.4. Answer: E. Quinine leads to eighth cranial nerve dysfunction, which causes tinnitus and deafness. Tinnitus is the most common symptom found in patients with cinchonism. This is an important diagnostic finding because of the limited differential diagnosis of tinnitus, which includes salicylates, loop diuretics, and aminoglycosides. In patients with cinchonism, the tinnitus and hearing impairment usually resolve within 48-72 hours and permanent hearing impairment is unlikely.

Roche RJ, et al. Quinine induces reversible high-tone hearing loss. *Br J Clin Pharmacol.* 1990;29:780-782.

55.5. Answer: D. Quinine and quinidine both block cardiac sodium channels with resultant QRS complex widening and impaired contraction. Sodium bicarbonate is safely used to treat conduction disturbances from quinine toxicity. All the other choices will worsen intraventricular conduction delays. Since cinchona alkaloids also prolong the QT interval, the potassium concentration must be followed and corrected as needed because hypertonic sodium bicarbonate will lower the serum potassium concentration and exacerbate QT interval prolongation.

Wasserman F, et al. Successful treatment of quinidine and procainamide intoxication. *N Engl J Med.* 1958;259:797-802.

55.6. Answer: D. Diazepam and epinephrine reduce the mortality from chloroquine overdose. The treatment bundle includes the administration of these two medications in conjunction with early intubation and aggressive cardiovascular and neurologic support.

Riou B, et al. Treatment of severe chloroquine poisoning. *N Engl J Med.* 1988;318:1-7.

55.7. Answer: A. Hypokalemia occurs in patients with chloroquine and quinidine overdoses. The mechanism is believed to be an intracellular shift of potassium, as opposed to a total body deficit. Data suggest that hypokalemia is protective against cardiac toxicity and prolongs survival. However, as severe hypokalemia is associated with lethal dysrhythmias, if patients have significant electrocardiographic changes, it is reasonable to supplement the potassium. It is important to monitor for rebound hyperkalemia as chloroquine toxicity resolves and redistribution of intracellular potassium occurs. Hypoglycemia, not hyperglycemia, also occurs with chloroquine overdoses.

Brandfonbrener M, et al. The effect of serum potassium concentration on quinidine toxicity. *J Pharmacol Exp Ther.* 1966;154:250-254.

Meeran K, Jacobs MG. Chloroquine poisoning. Rapidly fatal without treatment. *BMJ.* 1993;307:49-50.

55.8. Answer: C. Mefloquine is commonly associated with neuropsychiatric symptoms. Up to 40% of patients who are prescribed mefloquine develop insomnia and very vivid dreams. Other symptoms include dizziness, headache, vertigo, fatigue, and mood alteration. Women are more predisposed to the neuropsychiatric side effects of mefloquine. Other predisposing factors include a history of neuropsychiatric disorders and exposure to mefloquine within the past 2 months.

Schlagenhauf P. Mefloquine for malaria chemoprophylaxis 1992-1998: A review. *J Travel Med.* 1999;6:122-133.

van Riemsdijk MM, et al. Atovaquone plus chloroguanide versus mefloquine for malaria prophylaxis: A focus on neuropsychiatric adverse events. *Clin Pharmacol Ther.* 2002;72:294-301.

55.9. Answer: E. Primaquine causes red blood cell (RBC) oxidant stress and resultant hemolysis or methemoglobinemia. This occurs both in patients who are given high doses of primaquine as well as in patients who have underlying glucose-6-phosphate dehydrogenase (G6PD) deficiency.

Luzzi GA, Peto TE. Adverse effects of antimalarials. An update. *Drug Saf.* 1993;8:295-311.

Taylor WR, White NJ. Antimalarial drug toxicity: A review. *Drug Saf.* 2004;27:25-61.

55.10. Answer: E. Quinine is the most common cause of drug-induced thrombotic microangiopathy syndrome and is also a common cause of drug-induced thrombocytopenia. Thrombocytopenia rarely occurs after ingestion of very small amounts of quinine, such as what is found in tonic drinks, a phenomenon referred to as cocktail purpura. Other antimalarials that are associated with thrombocytopenia include mefloquine and dapsone.

George JN, et al. After the party's over. *N Engl J Med.* 2017;376:74-80.

Taylor WR, White NJ. Antimalarial drug toxicity: A review. *Drug Saf.* 2004;27:25-61.

Antituberculous Medications

QUESTIONS

56.1. A 42-year-old man presents to the emergency department for evaluation of painless blurry vision. On examination, he has a loss of peripheral vision. He is currently prescribed a medication to treat tuberculosis. The pathophysiology of his symptoms results from the inactivation of which of the following metals?
A. Copper
B. Iron
C. Magnesium
D. Calcium
E. Cobalt

56.2. A 42-year-old woman is prescribed isoniazid (INH) as part of an antituberculosis regimen. Genetic testing reveals that she is a phenotypically slow acetylator. What implications does this have for her risk of INH toxicity?
A. Her risks of peripheral neuropathy and hepatotoxicity are both higher
B. Her risks of peripheral neuropathy and hepatotoxicity are both lower
C. Her risk of peripheral neuropathy is higher and her risk of hepatoxicity is unchanged
D. Her risk of peripheral neuropathy is lower and her risk of hepatoxicity is higher
E. Her risk of peripheral neuropathy is unchanged and her risk of hepatoxicity is lower

56.3. A 26-year-old woman presents to the emergency department for further evaluation of a headache. Her only past medical history is tuberculosis, for which she is currently receiving treatment. Her physical examination is unrevealing. A lumbar puncture is performed, and xanthochromia is visualized. A cerebral angiogram reveals no aneurysm and no source of intracranial hemorrhage. Use of which of the following antituberculosis medications would best explain this presentation?
A. Isoniazid
B. Ethambutol
C. Rifampin
D. Ethionamide
E. Pyrazinamide

56.4. A 63-year-old man presents to the emergency department with progressive blurred vision and eye pain. His red-green discrimination and peripheral vision are intact. He is currently undergoing treatment for tuberculosis. Which of the following conditions increased his risk of developing this toxicity?
A. Copper deficiency
B. Concomitant treatment for HIV
C. Supratherapeutic salicylate usage
D. Slow acetylation
E. Concomitant pyrazinamide treatment

56.5. Which of the following statements regarding the treatment of isoniazid-induced seizures is correct?
A. Diazepam worsens isoniazid-induced seizures
B. Pyridoxine should be infused over 3-6 hours
C. If the amount of isoniazid ingested is known, pyridoxine should be given in a gram-for-gram dose
D. If the amount of isoniazid ingested is unknown, 50 g of pyridoxine is the usual recommended dose in adults
E. Pyridoxine should be given slowly due to its fat solubility

56.6. A 22-year-old man presents to the emergency department with seizures after eating a *Gyromitra* mushroom. His seizures resolve after a single dose of pyridoxine. Unfortunately, a medication error occurs, and a continuous infusion of pyridoxine is maintained for 3 days. A rapid response team is called to the patient's room after he develops which of the following toxicities?
A. A rectal temperature of 109 °F (42.8 °C)
B. Loss of sensation in both of his legs
C. Polymorphic ventricular tachycardia
D. Hematemesis
E. Facial droop

56.7. A 47-year-old man presents to the emergency department with new paranoid delusions and suicidal ideation. His family notes that he was more irritable at home and has been sleeping more than usual. The patient started a new medication to treat his tuberculosis 7 days prior to presentation. Which of the following antituberculosis medications best explains his presentation?
A. Isoniazid
B. Rifampin
C. Pyrazinamide
D. Bedaquiline
E. Cycloserine

56.8. A 42-year-old woman with a past medical history of a kidney transplant presents to the emergency department for further evaluation of a rising creatinine. She

is diagnosed with acute graft rejection. She was also recently diagnosed with tuberculosis and started on a medication. Which of the following medications contributed to her graft rejection?
A. Rifampin
B. Cycloserine
C. Isoniazid
D. Capreomycin
E. Ethambutol

56.9. A 27-year-old woman presents to the emergency department for evaluation of abdominal pain. She had a recent positive screening QuantiFERON, for which she has been taking isoniazid (INH) and pyridoxine for the past 5 weeks. Her laboratory analysis demonstrates an aspartate aminotransferase (AST) of 307 IU/L, alanine aminotransferase (ALT) of 321 IU/L, alkaline phosphates of 190 IU/L, INR of 1.1, and total bilirubin of 2.3 mg/dL (39.3 micromol/L). What is the most appropriate next step?
A. Increase the dose of pyridoxine
B. Decrease the dose of INH
C. Order genetic testing to determine acetylator status
D. Discontinue the INH and repeat liver function tests in 2 weeks
E. Reassurance and repeat liver function tests in 1 week

56.10. A 56-year-old man with a history of multidrug-resistant tuberculosis (MDR-TB) presents to the emergency department for evaluation of an abscess on his left buttock. On review of systems, he describes ringing in his ears and hearing loss. Which of the following antituberculosis medications best explains his presentation?
A. Rifampin
B. Cycloserine
C. Isoniazid
D. Capreomycin
E. Ethambutol

ANSWERS

56.1. Answer: A. This patient is taking ethambutol to treat his tuberculosis. Chronic ethambutol use leads to ocular toxicity. Patients present with painless blurry vision, scotomas around the blind spot in the central field, decreased perception of color, and loss of peripheral vision. Ethambutol is a strong metal chelator, inactivating zinc and copper. This inactivation is related to the induction of vacuoles in the retinal cells with resultant changes in cell permeability and cell death.

Kozak SF, et al. The role of copper on ethambutol's antimicrobial action and implications for ethambutol-induced optic neuropathy. *Diagn Microbiol Infect Dis.* 1998;30:83-87.

56.2. Answer: C. *N*-Acetyltransferase type 2 (NAT2) metabolizes isoniazid (INH), and genetic polymorphisms account for three phenotypes: fast, intermediate, and slow acetylators. Slow acetylators are at increased risk of developing peripheral neuropathy, but there is no significant association between variations in polymorphisms and hepatotoxicity.

Yamada S, et al. Genetic variations of NAT2 and CYP2E1 and isoniazid hepatotoxicity in a diverse population. *Pharmacogenomics.* 2009;10:1433-1445.

Goel UC, et al. Isoniazid-induced neuropathy in slow versus rapid acetylators. *J Assoc Physicians India.* 1992;40:671-672.

56.3. Answer: C. Rifampin imparts a reddish color to all body fluids, including urine and cerebrospinal fluid (CSF). This red discoloration of the CSF is occasionally erroneously identified as xanthochromia. The red-colored fluid also interferes with certain colorimetric tests, including the bilirubin assay. The red discoloration to the skin is partially removed by scrubbing.

Holdiness MR. A review of the Redman syndrome and rifampicin overdosage. *Med Toxicol Adverse Drug Exp.* 1989;4:444-451.

Holdiness MR. Neurological manifestations and toxicities of the antituberculosis drugs. A review. *Med Toxicol.* 1987;2:33-51.

56.4. Answer B. This patient developed uveitis from rifampin usage. As compared to the ocular toxicity caused by ethambutol and isoniazid, rifampin causes painful visual symptoms. Color discrimination and peripheral vision are preserved with rifampin-associated ocular toxicity. Protease inhibitors exacerbate the uveitis caused by rifampin, likely secondary to elevated serum rifampin concentrations. Rifampin should not routinely be administered to patients who are prescribed protease inhibitors. Rifampin alters the metabolism of pyrazinamide and increases the risk of hepatotoxicity.

Burman WJ, et al. Therapeutic implications of drug interactions in the treatment of human immunodeficiency virus-related tuberculosis. *Clin Infect Dis.* 1999;28:419-429.

56.5. Answer: C. Isoniazid (INH) induces a functional pyridoxine deficiency, which results in a decrease in gamma-aminobutyric acid (GABA) concentration and refractory seizures. The seizures should be treated with pyridoxine and benzodiazepines. If the amount of ingested INH is unknown, 70 mg/kg of pyridoxine (to a maximum of 5 g) should be administered. This dose is repeated if seizures recur or if coma is prolonged. If the amount of isoniazid ingested is known, pyridoxine should be administered in a gram-for-gram dose with the first dose being no greater than the maximal empiric dose (70 mg/kg up to 5 g in an adult). Pyridoxine should be administered at a rate of 1 g every 2-3 minutes. If sufficient intravenous pyridoxine is not available, crushed pyridoxine tablets should be administered with fluids through a nasogastric tube.

Brown CV. Acute isoniazid poisoning. *Am Rev Respir Dis.* 1972; 105:206-216.

Wason S, et al. Single high-dose pyridoxine treatment for isoniazid overdose. *JAMA.* 1981;246:1102-1104.

56.6. Answer: B. Pyridoxine is associated with peripheral neuropathy in patients taking daily doses of >200 mg for a month. Peripheral neuropathy also develops in patients who receive massive doses of pyridoxine, as occurred in this case. The neuropathy is a sensory neuropathy with associated ataxia. The treatment is primarily supportive; however, symptoms persist in certain patients despite discontinuation of the pyridoxine.

Albin R, et al. Acute sensory neuropathy-neuronopathy from pyridoxine overdose. *Neurology.* 1987;37:1729-1732.

Schaumburg H. Sensory neuropathy from pyridoxine abuse. *N Engl J Med.* 1984;310:198.

56.7. Answer: E. Cycloserine is a partial agonist of N-methyl-D-aspartate (NMDA) and the glycine receptor. This leads to somnolence, headache, tremor, dysarthria, confusion, and irritability. Some patients also develop suicidal ideation, paranoid delusions, and depression. Toxicity develops within 2 weeks of initiating the medication and resolves upon discontinuation. This medication should be avoided in patients who have a known history of psychiatric illness or a seizure disorder.

Kwon H-M, et al. Cycloserine-induced encephalopathy: Evidence on brain MRI. *Eur J Neurol.* 2008;15:e60-e61.

56.8. Answer: A. Rifampin is a P-glycoprotein inducer, which affects the clearance of several drugs. Rifampin is also a potent inducer of CYP enzymes, specifically CYP1A2, CYP2C9, CYP2C19, and CYP3A4. As a result, rifampin use is associated with acute graft rejection in transplanted patients because it decreases concentrations of drugs such as tacrolimus and myocphenolate. Rifampin also leads to methadone withdrawal, difficulty controlling phenytoin concentrations, and unplanned pregnancy because of its effects on oral contraceptives.

Yew WW. Clinically significant interactions with drugs used in the treatment of tuberculosis. *Drug Saf.* 2002;25:111-133.

56.9. Answer: D. This patient developed isoniazid (INH)-induced hepatotoxicity while being treated for latent tuberculosis (TB). This is an idiosyncratic reaction that is partially explained by direct drug toxicity and toxic metabolites formed via acetylation/oxidation. The metabolites most likely responsible for the INH hepatotoxicity are acetylhydrazine and hydrazine. Pyridoxine supplementation prevents INH-associated peripheral neuropathy but does not alter the incidence of hepatotoxicity. Genetic testing for acetylation status is not an effective use of time or money given the complex interactions and incompletely understood mechanism of INH-induced hepatotoxicity. Reassurance in this case is likely insufficient. Hepatotoxicity resulting from therapeutic INH treatment mandates termination of therapy. Once the liver injury has resolved, INH is safe to be reinstituted if the liver function tests are closely monitored afterward.

Singh J, et al. Hepatotoxicity due to antituberculosis therapy. Clinical profile and reintroduction of therapy. *J Clin Gastroenterol.* 1996;22:211-214.

56.10. Answer: D. Capreomycin is poorly absorbed orally and therefore must be administered intramuscularly. It leads to sterile abscesses at the injection sites. Chronic use of capreomycin also leads to tinnitus and hearing loss. Screening with audiometry is recommended.

Reisfeld B, et al. A physiologically based pharmacokinetic model for capreomycin. *Antimicrob Agents Chemother.* 2012;56:926-934.

57

Antidysrhythmics

57.1. A 26-year-old man is diagnosed with hypertrophic obstructive cardiomyopathy (HOCM) and is started on disopyramide. Which of the following statements is most accurate?
A. Disopyramide causes muscarinic toxicity at therapeutic concentrations
B. QT interval prolongation is unlikely with disopyramide
C. Disopyramide causes hypoglycemia in overdose
D. Disopyramide has a positive inotropic effect
E. QRS complex prolongation is unlikely to occur

57.2. Conduction disturbances associated with flecainide, quinidine, and procainamide toxicity have been successfully treated with which of the following medications?
A. Tocainide
B. Magnesium sulfate
C. Dobutamine
D. Sodium bicarbonate
E. Lidocaine

57.3. A 59-year-old man with a history of atrial fibrillation treated with warfarin presents to the emergency department with headache, nausea, and emesis. He is found to have an intracranial hemorrhage, and his international normalized ratio (INR) is 6.2. He has recently switched antidysrhythmics. A switch to which of the following xenobiotics most likely occurred?
A. Amiodarone
B. Digoxin
C. Metoprolol
D. Atenolol
E. Diltiazem

57.4. A 24-year-old woman undergoes tumescent liposuction at an outpatient surgical clinic. Two hours after completion of the procedure, she complains of dizziness, has a rapid decline in her mental status, and then has a generalized tonic-clonic seizure. This is followed by a cardiac arrest. Advanced cardiac life support is initiated, and she is transferred to a tertiary center. An electrocardiogram performed prior to her cardiac arrest demonstrates a wide QRS complex. What class of antidysrhythmic caused her presentation?
A. IA
B. IB
C. IC
D. II
E. III

57.5. Which class of antidysrhythmics will have the *least* effect on an electrocardiogram at therapeutic concentrations?
A. IA
B. IB
C. II
D. III
E. IV

57.6. A 27-year-old man presents to the emergency department with a known tricyclic antidepressant overdose. His QRS complex is 140 msec on an electrocardiogram (ECG). The patient develops ventricular tachycardia. Which class of antidysrhythmics would be reasonable to administer in this patient?
A. IB
B. IC
C. II
D. III
E. IV

57.7. A 3-year-old boy is brought into the emergency department because he ingested his grandfather's antidysrhythmic. His electrocardiogram demonstrates a markedly prolonged QRS complex, a prolonged PR interval, and minimal QT prolongation. Which of the following antidysrhythmics did he ingest?
A. Flecainide
B. Propafenone
C. Amiodarone
D. Digoxin
E. Disopyramide

57.8. A 67-year-old woman with a past medical history of emphysema on supplemental home oxygen therapy presents to the emergency department with significantly worsening cough, shortness of breath, hemoptysis, and increasing oxygen requirements. She has a bronchioalveolar lavage performed, which demonstrates an interstitial pneumonitis with many macrophages and a finely vacuolated foamy cytoplasm. Which antidysrhythmic has she been taking for the last 3 years?
A. Flecainide
B. Propafenone
C. Amiodarone
D. Digoxin
E. Disopyramide

57.9. A 67-year-old man presents to the emergency department with decompensated heart failure. He develops refractory ventricular tachycardia and is initiated on intravenous lidocaine therapy. Which of the following options is the most important impact his congestive heart failure (CHF) will have on the pharmacokinetics of lidocaine?
A. CHF decreases hepatic clearance of lidocaine
B. CHF decreases renal clearance of lidocaine
C. CHF increases the volume of distribution of lidocaine
D. CHF decreases the protein binding of lidocaine
E. CHF increases the fraction of ionized lidocaine

57.10. Which of the following options is an active metabolite of procainamide that leads to prolongation of the cardiac action potential and accumulates in patients with impaired kidney function?
A. Monoethylglycylxylidide (MEGX)
B. Flecainide
C. Glycine xylidide (GX)
D. *N*-Acetylprocainamide (NAPA)
E. 2-Oxoquinidione

ANSWERS

57.1. Answer: C. Disopyramide is a type IA antidysrhythmic with use-dependent sodium channel blockade, potassium channel blockade, potassium-ATP channel blockade in the pancreas, and negative inotropic properties. Hyperinsulinemic hypoglycemia occurs at toxic concentrations. Disopyramide has clinically relevant antimuscarinic effects at therapeutic doses. Negative inotropic effect of disopyramide makes it a poor choice in patients with impaired cardiac output but ideal in the setting of HOCM.

Sherrid MV, et al. Multicenter study of the efficacy and safety of disopyramide in obstructive hypertrophic cardiomyopathy. *J Am Coll Cardiol.* 2005;45:1251-1258.

57.2. Answer: D. Sodium bicarbonate improves intraventricular conduction in patients who have toxicity from sodium channel–blocking antidysrhythmics. Alkalinization reduces the binding of these antidysrhythmics to the fast sodium channels in the Purkinje fibers. The sodium alone is capable of improving conduction by increasing the extracellular sodium concentration.

Kim SY, Benowitz NL. Poisoning due to class IA antiarrhythmic drugs, quinidine, procainamide and disopyramide. *Drug Safety.* 1990; 5:393-420.

Wasserman F, et al. Successful treatment of quinidine and procainamide intoxication. *N Engl J Med.* 1958;259:797-802.

57.3. Answer: A. Amiodarone competes with warfarin for P-glycoprotein binding, leading to elevated warfarin concentrations. As patients are being switched to amiodarone as therapy, they will need adjustment of their warfarin dosing and should be monitored frequently.

Sanoski CA, Bauman JL. Clinical observations with the amiodarone/warfarin interaction dosing relationships with long term therapy. *Chest.* 2002;121:19-23.

57.4. Answer: B. This patient was undergoing tumescent liposuction, which involves injecting large volumes of dilute lidocaine to distend subcutaneous fat prior to liposuction. Lidocaine is a type IB antidysrhythmic. Toxicity is immediate or delayed and is sometimes fatal.

Rao RB, et al. Deaths related to liposuction. *N Engl J Med.* 199913; 340:1471-1475.

Mrad S, et al. Cardiac arrest following liposuction: A case report of lidocaine toxicity. *Oman Med J.* 2019;34:341-344.

57.5 Answer: B: Class IB antidysrythmics have no effect on the electrocardiogram (ECG) at therapeutic doses. Class IB antidysrhythmics have their highest affinity for inactivated sodium channels and demonstrate rapid "on-off" metabolism. They bind to the sodium channel primarily during the late electrical systole. All class IB antidysrhythmics do not bind to activated sodium channels and in therapeutic doses they do not affect the rate of rise of phase 0 of the action potential or V_{max}. This distinction is important to remember, as clinicians often refer to ECG abnormalities as an aid in the diagnosis of antidysrhythmic overdoses.

Bennett PB, et al. Competition between lidocaine and one of its metabolites, glycylxylidide, for cardiac sodium channels. *Circulation.* 1988;78;692-700.

57.6. Answer: A. Patients have a potential benefit from sodium channel blockers with short channel recovery times, such as those from class IB. Class IC antidysrhythmics demonstrate toxicity similar to that of the tricyclic antidepressants, with binding times of 10 seconds or more to the cardiac sodium channel. They would further exacerbate tricyclic antidepressant toxicity.

Foianini A, et al. What is the role of lidocaine or phenytoin in tricyclic antidepressant-induced cardiotoxicity? *Clin Toxicol.* 2010;48:325-330.

57.7. Answer: A. Flecainide is a class IC antidysrhythmic with a characteristic constellation of electrocardiographic findings including a prolonged QRS and a prolonged PR, with minimal QT prolongation. The QRS complex has

significant prognostic utility; a QRS duration that is >200 msec is predictive of the need for mechanical circulatory support.

Valentino MA, et al. Flecainide toxicity: A case report and systematic review of its electrocardiographic patterns and management. *Cardiovasc Toxicol.* 2016;17:260-266.

57.8. Answer: C. Amiodarone causes a pneumonitis that develops in 5% of patients who take this medication. It typically develops after years of treatment. It is dose related, and patients prescribed doses >400 mg/day are at a higher risk. Oxygen therapy also increases the risk of developing the pneumonitis. When amiodarone-induced pulmonary toxicity is diagnosed early, the prognosis is favorable. However, if the diagnosis is delayed, it leads to pulmonary fibrosis and death.

Camus P, et al. Amiodarone pulmonary toxicity. *Clin Chest Med.* 2004;25:65-75.

Wolkove N, Baltzan M. Amiodarone pulmonary toxicity. *Can Respir J.* 2009;16:43-48.

57.9. Answer: A. Although CHF alters the volume of distribution and protein binding of lidocaine, reduced hepatic perfusion is most significant. Lidocaine is a drug with a high-extraction ratio, which means that its metabolism and clearance are highly dependent on hepatic blood flow. CHF significantly reduces hepatic blood flow and drug clearance.

Prescott LF, et al. Impaired lidocaine metabolism in patients with myocardial infarction and cardiac failure. *Br Med J.* 1976;1:939-941.

57.10 Answer: D. Procainamide undergoes hepatic biotransformation by acetylation to *N*-acetylprocainamide (NAPA), the rate of which is genetically determined. Slow acetylators are at risk of developing drug-induced systemic lupus erythematosus (SLE). Elevated procainamide concentrations lead to sodium channel blockade and dysrhythmias while accumulation of NAPA leads to QT interval prolongation and risk for torsade de pointes. Both procainamide and NAPA are renally eliminated and accumulate in patients with chronic kidney disease.

Low CL, et al. Relative efficacy of hemoperfusion, hemodialysis and CAPD in the removal of procainamide and NAPA in a patient with severe procainamide toxicity. *Nephrol Dial Transplant.* 1996;11:881-884.

Antithrombotics

QUESTIONS

58.1. A 70-year-old man is brought into the emergency department after sustaining an intracranial hemorrhage. He has a history of atrial fibrillation and is prescribed warfarin. Which of the following treatments is indicated?
A. Prothrombin complex concentrate
B. Andexanet alfa
C. Idarucizumab
D. Desmopressin
E. Protamine sulfate

58.2. Which of the following xenobiotics is an appropriate treatment option in the management of warfarin-induced coagulopathy in patients with a history of heparin-induced thrombocytopenia (HIT)?
A. Prothrombin complex concentrate
B. Factor eight inhibitor bypassing activity
C. Andexanet alfa
D. Protamine sulfate
E. Idarucizumab

58.3. A 2-year-old boy presents to the emergency department 3 hours after ingesting five of his grandmother's rivaroxaban pills. He is entirely asymptomatic with a normal physical examination. Which of the following treatment options would be best in the management of this patient's overdose?
A. Immediately discharge the patient home
B. Administer oral activated charcoal
C. Administer oral vitamin K
D. Administer prothrombin complex concentrate
E. Administer factor eight inhibitor bypassing activity

58.4. A 3-year-old girl presents to the emergency department after a single unsupervised ingestion of brodifacoum while visiting a relative's house. Which laboratory studies would be most appropriate?
A. Obtain an international normalized ratio (INR) at baseline and 48 hours after exposure
B. Obtain an INR at 48 hours after exposure
C. Obtain a partial thromboplastin time (PTT) at baseline and 48 hours after exposure
D. Obtain a PTT at 48 hours after exposure
E. Obtain a factor V concentration immediately

58.5. A 67-year-old man has a 500-mL bag containing 50,000 units of heparin unintentionally infused while in the hospital. One hour after the mistake is discovered, his partial thromboplastin time (PTT) is reported as >150 seconds. The patient is asymptomatic with normal vital signs and no signs of bleeding. Which therapy would be the most appropriate for this patient?
A. Infuse tranexemic acid intravenously
B. Infuse protamine intravenously and then repeat the PTT
C. Perform an exchange transfusion on the patient
D. Administer prothrombin complex concentrate intravenously and repeat the PTT
E. Observe the patient for bleeding and then repeat the PTT

58.6. A 65-year-old woman presents to the emergency department with melena. Her hemoglobin is 5 g/dL lower than her baseline. Further history reveals that the patient had overdosed on enoxaparin in a suicide attempt. Which of the following initial treatments is reasonable to administer for this patient?
A. Idarucizumab
B. Fresh frozen plasma
C. Protamine sulfate
D. Prothrombin complex concentrate
E. Vitamin K

58.7. A 50-year-old man presents to the emergency department with life-threatening bleeding after an intentional overdose of dabigatran. Which of the following treatments is indicated?
A. Prothrombin complex concentrate
B. Idarucizumab
C. Andexanet alfa
D. Protamine sulfate
E. Desmopressin

58.8. Low-molecular-weight heparins differ from unfractionated (conventional) heparin in which of the following ways?

A. They have a lower bioavailability
B. They have targeted activity against factor X
C. It is difficult to achieve adequate anticoagulation with fixed dosing
D. They have a lower incidence of bleeding complications
E. They are monitored by the partial thromboplastin time (PTT)

58.9. Which of the following adverse effects is associated with intravenous vitamin K administration?
A. Non-immune hypersensitivity (anaphylactoid) reaction
B. White clot syndrome
C. Thrombocytopenia
D. Arthralgias
E. Risk of HIV transmission

58.10. Which of the following options differentiates postoperative thrombocytopenia from heparin-induced thrombocytopenia (HIT)?
A. It is associated with white clot syndrome
B. It occurs because of platelet consumption
C. It is associated with hyperkalemia
D. It is associated with osteoporosis
E. Patients often present with hemorrhagic complications

ANSWERS

58.1. Answer: A. The US Food and Drug Administration (FDA) approved factor replacement with four-factor prothrombin complex concentrate (PCC) as first-line treatment for major bleeding in the setting of vitamin K antagonist–induced coagulopathy. The dosing of PCC is based on the international normalized ratio (INR) and body weight. The typical doses range between 25 and 50 units/kg with the largest dose based on a maximum weight of 100 kg.

Holbrook A, et al. Evidence-based management of anticoagulant therapy: Antithrombotic therapy and prevention of thrombosis, 9th ed: American College of Chest Physicians Evidence-Based Clinical Practice Guidelines. *Chest.* 2012;141(2 suppl):e152S-e184S.

58.2. Answer: B. Most forms of prothrombin complex concentrate (PCC) contain small amounts of heparin. These heparin-containing PCCs are contraindicated in patients with a history of HIT. In patients with HIT, factor eight inhibitor bypassing activity (FEIBA), an activated prothrombin complex concentrate that does not contain heparin, is recommended.

Baxalta US Inc. FEIBA (anti-inhibitor coagulant complex). http://www. shirecontent.com/PI/PDFs/FEIBA_USA_ENG.pdf. Accessed July 23, 2021.

58.3. Answer: B. Rivaroxaban absorption is decreased after activated charcoal administration, even when given up to 8 hours after a single oral dose of rivaroxaban. Absorption is decreased by 43% if activated charcoal is given within 2 hours of rivaroxaban ingestion and by 29% when given within 8 hours. This child is entirely asymptomatic with no active bleeding, so no other antidotal therapy is indicated at this time.

Ollier E, et al. Effect of activated charcoal on rivaroxaban complex absorption. *Clin Pharmacokinet.* 2017;56:793-801.

58.4. Answer: B. Brodifacoum, a rodenticide, is a long-acting vitamin K antagonist. Long-acting anticoagulant rodenticides are structurally and biochemically similar to warfarin. As such, these long-acting anticoagulants do not produce immediate changes in the INR. The optimum timing of laboratory studies in these patients is determined to be within 24-48 hours. Obtaining baseline INR testing is not cost effective and exposes the child to the discomfort of unnecessary phlebotomy. Factor V is not activated by vitamin K, so it is abnormal only in patients with liver disease.

Smolinske SC, et al. Superwarfarin poisoning in children: A prospective study. *Pediatrics* 1989;84:490-494.

58.5. Answer: E. One milligram of protamine binds 100 units of heparin. Since protamine infusion is associated with severe immune (anaphylaxis) and non-immune reactions, it is indicated only for the reversal of consequential heparin overdose. Although the 50,000 units of heparin might lead to significant bleeding, it has a short half-life and this patient is without symptoms. If reversal is required, excessive protamine might lead to worsening anticoagulation. The protamine dose should be based on the amount of heparin remaining using a 1-2 hour half-life, and be no >50 mg. Additional dosing is reasonable based on a repeat PTT and the clinical status of the patient. Exchange transfusion is performed in neonates with significant bleeding to remove heparin if protamine is contraindicated. Prothrombin complex concentrate is not usually used in the management of heparin-induced bleeding.

Holland CL, et al. Adverse reactions to protamine sulfate following cardiac surgery. *Clin Cardiol.* 1984;7:157-162.

58.6. Answer: C. Protamine sulfate partially reverses low-molecular-weight heparins (LMWHs), such as enoxaparin, dalteparin, and tinzaparin. There are reports of both success and failure of protamine administration to reverse LMWH-associated bleeding. Protamine is reasonable therapy for LMWH excess associated with hemorrhage, but complete reversal should not be expected, and caution is advised to limit the protamine dose.

Chawla L, et al. Incomplete reversal of enoxaparin toxicity by protamine: Implications of renal insufficiency, obesity and low molecular weight heparin sulfate content. *Obesity Surg.* 2004;14:695-698.

Garcia DA, et al. Parenteral anticoagulants: Antithrombotic therapy and prevention of thrombosis, 9th ed: American College of Chest Physicians Evidence-Based Clinical Practice Guidelines. *Chest.* 2012;141(2 suppl):e24S-e43S.

58.7. Answer: B. Idarucizumab is a monoclonal antibody targeting dabigatran. In murine and human studies, idarucizumab administration resulted in normalization of a battery of functional clotting assays, including clotting time, activated partial thromboplastin time (aPTT), and thrombin time (TT). In a prospective study containing 90 patients who received 5 g of intravenous idarucizumab for urgent reversal of dabigatran-induced coagulopathy, reversal of coagulopathy occurred in 100% of patients despite 18 deaths in the study population. While there are significant limitations to many of the studies that evaluate idarucizumab, it is reasonable to administer this antidote to a patient who has life-threatening bleeding following an overdose of dabigatran.

Van Ryn J, et al. An antibody selective to dabigatran safely neutralizes both dabigatran-induced anticoagulant and bleeding activity in in vitro and in vivo models. *J Thromb Haemost.* 2011;9:110.

Schiele F, et al. A specific antidote for dabigatran: Functional and structural characterization. *Blood.* 2013;121:3554-3562.

58.8. Answer: B. Low-molecular-weight heparins (LMWHs) differ from unfractionated heparin in that they have a greater bioavailability and they have targeted activity against factor Xa. Most patients achieve adequate anticoagulation with fixed dosing. As a result of their targeted factor Xa activity, LMWHs have minimal effect on the activated PTT, thus eliminating the need for and usefulness of monitoring the PTT. Unfortunately, although these properties make administration and monitoring of LMWHs easier than with conventional heparin, they do not eliminate or even reduce the risk of bleeding complications.

Bounameaux H, Goldhaber SZ. Uses of low-molecular-weight heparin. *Blood Rev.* 1995;9:213-219.

Green D, et al. Low molecular weight heparin: A critical analysis of clinical trials. *Pharmacol Rev.* 1994;46:89-109.

58.9. Answer: A. There are cases of death secondary to non-immune hypersenstivity reactions from the rapid intravenous administration of vitamin K; this is likely a result of the colloidal formulation of the preparation. When administered orally, vitamin K is virtually free of adverse effects, except for overcorrection of the INR for a patient requiring maintenance anticoagulation. White clot syndrome and thrombocytopenia are associated with heparin administration. Arthralgia is associated with prothrombin complex concentrate. While rare, there is a risk of HIV transmission with the transfusion of any blood products, including fresh frozen plasma.

Fiore L, et al. Anaphylactoid reactions to vitamin K. *J Thromb Thrombolysis.* 2001;11:175-183.

58.10. Answer: B. Postoperative thrombocytopenia occurs in the first 1 or 2 days after surgery and usually results from platelet consumption and improves by the third postoperative day. Heparin, on the other hand, stimulates platelets to release PF4, which subsequently complexes with heparin to provoke an IgG response, causing platelet aggregation and thrombocytopenia. White clot syndrome is associated with a more severe form of heparin-induced thrombocytopenia (HIT). Patients with HIT present with either hemorrhagic or thromboembolic complications. Heparin use is also associated with necrotizing skin lesions, hyperkalemia from aldosterone suppression, and osteoporosis (in patients on long-term therapy with unfractionated heparin). Some patients develop bone fractures if treated continuously for >3 months.

Warkentin TE, et al. Heparin-induced thrombocytopenia in patients treated with low-molecular-weight heparin or unfractionated heparin. *N Engl J Med*. 1995;332:1330-1335.

Hovanessian HC. New-generation anticoagulants: The low molecular weight heparins. *Ann Emerg Med*. 2012;34:768-779.

59

Beta Adrenergic Antagonists

QUESTIONS

59.1. Which of the following beta adrenergic antagonists is responsible for the majority of intentional overdoses and deaths?
A. Metoprolol
B. Propranolol
C. Carvedilol
D. Atenolol
E. Esmolol

59.2. A 65-year-old woman presents to the hospital after an intentional ingestion of her medication. Her initial heart rate is 35 beats/min and her blood pressure is 60/40 mmHg. Four hours later, she is found pulseless and her rhythm on the monitor is torsade de pointes. Which beta adrenergic antagonist is most likely responsible for her clinical presentation?
A. Labetalol
B. Sotalol
C. Propranolol
D. Nebivolol
E. Atenolol

59.3. Which of the following statements concerning myocardial contractility is true?
A. Intracellular sodium decreases contractility by preventing calcium influx
B. Intracellular sodium increases contractility by opening calcium release channels in the sarcoplasmic reticulum
C. Phosphorylating phospholamban increases contractility by opening calcium release channels in the sarcoplasmic reticulum

D. Blockade of outward potassium channels prolongs the action potential duration and decreases contractility
E. Beta adrenergic stimulation increases cyclic adenosine monophosphate (cAMP) concentrations, which in turn activate protein kinases

59.4. Which of the following statements concerning inotropes is true?
A. Glucagon increases cyclic adenosine monophosphate (cAMP) concentrations by stimulating beta adrenergic receptors
B. Amrinone increases cAMP concentrations by acting on a unique PDI receptor
C. Digoxin decreases intracellular sodium and hence increases intracellular calcium
D. Glucagon receptor stimulation increases protein kinase C activity
E. Milrinone increases cAMP concentrations by inhibiting its breakdown

59.5. A 19-year-old woman presents to the emergency department following an intentional overdose of her mother's medication. While in the hospital, she has a generalized tonic-clonic seizure. Her blood pressure at the time of the seizure is 110/70 mmHg. Which of the following beta adrenergic antagonists best explains her presentation?
A. Acebutolol
B. Labetalol
C. Nadolol
D. Propranolol
E. Sotalol

59.6. A 36-year-old man with a past medical history of hypertension and chronic kidney disease is initiated on hemodialysis. Which of the following beta adrenergic antagonists would be most affected by his new hemodialysis therapy?
A. Atenolol
B. Labetalol
C. Metoprolol
D. Propranolol
E. Timolol

59.7. Which of the following options best describes the role of beta$_3$ adrenergic receptors?
A. Increased contractility in the heart
B. Increased cardiac chronotropy
C. Increased cardiac relaxation
D. Prevents myocyte apoptosis
E. Increased cardioprotection in the failing heart

59.8. Which of the following beta adrenergic antagonists demonstrate intrinsic sympathomimetic activity?
A. Sotalol
B. Carvedilol
C. Pindolol

D. Betaxolol
E. Propranolol

59.9. A previously healthy 19-year-old man presents to the emergency department following an unintentional ingestion of three of his grandfather's metoprolol tablets. Which of the following therapies will this patient likely require?
A. Orogastric lavage
B. Glucagon
C. Calcium gluconate
D. High-dose insulin therapy
E. None of the above

59.10. Overdoses of beta adrenergic antagonists and calcium channel blockers share many features in common. Which of the following findings would be more suggestive of a beta adrenergic antagonist overdose?
A. Preserved mental status
B. Hypotension
C. Bradycardia
D. Hypoglycemia
E. Hypokalemia

ANSWERS

59.1. Answer: B. Propranolol is prescribed frequently for conditions such as anxiety, stress, and migraine prophylaxis. It is also the most frequent culprit in beta adrenergic antagonist–related deaths. Propranolol is more lethal than the other listed beta adrenergic antagonists due to its lipophilic and membrane-stabilizing properties. Other beta adrenergic antagonists with membrane-stabilizing effects include acebutolol and carvedilol.

Love JN, et al. Characterization of fatal beta blocker ingestion: A review of the American Association of Poison Control Centers data from 1985 to 1995. *J Toxicol Clin Toxicol.* 1997;35:353-359.

59.2. Answer: B. In addition to beta$_1$ and beta$_2$ adrenergic antagonism, sotalol also blocks potassium channels. Patients who overdose on sotalol present with bradycardia, hypotension, and a prolonged QT interval, which occasionally progresses to ventricular dysrhythmias and torsade de pointes.

Arstall MA, et al. Sotalol-induced torsade de pointes: Management with magnesium infusion. *Postgrad Med J.* 1992;68:289-290.

59.3. Answer: E. Beta adrenergic receptors are coupled to G$_S$ proteins. When catecholamines bind to the receptor, they activate adenylate cyclase (also known as adenylyl cyclase), leading to an increase in the formation of cAMP. Increased cAMP activates protein kinase A, which phosphorylates different sites in the cardiac myocyte, including the very important L-type calcium channel. Phosphorylation of the L-type calcium channel works to increase the permeability of this channel to calcium and to trigger the release of calcium from the sarcoplasmic reticulum. This is the main way that catecholamines act as positive inotropes. Digoxin, on the other hand, causes increased intracellular sodium through inhibition of the Na$^+$/K$^+$-ATPase pump, leading to increased intracellular calcium by inhibiting the extrusion of calcium by the calcium-sodium exchange pump. Phospholamban inhibits the sarcoplasmic calcium pump. This inhibition is removed by phosphorylation of phospholamban, resulting in greater sarcoplasmic calcium stores and thus greater contractility. Blocking outward potassium channels increases the action potential duration, but this increases contractility by prolonging the time that slow calcium channels remain open.

Barry WH, Bridge JHB. Intracellular calcium homeostasis in cardiac myocytes. *Circulation.* 1993;87:1806-1815.

59.4. Answer: E. Glucagon increases cAMP concentrations independently of the beta adrenergic receptor. Amrinone and milrinone decrease cAMP breakdown by inhibiting phosphodiesterase. There is no such thing as a PDI receptor. The primary inotropic action of digoxin is to inhibit the sodium-potassium exchange pump, resulting in increased intracellular sodium. This inhibits the extrusion of calcium and therefore increases contractility.

Yagami T. Differential coupling of glucagon and beta-adrenergic receptors with the small and large forms of the stimulatory G protein. *Mol Pharmacol.* 1995;48:849-854.

59.5. Answer: D. Of all the beta adrenergic antagonists, propranolol has the greatest lipid solubility and the greatest membrane-stabilizing effect. It is most likely to cause seizures in overdose. In patients who overdose on propranolol, seizures sometimes occur even with a normal blood pressure.

Buiumsohn A, et al. Seizures and intraventricular conduction defect in propranolol poisonings. A report of two cases. *Ann Intern Med.* 1979;91:860-862.

59.6. Answer: A. Atenolol has high water solubility (resulting in a low volume of distribution) and low protein binding. These properties mean that hemodialysis would impact serum concentrations of this medication. The other beta adrenergic antagonists have moderate to high lipid solubility and protein binding and are therefore unlikely to be removed by hemodialysis.

Saitz R, et al. Atenolol-induced cardiovascular collapse treated with hemodialysis. *Crit Care Med.* 1991;19:116-118.

59.7. Answer: E. There are three beta adrenergic receptors in the human body. Answer choices A-C describe the activity of the beta$_2$ adrenergic receptor under normal conditions. Answer choice D describes the activity of the beta$_2$ adrenergic receptor following chronic stimulation. The beta$_3$ adrenergic receptor is present in the heart and the endothelium and is believed to result in cardioprotection for the failing heart. When the heart fails, the compensatory response is an elevation of catecholamines, which help transiently. However, with chronic stimulation, the beta$_1$ and beta$_2$ adrenergic receptors become desensitized, leading to progression of heart failure. The beta$_3$ adrenergic receptors are not desensitized and, through the generation of nitric oxide, result in cardioprotection. Beta$_3$ adrenergic receptors are also responsible for metabolic regulation in adipose tissue. Ultimately, chronic beta$_3$ adrenergic receptor stimulation prevents maladaptive myocardial remodeling. Increasing evidence demonstrates that metoprolol and nebivolol, both beta$_1$ adrenergic antagonists, appear to upregulate beta$_3$ adrenergic receptors and improve cardiac function while carvedilol reduces beta$_3$ adrenergic receptor expression.

Emorine LJ, et al. Molecular characterization of the human beta 3-adrenergic receptor. *Science.* 1989;245:1118-1121.

Cannavo A, Koch WJ. Targeting β3-adrenergic receptors in the heart: Selective agonism and β-blockade. *J Cardiovasc Pharmacol.* 2017;69:71-78.

59.8. Answer: C. Pindolol, acebutolol, carteolol, and penbutolol are all beta adrenergic antagonists that have intrinsic sympathomimetic activity. Theoretically, the intrinsic sympathomimetic activity should avoid the dramatic decrease in resting heart rates that occurs with other beta adrenergic antagonists.

Frishman WH, Saunders E. Beta-Adrenergic blockers. *J Clin Hypertens.* 2011;13:649-653.

59.9. Answer: E. In otherwise healthy adults, an overdose of metoprolol is benign. With the exception of propranolol and sotalol, most healthy patients who overdose on beta adrenergic antagonists alone do well, and about one-third of patients are entirely asymptomatic. The risks of orogastric lavage in this scenario far outweigh the benefits. Patients who are resting and not dependent on their sympathetic stimulation to maintain cardiac output do not require the beta adrenergic stimulation. Therefore, it would be unlikely that glucagon, calcium gluconate, or high-dose insulin therapy would be needed in this scenario. In fact, when the poison center is called following a single pill ingestion of metoprolol, many of these patients are managed at home and not sent into the hospital.

Elkharrat D, et al. Beta-adrenergic receptor blockade: A self-limited phenomenon explaining the benignancy of acute poisoning with beta adrenergic inhibitors. Report of a series of 40 patients seen at the Fernand-Widal toxicology center, with a 0% mortality rate. *Semin Hop.* 1982;58:1073-1076.

59.10. Answer: D. Patients who are critically ill following either a beta adrenergic antagonist or calcium channel blocker overdose will be bradycardic and hypotensive. Calcium channel blockers demonstrate neuroprotective properties; therefore, patients who overdose on calcium channel blockers tend to have a preserved mental status. Beta adrenergic antagonist toxicity is associated with hyperkalemia not hypokalemia. Beta adrenergic antagonists interfere with glycogenolysis and gluconeogenesis and lead to hypoglycemia, which occurs more frequently in children.

Poterucha JT, et al. Frequency and severity of hypoglycemia in children with beta-blocker-treated long QT syndrome. *Heart Rhythm.* 2015;12:1815-1819.

Calcium Channel Blockers

QUESTIONS

60.1. In therapeutic dosing, which one of the following channels do calcium channel blockers antagonize?
  A. Voltage-sensitive L-type channels
  B. Voltage-sensitive T-type channels
  C. Receptor-activated S-type channels
  D. Receptor-activated T-type channels
  E. Naloxone-sensitive calcium channels

60.2. Which of the following proteins is involved in contraction coupling within the cardiac muscle cell?
  A. Tropomyosin
  B. Actin
  C. Calmodulin
  D. Myosin light chain kinase
  E. Myoglobin

60.3. Which of the following findings is more characteristic of a calcium channel blocker overdose as compared to a beta adrenergic antagonist overdose?
  A. Sinus bradycardia
  B. Hypotension
  C. Depressed mental status
  D. Hyperglycemia
  E. Nausea and vomiting

60.4. A 2-year-old girl presents to the emergency department 2 hours after a suspected ingestion of one of her grandmother's extended-release diltiazem tablets. She is entirely asymptomatic. Which of the following interventions would be reasonable to perform next in this patient?
  A. Orogastric lavage
  B. Oral activated charcoal administration
  C. Intravenous calcium gluconate administration
  D. Intravenous glucagon administration
  E. Discharge patient home with return precautions

60.5. A 27-year-old man presents to the emergency department following an intentional overdose of diltiazem. He is critically ill and is initiated on high-dose insulin therapy. Which of the following options is an expected side effect of this treatment regimen?
  A. Hypermagnesemia
  B. Hyperphosphatemia
  C. Hypokalemia
  D. Hyperglycemia
  E. Hypocalcemia

60.6. A 67-year-old woman presents to the emergency department with bradycardia and hypotension. Her medication list includes diltiazem; however, she has not changed the dose in years. Addition of which of the following new medications is a possible explanation for this patient's presentation?
  A. Fluoxetine
  B. Acetaminophen
  C. Levothyroxine
  D. Ciprofloxacin
  E. Metformin

60.7. Which of the following calcium channel blockers has the greatest potency for the myocardium?
   A. Verapamil
   B. Diltiazem
   C. Nifedipine
   D. Amlodipine
   E. Nicardipine

60.8. Which of the following calcium channel blocker treatments increases cardiac output through preventing the breakdown of cyclic adenosine monophosphate (cAMP) by phosphodiesterase (PDE) enzyme inhibition?
   A. Amrinone
   B. Glucagon
   C. Atropine
   D. Calcium gluconate
   E. Norepinephrine

60.9. A 37-year-old man presents to the emergency department following an intentional ingestion of an entire bottle of nifedipine. As part of the management of his toxicity, several grams of calcium gluconate are administered. Which of the following options is an adverse effect seen with this treatment regimen?
   A. Diarrhea
   B. Hypocalcemia
   C. Confusion
   D. Hyperphosphatemia
   E. Hypermagnesemia

60.10. A 56-year-old man presents after an intentional overdose of a bottle of diltiazem. He remains bradycardic to 25 beats/min and hypotensive to 40/10 mmHg despite receiving standard treatment options. A bedside echocardiogram demonstrates very poor cardiac contractility. Which of the following adjunctive therapies would be reasonable at this time?
   A. Hemodialysis
   B. Methylene blue
   C. Electrical pacing
   D. Venovenous extracorporeal membrane oxygenation
   E. Venoarterial extracorporeal membrane oxygenation

ANSWERS

60.1. Answer: A. Calcium channel blockers antagonize the voltage-sensitive L-type calcium channels in both the myocardium and vascular smooth muscle. These channels are opened upon cellular depolarization and allow influx of calcium to initiate muscular contraction.

> Katz AM. Calcium channel diversity in the cardiovascular system. *J Am Coll Cardiol.* 1996;28:522-529.

60.2. Answer: A. When calcium enters the myocardial cell and is released from the sarcoplasmic reticulum, it binds troponin C, which causes a conformational change that displaces troponin and tropomyosin from the actin. This allows actin and myosin to bind, resulting in a contraction. Myosin light chain kinase is found only in smooth muscle cells and is activated by calcium/calmodulin complex. Then myosin light chain kinase activates myosin, allowing it to bind to actin, and a contraction occurs.

> Adelstein RS, et al. Regulation of smooth muscle contractile proteins by calmodulin and cyclic AMP. *Fed Proc.* 1982;41:2873-2878.

> Katz A. Contractile proteins of the heart. *Physiol Rev.* 1970;50:63-167.

60.3. Answer: D. Calcium channel blocker toxicity results in blockade of L-type calcium channels in the pancreas, leading to decreased insulin release and resultant hyperglycemia.

Hyperglycemia is a prognostic sign in the cases of severe calcium channel blocker poisoning. Bradycardia and hypotension occur in both calcium channel blocker and beta adrenergic antagonist toxicity. A depressed mental status is more typical of a beta adrenergic antagonist; patients who overdose on calcium channel blockers often have a preserved mental status. Nausea and vomiting are not typical in calcium channel blocker toxicity.

> Levine M, et al. Assessment of hyperglycemia after calcium channel blocker overdoses involving diltiazem or verapamil. *Crit Care Med.* 2007;35:2071-2075.

60.4. Answer: B. We recommend 1 g/kg of activated charcoal in patients who present following an overdose of a calcium channel blocker. Charcoal adsorbs to calcium channel blockers. In patients who demonstrate significant signs of toxicity, multiple-dose activated charcoal is reasonable as a continuous presence of activated charcoal in the gastrointestinal tract adsorbs xenobiotics as they are liberated from extended-release formulations. Orogastric lavage is challenging in young children, and because this child is asymptomatic 2 hours after a suspected ingestion, the risks outweigh the benefits. While the patient is asymptotic with normal vital signs, given the significant toxicity associated with an extended-release diltiazem, we recommend 24-hour observation in a monitored setting. There is no indication to administer prophylactic antidotes such as calcium gluconate and glucagon in this patient.

Roberts D, et al. Diltiazem overdose: Pharmacokinetics of diltiazem and its metabolites and effect of multiple dose charcoal therapy. *J Toxicol Clin Toxicol*. 1991;29:45-52.

60.5. Answer: C. An anticipated effect of insulin therapy includes hypokalemia; this occurs because potassium is shifted from the extracellular space to the intracellular space. Often the degree of hypokalemia that occurs is clinically insignificant. Caution is needed when repleting potassium, as there is a risk of rebound hyperkalemia.

Holger JS, et al. High-dose insulin: A consecutive case series in toxin-induced cardiogenic shock. *Clin Toxicol*. 2011;49:653-658.

Greene SL, et al. Relative safety of hyperinsulinaemia/euglycaemia in the management of calcium channel blocker overdose: A prospective observational study. *Intensive Care Med*. 2007;33:2019-2024.

60.6. Answer: A. CYP3A4, which metabolizes most calcium channel blockers, is also responsible for the oxidation of numerous other xenobiotics. Inhibitors of CYP3A4, such as fluoxetine, cimetidine, and macrolide antibiotics, increase serum concentrations of diltiazem and lead to calcium channel blocker toxicity. The other listed choices do not have significant drug-drug interactions with diltiazem.

Quinn DI, Day RO. Drug interactions of clinical importance. An updated guide. *Drug Saf*. 1995;12:393-452.

60.7. Answer: A. The nondihydropyridine calcium channel blockers, such as verapamil and diltiazem, have the greatest potency for the myocardium, with verapamil being the most potent. The dihydropyridine calcium channel blockers, such as nifedipine, have little effect at the myocardium and have most of their effect at the peripheral vascular tissue. Therefore, dihydropyridine calcium channel blockers have the most potent vasodilatory effects as compared to nondihydropyridine calcium channel blockers.

Pitt B. Diversity of calcium antagonists. *Clin Ther*. 1997;19(suppl A):3-17.

60.8. Answer: A. Phosphodiesterase inhibitors, such as amrinone and milrinone, were used to treat patients with calcium channel blocker poisoning. They increase cardiac output by inhibiting the breakdown of cyclic adenosine monophosphate (cAMP) by inhibiting PDE, which increases intracellular cAMP concentrations. Unfortunately, these medications are not readily available in many emergency departments, and other antidotes such as calcium gluconate and high-dose insulin therapy are more effective and easier to use. As such, we do not recommend the routine use of PDE inhibitors in the management of calcium channel blocker toxicity.

Koury SI, et al. Amrinone as an antidote in experimental verapamil overdose. *Acad Emerg Med*. 1996;3:762-767.

60.9. Answer: C. The adverse effects of calcium gluconate include nausea, vomiting, constipation, ileus, hypercalcemia, hypophosphatemia, polyuria, polydipsia, nephrolithiasis, alteration in mental status, hyporeflexia, coma, and dysrhythmias. Calcium gluconate is used in the treatment of hypermagnesemia.

Turner JJO. Hypercalcaemia—presentation and management. *Clin Med (Lond)*. 2017;17:270-273.

60.10. Answer: E. Venovenous extracorporeal membrane oxygenation is used primarily for patients with refractory respiratory failure and is not adequate to treat the shock caused by severe calcium channel blocker toxicity. Venoarterial extracorporeal membrane oxygenation is recommended in severe circulatory shock and would be reasonable to perform in a patient with refractory calcium channel blocker toxicity. Unless there is another indication, hemodialysis is not useful in the routine management of patients with calcium channel blocker poisoning. Methylene blue assists more with vasodilatory shock, and there are reports of it being used successfully in the management of patients who overdosed on amlodipine. Unfortunately, patients who have severe calcium channel blocker toxicity frequently do not have appropriate capture with electrical pacing.

De Rita F, et al. Rescue extracorporeal life support for acute verapamil and propranolol toxicity in a neonate. *Artifi Organs*. 2011;35:416-420.

Weinberg RL, et al. Venoarterial extracorporeal membrane oxygenation for the management of massive amlodipine overdose. *Perfusion*. 2014;29:53-56.

Miscellaneous Antihypertensives and Pharmacologically Related Agents

61

QUESTIONS

61.1. A 63-year-old man with a past medical history of hypertension presents to the emergency department with isolated angioedema to both his lips and tongue. He has no rash, wheezing, or gastrointestinal symptoms. Which target of the implicated antihypertensive is responsible for the development of angioedema?
A. Leukotrienes
B. Prostaglandin D_2
C. Bradykinin
D. Histamine
E. Norepinephrine

61.2. In the patient in Question 61.1, which of the therapies below would best treat his symptoms?
A. Methylene blue
B. Naloxone
C. Fresh frozen plasma
D. Epinephrine
E. Diphenhydramine

61.3. Naloxone is a potential therapy in a patient poisoned with which of the following antihypertensives?
A. Prazosin
B. Captopril
C. Reserpine
D. Minoxidil
E. Nifedipine

61.4. Which of the following options contributes to the antihypertensive effect of clonidine?
A. Alpha$_1$ adrenergic antagonism
B. Imidazoline (I_1) agonism
C. I_2 agonism
D. Beta$_1$ adrenergic antagonism
E. Beta$_2$ adrenergic antagonism

61.5. A 62-year-old man with a past medical history of hypertension is admitted to the hospital for further management of cholecystitis. His clonidine is held while he is awaiting surgery, and 24 hours later, he develops a tremor, his heart rate rises to 135 beats/min, and his blood pressure is 220/98 mmHg. Which of the following therapies is indicated?
A. Esmolol
B. Labetalol
C. Clonidine
D. Hydralazine
E. Nicardipine

61.6. Which of the following clinical findings occurs early in a patient after a massive clonidine overdose?
A. Hypertension
B. Hyperthermia
C. Mydriasis
D. Tachypnea
E. Agitation

61.7. A 56-year-old man with a past medical history of diabetes presents to the hospital for evaluation of his worsening hyperglycemia. He is compliant with all of his medications. He was recently initiated on a new antihypertensive medication. Which of the following medications best explains his elevated blood glucose?
   A. Nifedipine
   B. Clonidine
   C. Hydrochlorothiazide
   D. Enalapril
   E. Hydralazine

61.8. A 67-year-old man presents to the hospital after an intentional ingestion of his prazosin. He is light-headed and has a syncopal episode in the emergency department. His blood pressure is 60/30 mmHg. Which of the following options would be the best initial treatment in the management of this patient?
   A. Norepinephrine
   B. Dopamine
   C. Dobutamine
   D. Milrinone
   E. Phenylephrine

61.9. A 36-year-old woman is prescribed hydralazine to treat her postpartum hypertension. Which of the following adverse effects is associated with daily hydralazine use?
   A. Lupuslike syndrome
   B. Polycythemia
   C. Diabetes insipidus
   D. Left ventricular fibrosis
   E. Hemorrhagic gastritis

61.10. An 89-year-old woman presents to the emergency department with headache, nausea, and vomiting. Her laboratory analysis reveals a sodium of 114 mEq/L. Chronic use of which of the following antihypertensives best explains this patient's presentation?
   A. Nifedipine
   B. Hydrochlorothiazide
   C. Diltiazem
   D. Clonidine
   E. Hydralazine

ANSWERS

61.1. Answer: C. Angiotensin-converting enzyme, in addition to metabolizing angiotensin I to angiotensin II, also degrades bradykinin. When inhibited, the resultant increase in bradykinin produces vasodilation, increased interstitial fluid, and possibly angioedema or a persistent cough. While angiotensin-converting enzyme inhibitors (ACEIs) work at all of the targets listed in the choices, the mechanism by which angioedema occurs is mainly through the inhibition of bradykinin and the degradation of substance P.

Israili ZH, Hall WD. Cough and angioneurotic edema associated with angiotensin-converting enzyme inhibitor therapy. *Ann Intern Med.* 1992;117:234-242.

Kostis WJ, et al. ACE inhibitor-induced angioedema: A review. *Curr Hypertens Rep.* 2018;20:55.

61.2. Answer: C. Fresh frozen plasma (FFP) contains kinase II, which acts as an angiotensin-converting enzyme (ACE) and leads to degradation of bradykinin. As angioedema secondary to angiotensin-converting enzyme inhibitors (ACEIs) is not an IgE-mediated effect, epinephrine, diphenhydramine, and corticosteroids are unlikely to be effective. Tranexamic acid (TXA) inhibits the conversion of plasminogen to plasmin, which is a necessary step in the formation of bradykinin. It is, therefore, also reasonable to administer TXA in the management of angioedema secondary to ACEI use. The

ACEI should be discontinued in this patient, and the use of further ACEIs or angiotensin II receptor blockers (ARBs) is contraindicated.

van den Elzen M, et al. Efficacy of treatment of non-hereditary angioedema. *Clin Rev Allergy Immunol.* 2018;54:412-431.

Wang K, et al. Tranexamic acid for ACE inhibitor induced angioedema: A case report. *Am J Emerg Med.* 2020:S0735-6757(20)30923-2.

61.3. Answer: B. Although naloxone is used as an antidote for clonidine poisoning, there is some evidence that it is also effective in reversing the hypotensive effects of an angiotensin-converting enzyme inhibitor (ACEI) overdose.

Millar JA, et al. Attenuation of the antihypertensive effect of captopril by the opioid receptor antagonist naloxone. *Clin Exp Pharmacol Physiol.* 1983;10:253-259.

Varon J, Duncan SR. Naloxone reversal of hypotension due to captopril overdose. *Ann Emerg Med.* 1991;20:1125-1127.

61.4. Answer: B. Clonidine exerts its antihypertensive effects through agonism at two different receptors: imidazoline$_1$ and alpha$_2$ adrenergic receptors. Both work synergistically to reduce sympathetic tone and inhibit sympathetic neurotransmission. The opioidlike effects that occur with clonidine overdoses are due to its action on I_2 receptors and through the release of beta-endorphins, which directly stimulate the opioid receptors.

Lowry JA, Brown JT. Significance of the imidazoline receptors in toxicology. *Clin Toxicol (Phila)*. 2014;52:454-469.

61.5. Answer: C. Clonidine is a centrally acting $alpha_2$ adrenergic agonist, and sudden discontinuation of this medication leads to a rebound sympathetic surge, including symptoms such as tremor, tachycardia, fever, agitation, and severe hypertension. Administering clonidine will relieve the symptoms of withdrawal. Benzodiazepines are also a reasonable alternative. Esmolol exacerbates the symptoms of clonidine withdrawal and leads to paradoxical hypertension. Beta adrenergic antagonists, such as labetalol, should be avoided in the treatment of clonidine withdrawal.

Bailey RR, Neale TJ. Rapid clonidine withdrawal with blood pressure overshoot exaggerated by beta-blockade. *Br Med J*. 1976;1:942-943.

61.6. Answer: A. Physical findings in a patient with a clonidine overdose include central nervous system depression, bradycardia, hypotension, hypothermia, and miosis. Paradoxically, hypertension occurs early in overdose due to nonspecific peripheral alpha adrenergic agonism and norepinephrine release. Typically, this hypertension is limited as the central sympatholytic effects become prominent and hypotension ensues.

Anderson FJ, et al. Clonidine overdose: Report of six cases and review of the literature. *Ann Emerg Med*. 1981;10:107-112.

61.7. Answer: C. Thiazide diuretics cause hyperglycemia primarily through their depletion of total body potassium stores. Because insulin release is dependent on transmembrane potassium, hypokalemia leads to a decrease in insulin release and a resultant hyperglycemia. The incidence of thiazide-associated hyperglycemia has decreased since the recommended dosage of hydrochlorothiazide has been lowered. Thiazide-associated hyperglycemia is treated with appropriate potassium supplementation.

Luna B, Feinglos MN. Drug-induced hyperglycemia. *JAMA*. 2001; 286:1945-1948.

61.8. Answer: E. Prazosin is a selective $alpha_1$ adrenergic antagonist that leads to arterial smooth muscle relaxation, vasodilation, and hypotension. Patients also develop central nervous system depression and coma following overdose. Phenylephrine would help to treat the peripheral vasodilation and is a reasonable initial vasopressor to use in the management of this patient.

Rygnestad TK, Dale O. Self-poisoning with prazosin. *Acta Med Scand*. 1983;213:157-158.

61.9. Answer: A. Chronic daily use of hydralazine is associated with hemolytic anemia, vasculitis, glomerulonephritis, and a lupuslike syndrome. Left ventricular, multifocal, subacute necrosis and eventual fibrosis are associated with chronic use of minoxidil.

Pettinger WA, Mitchell HC. Side effects of vasodilator therapy. *Hypertension*. 1988;11:36.

61.10. Answer: B. Thiazides are responsible for diuretic-induced hyponatremia. Hyponatremia develops as early as 14 days following initiation of therapy with this diuretic. This is associated with excess antidiuretic hormone, hypokalemia, and excess water intake. Risk factors for the development of diuretic-induced hyponatremia include female gender, older age, and malnutrition.

Sonnenblick M, et al. Diuretic-induced severe hyponatremia. Review and analysis of 129 reported patients. *Chest*. 1993;103:601-606.

Cardioactive Steroids

QUESTIONS

62.1. Which of the following mechanisms best explains the ability of digoxin to improve cardiac contractility?
A. The sodium-calcium transporter is indirectly stimulated to increase intracellular calcium
B. The sodium-calcium transporter is indirectly inhibited to increase intracellular calcium
C. Protein kinase is phosphorylated to enhance calcium channel function increasing intracellular calcium
D. The degradation of cyclic adenosine monophosphate is inhibited
E. The ryanodine receptor is inhibited

62.2. Which of the following properties explains the exceedingly low rate of allergic reactions to digoxin-specific antibody fragments?
A. The antibodies are enzymatically cleaved, separating the Fab and Fc fragments
B. The current antidote uses recombinant human technology
C. Patients are only treated once in a lifetime to reduce the risk of reaction
D. It is standard to pretreat patients with corticosteroids and antihistamines
E. The total dose of antidote is so small that an immune response is unlikely

62.3. A 29-year-old woman with no past medical history ingests "one bottle" of her mother's digoxin (0.25 mg) pills 1 hour before presenting to the hospital. She vomited once and has sinus bradycardia at 55 beats/min on her electrocardiogram (ECG). Which of the following potassium concentrations should prompt administration of digoxin-specific antibody fragments in the absence of any other signs or symptoms of toxicity?
A. 2.0 mEq/L
B. 2.5 mEq/L
C. 4.0 mEq/L
D. 4.5 mEq/L
E. 5.0 mEq/L

62.4. Which of the following complications is a concern when administering digoxin-specific antibody fragments to patients with end-stage kidney disease who require hemodialysis?
A. Patients successfully treated with digoxin-specific antibody fragments have recrudescent toxicity because the antibody-bound digoxin is not efficiently eliminated
B. The volume of distribution of digoxin is increased so that the dose of digoxin-specific antibody fragments will be underestimated
C. If hemodialysis is performed shortly after digoxin-specific antibody fragments are administered, unbound antibody fragments will be cleared by hemodialysis
D. Patients who require hemodialysis have a greater risk of allergic reactions due to the enzymes used to prepare hemodialysis filters
E. The protein binding of digoxin is decreased so that the dose of digoxin-specific antibody fragments will be underestimated

62.5. Which of the following electrocardiographic findings is **NOT** compatible with digoxin toxicity?
A. Sinus bradycardia
B. First-degree atrioventricular (AV) blockade
C. Atrial fibrillation with a rapid ventricular response
D. Ventricular tachycardia
E. Atrial tachycardia with high-degree AV blockade

62.6. A 22-year-old woman ingests a wild salad made from the leaves of lily of the valley (*Convallaria majalis*). She presents to the hospital 2 hours later with vomiting and is found to have a sinus bradycardia with a heart rate of 45 beats/min. Her serum potassium concentration is 6.5 mEq/L. The laboratory reports a digoxin concentration of 1.5 ng/mL. Which of the following methods is the best way to determine the appropriate dose of digoxin-specific antibody fragments?
A. Vials of digoxin-specific antibody fragments = Digoxin concentration (ng/mL) × Patient weight (kg)/100
B. Administer an empiric dose of 10 vials
C. Administer an empiric dose of 20 vials
D. Administer 1-2 vials and reassess the need for more clinically
E. Do not give digoxin-specific antibody fragments as they are unlikely to be effective

62.7. Which of the following plants contains a cardioactive steroid like digoxin?
A. Monk's hood (*Aconitum napellus*)
B. Red squill (*Urginea maritima*)
C. False hellebore (*Veratrum viride*)
D. Deadly nightshade (*Atropa belladonna*)
E. Japanese yew (*Taxus cuspidata*)

62.8. An 88-year-old (70-kg) woman with a history of hypertension, atrial fibrillation, and heart failure with a reduced ejection fraction (15%) is maintained on atenolol, digoxin, spironolactone, atorvastatin, and aspirin. She presents to the hospital complaining of weakness and lethargy after several days of diarrhea. She has a heart rate of 50 beats/min, which

is 100% paced on an electrocardiogram, her serum potassium is 5.2 mEq/L, and she has new prerenal acute kidney injury. The laboratory reports a digoxin concentration of 3.4 ng/mL. Treating with which of the following number of vials is the most reasonable course of action?
A. 1 vial
B. 2 vials
C. 5 vials
D. 10 vials
E. 15 vials

62.9. A 78-year-old man was maintained on a stable dose of digoxin for many years. He develops hand cellulitis after cutting himself in the garden. He has a history of severe penicillin allergy, so his primary care physician prescribes a 10-day course of erythromycin. The patient presents to the hospital after 1 week of therapy complaining of anorexia, weakness, and confusion. He has a digoxin concentration of 2.8 ng/mL and a new sinus bradycardia with a heart rate of 50 beats/min. What mechanism best explains his development of digoxin toxicity?
A. Erythromycin kills a gut bacterium that metabolizes digoxin prior to absorption
B. Erythromycin blocks P-glycoprotein, decreasing efflux into the intestines
C. Erythromycin inhibits metabolism of digoxin by CYP3A4
D. Erythromycin prevents phase II hepatic conjugation of digoxin
E. Erythromycin enhances enterohepatic circulation of digoxin

62.10. Which of the following diuretics is associated with a false-positive laboratory result for digoxin?
A. Chlorthalidone
B. Spironolactone
C. Furosemide
D. Hydrochlorothiazide
E. Metolazone

ANSWERS

62.1. Answer: B. Digoxin and other cardioactive steroids inhibit the activity of Na^+, K^+-ATPase, which in turn inhibits the sodium-calcium antiporter. This leads to an increase in intracellular calcium that ultimately enhances contractility by increasing calcium-dependent calcium release from the sarcoplasmic reticulum.

Blaustein MP. Physiological effects of endogenous ouabain: Control of intracellular Ca2+ stores and cell responsiveness. *Am J Physiol.* 1993;264(6 Pt 1):C1367-1387.

Eisner DA, Smith TW. The Na-K pump and its effect in cardiac muscle. In: Fozzard HA, ed. *The Heart and Cardiovascular System: Scientific Foundations.* 2nd ed. New York, NY: Raven Press; 1991:863-902.

62.2. Answer: A. Digoxin-specific antibody fragments significantly increased the safety of antibody therapy by almost completely eliminating allergic reactions. When the whole IgG molecule is cleaved, the Fc portion is eliminated. Since the Fc portion contains the sequence that is recognized by immune cells as foreign, the remaining Fab antidote is almost devoid of allergic manifestations and does not trigger any future immune response if it is needed again.

Butler VP Jr, et al. Effects of sheep digoxin-specific antibodies and their Fab fragments on digoxin pharmacokinetics in dogs. *J Clin Invest.* 1977;59:345-359.

62.3. Answer: E. In a study published in 1973, all adult patients with acute digitalis ingestions who had serum potassium concentrations >5.5 mEq/L died. Fifty percent of patients who had concentrations between 5.0 mEq/L and 5.5 mEq/L died. As this study was done prior to the availability of digoxin-specific antibody fragments, this criterion is now used to initiate therapy following acute digoxin ingestions. It is important to note that angiotensin-converting enzyme inhibitors (ACEIs) often lead to mild elevations of potassium and were not invented at the time the study was done; therefore, it is unclear if this rule applies to patients taking ACEIs.

Bismuth C, et al. Hyperkalemia in acute digitalis poisoning: Prognostic significance and therapeutic implications. *Clin Toxicol.* 1973;6:153-162.

62.4. Answer: A. In patients with normal kidney function, 60-80% of digoxin is eliminated renally and the remainder hepatically. Patients with complete kidney failure are still prescribed reduced doses of digoxin given intact hepatic clearance. Digoxin-specific antibodies bind to digoxin, and that complex is renally eliminated. Because both digoxin and antibody fragments are too large to be cleared by hemodialysis, the bound digoxin is slowly released as the combined product is degraded in the reticuloendothelial system. For some patients, the release is too large for hepatic clearance and toxicity recurs.

Rosen MR, et al. Electrophysiology and pharmacology of cardiac arrhythmias. IV. Cardiac antiarrhythmic and toxic effects of digitalis. *Am Heart J.* 1975;89:391-399.

62.5. Answer: C. Digoxin toxicity produces bradycardia from atrioventricular (AV) nodal blockade and a variety of tachydysrhythmias from increased atrial or ventricular automaticity. Common rhythms include slow rhythms, such as sinus bradycardia, that are initiated above the AV node, slower ventricular rhythms, rapid supranodal rhythms that

have slowed AV conduction (atrial tachycardia with high-degree AV block, slow atrial fibrillation), and rapid ventricular rhythms. As such, almost any rhythm except rapid atrial fibrillation, sinus tachycardia, and AV nodal reentrant tachycardia is consistent with digoxin toxicity.

Kelly RA, Smith TW. Recognition and management of digitalis toxicity. *Am J Cardiol.* 1992;69:108G-118G.

Rosen MR, et al. Electrophysiology and pharmacology of cardiac arrhythmias. IV. Cardiac antiarrhythmic and toxic effects of digitalis. *Am Heart J.* 1975;89:391-399.

62.6. Answer: D. The exact dosing of digoxin-specific antibody fragments in patients poisoned with other cardioactive steroids is unknown. Answer choice A, which would be appropriate for acute digoxin poisoning, is not applicable in this case. As the cost of antidote increases and the availability remains limited, the most reasonable approach is to plan for an empiric dose of 10-20 vials but to administer them slowly and reassess the need for repeated dosing based on clinical response. In unstable patients, a larger initial dose is reasonable.

Shumaik GM, et al. Oleander poisoning: Treatment with digoxin-specific Fab antibody fragments. *Ann Emerg Med.* 1988;17:732-735.

Safadi R, et al. Beneficial effect of digoxin-specific Fab antibody fragments in oleander intoxication. *Arch Intern Med.* 1995;155:2121-2125.

62.7. Answer: B. All the choices have some cardiac toxicity, but only red squill has a cardioactive steroid similar to digoxin. Many other plants, such as yellow and common oleander and lily of the valley, also contain cardioactive steroids. Toxicity is nearly identical to digoxin or digitoxin.

Tuncok Y, et al. Urginea maritima (squill) toxicity. *J Toxicol Clin Toxicol.* 1995;33:83-86.

62.8. Answer: A. The calculated number of vials of digoxin-specific antibody fragments to completely bind a presumed steady-state concentration of digoxin is as follows: Vials = Digoxin concentration (ng/mL) × Patient weight (kg)/100, which would be just over 2 vials in this patient. Since it is unclear that this patient is even suffering from digoxin toxicity, and that it is expected that her kidney function will recover with rehydration, and that the patient likely has a clinical benefit from her digoxin, it would be reasonable to administer a single vial of antidote and then reassess for signs of a clinical response. In clearly life-threating toxicity, we recommend full equimolar neutralizing doses.

Chan BS, et al. Efficacy and effectiveness of anti-digoxin antibodies in chronic digoxin poisonings from the DORA study (ATOM-1). *Clin Toxicol.* 2016;54:488-494.

Chan BS, et al. Clinical outcomes from early use of digoxin-specific antibodies versus observation in chronic digoxin poisoning (ATOM-4). *Clin Toxicol.* 2019;57:638-643.

62.9. Answer: A. Erythromycin is a complex drug that is responsible for many adverse drug interactions. It is both a P-glycoprotein inhibitor and a strong inhibitor of CYP3A4. Although digoxin is a substrate for P-glycoprotein, erythromycin does not alter its efflux. Only a very small portion of digoxin is metabolized by CYP3A4. Rather, erythromycin alters gut flora by removing a bacterium *Eggerthella lenta* (formerly known as *Eubacterium lentum*) that metabolizes digoxin prior to it reaching the systemic circulation. The net result is an increase in the bioavailability and the serum digoxin concentration increases.

Lindenbaum J, et al. Inactivation of digoxin by the gut flora: Reversal by antibiotic therapy. *N Engl J Med.* 1981;305:789-794.

Hughes J, Crowe A. Inhibition of P-glycoprotein-mediated efflux of digoxin and its metabolites by macrolide antibiotics. *J Pharmacol Sci.* 2010;113:315-324.

62.10. Answer: B. Several xenobiotics produce false-positive test results for digoxin. Conditions such as pregnancy, congestive heart failure, and kidney failure are associated with increased circulating concentrations of endogenous digoxin-like immunoreactive substance (EDLIS). These, like the plant-derived cardioactive steroids, are sufficiently similar in structure to cause false-positive results. Spironolactone has a steroidal structure that is also quite similar to digoxin and interferes with the assay.

Haddy FJ. Endogenous digitalis-like factor or factors. *N Engl J Med.* 1987;316:621-623.

Shilo L, et al. Endogenous digoxin-like immunoreactivity in congestive heart failure. *Br Med J (Clin Res Ed).* 1987;295:415-416.

Silber B, et al. Spironolactone-associated digoxin radioimmunoassay interference. *Clin Chem.* 1979;25:48-50.

Methylxanthines and Selective Beta₂ Adrenergic Agonists

63

QUESTIONS

63.1. A 22-year-old man is brought from a gym to the hospital due to nausea and vomiting. His vital signs are notable for a heart rate of 158 beats/min and a blood pressure of 140/30 mmHg. His electrolytes show a potassium of 2.9 mEq/L, a glucose of 256 mg/dL (14.2 mmol/L), and an anion gap of 26 mEq/L. What medication should be administered as part of his therapy?
A. Adenosine
B. Diltiazem
C. Calcium gluconate
D. Esmolol
E. Digoxin

62.2. An 18-year-old woman presents to the hospital after an intentional ingestion of her grandmother's theophylline. In triage, her vital signs are remarkable for a tachycardia to 160 beats/min, a respiratory rate of 28 breaths/min, and a blood pressure of 60/10 mmHg. She then has a generalized tonic-clonic seizure. Following stabilization, what intervention is indicated?
A. Hemodialysis
B. Whole bowel irrigation
C. Sedation with dexmedetomidine
D. Intravenous lipid emulsion therapy
E. Intravenous adenosine

63.3. A 16-year-old girl presents to the emergency department following an acute overdose of caffeine. Her blood pressure is 50/10 mmHg. What vasopressor should be initiated?
A. Epinephrine
B. Dopamine
C. Dobutamine
D. Isoproterenol
E. Phenylephrine

63.4. An 18-year-old college freshman presents to the student health center due to a gnawing, gradually worsening headache associated with nausea, yawning, irritability, and lethargy. He had just finished his last examination the day prior to presentation. His roommates are all entirely asymptomatic. The patient states he has had similar headaches in the past. On examination, he is afebrile, his neurologic examination is entirely within normal limits, and he has no nuchal rigidity. What is the most likely diagnosis?
A. A carbon monoxide exposure in his dormitory
B. A subarachnoid hemorrhage
C. Meningitis
D. Opioid withdrawal
E. Caffeine withdrawal

63.5. Which of the following statements about the metabolism of caffeine is correct?
A. Caffeine is primarily eliminated by glomerular filtration
B. In preterm infants, caffeine is metabolized in the liver to theophylline
C. Caffeine is secreted in large concentrations in breast milk
D. Caffeine induces microsomal enzyme activity
E. Caffeine is primarily metabolized by hydroxylation

63.6. Caffeine exerts its primary physiologic effects at which of the following receptors?
A. Adenosine
B. Muscarinic
C. Nicotinic
D. Dopaminergic
E. Serotonergic

63.7. A 67-year-old woman presents following an acute, intentional ingestion of theophylline. Which of the following laboratory abnormalities would be consistent with her overdose?
A. Hypokalemia
B. Respiratory acidosis
C. Hypoglycemia
D. Hyperchloremia
E. Hypernatremia

63.8. Which of the following options increases the metabolism of theophylline?
A. Congestive heart failure
B. Cigarette smoking
C. Erythromycin
D. Allopurinol
E. Influenza vaccine

63.9. Which of the following statements about caffeine and the gastrointestinal tract is correct?
A. Small doses of caffeine administered each day causes gastric erosions in animals
B. Caffeine increases secretion of both pepsin and gastric acid

C. Decaffeinated coffee is used to prevent stomach injury in patients with ulcers
D. Accumulated cAMP causes an increase in secretions in the stomach
E. Caffeine is a potent inhibitor of histamine type 2 (H_2) receptors in the stomach

63.10. A 6-year-old boy ingests several of his grandfather's theophylline pills. Which of the following gastrointestinal decontamination techniques best reduces the absorption of theophylline?
A. Induced emesis
B. Gastric lavage
C. Activated charcoal
D. Cathartics
E. Whole bowel irrigation

ANSWERS

63.1. Answer: D. The patient's hyperglycemia, hypokalemia, tachycardia, blood pressure remarkable for a wide pulse pressure, and gastrointestinal symptoms are all consistent with either methylxanthine or beta adrenergic agonist toxicity. Body builders frequently use caffeine supplements as part of their workout regimen and occasionally will also use clenbuterol, a beta adrenergic agonist. In patients who present with symptoms and laboratory findings consistent with either of these diagnoses, a trial of esmolol is recommended to treat their symptoms. Esmolol is a beta$_1$ selective beta adrenergic antagonist, whose short duration of action allows it to be a relatively safe way to test its efficacy. Adenosine is unlikely to be effective in methylxanthine toxicity since, in addition to nonselective inhibition of phosphodiesterase, methylxanthines also block central and peripheral adenosine receptors.

Seneff M, et al. Acute theophylline toxicity and the use of esmolol to reverse cardiovascular instability. *Ann Emerg Med*. 1990;19:671-673.

62.2. Answer: A. Although theophylline overdoses have become very rare in the United States, there are still patients who are prescribed this medication elsewhere. Theophylline is also available as a veterinary medication. In severe, life-threatening overdoses, hemodialysis should be performed. Since the indication for hemodialysis is removal of toxin, hypotension is

not an absolute contraindication, but the patient will likely require a vasopressor to tolerate the procedure.

Ghannoum M, et al. Extracorporeal treatment for theophylline poisoning: Systematic review and recommendations from the EXTRIP workgroup. *Clin Toxicol*. 2015;53:215-229.

63.3. Answer: E. The toxicity of methylxanthines is partially related to catecholamine release, in particular epinephrine, from inhibition of presynaptic adenosine receptors. The administration of a vasopressor that has further beta adrenergic agonist effect should be avoided. Because significant peripheral vasodilation occurs, an alpha adrenergic agonist, such as phenylephrine, should be the first-line pressor of choice.

Kearney TE, et al. Theophylline toxicity and the beta-adrenergic system. *Ann Intern Med*. 1985;102:766-769.

Higbee MD, et al. Stimulation of endogenous catecholamine release by theophylline: A proposed additional mechanism of action for theophylline effects. *J Allergy Clin Immunol*. 1982;70:377.

63.4. Answer: E. Caffeine use is very common world-wide. Many people increase their caffeine intake during times where they need to be more alert. College students will often drink more coffee during the semester, especially in preparation for final examinations. Fifty-two percent of patients who drank 2.5 cups of coffee a day experienced caffeine withdrawal following abstinence. While carbon monoxide should always be on the differential diagnosis for patients who present with headaches, the patient's roommates do not have any symptoms. The patient has experienced headaches like this in the past and the headache is gradual in onset, so a subarachnoid hemorrhage is less likely. He has no nuchal rigidity or fever, and again, he has had similar symptoms in the past, so meningitis is also less likely.

Silverman K, et al. Withdrawal syndrome after the double-blind cessation of caffeine consumption. *N Engl J Med*. 1992;327:1109-1114.

63.5. Answer: B. In preterm infants, caffeine is converted significantly to theophylline. Only 5% of caffeine is recovered in the urine unchanged. The primary metabolic pathway is demethylation. In adults, only about 3% of caffeine is converted to theophylline. Caffeine does not induce cytochrome P450 enzymes. Maternal consumption of caffeine in low doses does not lead to clinically relevant concentrations of caffeine in the breast milk.

Berlin CM, et al. Disposition of dietary caffeine in milk, saliva, and plasma of lactating women. *Pediatrics*. 1984;73:59-63.

Giacoia G, et al. Theophylline pharmacokinetics in premature infants with apnea. *J Pediatr*. 1976;89:829-832.

63.6. Answer: A. Caffeine is a nonselective adenosine receptor antagonist.

Fredholm BB, et al. Nomenclature and classification of purinoceptors. *Pharmacol Rev*. 1994;46:143-156.

63.7. Answer: A. Patients with acute theophylline toxicity have a respiratory alkalosis, metabolic acidosis, hypokalemia, hyperglycemia, and leukocytosis.

Shannon MW, Lovejoy FJ Jr. Hypokalemia after theophylline intoxication. The effects of acute vs. chronic poisoning. *Arch Intern Med*. 1989;149:2725-2729.

63.8. Answer: B. Theophylline is metabolized primarily by the enzyme CYP1A2. Cigarette smoking induces CYP1A2 and therefore increases the metabolism of theophylline. Historically, when patients with asthma who were prescribed theophylline abruptly stopped smoking, they would be at risk for developing theophylline toxicity. On the other hand, oral contraceptives decrease the clearance of theophylline, and women should be asked about oral contraceptive use prior to prescribing theophylline. Other drugs that decrease the metabolism of theophylline include ciprofloxacin, erythromycin, and clarithromycin.

Cusack B, et al. Theophylline kinetics in relation to age: The importance of smoking. *Br J Clin Pharmacol*. 1980;10:109-114.

63.9. Answer: B. Caffeine stimulates pepsin and gastric acid secretion. Peptic ulcer disease as well as heartburn are aggravated by caffeine ingestion. Both decaffeinated and regular coffee contain other stimulants of acid secretion, such as essential oils. Caffeine is a potent stimulator of the H$_2$ receptor in the stomach.

Cohen A. Pathogenesis of coffee-induced gastrointestinal symptoms. *N Engl J Med*. 1980;303:122-124.

63.10. Answer: C. Activated charcoal is the most effective therapy to reduce the absorption and subsequent area under the curve for theophylline by interfering with the enteroenteric circulation. With large doses or the use of modified-release preparations, multiple doses of activated charcoal are recommended when there are no contraindications.

Minton Na, et al. Prevention of drug absorption in simulated theophylline overdose. *Hum Exp Toxicol*. 1995;14:170-174.

Kulig KW, et al. Intravenous theophylline poisoning and multiple-dose charcoal in an animal model. *Ann Emerg Med*. 1987;16:842-846.

Local Anesthetics

QUESTIONS

64.1. Which of the following local anesthetics shares the same metabolite as cocaine?
A. Etidocaine
B. Prilocaine
C. Tetracaine
D. Ropivacaine
E. Lidocaine

64.2. Which of the following statements is true regarding the relationship between the structure of local anesthetics and their potency?
A. Shorter intermediate chain lengths are correlated with higher potency
B. The aromatic side of the anesthetic determines occupancy of the sodium channel
C. The pK_a of an anesthetic determines its duration of action
D. A high degree of protein binding increases toxicity risk
E. The lipophilic group on an anesthetic is the amine substituent

64.3. A 37-year-old man has a cardiac arrest while undergoing an elective orthopedic surgery performed with local anesthesia only. Which of the following therapies is indicated if the patient's cardiac toxicity persists despite standard advanced cardiac life support measures?
A. Intravenous lipid emulsion
B. Cardiopulmonary bypass
C. Lidocaine
D. Venoarterial extracorporeal membrane oxygenation
E. Phenytoin

64.4. Which of the following local anesthetics has the lowest minimum intravenous toxic dose?
A. Tetracaine
B. Etidocaine
C. Bupivacaine
D. Mepivacaine
E. Lidocaine

64.5. A 14-month-old boy presents to the emergency department with cyanosis. His oxygen saturation is 87% and does not improve significantly with supplemental oxygen. Which of the following local anesthetics is the most likely cause of his symptoms?
A. Bupivacaine
B. Lidocaine
C. Ropivacaine
D. Benzocaine
E. Cocaine

64.6. A 35-year-old woman presents to the emergency department with a tremor, palpitations, and an elevated blood pressure. She was at the dentist's office 30 minutes prior to presentation, where she only received local anesthesia. Which of the following xenobiotics best explains her presentation?
A. Lidocaine
B. Prilocaine
C. Tetracaine
D. Ropivacaine
E. Epinephrine

64.7. A 6-week-old boy is being treated with intravenous lidocaine as a treatment for neonatal seizures. Despite using the standard infusion rate, he develops cardiac toxicity from the lidocaine. On chart review, a new medication was added in error prior to him developing toxicity. Addition of which of the following medications best explains his lidocaine toxicity?
A. Ceftriaxone
B. Propranolol
C. Metoprolol
D. Digoxin
E. Famotidine

64.8. A 70-year-old man develops pain in his legs and buttocks following an elective surgery during which he received spinal anesthesia. What local anesthetic carries the highest risk of causing these symptoms?
A. Tetracaine
B. Lidocaine
C. Bupivacaine
D. Ropivacaine
E. Mepivacaine

64.9. A 27-year-old man is in the intensive care unit receiving intravenous lipid emulsion therapy. He becomes confused, diaphoretic, and tremulous. His serum blood glucose is 223 mg/dL (12.4 mmol/L). Which of the following interventions is the best next step in management?
A. Extracorporeal membrane oxygenation therapy
B. Dextrose bolus
C. High-dose insulin therapy
D. Hemodialysis
E. Sodium bicarbonate

64.10. Which of the following electrocardiographic findings is consistent with local anesthetic toxicity?
A. Notched P wave
B. Bidirectional ventricular tachycardia
C. Torsade de pointes
D. Increased QRS complex duration
E. Sinus bradycardia with frequent premature ventricular contractions

ANSWERS

64.1. Answer: C. Local anesthetics are divided into two classes based on their chemical structure, esters and amides. Para-aminobenzoic acid (PABA) is one of the metabolites of the ester local anesthetics, which include cocaine, tetracaine, procaine, and chloroprocaine.

Hino Y, et al. Sensitive and selective determination of tetracaine and its metabolite in human samples by gas chromatography-mass spectrometry. *J Anal Toxicol.* 2000;24:165-169.

64.2. Answer: D. Shorter intermediate chain lengths do not correlate with higher potency, aromatic side chains are responsible for lipophilicity, and the pK_a of an anesthetic is more closely related with the onset of action of local anesthetics (as it also loosely relates to lipophilicity). Protein binding increases toxicity risk by strengthening and lengthening the duration of time local anesthetics will bind with their receptors.

Covino BG, Giddon DB. Pharmacology of local anesthetic agents. *J Dent Res.* 1981;60:1454-1459.

64.3. Answer: A. This patient had an intravascular injection of bupivacaine during his orthopedic surgery, which led to a cardiac arrest. The American Society of Regional Anesthesia and Pain Medicine suggests dosing for a patient in cardiac arrest to be a 1.5 mL/kg bolus of 20% intravenous lipid emulsion administered over 1 minute while continuing chest compressions and airway management. This is followed by a continuous infusion of 0.25 mL/kg/min to run for 30-60 minutes. While the other answers are being studied as alternative management strategies, the current first-line therapy after basic airway and circulatory support in this scenario remains intravenous lipid emulsion.

Neal JM, et al. American Society of Regional Anesthesia and Pain Medicine checklist for managing local anesthetic systemic toxicity: 2012 version. *Reg Anesthes Pain Med.* 2012;37:16-18.

64.4. Answer: C. Because bupivacaine is designed to have a greater affinity and duration of action than the other listed local anesthetics, toxicity results from a smaller intravenous dose of bupivacaine than with other local anesthetics. In fact, the therapeutic index is so narrow that there is no acceptable indication for intravenous bupivacaine.

Scott DB. "Maximal recommended doses" of local anaesthetic drugs. *Br J Anaesth.* 1989;63:373-374.

64.5. Answer: D. Benzocaine, which is in many topical teething medications, is associated with methemoglobinemia. Benzocaine is initially metabolized to aniline and then further metabolized to phenylhydroxylamine and nitrobenzene, which are both potent oxidizers. While methemoglobinemia is occasionally reported with lidocaine, tetracaine, and prilocaine, it occurs much less frequently than with benzocaine.

Moore T, et al. Reported adverse event cases of methemoglobinemia associated with benzocaine products. *Arch Intern Med.* 2004;164:1192-1196.

64.6. Answer: E. This patient was administered lidocaine with epinephrine while at the dentist. While epinephrine is used commonly to decrease vascular absorption of the local anesthetic, prolong the duration of anesthetic effect, and decrease the risk of bleeding into the surgical field, it is not without significant adverse effects. Epinephrine, especially if injected intravascularly, leads to palpitations and tremors, local tissue ischemia, and, rarely, life-threatening reactions such as myocardial ischemia and hypertensive crises.

Yagiela JA. Intravascular lidocaine toxicity: Influence of epinephrine and route of administration. *Anesth Prog.* 1985;32:57-61.

64.7. Answer: B. Low-dose lidocaine is used in the treatment of refractory neonatal seizures; however, at higher concentrations, it is associated with an increased risk of cardiac toxicity. Newborns have an immature hepatic enzyme system and have prolonged elimination of amino amides. Propranolol and cimetidine decrease the clearance of lidocaine by inhibiting hepatic CYP450 enzymes, including CYP1A2 and CYP3A4, which are involved in lidocaine *N*-demethylation and 3-hydroxylation in humans.

Wang JS, et al. Involvement of CYP1A2 and CYP3A4 in lidocaine N-deethylation and 3-hydroxylation in humans. *Drug Metab Dispos.* 2000;28:959-965.

64.8. Answer: B. When used as part of spinal anesthesia, lidocaine is associated with painful, but self-limited, postanesthesia buttock and leg pain or dysesthesia, referred to as transient neurologic symptoms.

Zaric D, Pace NL. Transient neurologic symptoms (TNS) following spinal anaesthesia with lidocaine versus other local anaesthetics. *Cochrane Database Syst Rev.* 2009;2:CD003006.

64.9. Answer: B. Hyperlipidemia after using intravenous lipid emulsion (ILE) interferes with many laboratory studies, making them uninterpretable. Colorimetric methods are more prone to the effects of ILE than potentiometric methods. Glucose measurements by colorimetric method do not accurately report hypoglycemia. Centrifugation at 140,000 g for 10 minutes minimizes most interference. In this case, the patient's actual glucose concentration of 48.6 mg/dL (2.7 mmol/L) was falsely reported as 223 mg/dL (12.4 mmol/L).

Grunbaum AM, et al. Review of the effect of intravenous lipid emulsion on laboratory analyses. *Clin Toxicol (Phila).* 2016;54:92-102.

64.10. Answer: D. Lidocaine, bupivacaine, and other local anesthetics cause blockade of the fast sodium channels of the cardiac myocyte and lead to decreased maximum upstroke velocity of the action potential. This effect slows impulse conduction in the sinoatrial and atrioventricular nodes, the His-Purkinje system, and atrial and ventricular muscle. These changes are reflected in the electrocardiogram by increases in PR interval and QRS complex duration.

Clarkson C, Hondeghem LM. Mechanism for bupivicaine depression of cardiac conduction: Fast block of sodium channels during the action potential with slow recovery from block during diastole. *Anesthesiology.* 1985;62:396-405.

Finkelstein F, Kreeft J. Massive lidocaine poisoning. *N Engl J Med.* 1979;301:50.

Inhalational Anesthetics

QUESTIONS

65.1. A 29-year-old man presents to the emergency department with ataxia after several weeks of huffing the contents of whipped cream charger gas canisters. The generation of which ion is responsible for his symptoms?
- A. Fe^{2+}
- B. Fe^{3+}
- C. Co^{+}
- D. Co^{2+}
- E. Co^{3+}

65.2. A 46-year-old dentist huffs the anesthetic gas used in her office for several days. She develops distal extremity numbness, progressing to paresthesias, weakness, and ultimately truncal ataxia. If the first-line treatment for her toxicity is unavailable, what is a reasonable alternative?
- A. Methionine
- B. Pregabalin
- C. Neostigmine
- D. Botulinum antitoxin
- E. Pralidoxime

65.3. Which of the following factors increases the risk of developing halothane-induced hepatitis?
- A. Smoking
- B. Obesity
- C. Alcohol use disorder
- D. Diabetes mellitus
- E. Concurrent acetaminophen use

65.4. Methoxyflurane-induced kidney toxicity is mediated by which of the following mechanisms?
- A. Selective afferent arteriole vasoconstriction
- B. CYP2E1 metabolism leading to formation of a free radical by-product
- C. Antibodies to haptinized protein leading to hypersensitivity
- D. Acute tubular necrosis
- E. Inorganic fluoride released during biotransformation

65.5. Which of the following inhaled anesthetics reacts with the alkali component of carbon dioxide filters in anesthesia circuits to create a vinyl ether?
- A. Nitrous oxide
- B. Halothane
- C. Sevoflurane
- D. Desflurane
- E. Methoxyflurane

65.6. An anesthesiologist is preparing for her first case of the week and notices that the fresh gas flow valve on the anesthesia machine was open all weekend. If she proceeds with the case, her patient is at risk of developing elevated concentrations of which of the following?
- A. Methemoglobin
- B. Methemoglobin reductase
- C. Sulfhemoglobin
- D. Carboxyhemoglobin
- E. Oxyhemoglobin

65.7. A 52-year-old anesthesiologist is brought to the emergency room after a suicide attempt at work. He is obtunded, hypotensive, and hypothermic. His breath has a sweet, fruity odor. Ingestion of what toxin is most likely responsible for his presentation?
A. Carfentanil
B. Vecuronium
C. Phenylephrine
D. Sugammadex
E. Halothane

65.8. A 35-year-old man is admitted to the intensive care unit with tetanus. After 5 days of sedation, he develops marked leukopenia and megaloblastic erythropoiesis. Which of the following inhaled anesthetics is responsible for his findings?
A. Nitrous oxide
B. Halothane
C. Sevoflurane
D. Desflurane
E. Methoxyflurane

65.9. A 56-year-old man develops elevation of his aspartate aminotransferase (AST) to 92 IU/L and alanine aminotransferase (ALT) to 81 IU/L after a routine outpatient operation for a hernia repair, during which he was exposed to halothane gas for anesthesia. Which subsequent outcome is most likely?
A. Complete recovery
B. Chronic mild elevation of transaminases
C. Progression to acute hepatitis
D. Hepatic necrosis
E. Multiorgan system failure

65.10. A 3-year-old boy is sedated in the intensive care unit for 2 weeks with isoflurane. After sedation is weaned, which of the following sequelae is he at risk of developing?
A. Acute kidney injury
B. Psychomotor agitation
C. Nausea and emesis
D. Diplopia
E. Bradycardia

ANSWERS

65.1. Answer: D. Nitrous oxide, the compressed gas found in whipped cream charger canisters, converts the active cobalt moiety of methionine synthase, Co^+, to the inactive form, Co^{2+}. Methionine is critical for the generation of myelin, and inhibition of its synthesis leads to multiple neurologic symptoms, including numbness, paresthesias, weakness, and ataxia.

Nunn JF. Clinical aspects of the interaction between nitrous oxide and vitamin B12. *Br J Anaesth.* 1987;59:3-13.

65.2. Answer: A. Standard treatment for nitrous oxide toxicity is vitamin B_{12} (cyanocobalamin) supplementation. Methionine is used both as a second-line treatment and as an adjunct to cyanocobalamin.

Stacy CB, et al. Methionine in the treatment of nitrous-oxide-induced neuropathy and myeloneuropathy. *J Neurol.* 1992;239:401-403.

65.3. Answer: B. Halothane distributes to adipose tissue and subsequently slowly redistributes back to the systemic circulation, exposing the liver to toxic metabolites over time. Middle age and female sex are also risk factors. A genetic component likely contributes, as multiple cases are described among related individuals.

Abernethy DR, Greenblatt DJ. Pharmacokinetics of drugs in obesity. *Clin Pharmacokinet.* 1982;7:108-124.

Vaughan RW. Biochemical and biotransformation alterations in obesity. *Contemp Anesth Pract.* 1982;5:55-70.

65.4. Answer: E. Although the exact mechanism is unknown, methoxyflurane-induced kidney injury, which typically manifests as nephrogenic diabetes insipidus, is due to the release of inorganic fluoride and correlates to both dose of methoxyflurane and peak serum fluoride concentration. CYP2E1 generation of free radicals and a hypersensitivity reaction to haptinized proteins are proposed mechanisms of halothane-induced hepatotoxicity.

Taves DR, et al. Toxicity following methoxyflurane anesthesia. II. Fluoride concentrations in nephrotoxicity. *JAMA.* 1970;214:91-95.

Cousins MJ, Mazze RI. Methoxyflurane nephrotoxicity. A study of dose response in man. *JAMA.* 1973;225:1611-1616.

65.5. Answer: C. Sevoflurane reacts with the alkali component of carbon dioxide filters to create "Compound A" [$CF_2C(CF_3)OCH_2F$], a vinyl ether that is nephrotoxic to rats. The extent of toxicity is unclear, but studies show increases in urinary glucose and protein excretion after exposure to Compound A, although no increase in blood urea nitrogen, creatinine, or creatinine clearance occur.

Higuchi H, et al. Effects of sevoflurane and isoflurane on renal function and possible markers of nephrotoxicity. *Anesthesiology.* 1998;89:307-322.

65.6. Answer: D. Desflurane and isoflurane both contain a difluoromethoxy moiety that degrades to carbon monoxide, particularly in the presence of desiccated CO_2 filters found in anesthesia circuits. This results in elevated carboxyhemoglobin levels, in one case as high as 36% in an exposed patient. In this scenario, the CO_2 filter should be replaced before the case is started.

Berry PD, et al. Severe carbon monoxide poisoning during desflurane anesthesia. *Anesthesiology*. 1999;90:613-616.

65.7. Answer: E. Rapid absorption of halothane from the gastric mucosa is responsible for depressed levels of consciousness, hypotension, and hypothermia. Symptoms also include vomiting, bradypnea, and bradycardia. The key to this diagnosis is the sweet fruity odor of halothane that is present on the patient's breath.

Curelaru I, et al. A case of recovery from coma produced by the ingestion of 250 ml of halothane. *Br J Anaesth*. 1968;40:283-288.

Wig J, et al. Coma following ingestion of halothane. Its successful management. *Anaesthesia*. 1983;38:552-555.

65.8. Answer: A. Nitrous oxide disrupts the synthesis of methionine from 5-methyltetrahydrofolate. Methionine is critical for DNA synthesis, leading to bone marrow suppression in its absence. The treatment is folinic acid.

Lassen HC, et al. Treatment of tetanus; severe bone-marrow depression after prolonged nitrous-oxide anaesthesia. *Lancet*. 1956;270:527-530.

O'Sullivan H, et al. Human bone marrow biochemical function and megaloblastic hematopoiesis after nitrous oxide anesthesia. *Anesthesiology*. 1981;55:645-649.

65.9. Answer: A. Halothane-induced elevation of serum aminotransferases occurs in up to 20% of exposed individuals, most of whom make a complete recovery. Approximately 1 in 10,000 cases progress to acute hepatitis, and 1 in 35,000 progress to hepatic necrosis.

Anonymous. Summary of the national Halothane Study. Possible association between halothane anesthesia and postoperative hepatic necrosis. *JAMA*. 1966;197:775-788.

65.10. Answer: B. Psychomotor agitation occurs following use of isoflurane for long-term sedation and is likely mediated by neuronal apoptosis. Symptoms are far more common in patients under 4 years of age, and are generally reversible, abating after minutes to days.

Ariyama J, et al. Risk factors for the development of reversible psychomotor dysfunction following prolonged isoflurane inhalation in the general intensive care unit. *J Clin Anesth*. 2009;21:567-573.

Neuromuscular Blockers

66

QUESTIONS

66.1. An 83-year-old man is found unresponsive at home after his neighbors noted 1 week's worth of newspapers piled on his front step. He is intubated for airway protection; a paralytic medication is used to facilitate the procedure. The patient subsequently becomes bradycardic and then asystolic. What is the most likely underlying mechanism of this complication?
   A. Apnea
   B. Hypercapnia
   C. Hyperkalemia
   D. Cardiac tamponade
   E. Atrial perforation

66.2. A 39-year-old woman is undergoing elective surgery with general anesthesia. The surgery is aborted for inconsequential reasons, and her rocuronium paralysis is reversed in the operating room. She has an uneventful recovery and is discharged home. What precautions does this patient need to take over the following week to avoid potential adverse consequences?
   A. Decrease the dose of her warfarin
   B. Use secondary contraceptive modalities in addition to her oral contraceptive pills
   C. Avoid the intake of tyramine-containing foods
   D. Use abundant sun protection
   E. Avoid the use of alcohol

66.3. Which of the following options leads to a prolonged or potentiated effect of atracurium?
   A. Hypothermia
   B. Chronic use of pancuronium
   C. Hypomagnesemia
   D. Sepsis
   E. Respiratory alkalosis

66.4. Which of the following xenobiotics is used as a precipitating agent during a muscle biopsy to assess the susceptibility to developing malignant hyperthermia?
   A. Desflurane
   B. Succinylcholine
   C. Caffeine
   D. Theophylline
   E. Sevoflurane

66.5. Which of the following statements regarding reversal of neuromuscular blockade is correct?
   A. Pyridostigmine is used to reverse paralysis after succinylcholine
   B. Neostigmine is used to reverse paralysis after cisatracurium
   C. Atropine is used to reverse paralysis after rocuronium
   D. Glycopyrrolate is used to reverse paralysis after vecuronium
   E. Physostigmine is used to reverse paralysis after succinylcholine

66.6. Which of the following xenobiotics is metabolized by the same enzyme that metabolizes succinylcholine?
 A. Cocaine
 B. Acetaminophen
 C. Camphor
 D. Codeine
 E. Lorazepam

66.7. A 21-year-old man is undergoing an elective surgical procedure and develops masseter spasm and an elevated PCO_2. His rectal temperature is 98.6 °F (37 °C). Which of the following antidotes should be administered to this patient?
 A. Midazolam
 B. Cyproheptadine
 C. Bromocriptine
 D. Dantrolene
 E. No antidote is indicated at this time

66.8. Which of the following neuromuscular blockers is associated with an increased risk of seizures?
 A. Succinylcholine
 B. Pancuronium
 C. Vecuronium
 D. Atracurium
 E. Rocuronium

66.9. A 27-year-old man presents to the emergency department after a suicidal ingestion. He requires endotracheal intubation, and a neuromuscular blocker is used to assist in the procedure. Four hours later, he remains paralyzed. Which of the following ingestions best explains this patient's presentation?
 A. Gamma-butyrolactone
 B. Heroin
 C. Aldicarb
 D. Aconite
 E. Diltiazem

66.10. Which of the following mechanisms best explains how tetrodotoxin leads to skeletal muscle paralysis?
 A. Blocks acetylcholine (ACh) release from the presynaptic neuron by inhibiting the binding of ACh-containing vesicles to the neuronal membrane in the region of the synaptic cleft
 B. Blocks voltage-sensitive sodium channels, preventing action potential conduction in the motor neuron
 C. Modulation of postsynaptic ACh receptor activity at the neuromuscular junction (NMJ) through depolarizing (phase I blockade) and nondepolarizing (phase II blockade)
 D. Modulation of postsynaptic ACh receptor activity at the NMJ through nondepolarizing (phase II blockade)
 E. Inhibits the binding of glycine to the alpha-subunit of the glycinergic chloride channel

ANSWERS

66.1. Answer: C. Succinylcholine causes a transient elevation of serum potassium of approximately 0.5 mEq/L within minutes of administration, both in normal individuals and in patients with kidney failure. This patient was unresponsive on the ground for a long period of time and likely had a concomitant rhabdomyolysis. Succinylcholine should be avoided in patients who have any underlying condition that predisposes them to hyperkalemia.

Matthews JM. Succinylcholine-induced hyperkalemia and rhabdomyolysis in a patient with necrotizing pancreatitis. *Anesth Analg.* 2000;91:1552-1554.

66.2. Answer: B. Rocuronium is reversed with sugammadex, which binds progesterone in addition to neuromuscular blocking agents. Patients who are taking oral contraceptive pills should use a non–hormone-based contraceptive for at least 1 week following the administration of sugammadex.

Ahrishami A, et al. Sufammadex, a selective reversal medication for preventing postoperative residual neuromuscular blockade. *Cochrane Database Syst Rev.* 2009;4:CD007362.

Williams R, Bryant H. Sugammadex advice for women of childbearing age. *Anaesthesia.* 2018;73:133-134.

66.3. Answer: A. Many conditions potentiate the duration or intensity of nondepolarizing neuromuscular blocking agents (NDNMBs), such as hypothermia, respiratory acidosis, hypokalemia, hypocalcemia, hypermagnesemia, hypophosphatemia, shock, and liver or kidney failure. Acute sepsis and inflammatory conditions, on the other hand, are associated with mild resistance to the effects of NDNMBs.

Prielipp RC, Coursin DB. Applied pharmacology of common neuromuscular blocking agents in critical care. *New Horiz.* 1994;2:34-47.

66.4. Answer: C. The muscle biopsy was formally known as the caffeine halothane contracture test (CHCT), which exposes fresh living muscle, typically obtained from the thigh, to caffeine or halothane. A positive response to either of these confirms the diagnosis. Choices A, B, and E precipitate malignant hyperthermia in susceptible patients but are not used in the routine testing. Choice D has no role in testing for malignant hyperthermia.

Halliday NJ. Malignant hyperthermia. *J Craniofac Surg.* 2003;14: 800-802.

66.5. Answer: B. Rocuronium, cisatracurium, and vecuronium are nondepolarizing neuromuscular blockers, whereas succinylcholine is a depolarizing neuromuscular blocker. As such, increasing synaptic acetylcholine concentrations via neostigmine or physostigmine would improve strength. Muscle contraction is mediated by skeletal muscle nicotinic acetylcholine receptors, not muscarinic receptors.

Bevan DR, et al. Reversal of neuromuscular blockade. *Anesthesiology.* 1992;77:785-805.

66.6. Answer: A. Succinylcholine is hydrolyzed primarily by plasma cholinesterase (also known as butyryl cholinesterase and pseudocholinesterase) and to a slight extent by alkaline hydrolysis. Plasma cholinesterase is also involved in the metabolism of cocaine. Low plasma cholinesterase activity is associated with an increased risk of cocaine toxicity.

Hoffman RS, et al. Association between life-threatening cocaine toxicity and plasma cholinesterase activity. *Ann Emerg Med.* 1992;21:247-253.

66.7. Answer: D. Despite the name being malignant hyperthermia, an elevated temperature is not a universal finding, and in many patients, hyperthermia does not develop until much later in the disease course. The earliest sign of malignant hyperthermia is an elevated PCO_2 followed by tachycardia, hypertension, and skeletal and jaw muscle rigidity. Patients with suspected malignant hyperthermia should be treated immediately with dantrolene. The mortality from malignant hyperthermia improves from 64% to less than 5% with the prompt administration of this antidote.

Verburg MP, et al. In vivo induced malignant hyperthermia in pigs. I. Physiological and biochemical changes and the influence of dantrolene sodium. *Acta Anaesthesiol Scand.* 1984;28:1-8.

Larach MG, et al. Cardiac arrests and deaths associated with malignant hyperthermia in North America from 1987 to 2006: A report from the North American Malignant Hyperthermia Registry of the malignant hyperthermia association of the United States. *Anesthesiology.* 2008;108:603-611.

66.8. Answer: D. Metabolism of atracurium and cisatracurium generates laudanosine, which crosses the blood–brain and placental barrier and causes neuroexcitation, but lacks any neuromuscular blocking activity. In the central nervous system, laudanosine has an inhibitory effect at the gamma-aminobutyric acid, nicotinic acetylcholine, and opioid receptors. At high serum concentrations, in experimental animals, laudanosine causes dose-related neuroexcitation, myoclonic activity, and generalized seizures.

Chapple DJ, et al. Cardiovascular and neurological effects of laudanosine. Studies in mice and rats, and in conscious and anaesthetized dogs. *Br J Anaesth.* 1987;59:218-225.

Fodale V, Santamaria LB. Laudanosine, an atracurium and cisatracurium metabolite. *Eur J Anaesthesiol.* 2002;19:466-473.

66.9. Answer: C. This patient was intubated using succinylcholine following an overdose of aldicarb, a carbamate. The metabolism of succinylcholine lasts for several hours if the metabolism is significantly slowed because of inactivation of pseudocholinesterase, which occurs with both organic phosphorous and carbamate toxicity.

Kopman AF, et al. Prolonged response to succinylcholine following physostigmine. *Anesthesiology.* 1978;49:142-143.

66.10. Answer: B. Tetrodotoxin leads to skeletal muscle paralysis by blocking voltage-sensitive sodium channels, preventing action potential conduction in the motor neuron. Choice A describes the mechanism of how botulinum toxin leads to paralysis. Succinylcholine is the only depolarizing neuromuscular blocker in current clinical use, the remainder of the neuromuscular blockers used clinically are nondepolarizing neuromuscular blockers. Choice E describes the mechanism of toxicity of strychnine.

Ahasan HA, et al. Paralytic complications of puffer fish (tetrodotoxin) poisoning. *Singapore Med J.* 2004;45:73-74.

Antipsychotics

QUESTIONS

67.1. A 32-year-old man with a past medical history of schizophrenia is started on a new antipsychotic medication and develops increased salivation. Sialorrhea is a side effect of which of the following antipsychotics?
A. Quetiapine
B. Chlorpromazine
C. Clozapine
D. Haloperidol
E. Olanzapine

67.2. A 29-year-old man being treated with increasing doses of antipsychotics for worsening "agitation" might actually be suffering from which of the following side effects of these medications?
A. Tardive dyskinesia
B. Tardive dystonia
C. Parkinsonian tremor
D. Chorea
E. Akathisia

67.3. A 26-year-old man with a history of schizoaffective disorder presents to the emergency department with a temperature of 101.5 °F (38.6 °C), malaise, vomiting, and myalgias. On examination, he is tachycardic to 120 beats/min with no detectable murmur. The remainder of his examination is notable for jugular venous distension and bibasilar rales. What medication was newly added to his regimen 18 days prior to onset of symptoms?
A. Clozapine
B. Olanzapine
C. Fluphenazine
D. Aripiprazole
E. Risperidone

67.4. Which of the following antipsychotics was withdrawn from the US market in 1998 due to QT prolongation?
A. Ziprasidone
B. Bifeprunox
C. Amisulpride
D. Sertindole
E. Asenapine

67.5. A 24-year-old man with a past medical history of epilepsy is diagnosed with schizophrenia. His psychiatrist is considering options for treatment. Although many antipsychotics lower the seizure threshold, which of the following poses the highest risk of inducing seizures?
A. Chlorpromazine
B. Thioridazine
C. Haloperidol
D. Risperidone
E. Pimozide

67.6. A 28-year-old woman with a past medical history of schizophrenia presents to the emergency department with throat pain, stridor, and dysphonia. She was recently started on haloperidol 8 days prior to presentation. Which extrapyramidal syndrome is she experiencing?
A. Akathisia
B. Dystonia
C. Neuroleptic malignant syndrome
D. Tardive dyskinesia
E. Parkinsonism

67.7. A 24-year-old man with a past medical history of schizophrenia presents to the emergency department with a protrusion of his tongue. A medication is administered, and his symptoms resolve entirely. What is the mechanism of action of the treatment he was given?
A. Histaminergic
B. Beta adrenergic blockade
C. Dopaminergic
D. Muscarinic
E. Anticholinergic

67.8. Neuroleptic malignant syndrome (NMS) is a life-threatening condition associated with autonomic instability, altered mental status, hyperthermia, and rigidity. How is NMS best distinguished from either anticholinergic toxicity or serotonin toxicity?
A. Elevated temperature
B. Mental status
C. Creatinine kinase elevation
D. Medication history
E. Tachycardia

67.9. Which medication is considered first-line in the treatment of neuroleptic malignant syndrome (NMS)?
A. Dantrolene
B. Midazolam
C. Bromocriptine
D. Physostigmine
E. Cyproheptadine

67.10. A 29-year-old man is hospitalized in an intensive care unit with severe neuroleptic malignant syndrome (NMS) that is refractory to medications. Which treatment option could be initiated as an adjunctive therapy?
A. Extracorporeal removal
B. Urinary acidification
C. Electroconvulsive therapy
D. Cyproheptadine
E. Hyperbaric oxygen

ANSWERS

67.1. Answer C. While clozapine binds avidly to the M_1 muscarinic receptor causing antimuscarinic effects, its nor-clozapine metabolite activates the M_1 receptor, which produces sialorrhea at therapeutic doses. In addition to antimuscarinic effects, clozapine also antagonizes many serotonin receptors, including $5\text{-}HT_{2A}$, $alpha_1$ adrenergic, $alpha_2$ adrenergic, and H_1 histamine receptors.

Richelson E. Receptor pharmacology of neuroleptics: Relation to clinical effects. *J Clin Psychiatry*. 1999;60(suppl 10):5-14.

67.2. Answer: E. Akathisia is a form of involuntary motor restlessness that results in an inability to remain still for any sustained period. It is one of the most common of the extrapyramidal side effects of antipsychotics and typically occurs within days to 3 months of starting oral antipsychotic, and often within minutes of certain intravenous (IV) medications. Patients with akathisia do not manifest any particular movement and often merely seem restless, making it easy to confuse this entity with psychotic agitation. Because this is a common and very troubling symptom to many patients, it is important to consider akathisia in the differential diagnosis of agitation in any patient on antipsychotics.

Braude WM, et al. Clinical characteristics of akathisia. A systematic investigation of acute psychiatric inpatient admissions. *Br J Psychiatry*. 1983;143:139-150.

Chauhan G, et al. Metoclopramide-induced akathisia. *J Anaesthesiol Clin Pharmacol*. 2012;28:548-549.

67.3. Answer: A. Clozapine is an atypical antipsychotic that helps improve both the positive and negative symptoms of schizophrenia. While it is an effective antipsychotic, it is not prescribed first-line due to two potentially life-threatening effects: agranulocytosis and myocarditis. It was withdrawn from the market in 1974 due to these toxicities but reinstated in the 1990s with strict monitoring parameters.

Miller DD. Review and management of clozapine side effects. *J Clin Psychiatry*. 2000;61(suppl 8):14-17.

Khokhar JY, et al. Unique effects of clozapine: A pharmacological perspective. *Adv Pharmacol*. 2018;82:137-162.

67.4. Answer: D. Sertindole was withdrawn from the US market in 1998 as up to 7.8% of patients taking sertindole developed prolongation of the QT interval to greater than 500 msec. Additionally, there are reports of torsade de pointes secondary to sertindole. Comparatively, ziprasidone is known to cause QT prolongation in only about 0.06% of patients.

Wenzel-Seifert K, et al. QTc prolongation by psychotropic drugs and the risk of torsade de pointes. *Dtsch Arztebl Int*. 2011;108:687-693.

67.5. Answer: A. Clozapine and chlorpromazine antagonize GABA$_A$, which lowers the seizure threshold. Additional factors are likely involved and still need elucidation. All the listed choices lower the seizure threshold, but clozapine and chlorpromazine pose the highest risk. The risk of developing seizures increases in a dose-dependent fashion.

Pisani F, et al. Effects of psychotropic drugs on seizure threshold. *Drug Saf.* 2002;25:91-110.

Omori Y, et al. Clozapine-induced seizures, electroencephalography abnormalities, and clinical responses in Japanese patients with schizophrenia. *Neuropsychiatr Dis Treat.* 2014;10:1973-1978.

Górska N, et al. Antipsychotic drugs in epilepsy. *Neurol Neurochir Pol.* 2019;53:408-412.

67.6. Answer: B. All the listed extrapyramidal syndromes occur either immediately after initiation of an antipsychotic or present in a delayed fashion. Dystonia refers to involuntary contractions of the muscles. While it is distressing, it is typically benign. The exception is when the dystonia involves the laryngeal muscles, as in this patient, when it is life threatening.

Fines RE, et al. Acute laryngeal dystonia related to neuroleptic agents. *Am J Emerg Med.* 1999;17:319-320.

Christodoulou C, Kalaitzi C. Antipsychotic drug-induced acute laryngeal dystonia: Two case reports and a mini review. *J Psychopharmacol.* 2005;19:307-311.

67.7. Answer: E. Acute dystonia presents as spasmodic torticollis, facial grimacing, protrusion of the tongue, and oculogyric crisis. It is best treated with an anticholinergic medication, such as benztropine or diphenhydramine. Multiple doses are often needed as the duration of action of Benztropine is shorter than the duration of action of most antipsychotics. Propranolol and clonazepam are often used in the treatment of akathisia if a dose reduction or switch to an alternate antipsychotic is not indicated.

Corre KA, et al. Extended therapy for acute dystonic reactions. *Ann Emerg Med.* 1984;13:194-197.

Meyer J. Chapter 16 Pharmacologic management of psychosis and mania. In Goodman & Gilman 13th ed.

67.8. Answer: D. The diagnosis of NMS is challenging as it is an uncommon disorder with an insidious onset. It has several features that overlap with anticholinergic and serotonin toxicity, including altered mental status, hyperthermia, and neuromuscular abnormalities. Neuroleptic malignant syndrome should be considered in patients who have a recent initiation of an antidopaminergic medication, increase in dose of their antipsychotic medication, or withdrawal of dopamine agonism. Neuroleptic malignant syndrome is also typically slower in onset as compared to either serotonin toxicity or anticholinergic toxicity.

Perry PJ, Wilborn CA. Serotonin syndrome vs neuroleptic malignant syndrome: A contrast of causes, diagnoses, and management. *Ann Clin Psychiatry.* 2012;24:155-162.

67.9. Answer: B. Neuroleptic malignant syndrome is a life-threatening condition associated with hyperthermia and rigidity. Benzodiazepines are considered first-line due to their ability to act rapidly to treat agitation and rigidity. Patients who are severely hyperthermic should also be rapidly cooled using ice water immersion. Although often recommended as adjuncts for severe NMS, the benefits of dantrolene and bromocriptine are debated and reserved for patients who are resistant to supportive care and benzodiazepines.

Reulbach U, et al. Managing an effective treatment for neuroleptic malignant syndrome. *Crit Care.* 2007;11:R4.

67.10. Answer: C. In a case series of five patients, the use of several electroconvulsive therapy (ECT) sessions resulted in resolution of symptoms of NMS. It is unclear whether resolution was due to ECT or NMS just running its course. Therefore, although the benefit of ECT is not proven, based on small studies, it is considered as an adjunct in severe and refractory cases.

Nisijima K, Ishiguro T. Electroconvulsive therapy for the treatment of neuroleptic malignant syndrome with psychotic symptoms: A report of five cases. *J ECT.* 1999;15:158-163.

Cyclic Antidepressants

68

QUESTIONS

68.1. A 16-year-old girl is found in her bedroom following an intentional overdose of amitriptyline. Her electrocardiogram (ECG) demonstrates an R wave at the terminal end of the QRS complex in lead AVR and a measured QRS complex of 140 msec. Which of the following therapeutic interventions is most effective in narrowing her QRS complex?
A. Acetazolamide
B. Intravenous hypertonic saline
C. Intravenous hypertonic sodium bicarbonate
D. Hyperventilation
E. Intravenous lidocaine

68.2. A 22-year-old man has a generalized tonic-clonic seizure following a large cyclic antidepressant overdose. Which of the following xenobiotics is safe to use to treat his seizures?
A. Lorazepam
B. Phenobarbital
C. Phenytoin
D. Lorazepam and phenobarbital
E. Lorazepam, phenobarbital, and phenytoin

68.3. A 22-year-old man presents to the hospital following an overdose of a tricyclic antidepressant. His electrocardiogram (ECG) shows a QRS complex that is 80 msec, long and his physical examination is unremarkable. He undergoes gastrointestinal decontamination with 50 g of oral activated charcoal. Assuming he remains asymptomatic, how long should he be observed prior to being deemed medically stable for transfer to the psychiatry service?
A. 2 hour
B. 4 hours
C. 6 hours
D. 12 hours
E. 24 hours

68.4. Amoxapine differs from the other cyclic antidepressants in that it causes a higher incidence of which of the following events in overdose?
A. Sinus tachycardia
B. Ventricular tachycardia
C. Respiratory depression
D. Seizures
E. Coma

68.5. A 29-year-old woman presents to the emergency department (ED) critically ill following an intentional ingestion of amitriptyline. She has already received activated charcoal in the ambulance. Her QRS complex on her electrocardiogram is 170 msec, and the physician taking care of her is concerned that she will progress to an unstable cardiac rhythm. In addition to hypertonic sodium bicarbonate, which of the following antidysrhythmics is safe to administer?
A. Quinidine
B. Sotalol
C. Propranolol
D. Disopyramide
E. Lidocaine

68.6. Which of the following electrocardiographic changes is highly predictive of seizures in patients with acute ingestions of first-generation tricyclic antidepressants?
A. Right bundle branch block pattern
B. Prolonged PR interval
C. A QT interval >480 msec
D. A QRS complex in the limb lead >100 msec
E. An S wave in leads I and aVL

68.7. Which of the following statements about the pharmacokinetics of the cyclic antidepressants is correct?
A. The volume of distribution is 2-5 L/kg
B. The cyclic antidepressants are 60% protein bound
C. The cyclic antidepressants do not partition well into fat
D. A very small percentage of the ingested dose is excreted unchanged in the urine
E. The cyclic antidepressants largely bind to albumin

68.8. Which of the following antidepressants has the most anticholinergic activity?
A. Amitriptyline
B. Doxepin
C. Fluoxetine
D. Maprotiline
E. Amoxapine

68.9. A 69-year-old man presents to health care after being found on the ground. A ventricular dysrhythmia was documented by paramedics, and he was defibrillated prior to arrival in the hospital. In the emergency department, his electrocardiogram (ECG) demonstrates a Brugada pattern. As part of his medical laboratory screening, a qualitative tricyclic antidepressant screen is ordered, and it returns as detectable. The patient states that he is not prescribed a cyclic antidepressant. Which of the following medications is he taking that would explain this result?
A. Carbamazepine
B. Lithium
C. Ibuprofen
D. Cannabidiol
E. Fentanyl

68.10. A patient is in the hospital following a consequential tricyclic antidepressant overdose. He was treated with hypertonic sodium bicarbonate boluses and was placed on a sodium bicarbonate infusion. His electrocardiogram (ECG) and vital signs have now normalized. How long should he be monitored in the hospital following termination of sodium bicarbonate therapy?
A. 2 hour
B. 4 hours
C. 6 hours
D. 12 hours
E. 24 hours

ANSWERS

68.1. Answer: C. Hypertonic sodium bicarbonate narrows the QRS complex by two mechanisms. Alkalinization of the blood to a pH of 7.50-7.55 reduces the binding of the tricyclic antidepressant (TCA) to the sodium channel, while the sodium in the hypertonic sodium bicarbonate increases the sodium gradient to enhance sodium flow through the sodium channel. The administration of hypertonic sodium bicarbonate is more effective than the administration of hypertonic saline or hyperventilation. Acetazolamide would worsen toxicity by causing acidemia. Lidocaine is beneficial in treating ventricular dysrhythmias but does not reliably reduce the duration of intraventricular conduction.

Bessen HA, et al. Effect of respiratory alkalosis in tricyclic antidepressant overdose. *West J Med.* 1983;139:373-376.

Pentel PR, Benowitz NL. Tricyclic antidepressant poisoning—management of arrhythmias. *Med Toxicol.* 1986;1:101-121.

Sasyniuk BI, et al. Experimental amitriptyline intoxication: Treatment of cardiac toxicity with sodium bicarbonate. *Ann Emerg Med.* 1986;15:1052-1059.

68.2. Answer: D. The mechanism for cyclic antidepressant–induced seizures is unclear but likely multifactorial. Seizures that occur secondary to cyclic antidepressant overdose typically respond well to benzodiazepines. If seizures are refractory to benzodiazepines, then barbiturates or propofol would be recommended. In cyclic antidepressant overdose, phenytoin is contraindicated because it is ineffective in treating the associated seizures and, more importantly, it exacerbates ventricular dysrhythmias.

Beaubien AR, et al. Antagonism of imipramine poisoning by anticonvulsants in the rat. *Toxicol Appl Pharmacol.*1976;38:1-6.

Callaham M, et al. Phenytoi prophylaxis of cardiotoxicity in experimental amitriptyline poisoning. *J Pharmacol Exp Ther.* 1988;245:216-220.

68.3. Answer: C. Most patients who develop signs of toxicity after a cyclic antidepressant overdose do so within the first 1-2 hours following the ingestion. If a patient is entirely asymptomatic with normal vital signs, a narrow QRS complex (<100 msec), and has received appropriate gastrointestinal decontamination with activated charcoal, then observation for 6 hours is adequate prior to being deemed medically stable to receive psychiatric treatment.

Banahan BF Jr, Schelkun PH. Tricyclic antidepressant overdose: Conservative management in a community hospital with cost-saving implications. *J Emerg Med.* 1990;8:451-454.

68.4. Answer: D. The incidence of seizures with amoxapine is nine times greater than with the first-generation tricyclic antidepressants. The mechanism is unclear. The incidence of cardiac toxicity from amoxapine appears to be lower than with the other tricyclic antidepressants.

Litovitz TL, Troutman WG. Amoxapine overdose: Seizures and fatalities. *JAMA.* 1983;250:1069-1071.

68.5. Answer: E. Lidocaine is used to treat ventricular dysrhythmias in patients with cyclic antidepressant overdoses who are unresponsive to hypertonic sodium bicarbonate. All the other antidysrhythmics tend to further slow intraventricular conduction (disopyramide and quinidine) or exacerbate hypotension (sotalol and propranolol) and should be avoided. Sotalol has the added increased risk of prolongation of the QT interval.

Langou RA, et al. Cardiovascular manifestations of tricyclic antidepressant overdose. *Am Heart J.* 1980;100:458-464.

68.6. Answer: D. Seizures occur in 30% of patients with a QRS complex >100 msec, and dysrhythmias occur in 50% of patients with a QRS complex >160 msec. Patients do not develop these clinical manifestations if their QRS interval is <100 msec.

Boehnert M, Lovejoy FH Jr. Value of the QRS duration versus the serum drug level in predicting seizures and ventricular arrhythmias after an acute overdose of tricyclic antidepressants. *N Engl J Med.* 1985;313:474-479.

68.7. Answer: D. Less than 10% of the cyclic antidepressants are cleared unchanged by the kidneys. The volume of distribution is very large and usually in the range of 10-50 L/kg. The protein binding is greater than 85%, with most of the drug binding to alpha-1-acid glycoprotein. The cyclic antidepressants are very lipophilic and are poorly water soluble.

Frommer DA, et al. Tricyclic antidepressant overdose: A review. *JAMA.* 1987;257:521-526.

68.8. Answer: A. Amitriptyline has the greatest anticholinergic activity of the listed cyclic antidepressants. Clomipramine and trimipramine are other antidepressants with potent anticholinergic activity. Doxepin, maprotiline, and amoxapine have significantly less anticholinergic activity. The selective serotonin reuptake inhibitors (SSRIs), with the exception of paroxetine, have no anticholinergic activity.

Burks JS, et al. Tricyclic antidepressant poisoning: Reversal of coma, choreathetosis and myoclonus by physostigmine. *JAMA.* 1974;230:1405-1407.

68.9. Answer: A. The qualitative tricyclic antidepressant screen is, unfortunately, not a reliable test. There are many false positives, including carbamazepine, cyclobenzaprine, cyproheptadine, diphenhydramine, hydroxyzine, and quetiapine. It is more important to use the patient's history, physical examination, and ECG to help decide the severity of illness and necessary therapeutic interventions.

Moeller KE, et al. Clinical interpretation of urine drug tests: What clinicians need to know about urine drug screens. *Mayo Clin Proc.* 2017;92:774-796.

68.10. Answer: E. Although the data are limited, the current recommendation is to observe patients for 24 hours after termination of therapy.

Shannon MW. Duration of QRS disturbances after severe tricyclic antidepressant intoxication. *J Toxicol Clin Toxicol.* 1992;30:377-386.

Serotonin Reuptake Inhibitors and Atypical Antidepressants

69

QUESTIONS

69.1. A 17-year-old girl presents to the emergency department 4 hours after an intentional overdose of citalopram. She is asymptomatic with an entirely normal physical examination. How long should this patient be observed in the hospital?
A. This patient could have been managed at home
B. She should be medically cleared and transferred to psychiatry now
C. 8 hours
D. 12 hours
E. 24 hours

69.2. Although uncommon, the use of selective serotonin reuptake inhibitors (SSRIs) causes hyponatremia by the development of the syndrome of inappropriate antidiuretic hormone (SIADH). Which of the following options is a risk factor for this adverse effect?
A. Polymorphism of CYP2D6
B. Age older than 65
C. Male sex
D. Obesity
E. Decreased water intake

69.3. A 46-year-old man with a major depressive disorder is taking fluoxetine and continues to experience severe depression, despite medication compliance. His physician switches him to phenelzine. Two days later, he presents to the hospital with agitation, hyperthermia, and rigidity. What is the most likely explanation for this patient's presentation?
A. Pharmacy dispensing error
B. Intentional overdose of phenelzine
C. Polymorphism of CYP2E1
D. Failure to discontinue fluoxetine
E. Presence of active metabolites

69.4. Treatment of a patient with serotonin toxicity should be aimed at correcting which of the following physical examination findings first?
A. Tremor
B. Clonus
C. Rigidity
D. Altered mental status
E. Diarrhea

69.5. Which of the following antidotes is the most reasonable adjunct in the management of a patient with serotonin toxicity?
A. Cyproheptadine
B. Dantrolene
C. Flumazenil
D. Bromocriptine
E. Physostigmine

69.6. A 22-year-old man ingests a friend's medication in a suicide attempt. Four hours later, he experiences a painful, prolonged erection. Priapism is a known side effect of which of the following medications?
A. Mirtazapine
B. Vortioxetine
C. Escitalopram
D. Trazodone
E. Paroxetine

69.7. The marketing of nefazadone in the United States (US) was discontinued in 2003 due to severe side effects. Which organ system is the principal site of the major toxicity caused by nefazodone?
A. Liver
B. Genitourinary
C. Hematopoietic
D. Nervous
E. Cardiac

69.8. A 38-year-old woman with a history of tobacco use is started on bupropion to aid in smoking cessation. She misunderstands the prescription and takes 450 mg/day rather than 150 mg. She is referred to the emergency department after calling the poison control center due to an increased risk of which of the following toxicities?
A. Urinary retention
B. Sexual dysfunction
C. Cardiac dysrhythmia
D. Status epilepticus
E. Respiratory depression

69.9. A 36-year-old man is admitted to the intensive care unit after an intentional overdose of bupropion. The QRS complex is prolonged at 220 msec. What is the underlying pathophysiology of this conduction delay?

A. Intracellular gap junction blockade
B. Potassium blockade (I_{kr})
C. Hypocalcemia
D. Sodium channel blockade
E. Sodium channel opening

69.10. A 28-year-old woman presents to the emergency department for further evaluation of a pins and needles sensation, electric shocks, dizziness, anxiety, and gastrointestinal symptoms. She notes the symptoms began following cessation of venlafaxine. What is the appropriate management for this patient's symptoms?
A. 24-hour observation
B. Restarting venlafaxine
C. Admission to an intensive care unit
D. Chlordiazepoxide taper
E. Reassurance

ANSWERS

69.1. Answer: E. Patients who overdose on citalopram or escitalopram develop seizures soon after their ingestion. QT interval prolongation, however, is reported to occur as late as 24 hours after an overdose. This delay is likely due to the metabolite, didesmethylcitalopram, causing I_{kr} blockade.

Grundemar L, et al. Symptoms and signs of severe citalopram overdose. *Lancet*. 1997;349:1602.

69.2. Answer: B. Risk factors for the development of SIADH secondary to SSRI use include age older than 65, low body weight, concomitant use of diuretics, female sex, and polydipsia. Mutations of CYP2D6 are not associated with an increased risk of hyponatremia.

Kirby D, Ames D. Hyponatraemia and selective serotonin re-uptake inhibitors in elderly patients. *Int J Geriatr Psychiatry*. 2001;16:484-493.

Stedman CAM, et al. Cytochrome P450 2D6 genotype does not predict SSRI (fluoxetine or paroxetine) induced hyponatraemia. *Hum Psychopharmacol*. 2002;17:187-190.

69.3. Answer: E. This patient's presentation is consistent with serotonin toxicity, which occurred because there was insufficient time to clear the active metabolites of fluoxetine prior to the initiation of a monoamine oxidase inhibitor (phenelzine). In patients who are chronically taking fluoxetine, clearance of the active metabolite, norfluoxetine, takes up to 16 days.

DeVane CLJ. Pharmacokinetics of the selective serotonin reuptake inhibitors. *Clin Psychiatry*. 1992;53(Suppl):13-20.

69.4. Answer: C. Rigidity in serotonin toxicity leads to hyperthermia, which must be addressed immediately and is life threatening. If a patient has a temperature greater than 105 °F(40.6 °C) because of rigidity, emergent treatment of the elevated temperature is indicated using ice water immersion until the patient's temperature is below 101 °F (38.3 °C). The rigidity usually improves with benzodiazepines alone; however, in rare cases of severe and resistant muscle rigidity, neuromuscular blockade is recommended.

Boyer EW, Shannon M. The serotonin syndrome. *N Engl J Med*. 2005;352:1112-1120.

69.5. Answer: A. Cyproheptadine is an antihistamine with antagonism at the 5-HT$_{1A}$ and 5-HT$_{2A}$ receptors. As an oral medication, cyproheptadine is used in mild cases of serotonin toxicity or in severe cases after enteral access is established.

Graudins A, et al. Treatment of the serotonin syndrome with cyproheptadine. *J Emerg Med*. 1998;16:615-619.

69.6. Answer: D. Adverse effects from trazodone following an overdose include orthostatic hypotension, seizures, central nervous system depression, and ventricular dysrhythmias. Trazodone also rarely causes priapism, both with therapeutic use and in overdose.

Hanno PM, et al. Trazodone-induced priapism. *Br J Urol*. 1988;61:94.

69.7. Answer: A. Nefazodone is an antidepressant that caused severe hepatotoxicity including hepatitis, jaundice, and hepatocellular necrosis. Most cases of hepatotoxicity occurred during the first 4 months of treatment.

Choi S. Nefazodone (Serzone) withdrawn because of hepatotoxicity. *CMAJ.* 2003;169:1187.

69.8. Answer: D. In overdose, bupropion causes seizures and occasionally status epilepticus. With therapeutic use, chronic doses >450 mg/day are also associated with an increased risk of seizures.

Johnston JA, et al. A 102-center prospective study of seizure in association with bupropion. *J Clin Psychiatry.* 1991;52:450-456.

69.9. Answer: A. Bupropion is a cardiotoxic xenobiotic that produces QRS complex widening as well as QT interval prolongation. The QRS widening associated with bupropion toxicity is not always responsive to sodium bicarbonate. The mechanism of the QRS widening caused by bupropion was assessed using animal models and is due to a deficiency in intracellular communication via gap junctions.

Caillier B, et al. QRS widening and QT prolongation under bupropion: A unique cardiac electrophysiological profile. *Fundam Clin Pharmacol.* 2012;26:599-608.

69.10. Answer: B. This patient has selective serotonin reuptake inhibitor (SSRI) discontinuation syndrome; while it is not life threatening, it is uncomfortable. Management includes restarting the SSRI (if not contraindicated) and then tapering the medication more gradually.

Wilson E, Lader M. A review of the management of antidepressant discontinuation symptoms. *Ther Adv Psychopharmacol.* 2015;5:357-368.

QUESTIONS

70.1. A 37-year-old woman presents to the hospital 2 hours after an ingestion of 50 sustained-release lithium tablets. She vomited once at home and has a notable tremor of her outstretched hands. Which of the following options would be the best modality to reduce her ongoing absorption the lithium?
A. Single-dose activated charcoal
B. Multiple-dose activated charcoal
C. Oral sorbitol
D. Whole bowel irrigation
E. Oral sodium bicarbonate

70.2. Which of the following options best describes lithium elimination?
A. Lithium is freely filtered by the kidney
B. Lithium is freely filtered and actively secreted in the renal tubules
C. Lithium is freely filtered then resorbed in the renal tubules
D. Lithium is conjugated in the liver and undergoes biliary elimination
E. Lithium is eliminated almost equally by both the liver and the kidneys

70.3. A 28-year-old woman develops polyuria and polydipsia after 10 months of lithium therapy. On examination, she is tachycardic (135 beats/min) and lethargic. She has a serum sodium of 162 mEq/L with a urine omolality of 200 mOsm/kg. Following cessation of her lithium dosing and restoration of her intravascular volume, which of the following therapies is indicated?

A. Hemodialysis
B. Amiloride
C. A continuous infusion of 0.9% sodium chloride
D. Desmopressin
E. Furosemide

70.4. A 42-year-old man has been on a stable dose of lithium for many years. Addition of which of the following new xenobiotics to his regimen would warrant more frequent monitoring of his lithium concentration?
A. Enalapril for newly diagnosed hypertension
B. Meloxicam for severe osteoarthritis of the knee
C. Topiramate for prophylaxis against headaches
D. Theophylline as add-on therapy for severe asthma
E. All of the above

70.5. A 47-year-old man has been taking lithium for years without difficulty. He presents to the emergency department because he is progressively more weak and tired. His laboratory analysis demonstrates normal kidney function, a normal sodium concentration, and a therapeutic lithium concentration. Which of the following tests will be most helpful?
A. Creatine phosphokinase
B. Ammonia
C. Aspartate aminotransferase
D. Thyroid-stimulating hormone
E. Cortisol

70.6. Which of the following options best describes the mechanism by which lithium treats bipolar depression?

A. Serotonin reuptake blockade

B. Serotonin receptor agonism

C. Blockade of the dopamine 5 (D_5) receptor

D. Inhibition of neuronal adenylate cyclase

E. Inhibition of glycogen synthase kinase 3 beta (GSK-3 beta)

70.7. Lithium use in pregnancy is associated with which of the following abnormalities in the newborn?

A. Myocardial abnormalities

B. Craniofacial dysmorphism

C. Short stature

D. Solitary kidney

E. Deafness

70.8. Which of the following options is likely to produce a falsely elevated lithium concentration?

A. Lipemia

B. Sampling in the wrong tube

C. Hemolysis

D. Hyperbilirubinemia

E. Isopropanol ingestion

70.9. A 16-year-old (40-kg) girl with a history of depression takes an unknown quantity of someone else's lithium in a suicide attempt. She is brought to the hospital approximately 3 hours later because of vomiting and diarrhea. She is awake and alert with a completely normal physical examination. Which of the following options would be an indication to perform hemodialysis in this patient?

A. An ingested dose >6 mEq/kg

B. A sodium of 158 mEq/L

C. A blood urea nitrogen (BUN) of 30 mg/dL (11 mmol/L) with a creatinine of 0.9 mg/dL (80 microm/L)

D. A lithium concentration of 5.5 mEq/L

E. An electrocardiogram (ECG) with diffuse ST- and T-wave abnormalities

70.10. A 27-year-old man takes lithium for his bipolar disorder. Although there is no history of overdose, his family notes that he has not been himself over the last few days. The patient is awake and oriented and has dysarthria and a tremor. Which of the following would be the best indicator to perform hemodialysis?

A. A lithium concentration of 3.8 mEq/L

B. A lithium concentration of 2.8 mEq/L

C. A creatinine concentration of 3.2 mg/dL (283 micromol/L)

D. A urine lithium concentration less than 10 mEq/L

E. An electrocardiogram (ECG) with diffuse ST- and T-wave abnormalities

ANSWERS

70.1. Answer: D. Lithium is not adsorbed to activated charcoal. While sorbitol is an option, it leads to salt and water depletion, which reduces the elimination of lithium by the kidney. In one study, oral sodium bicarbonate lowered lithium concentrations in volunteers, but this was likely the result of sodium loading causing enhanced elimination, not preventing absorption. Whole bowel irrigation (WBI) with polyethylene glycol electrolyte lavage solution (PEG-ELS) produces rapid bowel emptying without significant fluid or electrolyte balances and is the best option here. In a human volunteer study, WBI with PEG-ELS significantly reduced lithium absorption.

Smith SW, et al. Whole-bowel irrigation as a treatment for acute lithium overdose. *Ann Emerg Med.* 1991;20:536-539.

70.2. Answer: C. Lithium elimination is almost entirely dependent on kidney function. There is no metabolism, biotransformation, or liver involvement. After free filtration, lithium is resorbed in the renal tubules along with sodium.

Thus, in sodium-avid conditions, lithium elimination is greatly reduced.

Boer WH, et al. Evaluation of the lithium clearance method: Direct analysis of tubular lithium handling by micropuncture. *Kidney Int.* 1995;47:1023-1030.

Thomsen K, Shirley DG. A hypothesis linking sodium and lithium reabsorption in the distal nephron. *Nephrol Dial Transplant.* 2006;21:869-880.

70.3. Answer: B. This patient's symptoms and laboratory findings are consistent with diabetes insipidus (DI), which is a common and unfortunate adverse effect of lithium therapy. Patients who maintain intake of dilute fluids will continue to have polyuria but maintain normal or near normal sodium concentrations. When dilute fluid intake falls behind loss of dilute urine, the serum sodium increases. Volume status always takes precedence over sodium concentration; therefore, when patients are hypotensive or tachycardic, volume status should be restored prior to addressing the sodium concentration. While hemodialysis removes lithium and improves the sodium, this effect will be transient. It takes time for aquaporin expression in the renal tubules to return to normal. Continuous infusion of 0.9% saline will likely not lower the serum sodium, as dilute urine will continue to occur. Desmopressin (DDAVP) is the drug of choice for central DI, but is unlikely to be helpful here because the kidney is resistant to normal stimuli (nephrogenic DI). Amiloride and acetazolamide reduce polyuria and are shown to be effective in lithium-induced DI. Loop diuretics are generally not effective.

Bedford JJ, et al. Amiloride restores renal medullary osmolytes in lithium-induced nephrogenic diabetes insipidus. *Am J Physiol Renal Physiol.* 2008;294:F812-F820.

Gordon CE, et al. Acetazolamide in lithium-induced nephrogenic diabetes insipidus. *N Engl J Med.* 2016;375:2008-2009.

70.4. Answer: E. Lithium balance is susceptible to multiple drug interactions. Any new xenobiotic that decreases renal perfusion or alters renal sodium handling has the potential to alter lithium clearance. For many of these xenobiotics, chronic therapy is necessary. A short course of a few days of a nonsteroidal antiinflammatory drug has less of a risk than an expected prolonged course of therapy. In addition, drugs like theophylline increase the renal elimination of lithium. If in doubt, it is reasonable to monitor concentrations more frequently to be certain the patient remains in the therapeutic range.

Geisler A, Schou J. Adverse drug reactions to lithium. *Adverse Drug Reaction Bulletin.* 2001;206:787-790.

70.5. Answer: D. Lithium is concentrated in the thyroid gland, where it competes for the synthesis and transport of thyroid hormones and decreases the peripheral conversion of T_4 to T_3. Chronic lithium use is associated with hypothyroidism. There is no significant effect on adrenal function, liver function, or muscle integrity.

Bou Khalil R, Richa S. Thyroid adverse effects of psychotropic drugs: A review. *Clin Neuropharmacol.* 2011;34:248-255.

Gau C-S, et al. Association between mood stabilizers and hypothyroidism in patients with bipolar disorders: A nested, matched case-control study. *Bipolar Disord.* 2010;12:253-263.

Kibirige D, et al. Spectrum of lithium induced thyroid abnormalities: A current perspective. *Thyroid Res.* 2013;6:3.

70.6. Answer: E. Despite >50 years of clinical use and investigation, the exact mechanism of action of lithium in mood disorders remains elusive. It is certain that there are no significant direct interactions with other neurotransmitter function or binding. The effects of lithium are most likely mediated by the complex interactions with secondary and tertiary intracellular modulators. One of the most popular current theories involves inhibition of GSK-3-beta. Other proposed targets include myoinositol diacylglycerol (DAG) and inositol 1,4,5-trisphosphate (IP_3).

Beaulieu J-M, et al. Akt/GSK3 signaling in the action of psychotropic drugs. *Annu Rev Pharmacol Toxicol.* 2009;49:327-347.

Jope RS. Glycogen synthase kinase-3 in the etiology and treatment of mood disorders. *Front Mol Neurosci.* 2011;4:16.

70.7. Answer: A. Lithium use in pregnancy is associated with several congenital cardiac malformations, especially Ebstein abnormality. This association is largely supported by retrospective analyses and not established by well-controlled prospective data. Ideally, patients who are planning on becoming pregnant should be switched to alternative therapies prior to conception.

Dodd S, Berk M. The pharmacology of bipolar disorder during pregnancy and breastfeeding. *Expert Opin Drug Saf.* 2004;3:221-229.

Patorno E, et al. Lithium use in pregnancy and the risk of cardiac malformations. *N Engl J Med.* 2017;376:2245-2254.

Yacobi S, Ornoy A. Is lithium a real teratogen? What can we conclude from the prospective versus retrospective studies? A review. *Isr J Psychiatry Relat Sci.* 2008;45:95-106.

70.8. Answer: B. Some phlebotomy tubes are anticoagulated with lithium heparin. This will cause false positve results in patients not taking lithium and supratherapeutic concentrations in patients who are taking stable doses of lithium. Lipemia, hemolysis, hyperbilirubinemia, and acetone from isopropanol ingestion all interfere with other tests but do not alter lithium concentrations.

Lee DC, Klachko MN. Falsely elevated lithium levels in plasma samples obtained in lithium containing tubes. *J Toxicol Clin Toxicol.* 1996;34:467-469.

70.9. Answer: D. Although the ingested dose would suggest the potential for serious toxicity and predict a maximal concentration of approximately 6 mEq/L, this is a worst-case scenario. Patients often fail to reach predicted concentrations because of poor absorption (vomiting and diarrhea) and competing elimination during the absorptive phase. While this is concerning, it is usually insufficient to replace an actual measured concentration. Hypernatremia could result from fluid loses or diabetes insipidus and should be corrected with dilute fluids rather than hemodialysis. Similarly, the elevated BUN with a normal creatinine suggests salt and water depletion. Diffuse electrocardiographic changes are common in patients with lithium toxicity but do not have prognostic implications. For this patient, a lithium concentration of 5.5 mEq/L is an indication for hemodialysis independent of any other physical or laboratory findings.

Decker BS, et al. Extracorporeal treatment for lithium poisoning: Systematic review and recommendations from the EXTRIP Workgroup. *Clin J Am Soc Nephrol.* 2015;10:875-887.

70.10. Answer: C. Lithium elimination is enhanced by hemodialysis. According to the Extracorporeal Treatments

in Poisoning Workgroup, this patient's impaired kidney function is the single indication to begin hemodialysis. A high lithium concentration or an altered mental status would be other indications. There is no known role for urinary lithium concentrations. Diffuse ECG changes are common in patients with lithium toxicity but do not have prognostic implications.

Decker BS, et al. Extracorporeal treatment for lithium poisoning: Systematic review and recommendations from the EXTRIP Workgroup. *Clin J Am Soc Nephrol.* 2015;10:875-887.

Monoamine Oxidase Inhibitors

71

QUESTIONS

71.1. A 72-year-old man with a past medical history of Parkinson disease presents to the emergency department for further evaluation of abdominal pain and urinary retention. A urine drug screen is inadvertently ordered and returns positive for methamphetamine. Which of the following xenobiotics most likely caused this positive urine drug screen?
A. Levodopa/carbidopa
B. Ropinirole
C. Selegiline
D. Methamphetamine
E. Olanzapine

71.2. A 22-year-old woman presents to the emergency department after an intentional overdose of her monoamine oxidase inhibitor (MAO-I). Her blood pressure is 220/110 mmHg. Which of the following medications would be a reasonable choice to treat her blood pressure?
A. Esmolol
B. Metoprolol
C. Amlodipine
D. Diltiazem
E. Phentolamine

71.3. Tyramine precipitates a hypertensive crisis in patients on monoamine oxidase inhibitors (MAO-Is) through which of the following mechanisms?
A. Potentiation of the activity of endogenous catecholamines
B. Direct binding to postsynaptic alpha adrenergic receptors
C. Blockade of beta adrenergic receptors producing unopposed alpha adrenergic effects
D. Release of stored norepinephrine
E. Blockade of catechol-*O*-methyltransferase

71.4. Which of the following characteristics best describes monoamine oxidase inhibitor (MAO-I) overdoses?
A. Potentially delayed onset of symptoms
B. Hypothermia
C. Sedation
D. Anticholinergic toxicity
E. Availability of an antidote

71.5. Which of the following vasopressors should be avoided in patients who are hypotensive following an overdose of monoamine oxidase inhibitors (MAO-Is)?
A. Dopamine
B. Epinephrine
C. Norepinephrine
D. Vasopressin
E. Phenylephrine

71.6. A 56-year-old woman presents to the emergency department seizing after an overdose of her phenelzine. She continues to seize despite receiving two appropriate doses of lorazepam. Which of the following medications should be added to terminate her seizure?
A. Midazolam
B. Phenytoin
C. Valproic acid
D. Pyridoxine
E. Magnesium

71.7. A 65-year-old woman presents to the emergency department with a headache after eating pickled tuna. Her heart rate is 125 beats/min and blood pressure is 190/90 mmHg. Which of the following medications best explains her presentation?
A. Moclobemide
B. St. John's wort
C. Tranylcypromine
D. Selegiline
E. Rasagiline

71.8. A 36-year-old woman presents to the hospital with right lower quadrant pain and is diagnosed with appendicitis. She has a history of severe depression and is prescribed tranylcypromine. Which of the following analgesics would be safe to administer to this patient?

A. Morphine
B. Meperidine
C. Pentazocine
D. Tramadol
E. Tapentadol

71.9. A 64-year-old woman presents to the emergency department 20 minutes following an intentional overdose of her entire bottle of tranylcypromine. She is asymptomatic and her vital signs are normal. Which of the following options would be a reasonable next management step in this patient?
A. Orogastric lavage
B. Whole bowel irrigation
C. Empiric phenobarbital administration
D. Placement of ice packs to groin and axillae
E. Immediate endotracheal intubation using succinylcholine and etomidate

71.10. When switching from one first-generation monoamine oxidase inhibitor (MAO-I) to another, how long of a waiting period is recommended?
A. No waiting period needed
B. 3 days
C. 7 days
D. 14 days
E. 30 days

ANSWERS

71.1. Answer: C. Selegiline is metabolized to methamphetamine and is detected by many standard urine drug screens at therapeutic doses. Amantadine, another medication used in the treatment of Parkinson disease, also causes a positive methamphetamine screen. While methamphetamine use would be detected by a positive urine drug screen, it would be less likely to be the cause of this patient's presentation. The other xenobiotics on this list do not cross-react with methamphetamine.

Shin I, et al. Detection of l-methamphetamine and l-amphetamine as selegiline metabolites. *J Anal Toxicol.* 2021;45:99-104.

72.2. Answer: E. Phentolamine is appropriate to treat the severe hypertension caused by an overdose of an MAO-I. Other reasonable antihypertensives include nicardipine, nitroprusside, and nitroglycerin to allow for rapid titration. Oral antihypertensives and longer acting parenteral antihypertensives should be used with caution, as patients who overdose on MAO-Is are at risk of developing hypotension later in their clinical course.

Cockhill LA, Remick RA. Blood pressure effects of monoamine oxidase inhibitors—the highs and lows. *Can J Psychiatry.* 1987;32:803-808.

71.3. Answer: D. Tyramine, a monoamine derived from food, causes the release of norepinephrine from storage vesicles. There are two monoamine oxidase (MAO) isoforms: MAO-A is concentrated in the intestines and liver, and MAO-B is concentrated in the basal ganglia and brain. Because nonselective MAO-Is inhibit both isoforms of MAO, inhibition of intestinal and hepatic degradation of biogenic amines occurs and leads to absorption of undigested tyramine from the gut.

Da Prada M, et al. On tyramine, food, beverages and the reversible MAO inhibitor moclobemide. *J Neural Transm.* 1988;26(suppl):31-56.

71.4. Answer: A. While the onset of monoamine oxidase inhibitor (MAO-I) toxicity occurs rapidly in many cases, delays as late as 32 hours following ingestion are reported. Hyperthermia and agitation are characteristic. MAO-Is have no anticholinergic effects. No known antidote exists.

Linden CH, Rumack BH. Monoamine oxidase inhibitor overdose. *Ann Emerg Med.* 1984;13:1137-1144.

71.5. Answer: A. Dopamine is contraindicated in patients who are hypotensive following an MAO-I overdose. Most of the alpha adrenergic receptor–mediated vasoconstriction from dopamine is due to norepinephrine release, which is impaired because of MAO-I–induced dopamine-beta-hydroxylase inhibition. In the presence of impaired norepinephrine release, unopposed dopamine-induced vasodilation from peripheral dopamine and beta adrenergic receptors paradoxically lowers the blood pressure more. Patients who are hypotensive following an MAO-I overdose should be treated with intravenous fluid and direct-acting vasopressors, such as epinephrine and norepinephrine.

Braverman B, et al. Vasopressor challenges during chronic MAOI or TCA treatment in anesthetized dogs. *Life Sci.* 1987;40:2587-2595.

71.6. Answer: D. Phenelzine is a hydrazine-derived monoamine oxidase inhibitor (MAO-I) that depletes endogenous pyridoxine. In patients who present with status epilepticus that does not respond to benzodiazepines, we recommend that they be treated empirically with 70 mg/kg of pyridoxine (maximum dose of 5 g in adults).

Stewart JW, et al. Phenelzine-induced pyridoxine deficiency. *J Clin Psychopharmacol.* 1984;4:225-226.

71.7. Answer: C. Tranylcypromine is a first-generation monoamine oxidase inhibitor and causes nonspecific blockade of both monoamine oxidase A and B. This inhibition is irreversible and lasts until new monoamine oxidase is synthesized, a process that takes as long as 3 weeks. Patients who are prescribed monoamine oxidase inhibitors must be placed on a restrictive diet to ensure no adverse events occur from undigested tyramine. Foods rich in tyramine include aged cheese, fermented sausage, red wines, and picked meats. Selegiline and rasagiline inhibit monoamine oxidase B specifically so are less likely to cause this interaction. St. John's wort has some mild monoamine oxidase inhibition, but it is fairly weak, and this food interaction is less common. Moclobemide is a third-generation monoamine

oxidase inhibitor that was developed to specifically combat the limitations of first-generation monoamine amine oxidase inhibitors.

Folks DG. Monoamine oxidase inhibitors: Reappraisal of dietary considerations. *J Clin Psychopharmacol.* 1983;3:249-252.

71.8. Answer: A. Monoamine oxidase inhibitors (MAO-Is) are associated with many adverse drug interactions. Patients who are administered medication with serotonergic properties are at risk of developing serotonin toxicity. First-generation MAO-Is, such as tranylcypromine, also have extensive inhibitory effects on CYP2C9, CYP2C19, and CYP2D6. Medications that are contraindicated include dextromethorphan, meperidine, pentazocine, tramadol, and tapentadol. Morphine, oxycodone, buprenorphine, acetaminophen, aspirin, and nonsteroidal antiinflammatory drugs are safe analgesic options.

Gillman PK. Monoamine oxidase inhibitors, opioid analgesics and serotonin toxicity. *Br J Anaesth.* 2005;95:434-441.

71.9. Answer: A. Monoamine oxidase inhibitor (MAO-I) overdoses are associated with a very high morbidity and mortality. There is no effective antidote, and this patient presented soon after her overdose; therefore, gastrointestinal decontamination with orogastric lavage is reasonable. If patients present later, then activated charcoal would be reasonable. Whole bowel irrigation has limited utility in these patients. Hyperthermia is certainly a huge contributor to the morbidity and mortality associated with MAO-I overdoses; however, the best option is to place patients whose temperatures are >106 °F (41.1 °C) in an ice bath. If patients who overdose on an MAO-I require intubation, succinylcholine should be avoided, as there is a risk of worsening hyperkalemia in the setting of rhabdomyolysis.

Kulig K, et al. Management of acutely poisoned patients without gastric emptying. *Ann Emerg Med.* 1985;14:562-567.

71.10. Answer: D. First-generation, irreversible monoamine oxidase inhibitors (MAO-Is) have durations of effect that far surpass their pharmacologic half-lives. When switching from one first-generation MAO-I to another MAO-I, a selective serotonin receptor inhibitor (SSRI), or a cyclic antidepressant, a waiting period of 2-3 weeks is recommended to minimize the likelihood of adverse drug interactions.

True L, et al. Switching monoamine oxidase inhibitors. *Drug Intell Clin Pharm.* 1985;19:825-827.

Sedative–Hypnotics

72

QUESTIONS

72.1. A 32-year-old man is brought into the emergency department due to a suspected overdose. Witnesses reported the patient exhibited slurred speech and loss of coordination prior to collapsing. Once at the hospital, the doctor notices a fruity aroma coming from the patient and the electrocardiogram shows non-sustained ventricular tachycardia. Which medication should be administered to treat the cardiac toxicity?
A. Epinephrine
B. Chloral hydrate
C. Amiodarone
D. Lorazepam
E. Esmolol

72.2. Alkalinization of the urine with intravenous hypertonic sodium bicarbonate will enhance urinary excretion of which of the following barbiturates?
A. Amobarbital
B. Butabarbital
C. Secobarbital
D. Phenobarbital
E. Pentobarbital

72.3. A 26-year-old man presents to the hosptial with a depressed mental status after an intentional overdose of chloral hydrate. A serum ethanol concentration obtained approximately 2 hours after presentation is 248 mg/dL (53.8 mmol/L). Which of the following best explains why the patient remains obtunded 8 hours later?

A. Central inhibition of the glycine receptor
B. Direct competition by chloral hydrate for both alcohol and aldehyde dehydrogenase
C. A decrease in the reduced form of nicotinamide adenine dinucleotide (NADH)
D. Increased production of urochloralic acid
E. Buildup of trichloroacetic acid

72.4. A 52-year-old woman is in the intensive care unit for the management of severe ethanol withdrawal. She is being treated with intravenous (IV) benzodiazepines, hydration, and appropriate thiamine supplementation. While in the intensive care unit, she develops hypotension, a new metabolic acidosis, and an elevated lactate concentration. Which of the following is likely responsible?
A. Methanol
B. Isopropyl alcohol
C. Propylene glycol
D. Excess thiamine administration
E. Benzyl alcohol

72.5. A 23-year-old woman presents to the emergency department with a depressed mental status after an intentional oral overdose of lorazepam. Which of the following should be performed as part of her medical care?
A. Immediate orogastric lavage
B. Activated charcoal administration via a nasogastric tube
C. Administration of flumazenil
D. Obtaining a serum acetaminophen concentration
E. Obtaining a urine toxicology screen

72.6. A 28-year-old woman is being evaluated by an obstetrician after a positive home pregnancy test. The patient is very upset as she has been compliant with her oral contraceptive medication. Which of the following newly prescribed medications explains her pregnancy?
A. Phenobarbital
B. Lorazepam
C. Baclofen
D. Zolpidem
E. Clonazepam

72.7. A 17-year-old woman presents to the emergency department after an intentional overdose of a bottle of "nerve tonic" she found in her grandmother's attic. She has an altered sensorium and her laboratory results are notable for an elevated chloride concentration of 152 mEq/L and an anion gap of −14. Which of the following xenobiotics explains her presentation?
A. Meprobamate
B. Bromocarpine
C. Laudanum
D. Gabapentin
E. Amitriptyline

72.8. A 52-year-old man presents to the emergency department following an intentional overdose of his own medication. On physical examination, he has a depressed mental status, appears cyanotic, and has an oxygen saturation of 87% despite receiving 100%

oxygen via a facemask. A methemoglobin concentration results at >30%. What sedative-hypnotic best explains his presentation?
A. Zolpidem
B. Zaleplon
C. Zopiclone
D. Meprobamate
E. Melatonin

72.9. A 34-year-old woman presents to health care with recurrent generalized tonic-clonic seizures. She is currently being managed in the intensive care unit where she develops green urine. What is the likely cause of this finding?
A. *Klebsiella pneumoniae* urinary tract infection
B. Propofol infusion
C. Hydroxocobalamin infusion
D. Myoglobinuria
E. Phenazopyridine administration

72.10. A 26-year-old woman who is intubated in the intensive care unit develops a bradycardia to 41 beats/min. Which of the following medications most likely led to this finding?
A. Lorazepam
B. Propofol
C. Etomidate
D. Ketamine
E. Dexmedetomidine

ANSWERS

72.1. Answer: E. Chloral hydrate has a toxidrome like other sedative–hypnotics, causing respiratory depression and central nervous system (CNS) depression. Chloral hydrate causes a distinctive odor on the breath described as aromatic, fruity, or pearlike and leads to the development of cardiac dysrhythmias, most classically ventricular tachycardia and ventricular fibrillation. Chloral hydrate increases the susceptibility of the myocardium to catecholamines. If chloral hydrate is suspected to be the cause of the dysrhythmias, epinephrine should be avoided as it exacerbates the abnormal cardiac rhythm, and instead, a beta adrenergic antagonist, such as propranolol or esmolol, should be administered.

Zahedi A, et al. Successful treatment of chloral hydrate cardiac toxicity with propranolol. *Am J Emerg Med.* 1999;17:490-491.

72.2. Answer: D. Alkalinization with sodium bicarbonate will enhance the urinary excretion of phenobarbital because it has a pK_a that is relatively lower than the other barbiturates and, unlike the other barbiturates, undergoes significant renal elimination. However, alkalinization is less efficient at increasing total body clearance than multiple-dose activated charcoal. In patients with severe phenobarbital poisoning, hemodialysis is indicated.

Frenia M, et al. Multiple-dose activated charcoal compared to urinary alkalinization for the enhancement of phenobarbital elimination. *J Tox Clin Tox.* 1996;34:169-175.

Proudfoot AT, et al. Position paper on urine alkalinization. *J Toxicol Clin Toxicol.* 2004;42(1):1-26.

Mactier R, et al. Extracorporeal treatment for barbiturate poisoning: Recommendations from the EXTRIP Workgroup. *Am J Kidney Dis.* 2014;64:347-358.

72.3. Answer: B. Ethanol and chloral hydrate have synergistic pharmacodynamic and pharmacokinetic effects that cause prolonged sedation when taken concurrently. Chloral hydrate competes for both alcohol and aldehyde dehydrogenase and leads to a prolonged half-life of ethanol. Ethanol metabolism generates NADH, which is a cofactor enhancing the metabolism of chloral hydrate to trichloroethanol, an active metabolite.

Sellers EM, et al. Interaction of chloral hydrate and ethanol in man. II. Hemodynamics and performance. *Clin Pharmacol Ther.* 1972;13:50-58.

72.4. Answer: C. Certain intravenous sedative–hypnotics, such as lorazepam, diazepam, and phenobarbital, contain the diluent propylene glycol. Following prolonged infusion of lorazepam, the propylene glycol leads to hyperosmolarity, an anion gap metabolic acidosis, an elevated lactate concentration, and, rarely, hypotension. Although a toxic alcohol should always be on the differential diagnosis in a patient with a high anion gap, methanol does not typically lead to an elevated lactate. Isopropyl alcohol is usually tolerated well and leads to an elevated osmolar gap with a normal anion gap. Thiamine is benign and is associated with almost no adverse effects. Benzyl alcohol is associated with neonatal gasping syndrome.

Reynolds HN, et al. Hyperlactatemia, increased osmolar gap, and renal dysfunction during continuous lorazepam infusion. *Crit Care Med.* 2000;28:1631-1634.

72.5. Answer: D. It is important to obtain a serum acetaminophen concentration on all patients who present following an intentional overdose. Isolated oral benzodiazepine overdoses are benign, and usually only supportive care is needed. The risks of orogastric lavage far outweigh the benefits in this case. Given that this patient has a depressed mental status, activated charcoal should be avoided as there is a risk of aspiration. In a patient who is potentially benzodiazepine dependent, there is a risk of precipitating life-threatening withdrawal with flumazenil, and it should not be used routinely. A urine toxicology screen is generally not helpful in the management of the acutely poisoned patient.

Ashbourne JF, et al. Value of rapid screening for acetaminophen in all patients with intentional drug overdose. *Ann Emerg Med.* 1989;18:1035-1038.

72.6. Answer: A. Phenobarbital is a strong inducer of numerous cytochrome P450 enzymes. Furthermore, phenobarbital increases sex hormone–binding globulin (SHBG) concentration, which reduces free progestin concentrations. As a result, many estrogen-based oral contraceptives will lose their efficacy.

van de Kerkhof EG, et al. Induction of metabolism and transport in human intestine: Validation of precision-cut slices as a tool to study induction of drug metabolism in human intestine in vitro. *Drug Metab Dispos.* 2008;36:604-613.

Mansour V, et al. Oral contraceptives are susceptible to several interactions. *Pharmacy Times.* 2019;85:5. https://www.pharmacytimes.com/view/oral-contraceptives-are-susceptible-to-several-interactions.

Lynch T, Price A. The effect of cytochrome P450 metabolism on drug response, interactions, and adverse effects. *Am Fam Physician.* 2007; 76:391-396.

72.7. Answer: B. Bromocarpine was once used as a nerve tonic and was associated with bromide toxicity. Due to the interference of bromide with chloride in certain analyzers, bromide toxicity leads to a spuriously elevated chloride concentration and a resultant narrow or negative anion gap. Patients with bromism classically present with neurologic symptoms, including headache, confusion, hallucinations, and coma.

Carney MW. Five cases of bromism. *Lancet.* 1971;2:523-524.

Yamamoto K, et al. False hyperchloremia in bromism. *J Anesth.* 1991;5:88-91.

72.8. Answer: C. Zolpidem, zaleplon, and zopiclone are oral medications that are prescribed for sleep. They have receptor specificity and bind specifically to the benzodiazepine site subtype in the brain that contains the $GABA_A$ alpha$_1$ subunit. Because of this specificity, they act by decreasing sleep latency and do not cause other effects such as anxiolysis, antiepileptic activity, or muscle relaxation. As a sleep aid, they help to shorten sleep latency. Zopiclone is unique among this drug class in that it causes methemoglobinemia.

Fung HT, et al. Two cases of methemoglobinemia following zopiclone ingestion. *Clin Toxicol.* 2008;46:167-170.

72.9. Answer: B. Green urine occurs following propofol infusions. Although it is startling, it is a benign finding and resolves as the propofol infusion is discontinued. Other causes of green urine include amitriptyline, methylene blue, promethazine, and methocarbamol. *Klebsiella* causes purple urine, hydroxocobalamin causes the urine to turn a red color, myoglobinuria is classically a tea color, and phenazopyridine causes the urine to turn orange.

Barbara DW, Whalen FX Jr. Propofol induction resulting in green urine discoloration. *Anesthesiology.* 2012;116:924.

72.10. Answer: E. Dexmedetomidine is used often in the intensive care unit as a sedative. It acts as a central alpha$_2$ adrenergic agonist and leads to a decrease in the release of catecholamines. Its mechanism of action resembles that of clonidine, and like clonidine, it causes bradycardia and hypotension.

Chrysostomou C, et al. Dexmedetomidine: Sedation, analgesia and beyond. *Expert Opin Drug Metab Toxicol.* 2008;4:619-627.

Amphetamines

73.1. The addition of a halogen group (eg, iodine or bromine) to the phenylethylamine backbone of an amphetamine results in which of the following changes?
A. Increased potency and neurotoxicity
B. Enhanced hallucinogenic and serotonergic activity
C. Enhanced lipophilicity and faster penetration of the blood–brain barrier
D. Increased polarity and decreased penetration of the blood–brain barrier
E. Conversion from renal elimination to hepatic metabolism

73.2. Which of the following mechanisms best describes how amphetamines produce a sympathomimetic toxic syndrome?
A. Direct actions on the alpha and beta adrenergic receptors
B. Block the reuptake of catecholamines
C. Increase presynaptic cytoplasmic concentrations of catecholamines
D. Inhibition of catecholamine-O-methyltransferase (COMT)
E. Increase the sensitivity of adrenergic receptors to endogenous catecholamines

73.3. A 47-year-old man with depression, hypertension, and hyperlipidemia is brought to the hospital for altered mental status. His vital signs are blood pressure, 156/86 mmHg; pulse, 72 beats/min; respirations, 12 breaths/min; temperature, 98.6 °F (37.0 °C); and oxygen saturation, 96% on room air. A urine drug screen is reported as positive for amphetamines. Which of his maintenance medications was likely responsible for this false-positive result?
A. Amlodipine
B. Furosemide
C. Clonazepam
D. Bupropion
E. Atorvastatin

73.4. Which of the following amphetamines is often substituted for ecstasy [XTC or 3,4-methylenedioxy-methamphetamine (MDMA)] and is associated with a higher fatality rate?
A. Para-methoxyamphetamine
B. Methamphetamine
C. Methcathinone
D. 2,5-Dimethoxy-4-methylamphetamine (DOM or STP)
E. 1-(8-Bromobenzo[1,2-b;4,5-b]difuran-4-yl)-2-aminopropane (Bromo-dragonFLY)

73.5. Which of the following choices is likely responsible for the dental abnormalities that occur in chronic methamphetamine users?
A. Poor oral hygiene
B. High intake of sugar-containing beverages
C. Bruxism
D. Dry mouth
E. All of the above

73.6. A 21-year-old woman presents to the hospital with headache and confusion after MDMA at a party. She has a serum sodium of 111 mEq/L (111 mmol/L). Which of the following mechanisms best explains the etiology for her hyponatremia?
  A. Excessive water ingestion to prevent hyperthermia
  B. Increased release of vasopressin
  C. Decreased degradation of vasopressin
  D. Increased renal sensitivity to vasopressin
  E. Direct vasopressin receptor activation

73.7. Potent hallucinogenic amphetamines such as Bromo-dragonFLY are associated with which of the following clinical manifestations that are **not** typical of other amphetamines?
  A. Myocarditis
  B. Hepatotoxicity
  C. Peripheral vasospasm
  D. Acute kidney injury
  E. Hyperthermia

73.8. A 44-year-old man presents with severe and prolonged toxicity after a large intentional ingestion of methamphetamine. Which of the following therapies would theoretically best enhance elimination of this xenobiotic?
  A. Hemodialysis
  B. Multiple-dose activated charcoal (MDAC)
  C. Urinary alkalinization
  D. Urinary acidification
  E. Cholestyramine

73.9. A 24-year-old (75-kg) woman presents to the hospital with severe psychomotor agitation after using "bath salts." Her vital signs are: blood pressure, 186/90 mm Hg; pulse, 158 beats/min; respirations, 30 breaths/min; temperature, 101.2 °F (38.4 °C); and oxygen saturation, 98% on room air. Which of the following medications and routes is the most reasonable to rapidly control her behavior?
  A. Lorazepam 2-4 mg intramuscularly
  B. Olanzapine 7.5 mg sublingually
  C. Diazepam 10 mg intramuscularly
  D. Droperidol 0.625 mg intramuscularly
  E. Midazolam 5-10 mg intramuscularly

73.10. A 26-year-old man is brought to the hospital by friends for evaluation after using amphetamines for days. He is lethargic but oriented when stimulated. His vital signs are: blood pressure, 122/60 mmHg; pulse, 68 beats/min; respirations, 10 breaths/min; temperature, 98.6 °F (37.0 °C); oxygen saturation, 99% on room air; and point-of-care glucose, 88 mg/dL (4.9 mmol/L). Which of the following interventions is indicated?
  A. Computed tomography (CT) of the head
  B. Lumbar puncture
  C. Low-dose bupropion
  D. Venlafaxine
  E. Observation and referral for drug treatment

ANSWERS

73.1. Answer: A. The addition of a halogen group, such as iodine or bromine, increases the potency and neurotoxicity of the compound compared to non-halogenated compounds. Choice B occurs when there is a substitution at the para position of the phenyl ring. Choice C occurs when an extra methyl group is added to the terminal amine. Choice D occurs when a ketone group is added to the beta position. Recognizing these modifications allows clinicians to predict the effects of different amphetamines.

Harvey JA. Neurotoxic action of halogenated amphetamines. *Ann N Y Acad Sci.* 1978;305:289-304.

Luethi D, et al. Para-halogenation affects monoamine transporter inhibition properties and hepatocellular toxicity of amphetamines and methcathinones. *Front Pharmacol.* 2019;10:438.

73.2. Answer: C. Amphetamines are complex xenobiotics with multiple mechanisms of action. They enter the cell either by using the reuptake mechanism or through passive diffusion, but do not significantly block reuptake the way cocaine does. They are weak inhibitors of monoamine oxidase, but do not alter the activity of COMT. Amphetamines do not directly interact with adrenergic receptors. Instead, they enter presynaptic storage vesicle and buffer the pH gradient that holds catecholamines in place. This increases free cytoplasmic concentrations of catecholamines, resulting in increased release.

Sulzer D, et al. Amphetamine redistributes dopamine from synaptic vesicles to the cytosol and promotes reverse transport. *J Neurosci.* 1995;15(5 Pt 2):4102-4108.

Sulzer D, et al. Weak base model of amphetamine action. *Ann N Y Acad Sci.* 1992;654:525-528.

73.3. Answer: D. The urine drug assays used to test for amphetamines are susceptible to many false-positive and false-negative tests. False-negative results occur for either highly modified compounds or those that are so potent that their urine concentrations are exceedingly low. Although many false-positive results are unpredictable, bupropion and pseudophedrine have amphetaminelike structures, whereas selegiline is metabolized to amphetamine and methamphetamine.

Shin I, et al. Detection of l-methamphetamine and l-amphetamine as selegiline metabolites. *J Anal Toxicol*. 2021;45:99-104.

Moeller KE, et al. Clinical interpretation of urine drug tests: What clinicians need to know about urine drug screens. *Mayo Clin Proc*. 2017;92:774-796.

73.4. Answer: A. Substitution, contamination, and adulteration are common in the illicit drug market. MDMA is highly sought after but often unavailable because of law enforcement efforts. There are many reports of para-methoxyamphetamine being sold as MDMA at concerts with associated fatalities, although the etiology of the excess fatalities is unclear.

Ling LH, et al. Poisoning with the recreational drug paramethoxyamphetamine ("death"). *Med J Aust*. 2001;174:453-455.

Lurie Y, et al. Severe paramethoxymethamphetamine (PMMA) and paramethoxyamphetamine (PMA) outbreak in Israel. *Clin Toxicol (Phila)*. 2012;50:39-43.

Martin TL. Three cases of fatal paramethoxyamphetamine overdose. *J Anal Toxicol*. 2001;25:649-651.

73.5. Answer: E. There is a strong association between methamphetamine use and poor oral hygiene. The etiology is felt to be multifactorial with all the choices listed being contributory.

Clague J, et al. Mechanisms underlying methamphetamine-related dental disease. *J Am Dent Assoc*. 2017;148:377-386.

De-Carolis C, et al. Methamphetamine abuse and "meth mouth" in Europe. *Med Oral Patol Oral Cir Bucal*. 2015;20:e205-210.

73.6. Answer: B. Amphetamines with enhanced hallucinogenic properties, such as MDMA (also known as XTC or ecstasy), are associated with hyponatremia. Based on human volunteer studies, the mechanism is due to the release of vasopressin. Mildly hyponatremic patients should be treated with fluid restriction. Patients with altered mental status or seizures in the setting of hyponatremia should be treated with 3% sodium chloride.

Henry JA, et al. Low-dose MDMA ("ecstasy") induces vasopressin secretion. *Lancet*. 1998;351:1784.

73.7. Answer: C. Severe peripheral vasospasm resulting in gangrene is reported with these ultrapotent hallucinogenic amphetamines. This effect is most likely mediated by serotonin excess and resembles some of the effects reported with ergots and ergot derivatives. Vasodilatory therapy with phentolamine or a calcium channel blocker, such as nicardipine, is reasonable.

Andreasen MF, et al. A fatal poisoning involving Bromo-Dragonfly. *Forensic Sci Int*. 2009;183:91-96.

Thorlacius K, et al. [Bromo-dragon fly—life-threatening drug. Can cause tissue necrosis as demonstrated by the first described case]. *Lakartidningen*. 2008;105:1199-1200.

Walterscheid JP, et al. Pathological findings in 2 cases of fatal 25I-NBOMe toxicity. *Am J Forensic Med Pathol*. 2014;35:20-25.

73.8. Answer: D. Amphetamines are weak bases that are ion trapped in acid urine. This technique enhances elimination, however, urinary acidification requires systemic acidification and is rarely, if ever, done. In addition to the risks of serum acidification, urinary acidification exacerbates myoglobinuric kidney injury by increasing ferrihemate formation. Hemodialysis is unlikely to be beneficial because most amphetamines have large volumes of distribution. There are no good human data on the use of MDAC or cholestyramine in amphetamine poisoning.

Beckett AH, Rowland M. Urinary excretion kinetics of amphetamine in man. *J Pharm Pharmacol*. 1965;17:628-639.

Beckett AH, et al. Influence of urinary pH on excretion of amphetamine. *Lancet*. 1965;1:303.

73.9. Answer: E. There are no data to suggest that one particular drug offers a clear advantage in agitated patients with amphetamine toxicity, so the optimal choice is the one that produces the most rapid effect. Ideally, an intravenous medication is preferred because of instantaneous and complete absorption, but in many agitated patients, other routes are safer for the staff and turn out to be quicker because intravenous access is often challenging. Diazepam should never be given intramuscularly because its absorption is erratic. Midazolam acts rapidly while the peak sedative effect of lorazepam is delayed 15-20 minutes. The oral and sublingual routes are reasonable in cooperative patients but not easily accomplished in patients with severe agitation. Droperidol is recommended by many authors, but the listed antiemetic dose is likely inadequate, and 2.5-mg or 5-mg doses are commonly used.

Connors NJ, et al. Antipsychotics for the treatment of sympathomimetic toxicity: A systematic review. *Am J Emerg Med.* 2019;37:1880-1890.

Martel ML, et al. Randomized double-blind trial of intramuscular droperidol, ziprasidone, and lorazepam for acute undifferentiated agitation in the emergency department. *Acad Emerg Med.* 2021;28:421-434.

73.10. Answer: E. Following sustained amphetamine use, patients present with either acute psychotic reactions or complete exhaustion. Exhaustion is characterized by unremarkable vital signs and no serious abnormal physical findings. Patients will express depression and craving for amphetamines, which are best treated initially with non-pharmacologic interventions.

Kokkinidis L, et al. Amphetamine withdrawal: A behavioral evaluation. *Life Sci.* 1986;38:1617-1623.

Shoptaw SJ, et al. Treatment for amphetamine withdrawal. *Cochrane Database Syst Rev.* 2009;2:CD003021.

Cannabinoids

74.1. For which of the following conditions is marijuana use demonstrated to be superior to a United States (US) Food and Drug Administration (FDA) approved pharmaceutical based on a well-designed randomized controlled trial?
A. Asthma
B. Glaucoma
C. Epilepsy
D. Chronic pain
E. None of the above

74.2. Which of the following options best describe cannabinoid receptors?
A. CB_1 receptors are primarily involved in inflammation and cellular immunity
B. CB_2 receptors are highly localized to the frontal cortex of the brain
C. CB_1 and CB_2 receptors are postsynaptic modulators of other neurotransmitter responses
D. CB_1 receptor stimulation decreases cyclic adenosine monophosphate (cAMP), decreases calcium influx, and increases potassium efflux
E. Synthetic cannabinoids sold as marijuana substitutes bind exclusively to CB_2 receptors and are more potent agonists than tetrahydrocannabinol (THC)

74.3. Which of the following options is the primary psychoactive substance in marijuana?
A. Cannabidiol
B. Delta-9-tetrahydrocannabinol
C. Cannabichromene
D. Dronabinol
E. Delta-6-tricannabinol

74.4. Which physical examination finding is most suggestive of acute marijuana use?
A. Dysmetria
B. Bradycardia
C. Piloerection
D. Postural hypotension
E. Conjunctival injection

74.5. A 29-year-old man presents to the emergency department with abdominal pain and vomiting. He has taken several hot showers over the course of the day as that is the only way he gets relief from his pain. He has a history of frequent marijuana use. Which of the following medications will best help to relieve his symptoms?
A. Morphine
B. Ondansetron
C. Marijuana
D. Haloperidol
E. Diphenhydramine

74.6. Which of the following options is true regarding screening for tetrahydrocannabinol (THC) metabolites in urine?
A. It is not routinely performed on drug abuse screens
B. Confirmation is performed with immunoassay techniques
C. The threshold for a positive test is a concentration of 5 ng/mL
D. The results are dependent on patterns of individual usage
E. It is blocked by high doses of vitamin C

74.7. When compared to marijuana use, which of the following findings seems to be more commonly reported with synthetic cannabinoid use?
A. Acute kidney injury
B. Bradycardia
C. Tachycardia
D. Seizures
E. All of the above

74.8. Which of the following options is true regarding passive inhalation of marijuana?
A. It does not cause a positive urine test
B. It does not cause psychological responses
C. It causes a positive screening test but negative confirmatory test
D. It causes positive test results
E. It is not associated with physiologic responses

74.9. Prenatal use of marijuana is associated with which of the following options?
A. A withdrawal syndrome in the neonate
B. Complications similar to those associated with alcohol use
C. Consistent low birth weight
D. Neurobehavioral problems in the child
E. No measurable changes in male offspring

74.10. Which of the following options best describes a pharmacokinetic property of delta-9-tetrahydrocannabinol?
A. It concentrates in human breast milk
B. It is poorly protein bound
C. It is excreted primarily unchanged in the urine
D. It is distributed primarily in the body water
E. It is found in high concentration in the cerebrospinal fluid (CSF)

ANSWERS

74.1. Answer: E. Many studies assess the use of marijuana in a variety of medical conditions, including the ones above. There are no well-designed randomized trials that show either equivalency or superiority of marijuana to US FDA approved pharmaceuticals in any medical condition. In fact, most trials show clear inferiority. While some components of marijuana show promise as novel pharmaceuticals, most studies are fairly disappointing.

National Academies of Sciences, Engineering, and Medicine; Health and Medicine Division; Board on Population Health and Public Health Practice; Committee on the Health Effects of Marijuana. *An Evidence Review and Research Agenda. The Health Effects of Cannabis and Cannabinoids: The Current State of Evidence and Recommendations for Research.* Washington, DC: National Academies Press; 2017.

74.2. Answer: D. CB_1 cannabinoid receptors are widely distributed in the brain and modulate a variety of other neurotransmitters. Their relative absence in the brain stem explains why consciousness and vital signs are minimally affected. CB_2 receptors are involved in inflammation and pain. Both receptors are located on the presynaptic neurons and stimulation results in hyperpolarization and decreases the release of other neurotransmitters.

Seely KA, et al. Marijuana-based drugs: Innovative therapeutics or designer drugs of abuse? *Mol Interv.* 2011;11:36-51.

74.3. Answer: B. Delta-9-tetrahydrocannabinol (THC) is used to establish the potency of cannabis products and is the primary psychoactive substance in marijuana. Over 400 compounds have been identified in marijuana, but most have little or no psychoactive effect.

Hawks RL. The constituents of cannabis and the disposition and metabolism of cannabinoids. In: Hawks RL, ed. *The Analysis of Cannabinoids in Biological Fluids.* NIDA Research Monograph 42. Washington, DC: USDHHS, USGPO; 1982:125-317.

Joyce CRB, Curry SH. *The Botany and Chemistry of Cannabis.* London: J&A Churchill; 1970:1-60.

74.4. Answer: E. The effects of marijuana use on vital signs and physical examination findings are highly variable and generally mild. In volunteer studies, increases in both blood pressure and heart rate are minor. Piloerection is characteristic of opioid withdrawal. Conjunctival injection is fairly common, although it is of little clinical relevance other than for diagnosis.

Beaconsfield P, et al. Marihuana smoking. Cardiovascular effects in man and possible mechanisms. *N Engl J Med.* 1972;287:209-212.

74.5. Answer: D. This patient is experiencing cannabinoid hyperemesis syndrome (CHS). This syndrome consists of nausea, vomiting, and abdominal pain that is relieved by hot showers. CHS is thought to be caused by dysfunction of pain perception and an excess of substance P release. Dopamine antagonists, such as haloperidol, improve the symptoms caused by CHS. Capsaicin, which leads to depletion of substance P, is also used in the treatment of CHS. Opioids and antiemetics alone are not effective. Patients should be counseled regarding avoidance of further marijuana use as symptoms will recur with recurrent exposure.

Simonetto DA, et al. Cannabinoid hyperemesis: A case series of 98 patients. *Mayo Clin Proc.* 2012;87:114-119.

74.6. Answer: D. Immunoassay screening followed by confirmation with gas chromatography–mass spectrometry (GC-MS) is very accurate at detecting THC in urine. The duration of detection varies according to the pattern of use and body composition of the user. The confirmation cut off is 15 ng/mL, although concentrations as low as 2 ng/mL are often detected.

Ellis GM, et al. Excretion patterns of cannabinoid metabolites after last use in a group of chronic users. *Clin Pharmacol Ther.* 1985;38:572-578.

Schwartz RH, Hawks RL. Laboratory detection of marijuana use. *JAMA.* 1985;254:788-792.

74.7. Answer: E. Synthetic cannabinoids are not synthetic tetrahydrocannabinol (THC); they are a diverse group of chemical compounds that only share their ability to bind to cannabinoid receptors. As such, with each new generation of synthetic cannabinoids, a variety of clinical finding are noted that appear distinct from THC use.

Centers for Disease Control and Prevention (CDC). Acute kidney injury associated with synthetic cannabinoid use—multiple states, 2012. *MMWR Morb Mortal Wkly Rep.* 2013;62:93-98.

Lapoint J, et al. Severe toxicity following synthetic cannabinoid ingestion. *Clin Toxicol.* 2011;49:760 764.

74.8. Answer: D. Passive inhalation of marijuana smoke has been used as a legal defense against a positive urine drug screen. Studies show that depending on the concentration of smoke in the area where it is inhaled and the amount of time the person is present, urine drug screens are positive for days after exposure.

Chiang CN, Barnett G. Marijuana pharmacokinetics and pharmacodynamics. In: Redda KK, et al, eds. *Cocaine, Marijuana, Designer Drugs: Chemistry, Pharmacology, and Behavior.* Boca Raton, FL: CRC Press; 1989:113-126.

Cone EJ, et al. Passive inhalation of marijuana smoke: Urinalysis and room air levels of delta-9-tetrahydrocannabinol. *J Anal Toxicol.* 1987;11:89-96.

74.9. Answer: D. Pregnancy outcome studies of drug abuse are difficult to perform due to many confounding variables including nutrition, prenatal care, tobacco usage, and alcohol and other drug usage. Birth weight has varied between low and high depending on the amount of marijuana smoked. Most of the data points to neurobehavioral disorders appearing at different developmental milestones starting around 3 years of age.

Fried PA. Behavioral outcome in preschool and school-age children exposed prenatally to marijuana: A review and speculative interpretation. In: Wetherington CL, et al, eds. *Behavioral Studies of Drug-Exposed Offspring: Methodological Issues in Human and Animal Research.* NIDA Research Monograph 164. Washington, DC: USDHHS, USGPO; 1996:242-260.

Richardson GA, et al. The impact of prenatal marijuana and cocaine use on the infant and child. *Clin Obstet Gynecol.* 1993;36:302-318.

74.10. Answer: A. Tetrahydrocannabinol (THC) is hydrophobic and is stored in lipid tissue. The high fat content of breast milk makes it an ideal vehicle for storing and transporting THC. Neonatal exposure during the first month is associated with decreased motor development at 1 year.

Astley SJ, Little RE. Maternal marijuana use during lactation and infant development at one year. *Neurotoxicol Teratol.* 1990;12:161-168.

Perez-Reyes M, Wall ME. Presence of delta-9-tetrahydrocannabinol in human milk. *N Engl J Med.* 1982;307:819-820.

Cocaine

QUESTIONS

75.1. In an animal model of cocaine toxicity, treatment of which of the following parameters is best associated with survival?
A. Hypertension
B. Tachycardia
C. Hyperthermia
D. Hyperventilation
E. Acidosis

75.2. Which of the following options best describes the direct effect of cocaine on the heart?
A. Positive inotrope and chronotrope
B. Type IA and IC antidysrhythmic
C. Type II antidysrhythmic
D. Type IB antidysrhythmic
E. Type IV antidysrhythmic

75.3. Which of the following xenobiotics will prolong the metabolism of cocaine?
A. Bupivacaine
B. Pancuronium
C. Chlorpyrifos
D. Tetracycline
E. Metoprolol

75.4. Which of the following options is required to produce rhabdomyolysis in the setting of cocaine use?
A. Hyperthermia
B. Psychomotor agitation
C. Hypertension
D. Tachycardia
E. None of the above

75.5. Which of the following xenobiotics is commonly found as a cocaine adulterant?
A. Thallium
B. Sugar
C. Phenytoin
D. Strychnine
E. Scopolamine

75.6. A 22-year-old man presents to the hospital with a chief complaint of "not feeling well." Within 10 minutes of presentation, his electrocardiogram (ECG) progresses to a wide-complex tachycardia and his blood pressure falls. Shortly thereafter, a package is seen coming out of his rectum. What medication should be administered?
A. Sodium bicarbonate
B. Epinephrine
C. Atropine
D. Esmolol
E. Amiodarone

75.7. A 36-year-old man develops chest pain approximately 10 hours after being at a party. He had insufflated cocaine and drank several shots of vodka. Which of the following options is the likely cause of his delayed symptoms?
A. Benzoylecogonine
B. Cocaethylene
C. Norcocaine
D. Ecgonine methyl ester
E. Pseudocholinesterase

75.8. A 31-year-old woman is brought into the emergency department with crushing substernal chest pressure. Her electrocardiogram (ECG) shows ST segment elevation with a narrow QRS complex. Her blood pressure is 210/100 mmHg, her heart rate is 138 beats/min, and her temperature is 101.1 °F (38.4 °C) rectally. Aspirin (325 mg orally), diazepam (10 mg intravenously), and sublingual nitroglycerin (0.4 mg) are administered with no improvement in her pain. What medication should be administered next?
A. Phentolamine
B. Sodium bicarbonate
C. Lidocaine
D. Amiodarone
E. Esmolol

75.9. A 32-year-old man with a history of substance-use disorder presents to the emergency department with a purple discoloration to his left ear. A vasculitis is suspected. Which of the following xenobiotics is the likely culprit?

A. Levamisole
B. Caffeine
C. Diltiazem
D. Hydroxyzine
E. Phenacetin

75.10. A 54-year-old man presents to the emergency department with sudden-onset tearing chest pain radiating to his back shortly after insufflating cocaine. His blood pressure is 220/110 mmHg and his heart rate is 138 beats/min. His electrocardiogram shows a narrow-complex tachycardia with normal intervals. A computed tomography (CT) scan of his chest demonstrates a dissection of his ascending aorta. Which of the following therapies should be performed as part of the management of this patient?
A. Administration of intramuscular haloperidol
B. Administration of intravenous labetolol
C. Administration of sodium bicarbonate
D. Administration of intravenous nicardipine
E. Administration of intravenous amiodarone

ANSWERS

75.1. Answer: C. When conscious dogs were given cocaine, all interventions that corrected hyperthermia (diazepam, cooling) improved survival. Interventions that corrected hypertension and tachycardia (propranolol) or acidosis (bicarbonate) tended to have no beneficial effect or even worsen toxicity. This experiment has been replicated in other models and serves as the basis for current treatment regimens.

Catravas JD, Waters IW. Acute cocaine intoxication in the conscious dog: Studies on the mechanism of lethality. *J Pharmacol Exp Ther*. 1981;217:350-356.

75.2. Answer: B. Numerous studies demonstrate that the direct effect of cocaine on the myocardium is blockade of phase 0 (rapid sodium influx) and phase 3 (delayed potassium rectifier) current, similar to the type IA and IC antidysrhythmics. This mechanism has important implications with regard to treatment of patients with cocaine-induced wide-complex dysrhythmias. The positive inotropic and chronotropic effects are indirect in that they result from increases in epinephrine and norepinephrine and not cocaine directly.

Bauman JL, et al. Cocaine-related sudden cardiac death: A hypothesis correlating basic science and clinical observations. *J Clin Pharmacol*. 1994;34:902-911.

Winecoff AP, et al. Reversal of the electrocardiographic effects of cocaine by lidocaine. Part 1. Comparison with sodium bicarbonate and quinidine. *Pharmacotherapy*. 1994;14:698-703.

75.3. Answer: C. A significant portion of cocaine is metabolized by plasma cholinesterase to form ecgonine methyl ester. The organic phosphorous insecticide chlorpyrifos prolongs the effect of cocaine by inhibiting plasma cholinesterase. There are reports of patients taking advantage of this phenomenon by purposefully co-ingesting an organic phosphorous compound with cocaine. Succinylcholine is also metabolized by plasma cholinesterase, and if it is used as a neuromuscular blocker in a patient who had recently used cocaine, both the paralysis and the effects of cocaine are prolonged. Pancuronium, on the other hand, is not metabolized by this pathway. All of the other answers are not metabolized by plasma cholinesterase.

Herschman Z, Aaron C. Prolongation of cocaine effect. *Anesthesiology*. 1991;74:631-632.

Stewart DJ, et al. Hydrolysis of cocaine in human plasma by cholinesterase. *Life Sci*. 1977;20:1557-1564.

75.4. Answer: E. Rhabdomyolysis typically occurs in the setting of acute cocaine toxicity that includes abnormal vital signs and psychomotor agitation. However, the direct vasospastic effects of cocaine are sufficient to produce rhabdomyolysis in the absence of any of these findings.

> Zamora-Quezada JC, et al. Muscle and skin infarction after free-basing cocaine (crack). *Ann Intern Med*. 1988;108:564-566.

75.5. Answer: B. Xenobiotics that are commonly used to adulterate cocaine have physical or pharmacologic properties that are similar to cocaine: white powders (starch, sugar, talc), sympathomimetics, and local anesthetics. Although thallium, phenytoin, scopolamine, and strychnine contamination are reported, these are rare events.

> Insley BM, et al. Thallium poisoning in cocaine users. *Am J Emerg Med*. 1986;4:545-548.

> Shannon MW. Clinical toxicity of cocaine adulterants. *Ann Emerg Med*. 1988;17:1243-1247.

75.6. Answer: A. In patients who present to the emergency department with concealed drug packets, the greatest concern is for packet rupture and for a massive amount of cocaine to enter the circulation. Although cocaine causes tachycardia and hypertension, following a very large exposure, such as from a ruptured packet, patients develop bradycardia prior to progressing to cardiac arrest. Their ECG also shows a wide-complex rhythm with a very prominent R' in AVR because of the sodium channel–blocking effects of cocaine. If a patient has a wide-complex rhythm, then a trial of hypertonic sodium bicarbonate is indicated. If sodium bicarbonate does not resolve the dysrhythmia, then lidocaine is recommended.

> Kerns W 2nd, et al. Cocaine-induced wide complex dysrhythmia. *J Emerg Med*. 1997;15:321-329.

> Parker RB, et al. Comparative effects of sodium bicarbonate and sodium chloride on reversing cocaine-induced changes in the electrocardiogram. *J Cardiovasc Pharmacol*. 1999;34:864-869.

75.7. Answer: B. When cocaine is used concurrently with ethanol, a transesterification reaction occurs and a new compound, cocaethylene (also known as ethylbenzoylecgonine), is formed. Cocaethylene has a longer duration of action than cocaine. Benzoylecgonine is the metabolite of cocaine that standard urine drug screens detect. Norcocaine is a minor metabolite that occurs with cocaine *N*-demethylation in the liver. Ecgonine methyl ester occurs when cocaine is metabolized by plasma cholinesterase. Pseudocholinesterase is another name for plasma cholinesterase. Ecgonine methyl ester acts as a sedative, anticonvulsant, and protective metabolite of cocaine.

> Harris DS, et al. The pharmacology of cocaethylene in humans following cocaine and ethanol administration. *Drug Alcohol Depend*. 2003;72:169-182.

75.8. Answer: A. In patients who present with ST segment elevation following cocaine use, standard therapy should be initiated, including aspirin and nitroglycerin. As cocaine leads to an increased risk of coronary artery disease with plaque formation and rupture, patients who have ST segment elevation from cocaine use should also be evaluated by a cardiologist for emergent cardiac catheterization or thrombolysis if interventional cardiology is unavailable. However, the administration of the alpha adrenergic antagonist phentolamine concomitantly is indicated to relieve the hypertension and potentially relieve the vasospasm. Sodium bicarbonate and lidocaine are used if a patient has a wide-complex rhythm. Amiodarone currently has no role in the management of cocaine-induced dysrhythmias. Beta adrenergic antagonists are contraindicated in patients who manifest acute cocaine toxicity.

> Sand IC, et al. Experience with esmolol for the treatment of cocaine-associated cardiovascular complications. *Am J Emerg Med*. 1991;9:161-163.

> Hollander JE. Use of phentolamine for cocaine-induced myocardial ischemia. *N Engl J Med*. 1992;327:361.

75.9. Answer: A. While all the substances listed are adulterants of cocaine, levamisole is currently present in approximately 69% of the cocaine available in the United States. Levamisole leads to vasculitis and purpura, most commonly described on the tips of the ears. Levamisole also leads to neutropenia and agranulocytosis.

> Larocque A, Hoffman RS. Levamisole in cocaine: Unexpected news from an old acquaintance. *Clin Toxicol (Phila)*. 2012;50:231-241.

> Brunt TM, et al. Adverse effects of levamisole in cocaine users: A review and risk assessment. *Arch Toxicol*. 2017;91:2303-2313.

75.10. Answer: D. In patients who have an acute aortic dissection, controlling both the heart rate and blood pressure is paramount to their care. In non–cocaine-induced aortic dissection, an intravenous beta adrenergic antagonist to control the blood pressure is used. However, given this patient's recent cocaine use, there is a risk that the intravenous beta adrenergic antagonist could cause an unopposed alpha adrenergic effect and further worsen the heart rate and blood pressure. Therefore, the preferred agent to control this patient's heart rate and blood pressure would be a calcium channel blocker. When sedation is necessary in patients who have cocaine toxicity, the use of a benzodiazepine is recommended. Given this patient has narrow complexes on his electrocardiogram, there is no role for lidocaine at this time.

Boehrer JD, et al. Influence of labetalol on cocaine-induced coronary vasoconstriction in humans. *Am J Med*. 1993;94:608-610.

Ethanol

QUESTIONS

76.1. A 3-year-old boy (20 kg) ingests 50 mL of 100-proof vodka. What will the child's ethanol concentration be if all of the ethanol is immediately absorbed?
A. 20.8 mg/dL (4.5 mmol/L)
B. 41.6 mg/dL (9.0 mmol/L)
C. 208 mg/dL (45.2 mmol/L)
D. 416 mg/dL (90.3 mmol/L)
E. 520 mg/dL (112.9 mmol/L)

76.2. Alcoholic ketoacidosis (AKA) is best treated with which of the following options?
A. Rehydration, glucose, and thiamine
B. Sodium bicarbonate and rehydration
C. Pyridoxine, magnesium, and potassium
D. Glucose, potassium, naloxone, and pyridoxine
E. Fomepizole, pyridoxine, and dialysis

76.3. What is the first sign of thiamine (vitamin B_1) deficiency that develops within 1-2 weeks of its removal from the diet?
A. Dementia
B. Tachycardia
C. Ophthalmoplegia
D. Ataxia
E. Peripheral edema

76.4. Which of the following options is correct regarding alcoholic ketoacidosis (AKA)?
A. The serum lactate concentration is generally normal
B. The cellular redox state is low (ie, reduced)

C. The nitroprusside test is strongly positive
D. There is a normal anion gap metabolic acidosis
E. The serum glucose usually exceeds 300 mg/dL (16.7 mmol/L)

76.5. A 2-year-old girl is found unresponsive in the living room. A serum ethanol concentration is measured and is 85 mg/dL (18.5 mmol/L). What other test must be performed on this patient?
A. Serum blood glucose
B. Serum acetaminophen concentration
C. Serum salicylate concentration
D. Urine drug screen
E. Electrocardiogram

76.6. A 34-year-old woman presents to the emergency department for evaluation of palpitations. Her heart rate is 143 beats/min and her blood pressure is 128/80 mmHg. An electrocardiogram performed demonstrates a rapid atrial fibrillation. On further history, she states that she attended a large holiday party the prior evening. Her heart rate improves to 85 beats/min after a single dose of diltiazem. Which of the following medications should be initiated to treat her new atrial fibrillation?
A. 81 mg aspirin daily
B. Heparin infusion
C. Dabigatran daily
D. Rivaroxaban
E. No therapy indicated at this time

76.7. Which one of the following statements regarding ethanol metabolism is correct?

A. Acetate is converted to acetoacetate, which enters the citric acid cycle

B. Gluconeogenesis is impaired by the conversion of pyruvate to lactate

C. The microsomal ethanol oxidizing system (CYP2E1) is the main pathway for ethanol metabolism

D. Oxidation of ethanol to acetaldehyde by ADH requires $NADP^+$

E. Pyridoxine (vitamin B_6) is essential for the oxidation of acetaldehyde to acetate

76.8. A 54-year-old man with a history of alcohol use disorder is mandated by his job to have regular screening for continued ethanol use. Which of the following tests would provide the most useful information?

A. Cocaethylene

B. Hippuric acid

C. Phenol

D. Ethyl glucuronide

E. Benzoylecgonine

76.9. Which of the following vitamins is an essential cofactor for transketolase, pyruvate dehydrogenase, and alpha-ketoglutarate dehydrogenase?

A. Folate

B. Niacin

C. Pyridoxine

D. Riboflavin

E. Thiamine

76.10. A 27-year-old man is brought into the emergency department due to a concern of ethanol intoxication and "a smell of alcohol on his breath." His vital signs are a heart rate of 138 beats/min, a blood pressure of 128/80 mmHg, a respiratory rate of 28 breaths/min, oxygen saturation of 98% on room air, and a temperature of 98.6 °F (37 °C). On examination, he is minimally responsive with no obvious signs of trauma. What is the next step in management for this patient?

A. Observation

B. Breathalyzer assessment

C. Serum ethanol concentration

D. Serum salicylate concentration

E. Urine drug screen

ANSWERS

76.1. Answer: C. Fifty mL of 100-proof (50%) vodka is equivalent to 25 g or 25,000 mg. The blood ethanol concentration (in mg/dL) is derived by dividing the dose of ethanol (in mg) by the volume of distribution (in L/kg) multiplied by the weight (in kg) multiplied by 10. Thus, the blood concentration equals

$$25,000 \text{ mg}/(0.6 \text{ L/kg} \times 20 \text{ kg} \times 10 \text{ dL/L}) = 208 \text{ mg/dL}$$

$$208 \text{ mg/dL} \times 10 \text{ dL/L} \times 1 \text{ mmol}/46 \text{ mg} = 45.2 \text{ mmol/L}$$

Peterson C. Oral ethanol doses in patients with methanol poisoning. *Am J Hosp Pharm.* 1981;38:1024-1027.

76.2. Answer: A. Alcoholic ketoacidosis is best treated with rehydration, glucose, and thiamine. Exogenous insulin is usually unnecessary in patients without diabetes mellitus. Glucose administration stimulates insulin release and reduces the oxidation of fatty acids. Thiamine facilitates the entry of pyruvate into the citric acid cycle. Finally, hydration restores lost volume and enhances the excretion of organic acids.

Fulop M, Hoberman HD. Diabetic ketoacidosis and alcoholic ketosis. *Ann Intern Med.* 1979;91:796-797.

76.3. Answer: B. Tachycardia is the first manifestation of thiamine deficiency and occurs within 1-2 weeks after removal of thiamine from the diet.

Victor M, Adams RD. The effect of alcohol on the nervous system. In: Meritt HH, Hare CC, eds. *Metabolic and Toxic Diseases of the Nervous System.* Baltimore, MD: Williams & Wilkins; 1953:526-563.

76.4. Answer: B. One of the hallmarks of alcoholic ketoacidosis (AKA) is a high anion gap metabolic acidosis (occasionally with pH <6.80). The pathophysiology of AKA involves an overwhelmingly low cellular redox state such that most of the acetoacetate is reduced to beta-hydroxybutyrate. The nitroprusside test is used to detect the presence of ketones in serum and urine. The laboratory assay for ketones in a patient with AKA is often only mildly positive and substantially less than expected from the acid–base data because the nitroprusside reaction only detects molecules containing ketones such as acetone and acetoacetate and not beta-hydroxybutyrate. The diagnostic criteria for AKA should include a recent history of ethanol intake with a relative or absolute decline in ethanol consumption 24-72 hours before presentation, a history of vomiting, a blood glucose concentration <300 mg/dL (16.7 mmol/L), and a metabolic acidosis for which other causes are excluded by clinical observation or laboratory studies. Typically, the lactate concentration is elevated in AKA (occassionaly as high as 35 mmol/L) due to volume depletion and conversion of pyruvate to lactate to regenerate NAD⁺.

Fulop M. Alcoholic ketoacidosis. *Endocrinol Metab Clin North Am.* 1993;22:209-219.

Soffer A, Hamburger S. Alcoholic ketoacidosis: A review of 30 cases. *J Am Med Wom Assoc.* 1982;37:106-110.

76.5. Answer: A. Children, particular young children, have limited glycogen stores. Ethanol consumption following an overnight fast leads to profound hypoglycemia and, if not recognized and treated rapidly, will result in permanent neurologic disability. A careful history when evaluating a child who is hypoglycemic should include asking about alcoholic beverages in the home as well as other ethanol-containing products, such as mouthwashes. Children who have elevated ethanol concentrations, especially younger children, should be admitted overnight to the hospital to monitor for hypoglycemia as well as ensure a safe home environment.

Ernst AA, et al. Ethanol ingestion and related hypoglycemia in a pediatric and adolescent emergency department population. *Acad Emerg Med.* 1996;3:46-49.

76.6. Answer: E. "Holiday heart syndrome" is a syndrome in which patients who drink ethanol develop a cardiac dysrhythmia following an episode of large ethanol consumption. The most common dysrhythmia is atrial fibrillation, which usually reverts to normal sinus rhythm within 24 hours. The clinical course is benign and patients do not usually need to be initiated on antidysrhythmic medication or anticoagulation.

Greenspon AJ, Schaal SF. The "holiday heart": Electrophysiological studies of alcohol effects in alcoholics. *Ann Intern Med.* 1983;98:135-140.

76.7. Answer: B. Alcohol dehydrogenase (ADH) uses NAD⁺ as a hydrogen acceptor to oxidize ethanol to acetaldehyde, which it is further metabolized to acetate by aldehyde dehydrogenase (ALDH). Acetate is converted to acetyl coenzyme A, which enters the citric acid cycle and is metabolized to carbon dioxide and water. The ability of acetyl coenzyme A to enter the citric acid cycle is indirectly dependent on adequate thiamine stores. The metabolism of ethanol generates NADH and alters the redox (NAD⁺/NADH) ratio, thereby forcing the conversion of pyruvate to lactate and preventing gluconeogenesis.

Fulop M, Hoberman HD. Alcoholic ketosis. *Diabetes.* 1975;24:785-790.

76.8. Answer: D. Ethyl glucuronide and ethyl sulfate are nonoxidative direct ethanol metabolites and are excreted for a far longer time than ethanol. Testing for these metabolites is gaining popularity in certain settings to evaluate for continued ethanol use. Caution should be applied in interpreting ethyl glucuronide testing results. Ethyl glucuronide is sensitive to degradation or is synthesized by bacteria, such that infected urine results in either a false-positive or false-negative test result. Furthermore, unintentional exposures to ethanol, including mouthwash and hand sanitizers, are sufficient to cause a positive result for both ethyl glucuronide and ethyl sulfate. A common cutoff or reporting limit has yet to be determined for urinary ethyl glucuronide and ethyl sulfate when it is used as an ethanol biomarker.

Helander A. Biological markers in alcoholism. *J Neural Transm Suppl.* 2003;66:15-32.

Helander A, Dahl H. Urinary tract infection: A risk factor for false-negative urinary ethyl glucuronide but not ethyl sulfate in the detection of recent alcohol consumption. *Clin Chem.* 2005;51:1728-1730.

76.9. Answer: E. Thiamine (vitamin B₁) is an essential cofactor for transketolase, pyruvate dehydrogenase, and alpha-ketoglutarate dehydrogenase. Thiamine deficiency, commonly associated with alcohol use disorder, leads to a neurologic disorder known as Wernicke encephalopathy, which has a classic triad of oculomotor abnormalities, ataxia, and confusion. Thiamine deficiency also contributes to the development of (alcoholic ketoacidosis) AKA and a high output cardiac failure.

Lavoie J, Butterworth RF. Reduced activities of thiamine-dependent enzymes in brains of alcoholics in the absence of Wernicke's encephalopathy. *Alcohol Clin Exp Res.* 1995;19:1073-1077.

Butterworth RF, et al. Thiamine-dependent enzyme changes in the brains of alcoholics: Relationship to the Wernicke-Korsakoff syndrome. *Alcohol Clin Exp Res.* 1993;17:1084-1088.

76.10. Answer: D. The odor of alcohol on a patient's breath is very unreliable and should not be used as a definitive measure. In patients who present to the emergency department for evaluation of ethanol intoxication, it is important to perform a thorough physical examination to ensure no visible signs of trauma; in addition, a point-of-care blood glucose measurement should be taken, and close attention should be paid to vital signs. This patient is tachycardic and tachypneic, which warrants further evaluation to ensure other diagnoses are considered beyond just ethanol intoxication. In this case, a serum salicylate concentration resulted at 80 mg/dL (5.79 mmol/L). A urine drug screen will not be helpful here as it is neither sensitive nor specific. Although a serum ethanol concentration is often measured, it is important to not anchor on ethanol intoxication in a patient with abnormal vital signs. Breathalyzers are not reliable as they are associated with a falsely elevated value if a patient has ethanol in their mouth at the time of the test.

Moskowitz H, et al. Police officers' detection of breath odors from alcohol ingestion. *Accid Anal Prev*. 1999;31:175-180.

77

Alcohol Withdrawal

QUESTIONS

77.1. A 56-year-old man with alcohol use disorder is brought into the emergency department with vomiting and tremulousness. He is tachycardic, hypertensive, confused, and mildly agitated. He vomits multiple times during the examination. Which of the following options is the most appropriate initial treatment of his alcohol withdrawal?
  A. Lorazepam 2 mg intravenously
  B. Diazepam 10 mg intravenously
  C. Chlordiazepoxide 100 mg orally
  D. Phenobarbital 65 mg intravenously
  E. Fosphenytoin 20 mg/kg intravenously

77.2. What pathophysiologic changes cause the symptoms associated with alcohol withdrawal?
  A. Downregulation of gamma-aminobutyric acid (GABA)$_A$ receptors and *N*-methyl-D-aspartate (NMDA) receptors
  B. Upregulation of GABA$_B$ receptors
  C. Downregulation of kainate receptors
  D. Upregulation of NMDA receptors and downregulation of GABA$_A$ receptors
  E. Upregulation of kainate and NMDA receptors

77.3. A 49-year-old woman with alcohol use disorder presents to the emergency department after she stopped drinking alcohol because she sees cats jumping around her apartment. She knows that the cats are not truly there. She is alert and oriented, and her vital signs are within normal limits. What is her likelihood of developing delirium tremens (DTs)?
  A. These symptoms are related to alcohol withdrawal, but are neither positively nor negatively predictive of development of DTs
  B. These symptoms are positively predictive; one-third of patients with these hallucinations will go on to have DTs if left untreated
  C. These symptoms are negatively predictive because there is no autonomic instability
  D. These symptoms are not related to alcohol withdrawal, and she should have a psychiatric evaluation
  E. These symptoms describe DTs, and the patient now meets criteria for this diagnosis

77.4. A 38-year-old woman presents to the emergency department with mild alcohol withdrawal and is found to have a lactate concentration of 4.5 mmol/L. Where does the coenzyme she is deficient in act?
  A. The conversion of glucose to glucose-6-phosphate
  B. The pyruvate dehydrogenase complex
  C. Transportation of long-chain fatty acids across the mitochondrial membrane
  D. Complex I of the electron transport chain
  E. Complex IV of the electron transport chain

77.5. A 65-year-old man with alcohol use disorder presents to the emergency department with tachycardia and mild agitation. He also has marked ascites and gynecomastia. His laboratory studies are significant for thrombocytopenia and hypoalbuminemia. Which benzodiazepine is most appropriate to treat his alcohol withdrawal?

A. Midazolam
B. Diazepam
C. Lorazepam
D. Chlordiazepoxide
E. Clonazepam

77.6. A 50-year-old man with alcohol use disorder and prior episodes of delirium tremens (DTs) presents to the hospital with severe agitation. He has one 20-second generalized tonic-clonic seizure that stops spontaneously. His heart rate is 138 beats/min, his blood pressure is 174/110 mmHg, and his temperature is 100.5 °F (38.1 °C). He is admitted to the hospital and treated with intravenous benzodiazepines but does not improve. What further steps must be taken?

A. Obtain an electroencephalogram (EEG) to exclude nonconvulsive status epilepticus
B. Transition his regimen from benzodiazepines to dexmedetomidine
C. Add chlorpromazine to his other medications
D. Initiate labetalol for blood pressure control
E. Perform a lumbar puncture and treat based on the results

77.7. A 62-year-old woman with alcohol use disorder is admitted to the intensive care unit with delirium tremens. She is tachycardic, tremulous, and confused. She seized once in the emergency department. What is the most appropriate medication regimen to treat her alcohol withdrawal?

A. Scheduled dosing of lorazepam with a taper
B. Scheduled dosing of diazepam with a taper
C. Symptom-triggered dosing of lorazepam using the CIWA score
D. Symptom-triggered dosing of diazepam using the CIWA score
E. Symptom-triggered dosing of diazepam using the RASS score

77.8. Gabapentin shows promise for reducing craving in patients with alcohol use disorder. What is the proposed mechanism by which it does this?

A. Inhibition of voltage-gated calcium channels
B. Agonism at the $GABA_A$ receptor
C. Antagonism at the NMDA receptor
D. Agonism at the mu-opioid receptor
E. Inhibition of voltage-gated sodium channels

77.9. What is the most common presentation of an alcohol withdrawal seizure?

A. Status epilepticus with tonic-clonic movements
B. Nonconvulsive status epilepticus
C. A brief, generalized tonic-clonic seizure with a short post-ictal period
D. A brief, generalized tonic-clonic seizure with an extended post-ictal period
E. Multiple partial seizures

77.10. An increased serum concentration of which amino acid is associated with the development of alcohol withdrawal?

A. Glycine
B. Serine
C. Tryptophan
D. Homocysteine
E. Arginine

ANSWERS

77.1. Answer: B. Intravenous diazepam is the preferred medication for treatment of patients in moderate to severe alcohol withdrawal. Diazepam has a time to peak effect of minutes, allowing for rapid control without unintentional oversedation. Its active metabolites, desmethyldiazepam and oxazepam, extend its duration of action. Lorazepam has a longer time to peak effect than diazepam and does not have active metabolites. While it is hepatically metabolized, it is appropriate for patients with advanced liver disease because it has low hepatic clearance and no active metabolites. Oral chlordiazepoxide is an appropriate benzodiazepine for mild alcohol withdrawal, but patients with moderate to severe alcohol withdrawal, who are confused and are unable to tolerate oral medications, require intravenous therapy. Phenobarbital, while effective in binding gamma-aminobutyric acid (GABA)$_A$ receptors, has a higher risk of respiratory depression than benzodiazepines. The onset of action of phenobarbital is longer than that of diazepam, with clinical effects beginning in 20-40 minutes. Fosphenytoin has no role in the treatment of alcohol withdrawal. It does not regulate either GABA or N-methyl-D-aspartate (NMDA) receptors.

Ritson B, Chick J. Comparison of two benzodiazepines in the treatment of alcohol withdrawal: Effects on symptoms and cognitive recovery. *Drug Alcohol Depend.* 1986;18:329-334.

77.2. Answer: D. Alcohol stimulates the gamma aminobutyric acid (GABA)$_A$ receptor and inhibits the N-methyl-D-aspartate (NMDA) receptor. Continuous use results in downregulation of the GABA$_A$ receptor and upregulation of the excitatory NMDA receptor. These physiologic changes allow a person with alcohol tolerance to maintain a normal level of consciousness despite having sedating concentrations of ethanol in the brain. The binding site for ethanol is on the GABA$_A$ receptor, not the GABA$_B$ receptor. The kainate receptor, a different glutamate receptor, is not involved in the actions of ethanol.

> Brousse G, et al. Alteration of glutamate/GABA balance during acute alcohol withdrawal in emergency department: A prospective analysis. *Alcohol Alcohol.* 2012;47:501-508.

77.3. Answer: A. These symptoms describe alcoholic hallucinosis. Hallucinations are most often tactile or visual but are also auditory. Alcoholic hallucinosis is distinct from other manifestations of withdrawal in several ways. First, it need not be preceded by alcoholic tremulousness. Second, patients have a clear sensorium, unlike patients with DTs. While alcoholic hallucinosis is one manifestation of alcohol withdrawal, it is neither positively nor negatively predictive of the development of DTs.

> Glass IB. Alcoholic hallucinosis: A psychiatric enigma–1. The development of an idea. *Br J Addict.* 1989;84:29-41.

77.4. Answer: B. Thiamine is a required coenzyme in the pyruvate dehydrogenase complex, in which it facilitates the conversion of pyruvate to acetylcoenzyme A. It is also required in the citric acid cycle at the alpha-ketoglutarate complex and in the pentose phosphate pathway for transketolase.

> Kern D, et al. How thiamine diphosphate is activated in enzymes. *Science.* 1997;275:67-70.

77.5 Answer: C. This patient has multiple markers of advanced liver failure. Benzodiazepines that undergo hepatic metabolism or have active metabolites (chlordiazepoxide, midazolam, diazepam, and clonazepam) cause prolonged periods of sedation in patients with cirrhosis. Lorazepam does not have active metabolites.

> Wretlind M, et al. Disposition of three benzodiazepines after single oral administration in man. *Acta Pharmacol Toxicol (Copenh).* 1977;40 (Suppl 1): 28-39.

77.6. Answer: E. While these signs and symptoms are consistent with delirium tremens (DTs), they are also consistent with meningoencephalitis. Patients with alcohol use disorder who present with fever and disorientation without a clear infectious source should receive a lumbar puncture to exclude meningitis or encephalitis in addition to treatment for DTs. Dexmedetomidine is an alpha$_2$ adrenergic receptor agonist. It will treat this patient's tachycardia and hypertension but will not resolve the pathophysiology of alcohol withdrawal, which requires drugs that work on the gamma-aminobutyric acid (GABA) receptor. Similarly, labetalol is a beta adrenergic antagonist and does not work on the GABA receptor. Use of chlorpromazine is associated with a higher rate of seizures in patients with alcohol withdrawal.

> van Veen KE, et al. Bacterial meningitis in alcoholic patients: A population-based prospective study. *J Infect.* 2017;74:352-357.

77.7. Answer: E. Symptom-triggered therapy leads to shorter lengths of stay for patients with alcohol withdrawal. When using symptom-triggered therapy, symptoms are assessed using a clinical score, such as the Clinical Institute Withdrawal Assessment for Alcohol Scale (CIWA) or Richmond Agitation-Sedation Scale (RASS). While the CIWA is useful for patients in mild withdrawal, it requires participation from the patient and is therefore inadequate for patients with altered mental status.

> Saitz R, et al. Individualized treatment for alcohol withdrawal. A randomized double-blind controlled trial. *JAMA.* 1994;272:519-523.

77.8. Answer: A. While gabapentin is not helpful during acute withdrawal, literature supports its use in patients who continue to crave alcohol after the withdrawal period has ended. It inhibits the voltage-gated calcium channel, which inhibits the activity of glutamate, an excitatory neurotransmitter.

> Mason BJ, et al. Gabapentin treatment for alcohol dependence: A randomized clinical trial. *JAMA Intern Med.* 2014;174:70-77.

77.9. Answer: C. Alcohol withdrawal seizures are classically generalized, tonic-clonic, and brief. Patients quickly return to their baseline mental status. One-third of patients who present with an alcohol withdrawal seizure and are not appropriately treated progress to develop delirium tremens (DTs).

> Victor M, Brausch C. The role of abstinence in the genesis of alcoholic epilepsy. *Epilepsia.* 1967;8:1-20.

77.10. Answer: D. Elevated homocysteine concentrations are associated with the development of alcohol withdrawal, likely in the setting of folate deficiency, but cannot be used as a predictor for withdrawal. Interestingly, homocysteine acts as an excitatory neurotransmitter at the NMDA receptor, leading to seizures.

Bleich S, et al. Elevated homocysteine levels in alcohol withdrawal. *Alcohol Alcohol.* 2000;35:351-354.

Disulfiram and Disulfiramlike Reactions

QUESTIONS

78.1. Which of the following metabolites of disulfiram retains much of the same pharmacologic activity as the parent compound?
A. Thiocarboxylic acid
B. Diethylamide
C. Carbonyl sulfide
D. Diethyldithiocarbamate
E. Methyl mercaptan sulfate

78.2. Which is the most common adverse effect associated with chronic disulfiram therapy?
A. Hepatotoxicity
B. Nephrotoxicity
C. Neuropathy
D. Myopathy
E. Neutropenia

78.3. A 27-year-old man presents to the emergency department acutely intoxicated with ethanol. On examination, he is hypotensive to 60/30 mmHg despite an appropriate fluid challenge. A bedside echocardiogram demonstrates a reduced ejection fraction. A medication reconciliation reveals that he is prescribed disulfiram. Which of the following medications is reasonable to administer?
A. *N*-Acetylcysteine
B. Fomepizole
C. Glutathione
D. Flumazenil
E. Activated charcoal

78.4. A 22-year-old man presents to the emergency department with symptoms consistent with a disulfiram reaction. He has never been prescribed disulfiram. Which of the following mushrooms led to his presentation?
A. *Gyromitra ambigua*
B. *Clitocybe dealbata*
C. *Clitocybe dilatata*
D. *Coprinopsis atramentaria*
E. *Paxillus involutus.*

78.5. In the patient in Question 78.4, which constellation of symptoms did he develop that are consistent with a disulfiram-alcohol interaction?
A. Flushing, throbbing in the head and neck, headache, nausea, vomiting, hypotension, and tachycardia
B. Pruritus, dermatitis, headache, drowsiness, fatigue, impotence, and peripheral neuropathy
C. Hyperthermia, nausea, vomiting, diarrhea, bradycardia, diaphoresis, and lacrimation
D. Tachycardia, lethargy, abdominal pain, and a high anion gap metabolic acidosis
E. Tremor, tachycardia, seizures, coma, and hyperthermia

78.6. Which of the following adverse effects is more characteristic of the toxicity of disulfiram alone as compared to disulfiram without ethanol?
A. Optic neuritis
B. Facial erythema
C. Diaphoresis
D. Tachycardia
E. Hypotension

78.7. Which of the following xenobiotics interacts with ethanol to result in a disulfiramlike reaction?
A. Chloral hydrate
B. Chlorpropamide
C. Isoniazid
D. Niacin
E. Ranitidine

78.8. A 33-year-old man presents to the emergency department after an intentional overdose of disulfiram. He is hypotensive to 60/20 mmHg and fails an appropriate fluid challenge. Which of the following vasopressors should be avoided?
A. Dopamine
B. Dobutamine
C. Epinephrine
D. Norepinephrine
E. Phenylephrine

78.9. Which of the following mechanisms explains how disulfiram benefits patients with cocaine use disorder?
A. Irreversible inhibition of aldehyde dehydrogenase (ALDH)
B. Potent metal chelation
C. Inhibition of microsomal carboxylesterases and plasma cholinesterases
D. Inhibition of dopamine beta-hydroxylase (DBH)
E. The addition of a thiol moiety to cocaine

78.10. Which of the following neuropathies is consistent with disulfiram toxicity?
A. Foot drop
B. Wrist drop
C. Trigeminal neuralgia
D. Cranial nerve VII palsy
E. Guillian-Barré syndrome

ANSWERS

78.1. Answer: D. While all the choices listed are metabolites of disulfiram, only diethyldithiocarbamate is capable of slowing the metabolism of acetaldehyde.

Eneanya DI, et al. The actions and metabolic fate of disulfiram. *Annu Rev Pharmacol Toxicol.* 1981;21:575-579.

78.2. Answer: A. Hepatotoxicity is the most common adverse drug event associated with chronic disulfiram therapy. Neuropathy and myopathy are possible symptoms of acute and chronic disulfiram toxicity. Nephrotoxicity is not reported.

Forns X, et al. Disulfiram-induced hepatitis. Report of four cases and review of the literature. *J Hepatol.* 1994;21:853-857.

Enghusen Poulsen H, et al. Disulfiram therapy—adverse drug reactions and interactions. *Acta Psychiatr Scand Suppl.* 1992;369:59–65; discussion 65-56.

78.3. Answer: B. While fomepizole is not a true antidote for disulfiram or disulfiramlike reactions, it is reasonable to use in patients experiencing a severe disulfiram-ethanol reaction leading to cardiogenic or distributive shock. Fomepizole inhibits the enzyme alcohol dehydrogenase, which limits the progression of the disulfiram reaction by blocking ethanol metabolism to acetaldehyde. Symptomatic and supportive treatment is the mainstay of treatment.

Sande M, et al. Fomepizole for severe disulfiram-ethanol reactions. *Am J Emerg Med.* 2012;30:262 e263-265.

78.4. Answer: D. The mushroom *Coprinopsis atramentaria* contains the toxin coprine and cannot be safely ingested with alcohol. The metabolite of coprine, L-aminocyclopropanol, causes a disulfiramlike reaction when taken with ethanol.

Reynolds WA, Lowe FH. Mushrooms and a toxic reaction to alcohol: Report of four cases. *N Engl J Med.* 1965;272:630-631.

78.5. Answer: A. The symptoms that would be expected in a patient having a disulfiram reaction include flushing, throbbing in the head and neck, headache, nausea, vomiting, hypotension, and tachycardia.

Linden CH, et al. Disulfiram. *Topics Emerg Med.* 1984;6:30-37.

78.6. Answer: A. The toxic effects of disulfiram independent of ethanol include depression, lethargy, loss of libido, psychosis, delirium, meningeal signs, unilateral weakness, optic neuritis, and peripheral neuropathy. Unfortunately, these symptoms are often misdiagnosed as psychiatric illness or sequelae of alcoholism. Choices B-E are more characteristic of the disulfiram-ethanol reaction.

Enghusen Poulsen H, et al. Disulfiram therapy—adverse drug reactions and interactions. *Acta Psychiatr Scand Suppl.* 1992;369:59-65; discussion 65-56.

Knee ST, Razani J. Acute organic brain syndrome: A complication of disulfiram therapy. *Am J Psychiatry.* 1974;131:1281-1282.

78.7. Answer: B. Drug-ethanol interactions resulting in disulfiramlike reactions include carbamates, cephalosporins that contain the side chain *N*-methylthiotetrazole (nMTT), chloramphenicol, chlorpropamide, *Coprinopsis* mushrooms, thiuram, and tolbutamide.

Mergenhagen KA, et al. Fact versus fiction: A review of the evidence behind alcohol and antibiotic interactions. *Antimicrob Agents Chemother.* 2020;64:e02167-19.

78.8. Answer: A. Disulfiram inhibits dopamine beta-hydroxylase, which is responsible for converting dopamine to norepinephrine. A direct-acting adrenergic agonist, such as norepinephrine, should be used in patients who have refractory hypotension caused by disulfiram.

Musacchio JM, et al. Inhibition of dopamine-beta-hydroxylase by disulfiram in vivo. *J Pharmacol Exp Ther.* 1966;152:56-61.

78.9. Answer: D. One of the metabolites of disulfiram, diethyldithiocarbamate, inhibits dopamine beta-hydroxylase, which is the enzyme responsible for converting dopamine to norepinephrine. Inhibition of this enzyme results in increased concentrations of dopamine in the brain and periphery and decreased concentrations of norepinephrine and epinephrine. The increased concentration of dopamine is believed to be of therapeutic benefit in cocaine use disorder. Answer choice A is the mechanism by which disulfiram is of therapeutic benefit in alcohol dependency; answer choice B is the mechanism for nickel dermatitis; and answer choice C is a purported mechanism that explains pharmacokinetic increases in the plasma concentrations of cocaine. Disulfiram does not add a thiol moiety to cocaine.

Gaval-Cruz M, Weinshenker D. Mechanisms of disulfiram-induced cocaine abstinence: Antabuse and cocaine relapse. *Mol Interv.* 2009; 9:175-187.

78.10. Answer: A. Disulfiram is associated with a painful peripheral neuropathy. Patients present with distal weakness and foot drop. If the disulfiram is continued, the weakness and painful neuropathy progress proximally.

Frisoni GB, Di Monda V. Disulfiram neuropathy: A review (1971–1988) and report of a case. *Alcohol Alcohol.* 1989;24:429-437.

Hallucinogens

QUESTIONS

79.1. Which of the following options is responsible for the hallucinogenic properties of *Bufo alvarius* (Colorado River toad)?
A. Bufotenine
B. 5-Methoxydimethyl tryptamine
C. Alpha-methyltryptamine
D. Bufalin
E. Lysergic acid diethylamide

79.2. Ololiuqui refers to which naturally occurring lysergamide used in ancient Mexico?
A. *Argyreia nervosa*
B. *Lophophora Williamsii*
C. *Banisteriopsis caapi*
D. *Claviceps purpura*
E. *Turbina corymbosa*

79.3. Mescaline is a phenylethylamine that occurs naturally in which plant?
A. *Lophophora williamsii*
B. *Salvia divinorum*
C. *Mitragyna speciosa*
D. *Myristica fragrans*
E. *Argyreia nervosa*

79.4. Which of the following plants contains xenobiotics known to cause both antimuscarinic symptoms and hallucinations?
A. Susumber berry
B. Peruvian torch cactus
C. Angel's trumpet
D. Pacific yew
E. Ackee fruit

79.5. Most hallucinogens exert their hallucinogenic effects via which of the following receptors?
A. Serotonin
B. Gamma-hydroxybutyrate
C. Norepinephrine
D. Epinephrine
E. Opioid

79.6. Which of the following hallucinogens is the shortest acting?
A. Lysergic acid diethylamide
B. Nutmeg
C. Salvia
D. Jimsonweed
E. Peyote

79.7. A 30-year-old man ingests a *Panaeolus* mushroom and develops vomiting 30 minutes later followed by hallucinations. Which xenobiotic is responsible for this patient's symptoms?
A. Psilocybin
B. Lysergic acid diethylamide
C. Ibotenic acid
D. Muscimol
E. Muscazone

79.8. Ayahuasca is a hallucinogenic practice that is used by indigenous healers during religious ceremonies. What does ayahuasca contain?
A. Harmine alkaloids
B. Dimethyltryptamine (DMT)
C. Lysergic acid diethylamide (LSD)
D. Harmine alkaloids and DMT
E. Harmine alkaloids, DMT, and LSD

79.9. A 23-year-old woman presents to the emergency department very upset because she has recurrent visual hallucinations. The hallucinations get acutely worse after she drinks alcohol. She feels debilitated and is unable to leave her house as she is afraid that the hallucinations will recur. Which of the following choices likely contributed to her presentation?
A. Lysergic acid diethylamide
B. Nutmeg
C. Salvia
D. Jimsonweed
E. Peyote

79.10. A famous movie star posts a youtube video containing clips of her smoking the drug salvia. She appears giddy and is laughing uncontrollably. Which receptor does this substance act on?
A. Mu opioid receptor
B. Kappa opioid receptor
C. *N*-methyl-D-aspartate (NMDA) receptor
D. Acetylcholine receptor
E. Serotonin receptor

ANSWERS

79.1. Answer: B. 5-Methoxydimethyl tryptamine (5-MeO-DMT) is secreted from the parotid glands of *Bufo alvarius*. It is degraded by intestinal monoamine oxidase. In order to cause psychogenic effects, it must be extracted and either smoked or insufflated. Bufotenine is also produced by *Bufo alvarius* but does not cross the blood–brain barrier and mainly causes hypertension. Alpha-methyltryptamine is a synthetic tryptamine and is not naturally occurring. Bufalin, a type of bufadienolide produced by toad venom glands, is a cardioactive steroid causing digoxinlike toxicity.

Lyttle T. Misuse and legend in the "toad licking" phenomenon. *Int J Addict*. 1993;28:521-538.

79.2. Answer: E. *Turbina corymbosa* is a species of Morning Glory that was used by Aztecs in religious ceremonies. This was historically called by other names, such as *Rivea corymbosa*. The seeds of *T. corymbosa* contain lysergic acid hydroxyethylamide, as do other variants of morning glory such as *Ipomoea violacea*.

Isbell H, Gorodetzky CW. Effect of alkaloids of ololiuqui in man. *Psychopharmacologia*. 1966;8:331-339.

79.3. Answer: A. Peyote (*Lophophora williamsii*) is a cactus that contains mescaline, a hallucinogenic phenylethylamine. The "buttons" of the peyote plant are ingested and used in religious ceremonies in the Native American Church. In addition to sympathomimetic symptoms, mescaline also causes nausea, vomiting, and hallucinations. *Salvia divinorum*, *Mitragyna speciosa*, *Myristica fragrans*, and *Argyreia nervosa* are the scientific names for salvia, kratom, nutmeg, and woodrose, respectively.

Carstairs SD, Cantrell FL. Peyote and mescaline exposures: A 12-year review of a statewide poison center database. *Clin Toxicol*. 2010;48:350-353.

79.4. Answer: C. Angel's trumpet (*Brugmansia*) is a member of the Solanaceae family characterized by trumpet-shaped large white flowers. This plant contains belladonna alkaloids including scopolamine, hyoscyamine, and atropine, which are responsible for the antimuscarinic delirium. Other members of the belladonna alkaloid family include deadly nightshade (*Atropa belladonna*) and Jimsonweed (*Datura stramonium*). Susumber berry, Peruvian torch cactus, Pacific yew, and ackee fruit contain toxic xenobiotics but do not cause antimuscarinic delirium.

Kim Y, et al. Intoxication by angel's trumpet: Case report and literature review. *BMC Res Notes*. 2014;7:553.

79.5. Answer: A. There is a structural similarity among lysergamide, indolealkylamine, and phenylethylamine hallucinogens with serotonin. The hallucinations caused by these xenobiotics occur through central serotonin receptors. There are many different 5-HT receptor subtypes, and variations in affinity between subtypes explain the differences in the psychogenic properties of each xenobiotic.

Aghajanian GK, Marek GJ. Serotonin and hallucinogens. *Neuropsychopharmacology*. 1999;21:16S-23S.

79.6. Answer: C. The psychoactive effects of salvia (*Salvia divinorum*) when inhaled or ingested have a rapid peak in symptom onset of 5-10 minutes, and the duration of symptoms is brief, ranging between 20 minutes and 2 hours. In contrast, jimsonweed has a duration of action of 2-3 hours, whereas LSD, nutmeg, and peyote have a longer duration of action of 10-24 hours.

Siebert DJ. *Salvia divinorum* and salvinorin A: New pharmacologic findings. *J Ethnopharmacol*. 1994;43:53-56.

79.7. Answer: A. Psilocybin is a tryptamine found in *Psilocybe cyanescens, Panaeolus cyanescens, Conocybe cyanopus*, and *Gynophilus spectabilis* mushrooms. Other naturally occurring tryptamines include bufotenine and *N,N*-dimethyltryptamine; however, these are not found in mushrooms. Some members of the *Amanita* spp contain psychoactive components including ibotenic acid, muscimol, and muscazone; however, these are not tryptamines.

Schultes RE. Hallucinogens of plant origin. *Science.* 1969;163:245-254.

79.8. Answer: D. Dimethyltryptamine (DMT) is a monoamine, and when taken orally, it is metabolized by monoamine oxidase in the intestines. Harmine alkaloids are intentionally added to ayahuasca as they inhibit monoamine oxidase, which allows for absorption of DMT. This increases oral bioavailability, allowing the combination to be provided as a hallucinogenic beverage.

McKenna DJ. Clinical investigations of the therapeutic potential of ayahuasca: Rationale and regulatory challenges. *Pharmacol Ther.* 2004; 102:111-129.

79.9. Answer: A. Hallucinogen persisting perception disorder (HPPD) is a long-term complication of LSD use. It consists of recurrent perception symptoms that are experienced while the patient is initially intoxicated with the substance. These episodes lead to functional impairment. A characteristic finding is palinopsia, which is a continued visual perception of an object, even after it has left the visual field.

American Psychiatric Association. *Diagnostic and Statistical Manual of Mental Disorders.* 5th ed. Washington, DC: American Psychiatric Association; 2013.

79.10. Answer: B. Salvinorin A is the psychoactive component in *Salvia divinorum* (salvia). It is unique from the other hallucinogens in that it acts on the kappa opioid receptor. Stimulation of the kappa opioid receptor mediates euphoria and analgesia. Salvia does not lead to respiratory depression.

Yan F, Roth BL. Salvinorin A: A novel and highly selective kappa-opioid receptor agonist. *Life Sci.* 2004;75:2615-2619.

80

Gamma-Hydroxybutyric Acid (GHB)

QUESTIONS

80.1. A 27-year-old man presents to the emergency department (ED) sedated, with miotic pupils and bradypnea. His friends found him unresponsive at a party. They had all used the same amount of gamma-hydroxybutyric acid (GHB) earlier that evening. Which of the following xenobiotics is the patient also taking that best explains why he was more affected by the GHB as compared to his friends?
A. Acetaminophen
B. Dextromethorphan
C. Digoxin
D. Ibuprofen
E. Ritonavir

80.2. A 23-year-old man presents to the emergency department after ingesting gamma-hydroxybutyric acid (GHB) in a suicide attempt 1 hour prior to arrival. He denies other co-ingestions but rapidly becomes sedated and is intubated. What is the most appropriate gastrointestinal decontamination in this patient?
A. Orogastric lavage
B. Single-dose activated charcoal
C. Multiple-dose activated charcoal
D. Whole bowel irrigation
E. No gastrointestinal decontamination

80.3. A 22-year-old bodybuilder presents to the emergency department stating that she is withdrawing from gamma-hydroxybutyric acid (GHB). What medication could be used to treat her withdrawal?
A. Clonidine
B. Gabapentin

C. Naltrexone
D. Baclofen
E. Buprenorphine/naloxone

80.4. Why does illicit use of gamma-hydroxybutyric acid (GHB) occur among bodybuilders?
A. It improves resting heart rate
B. It acts as a stimulant to improve workouts
C. It potentially increases growth hormone
D. It has GABA$_B$ agonist effects
E. It has amnestic effects to "forget" workout pain

80.5. Which enzymes form gamma-hydroxybutyrate (GHB) from gamma-aminobutyric acid (GABA)?
A. GABA transaminase and succinic semialdehyde reductase
B. GABA decarboxylase and succinic semialdehyde reductase
C. GABA decarboxylase and succinic transaminase
D. Lactonase and succinic semialdehyde dehydrogenase
E. GABA transaminase and lactonase

80.6. Which of the following statements is true of gamma-hydroxybutyrate (GHB)?
A. It is a schedule II controlled substance
B. It is a schedule V controlled substance
C. It is an endogenous neurotransmitter
D. It is a third-line medication to treat attention deficit hyperactivity disorder
E. It is approved by the US Food and Drug Administration (FDA) for the treatment of fibromyalgia

80.7. A 6-year-old girl presents to the emergency department with bradypnea, miosis, increased salivation, and somnolence after ingesting a plastic toy bead. Her Australian grandmother found these beads in her attic and brought them as a present. Which of the following xenobiotics most likely caused this presentation?

A. Fentanyl
B. Oxycodone
C. Ethanol
D. 1,4-Butanediol
E. Gamma-butyrolactone

80.8. The activity of exogenous gamma-hydroxybutyric acid (GHB) occurs at which receptor site?

A. GHB receptor
B. $GABA_A$ receptor
C. $GABA_B$ receptor
D. Glutamate receptor
E. NMDA receptor

80.9. Gamma-hydroxybutyrate (GHB) toxicity in humans is associated with which of the following symptoms?

A. Mydriasis
B. Seizures
C. Urinary retention
D. Myoclonus
E. Hyperthermia

80.10. A 19-year-old woman presents to the emergency department requesting testing for gamma-hydroxybutyrate (GHB) as she was date-raped 7 hours ago. What testing should be performed?

A. Screening immunoassay followed by confirmatory specific gas chromatography–mass spectrometry of her whole blood
B. Gas chromatography–mass spectrometry of her urine
C. Whole blood spot testing
D. Urine metabolite screen for succinic acid
E. There is no confirmatory testing available for GHB if a patient presents >4 hours from time of ingestion

ANSWERS

80.1. Answer: E. In patients taking protease inhibitors, the first-pass metabolism of gamma-hydroxybutyric acid (GHB) is altered and low doses of GHB produce more toxic manifestations. The precise metabolic pathway is unknown, but this is likely a result of the interaction of protease inhibitors on the cytochrome P450 system.

Harrington RD, et al. Life-threatening interactions between HIV-1 protease inhibitors and the illicit drugs MDMA and gamma-hydroxybutyrate. *Arch Intern Med*. 1999;159:2221-2224.

Antoniou T, Tseng AL. Interactions between recreational drugs and antiretroviral agents. *Ann Pharmacother*. 2002;36:1598-1613.

80.2. Answer: E. GHB is rapidly absorbed from the gastrointestinal tract. Therefore, gastric lavage, single-dose activated charcoal, and whole bowel irrigation will likely not be effective in gastric decontamination. Furthermore, patients are only sedated for a brief time following this ingestion and generally do very well, even if they do need intubation for a brief period. It would be preferable to leave the patient's stomach empty to limit vomiting during or shortly after extubation.

Lettieri J, Fung HL. Absorption and first-pass metabolism of 14C-gamma-hydroxybutyric acid. *Res Commun Chem Pathol Pharmacol*. 1976;13:425-437.

Busardò FP, Jones AW. GHB pharmacology and toxicology: Acute intoxication, concentrations in blood and urine in forensic cases and treatment of the withdrawal syndrome. *Curr Neuropharmacol*. 2015;13:47-70.

80.3. Answer: D. GHB is both a precursor and degradation product of gamma-aminobutyric acid (GABA). The activity of endogenous GHB is mediated by the GHB receptor, while the activity of exogenous GHB is mediated by intrinsic activity at the $GABA_B$ receptor. Baclofen, which is a $GABA_B$ receptor agonist, is postulated to assist in the management of GHB withdrawal. Most patients also respond to benzodiazepines.

Floyd CN, et al. Baclofen in gamma-hydroxybutyrate withdrawal: Patterns of use and online availability. *Eur J Clin Pharmacol*. 2018; 74:349-356.

Snead OC 3rd, et al. In vivo conversion of gamma-aminobutyric acid and 1,4-butanediol to gamma-hydroxybutyric acid in rat brain. Studies using stable isotopes. *Biochem Pharmacol*. 1989;38:4375-4380.

80.4. Answer: C. In the 1980-1990s, bodybuilders promoted GHB as an anabolic supplement. This was believed to be due to an increase in growth hormone associated with onset of sleep. This led to an epidemic of GHB use.

Dyer JE, et al. Multistate outbreak of poisonings associated with illicit use of gamma hydroxybutyrate. *MMWR*. 1990;39:861-863.

Van Cauter E, et al. Simultaneous stimulation of slow-wave sleep and growth hormone secretion by gamma-hydroxybutyrate in normal young men. *J Clin Invest*. 1997;100:745-753.

80.5. Answer: A. GHB is formed from gamma-aminobutyric acid (GABA) by GABA transaminase and succinic semialdehyde reductase. GHB is also formed from gamma-butyrolactone by lactonases. 1,4-Butanediol forms gamma-hydroxybutyrate by alcohol dehydrogenase and aldehyde dehydrogenase.

Maitre M. The gamma-hydroxybutyrate signalling system in brain: Organization and functional implications. *Prog Neurobiol*. 1997;51:337-361.

80.6. Answer: C. GHB is an endogenous neurotransmitter. Exogenous GHB is both a schedule I and III controlled substance. It was made a schedule I drug in the United States in 2000 after the Hillory J. Farias and Samantha Reid Date-Rape Drug Prohibition Act was passed in 1999. Sodium oxybate, the salt form of GHB, sold under the trade name Xyrem, is a schedule III drug and is used in the treatment of narcolepsy. GHB is not used as a treatment for attention deficit hyperactivity disorder at this time. In 2010, the FDA declined to approve GHB for the treatment of fibromyalgia due to lack of evidence of efficacy and concerns for safety.

Office of the Federal Register. Federal Register. Schedules of Controlled Substances: Addition of gamma-hydroxybutyric acid to Schedule I. 21 CFR Part 1301. https://www.deadiversion.usdoj.gov/fed_regs/rules/2000/fr0313.htm.

Maitre M. The gamma-hydroxybutyrate signaling system in brain: Organization and functional implications. *Prog Neurobiol*. 1997;51:337-361.

80.7. Answer: D. In 2007, there was an epidemic of children in England and Australia who presented to health care with toxicity after ingesting toy beads marketed under the names Bindeez or Aquadots. 1,4-Butanediol (BD) was identified in the sticky surface material.

Gunja N, et al. Gamma-hydroxybutyrate poisoning from toy beads. *Med J Aust*. 2008;188:54-55.

Liechti ME, et al. Clinical features of gamma-hydroxybutyrate and gamma-butyrolactone toxicity and concomitant drug and alcohol use. *Drug Alcohol Depend*. 2006;81:323-326.

80.8. Answer: C. Exogenous GHB activity occurs at the $GABA_B$ receptor. Endogenous GHB activity occurs at the GHB receptor.

Snead OC 3rd. Evidence for a G protein-coupled gamma-hydroxybutyric acid receptor. *J Neurochem*. 2000;75:1986-1996.

Snead OC 3rd, Liu CC. Gamma-hydroxybutyric acid binding sites in rat and human brain synaptosomal membranes. *Biochem Pharmacol*. 1984;33:2587-2590.

80.9. Answer: D. Gamma-hydroxybutyric acid (GHB) is associated with myoclonus. Seizures are reported in animal models but not in humans.

Liechti ME, et al. Clinical features of gamma-hydroxybutyrate and gamma-butyrolactone toxicity and concomitant drug and alcohol use. *Drug Alcohol Depend*. 2006;81:323-326.

80.10. Answer: B. Gas chromatography–mass spectrometry (GC-MS) is the test of choice for both urine and serum GHB. GHB is typically detected in the urine above endogenous concentrations as long as 12 hours after an acute ingestion.

Brenneisen R, et al. Pharmacokinetics and excretion of gamma-hydroxybutyrate (GHB) in healthy subjects. *J Anal Toxicol*. 2004;28:625-630.

Inhalants

QUESTIONS

81.1. A 48-year-old man presents to the hospital with frequent bouts of lancinating pain to the right side of his face. He works as a mechanic in an autobody repair shop and reports that he is using a new solvent on oily car parts. Which of the following xenobiotics led to his symptoms?
A. Methylene chloride
B. Trichloroethylene
C. Toluene
D. Methanol
E. Isobutyl nitrite

81.2. A 26-year-old woman presents to the emergency department with profound, generalized weakness. Her laboratory evaluation is significant for a pH of 7.25 with an anion gap of 8. She explains that she used an inhalant recreationally for 3 months. Which metabolite will be present in her urine?
A. 2,5-Hexanedione
B. Phenol
C. Methyl hippuric acid
D. Hippuric acid
E. Benzo[a]pyrene

81.3. Which of the following mechanisms is responsible for the first- and second-degree burns of the upper airway that occur in patients who abuse inhalants?
A. Low pH
B. High pH
C. Defatting
D. Rapid expansion of gases
E. Reactive oxygen species resulting in cellular destruction

81.4. A 22-year-old woman presents to the emergency department because she is struggling to button her clothing and can no longer able to walk around her home without stumbling. This is especially worse in the dark. She reports that she inhales the propellant from over 100 whipped cream cannisters per day. What pathophysiology best explains her symptoms?
A. Irreversible oxidation of the cobalt ion of cyanocobalamin
B. Nutritional deficiency of cyanocobalamin
C. Nutritional deficiency of thiamine
D. Decreased concentration of homocysteine
E. Increased concentration of methylcobalamin

81.5. A 50-year-old man presents with painful, hypertrophic nodules in his bilateral wrists and knees. He has been inhaling a xenobiotic recreationally for several years while at work. Radiographs of the affected joints suggest a diagnosis. Which inhalant is most likely responsible?
A. Isobutyl nitrite
B. Carbon tetrachloride
C. Toluene
D. Difluoroethane
E. *n*-Hexane

81.6. A 37-year-old man presents to the emergency department with eye pain and bilateral central visual loss. On physical examination, he has elevated intraocular pressures. Which of the following xenobiotics led to this patient's presentation?
A. Methylene chloride
B. Trichloroethylene
C. Toluene
D. Methanol
E. Isobutyl nitrite

81.7. Which of the following toxicities is associated with chloroform inhalation?
A. Periportal hepatic necrosis
B. Lipid peroxidation of hepatic macromolecules
C. Distal renal tubular acidosis
D. Nephrotic syndrome
E. Megaloblastic anemia

81.8. What is the pathophysiology of the central nervous system effects of trichloroethane toxicity?
A. Stimulation of the N-methyl-D-aspartate (NMDA) receptor
B. Inhibition of the glycine receptor
C. Stimulation of the mu opioid receptor

D. Inhibition of the adenosine receptor
E. Stimulation of the gamma-aminobutyric acid type A (GABA$_A$) receptor

81.9. A 55-year-old man complains of paresthesias and weakness that started in his hands and feet but now also involve his arms and legs. He reports chronic exposure to adhesives. Which metabolic intermediate is responsible for his symptoms?
A. 1,1-Difluoroethane
B. 1,4-Butanediol
C. 2,5-Hexanedione
D. 1,1,1-Trichloroethane
E. Methyl-t-butyl ether

81.10. A 90-year-old European man who had a long career in a shoemaking shop presents with fatigue. He is diagnosed with chronic myelogenous leukemia. To which inhalant was he most likely exposed?
A. Benzene
B. Nitrous oxide
C. Acetone
D. Toluene
E. Methanol

ANSWERS

81.1. Answer: B. Trichloroethylene is a solvent used in degreasing solution. Exposure causes trigeminal neuralgia, flushing, and hepatotoxicity. Methylene chloride is metabolized to carbon monoxide in the body. Toluene causes weakness secondary to hypokalemia. The toxic metabolite of methanol, formic acid, is directly toxic to the optic nerve. Isobutyl nitrite causes methemoglobinemia.

Buxton PH, Hayward M. Polyneuritis cranialis associated with industrial trichloroethylene poisoning. *J Neurol Neurosurg Psychiatry*. 1967; 30:511-518.

81.2. Answer: D. This patient has hypokalemia-induced generalized weakness and a non-anion gap metabolic acidosis, consistent with toluene toxicity. Toluene causes a distal renal tubular acidosis, which is frequently associated with a normal anion gap. As the metabolite of toluene, hippuric acid, is eliminated as a hippurate ion, a hydrogen ion remains. However, sodium ions are also excreted more avidly, which sometimes causes extracellular volume contraction, a decreased glomerular filtration rate, and a high anion gap as the hippurate ions begin to accumulate.

Carlisle EJ, et al. Glue-sniffing and distal renal tubular acidosis: Sticking to the facts. *J Am Soc Nephrol*. 1991;1:1019-1027.

81.3. Answer: D. The upper airway burns are a result of thermal burns from rapid cooling of the gas as it expands on release from its pressurized container.

Albright JT, et al. Upper aerodigestive tract frostbite complicating volatile substance abuse. *Int J Pediatr Otorhinolaryngol*. 1999;49:63-67.

81.4. Answer: A. This patient has classic symptoms of nitrous oxide toxicity. Permanent oxidation of the cobalt ion of cyanocobalamin causes demyelination of the dorsal columns of the spinal cord. Patients experience paresthesias and numbness of the upper and lower extremities. These symptoms mimic a nutritional deficiency of cyanocobalamin. Without functional cyanocobalamin, serum homocysteine concentration increases because it cannot be converted to methionine. Nitrous oxide toxicity does not affect thiamine.

Layzer RB. Myeloneuropathy after prolonged exposure to nitrous oxide. *Lancet*. 1978;2:1227-1230.

81.5. Answer: D. The radiographic findings show skeletal fluorosis, a sequela of inhalation of fluorinated hydrocarbons such as 1,1-difluoroethane. Patients develop painful nodules in bones and joints and decreased joint mobility.

Chitkara M, et al. Multiple painless masses: Periostitis deformans secondary to fluoride intoxication. *Skeletal Radiol*. 2014;43:529-556.

81.6. Answer: E. The patient is presenting with "poppers retinopathy," which occurs in patients who abuse volatile alkyl nitrites. It is characterized by eye pain, elevated intraocular pressures, and bilateral vision loss. Optical coherence tomography demonstrates disruption of both the inner and outer segment layers of the fovea. The mainstay of therapy is abstinence from further alkyl nitrite use.

Vignal-Clermont C, et al. Poppers-associated retinal toxicity. *N Engl J Med*. 2010;363:1583-1585.

Pahlitzsch M, et al. Poppers maculopathy: Complete restitution of macular changes in OCT after drug abstinence. *Semin Ophthalmol*. 2016;31:479-484.

81.7. Answer: B. Halogenated hydrocarbons, especially carbon tetrachloride, cause hepatotoxicity. The literature describes both lipid peroxidation and centrilobular necrosis. Iron toxicity causes periportal necrosis. Toluene toxicity causes a non-anion gap metabolic acidosis resembling a distal renal tubular acidosis. Mercury toxicity leads to nephrotic syndrome. Nitrous oxide abuse leads to a megaloblastic anemia.

Baerg RD, Kimberg DV. Centrilobular hepatic necrosis and acute renal failure in "solvent sniffers". *Ann Intern Med*. 1970;73:713-720.

81.8. Answer: E. Trichloroethane, trichloroethylene, and toluene all bind at the GABA$_A$ receptor and increase the frequency of chloride channel opening comparably to ethanol.

Beckstead MJ, et al. Glycine and gamma-aminobutyric acid(A) receptor function is enhanced by inhaled drugs of abuse. *Mol Pharmacol*. 2000;57:1199-1205.

81.9. Answer: C. This patient reports a classic "dying-back" neuropathy, in which the longest axons are affected first. *n*-Hexane, a hydrocarbon found in adhesives, paints, and lacquers, is responsible for dying-back neuropathy via its toxic metabolite, 2,5-hexanedione. Exposure to methyl-*n*-butyl-ketone (MBK), not methyl-*t*-butyl ether, causes the same neuropathy as *n*-hexane due to the same metabolite (2,5-hexanedione).

Chang AP, et al. Focal conduction block in n-hexane polyneuropathy. *Muscle Nerve*. 1998;21:964-969.

81.10. Answer: A. Benzene is an International Agency for Research on Cancer (IARC) group I carcinogen known to cause leukemias and lymphomas. Benzene was associated with shoemaking. It was also found in glues and adhesives used in other occupations, before the United States banned most benzene-based products.

Travis LB, et al. Hematopoietic malignancies and related disorders among benzene-exposed workers in China. *Leuk Lymphoma*. 1994;14:91-102.

Nicotine

82.1. Which of the following options is true regarding nicotine pharmacokinetics?
  A. Renal excretion of nicotine accounts for a majority of nicotine elimination
  B. CYP2E1 is the major enzyme that is responsible for nicotine metabolism
  C. Nicotine induces CYP1A2 and accelerates the metabolism of drugs such as caffeine and clozapine
  D. Nicotine is a weak base and is more readily absorbed in an alkaline environment
  E. Nicotine metabolism is not affected by race or sex

82.2. The highest amount of nicotine content is found in which of the following options?
  A. One cigarette
  B. One cigar
  C. 1 g chewing tobacco
  D. One nicotine lozenge
  E. One nicotine patch

82.3. A mother calls the poison control center because her 3-year-old son ate a cigarette butt. How many ingested cigarette butts would warrant the child be sent into the hospital for monitoring?
  A. 1
  B. 3
  C. 5
  D. 7
  E. 9

82.4. A 2-year-old girl presents to the emergency department after she ate a whole cigarette. She has a single episode of vomiting. What is an acceptable observation time for this patient?
  A. 1 hour
  B. 4 hours
  C. 8 hours
  D. 12 hours
  E. 24 hours

82.5. Which of the following options best describes the pathophysiology of nicotine?
  A. Nicotine binds to muscarinic acetylcholine receptors in the brain and spinal cord
  B. After binding to its receptor, nicotine causes an influx of cations such as sodium and calcium
  C. Low doses of nicotine cause receptor blockade and manifestations of parasympathetic and neuromuscular blocking effects
  D. Nicotine-stimulated inhibition of dopamine in the mesolimbic area and nucleus accumbens is an important mediator of nicotine addiction
  E. Nicotine inhibits acetylcholine release at the nicotinic acetylcholine receptors

82.6. What is the most commonly reported symptom in patients with acute nicotine toxicity?
  A. Vomiting
  B. Tachycardia
  C. Paralysis
  D. Burning sensation
  E. Dizziness

82.7. Which laboratory test best reflects abstinence from tobacco products?
  A. Negative urinary cotinine
  B. Negative urinary nicotine
  C. Negative serum nicotine
  D. Negative 24-hour urine nicotine
  E. Negative urine ethyl glucuronide

82.8. A 24-year-old man is brought to the emergency department following a brief loss of consciousness while at a waterpipe ("hookah") bar. He is currently awake with a normal neurologic examination. His electrocardiogram is within normal limits. Which of the following therapies is indicated?
  A. Fomepizole
  B. Pralidoxime
  C. Hyperbaric oxygen therapy
  D. Activated charcoal
  E. Acidification of the urine

82.9. A 2-year-old girl is found unresponsive next to an empty bottle of e-cigarette refill liquid. On examination, she is tachycardic to 143 beats/min and has fasciculations. She is immediately intubated for airway protection. Which of the following therapies is indicated?
  A. Fomepizole
  B. Pralidoxime
  C. Hyperbaric oxygen therapy
  D. Activated charcoal
  E. Acidification of the urine

82.10. A 34 year old farmer presents to the emergency department following exposure to a nicotine based pesticide. Vital signs are blood pressure, 165/90 mmHg; heart rate, 120 beats/min; respiratory rate, 18 breaths/min; oxygen saturation, 99% on room air; and temperature, 99.0 °F (37.2 °C). The patient is nauseated and vomited twice while en route to the hospital. What is the most important next step?
  A. Obtain a chest radiograph
  B. Administer activated charcoal
  C. Obtain an electrocardiogram
  D. Undress the patient and decontaminate their skin
  E. Urinary acidification

ANSWERS

82.1. Answer: D. Nicotine is a weak base and is more readily absorbed in an alkaline environment. Metabolism of nicotine occurs primarily in the liver by CYP2A6 in addition to enzymes such as flavin monooxygenase. Renal excretion of unchanged nicotine accounts for 2-35% of total nicotine elimination, which is pH dependent. Although cigarette smoking induces CYP1A2 and accelerates the metabolism of drugs such as caffeine and clozapine, this is *not* an effect of nicotine. Nicotine metabolism is linked to race and sex, with Asians and African Americans metabolizing nicotine more slowly and women metabolizing nicotine more rapidly than men.

Benowitz N. Pharmacologic aspects of cigarette smoking and nicotine addiction. *N Engl J Med.* 1988;319:1318-1330.

82.2. Answer: E. A single nicotine patch contains up to 114 mg of nicotine. Although not designed to deliver this much nicotine, when used inappropriately (cut open, ingested), larger amount of nicotine are delivered than clinically intended. One cigarette contains 10-30 mg of nicotine. One cigar contains 15-30 mg of nicotine. One gram of chewing tobacco contains 6-8 mg of nicotine. Nicotine lozenges contains 2-4 mg of nicotine per lozenge.

Gupta S, et al. Bioavailability and absorption kinetics of nicotine following application of a transdermal system. *Br J Clin Pharmacol.* 1993;36:221-227.

Woolf A, et al. Childhood poisoning involving transdermal nicotine patches. *Pediatrics.* 1997;99:e4.

82.3. Answer: B. Children younger than 6 years old are at risk of developing nicotine toxicity if they ingest one full cigarette or three cigarette butts. When deciding whether to observe a patient at home or send them into the emergency department for further evaluation, an accurate assessment of the amount of nicotine ingested is needed.

Smolinske S, et al. Cigarette and nicotine chewing gum toxicity in children. *Hum Toxicol.* 1988;7:27-31.

Centers for Disease Control and Prevention (CDC). Ingestion of cigarettes and cigarette butts by children—Rhode Island, January 1994-July 1996. *MMWR Morb Mortal Wkly Rep.* 1997;46:125-128.

82.4. Answer: D. Nicotine is rapidly absorbed and metabolized. Patients with mild symptoms, such as the patient in this case, usually have complete resolution of their symptoms within 12 hours. Patients who ingest a nicotine patch should be observed for longer since the patch contains more than 100 mg and acts as a reservoir potentially leading to continued, delayed absorption.

Matsushima D, et al. Absorption and adverse effect following topical and oral administration of three transdermal nicotine products to dogs. *J Pharm Sci.* 1995;84:365-369.

82.5. Answer: B. Nicotine binds to the nicotinic acetylcholine receptors in the brain, spinal cord, autonomic ganglia, adrenal medulla, neuromuscular junctions, and chemoreceptors of the carotid and aortic bodies. Binding to this receptor results in an influx of cations (sodium and calcium) that causes downstream cell depolarization and subsequent neurotransmitter release. High doses of nicotine cause receptor blockade and parasympathetic symptoms and neuromuscular blocking effects. Nicotine-stimulated release of dopamine is a mediator of nicotine addiction.

Dani JA. Neuronal nicotinic acetylcholine receptor structure and function and response to nicotine. *Int Rev Neurobiol*. 2015;124:3-19.

Martin-Soelch C. Neuroadaptive changes associated with smoking: Structural and functional neural changes in nicotine dependence. *Brain Sci*. 2013;3:159-176.

Thesleft S. The mode of neuromuscular block caused by acetylcholine, nicotine, decamethonium and succinylcholine. *Acta Physiol Scand*. 1955; 34:218-231.

82.6. Answer: A. Although all the symptoms listed are reported, vomiting is the symptom most often reported in patients with acute nicotine toxicity. The vomiting helps to limit absorption in some patients by means of auto-decontamination. Nevertheless, induction of emesis is not recommended due to potential harm and it is unlikely to be of further benefit.

Benowitz N. Clinical pharmacology of nicotine: Implications for understanding, preventing, and treating tobacco addiction. *Clin Pharmacol Ther*. 2008;83:531-541.

82.7. Answer: A. Cotinine is the major inactive metabolite of nicotine—about 70% of circulating nicotine is metabolized to cotinine. Cotinine has an elimination half-life of about 20 hours (compared to nicotine, which is 1-4 hours) and is a more useful marker of exposure to nicotine. Urinary cotinine is used to assess abstinence from tobacco products given that it has a longer detection window than nicotine. Exposure to secondhand smoke causes detectable urinary cotinine. Urinary cotinine cannot be used to diagnose acute toxicity because it potentially reflects coincidental or chronic exposure. Urine ethyl glucuronide is a marker for ethanol consumption.

Acosta M, et al. Urine cotinine as an index of smoking status in smokers during 96-hr abstinence: Comparison between gas chromatography/mass spectrometry and immunoassay test strips. *Nicotine Tob Res*. 2004;6:615-620.

Sharma P, et al. Assessment of cotinine in urine and saliva of smokers, passive smokers, and nonsmokers: Method validation using liquid chromatography and mass spectrometry. *Ind J Psych*. 2019;61:270-276.

82.8. Answer: C. Waterpipes, also known as hookah or shisha, refer to the process of smoking tobacco through a pipe filled with water. The pipe is connected to a container holding tobacco, and using coal as a heat source, the user inhales the smoke produced. Unfortunately, in addition to nicotine, users are exposed to carbon monoxide and other carcinogens. In one report, a patient lost consciousness in a hookah bar and was found to have a carboxyhemoglobin of 33.8%. As this patient's examination and electrocardiogram are entirely normal, the greatest concern from a toxicologic perspective is carbon monoxide toxicity. Since this patient had an episode of loss of consciousness, hyperbaric therapy is indicated to protect against delayed neuropsychiatric symptoms.

Jacob III P, et al. Nicotine, carbon monoxide, and carcinogen exposure after a single use of a waterpipe. *Cancer Epidemiol Biomarkers Prev*. 2011;20:2345-2353.

Misek R, Patte C. Carbon monoxide toxicity after lighting coals at a hookah bar. *J Med Toxicol*. 2014;10:295-298.

82.9. Answer: D. Liquid nicotine is sold in concentrations as high as 3.6% as refills for electronic cigarettes. A 30-mL bottle contains >1 g of nicotine. As nicotine is absorbed rapidly from the gastrointestinal tract, gastric lavage will be of limited utility in most cases. Activated charcoal effectively adsorbs nicotine. As this patient is critically ill and intubated, 1 g/kg of activated charcoal should be administered to reduce absorption. Unfortunately, there is no antidote to nicotine. The mainstay of management is supportive care. Although urinary acidification enhances nicotine elimination, the risks outweigh the benefits, and it should not be done.

Chen BC, et al. Death following intentional ingestion of e-liquid. *Clin Toxicol*. 2015;53:914-916.

Noble MJ, et al. Unintentional pediatric ingestion of electronic cigarette nicotine refill liquid necessitating intubation. *Ann Emerg Med*. 2017;69:94-97.

82.10. Answer: D. Patients with dermal exposures to nicotine or nicotine-based pesticides should be undressed completely and have their skin washed with soap and copious amounts of water. This decontamination limits further personal and staff exposure to nicotine. Although a chest radiograph and an electrocardiogram are reasonable to obtain, they are not the essential next steps. Activated charcoal should not be administered to a vomiting patient who has had a dermal exposure to nicotine. Urinary acidification, although able to enhance the elimination of nicotine, is not recommended due to the potential risks outweighing the benefits.

Lavioe F, Harris T. Fatal nicotine ingestion. *J Emerg Med*. 1991;9:133-136.

Rogers A, et al. Catastrophic brain injury after nicotine insecticide ingestion. *J Emerg Med*. 2004;26:169-172.

Phencyclidine and Ketamine

QUESTIONS

83.1. Which of the following xenobiotics is most likely to cause a false-positive reaction on a urine screening immunoassay for phencyclidine?
A. Ketamine
B. Dextromethorphan
C. Amphetamine
D. Cocaine
E. Marijuana

83.2. Which of the following options best explains the effects of urine pH on phencyclidine elimination?
A. Alkalinization of the urine significantly increases phencyclidine elimination
B. Alkalinization of the urine significantly increases phencyclidine elimination but is of no clinical relevance
C. Acidification of the urine significantly increases phencyclidine elimination
D. Acidification of the urine significantly increases phencyclidine elimination but is of no clinical relevance
E. The is no effect of pH on urinary phencyclidine elimination

83.3. Chronic ketamine use is associated with dysfunction of which organ system?
A. Pulmonary
B. Cardiac
C. Hematologic
D. Genitourinary
E. Musculoskeletal

83.4. Phencyclidine and ketamine have multiple pharmacologic targets. Which of the following effects most likely accounts for the analgesia and anesthesia produced?
A. N-Methyl-D-aspartate (NMDA) antagonism
B. Opioid receptor agonism
C. Gamma-aminobutyric acid (GABA) agonism
D. Sigma receptor agonism
E. Monoamine oxidase (MAO) inhibition

83.5. A 27-year-old man presents to the emergency department with psychomotor agitation. Which of the following combinations of clinical findings would be most characteristic of phencyclidine or ketamine use?
A. Hypertension, bradycardia, nystagmus, normothermia
B. Hypotension, bradycardia, nystagmus, hyperthermia
C. Hypertension, tachycardia, nystagmus, hyperthermia
D. Hypotension, tachycardia, miosis, hyperthermia
E. Hypertension, tachycardia, anisocoria, hyperthermia

83.6. An 18-year-old woman presents to the emergency department minimally responsive following phencyclidine use. Her respiratory rate and depth are normal, and her airway protective reflexes are preserved. Which of the following decontamination options is indicated?
A. Single-dose activated charcoal
B. Multiple-dose activated charcoal
C. Continuous nasogastric suction
D. Single-dose activated charcoal followed by continuous nasogastric suction
E. No decontamination is preferable

83.7. Methoxetamine is a ketamine analogue that has emerged as a drug of abuse. Which of the following best distinguishes methoxetamine from ketamine?

A. Methoxetamine has less hepatotoxicity than ketamine

B. Methoxetamine has less nephrotoxicity than ketamine

C. Ketamine is metabolized by CYPs 2B6, 3A4, and 2C9, while methoxetamine is predominately metabolized by CYP1A2

D. The kinetics of methoxetamine produce a more intense high with a shorter duration of effect compared to ketamine

E. Both drugs are clinically and pharmacologically similar

83.8. A 16-year-old, 60-kg boy is brought to the hospital from a club. He is unresponsive, his eyes are open, and he has a blank stare. His respirations are preserved. According to friends, he went into a "K-hole" after using ketamine. Intravenous access is obtained, a rapid glucose is normal, and the patient is attached to a cardiac monitor with continuous pulse oximetry. About 2 hours later, he awakens and starts talking incoherently and thrashing in the bed. Which of the following therapies is indicated?

A. Lorazepam 2 mg intravenously

B. Haloperidol 10 mg intravenously

C. Midazolam 2 mg intravenously

D. Olanzapine 5 mg sublingually

E. Diazepam 10 mg intramuscularly

83.9. Which of the following effects is reported in chronic phencyclidine users following cessation of use?

A. Lack of energy

B. Psychosis

C. Diaphoresis

D. Tremor

E. Chest pain

83.10. Which of the following pharmacologic properties most likely accounts for the prolonged clinical effect of phencyclidine?

A. Saturable renal elimination

B. Enterohepatic recirculation

C. Prolonged gastrointestinal absorption

D. High lipid solubility

E. Low protein binding

ANSWERS

83.1. Answer: B. False-positive testing results on a urine screening immunoassay vary among manufacturers. Many current tests will give a positive result with other arylcyclohexylamine derivatives that are used as a phencyclidine substitute. Although ketamine shares chemical and structural similarities to phencyclidine, most testing platforms distinguish the two molecules. Dextromethorphan is the most clinically significant cross-reactant, in that dextromethorphan toxicity resembles phencyclidine toxicity and dextromethorphan is found in many nonprescription cold and cough remedies. A false-positive phencyclidine test could have serious implications in a child with an unsupervised ingestion of a dextromethorphan-containing cough remedy.

Warner A. Dextromethorphan: Analyte of the month. In: Service Training and Continuing Education. *Clinical Chemistry*. Vol 14. Washington, DC: 1993;27-28.

Schier J. Avoid unfavorable consequences: Dextromethorpan can bring about a false-positive phencyclidine urine drug screen. *J Emerg Med*. 2000;18:379-381.

Rengarajan A, Mullins ME. How often do false-positive phencyclidine urine screens occur with use of common medications? *Clin Toxicol (Phila)*. 2013;51:493-496.

83.2. Answer: D. Phencyclidine becomes ionized in acidic urine and therefore is not reabsorbed. Decreasing the urine pH increases phencyclidine clearance four-fold. A minority of phencyclidine is eliminated in the urine as the parent drug, so even this large increase in clearance is of little clinical relevance. As such, the risks of acidification outweigh the benefits, and it is not recommended.

Aronow R, et al. Clinical observations during phencyclidine intoxication and treatment based on ion-trapping. *NIDA Res Monogr*. 1978:218-228.

Cook CE, et al. Phencyclidine disposition after intravenous and oral doses. *Clin Pharmacol Ther*. 1982;31:625-634.

83.3. Answer: D. Chronic ketamine use produces an ulcerative cystitis that results in a small shrunken bladder and, often, straightening and reflux of the ureters. Patients typically complain of symptoms consistent with a urinary tract infection, but have sterile urine cultures.

Shahani R, et al. Ketamine-associated ulcerative cystitis: A new clinical entity. *Urology*. 2007;69:810-812.

83.4. Answer: A. Except for not interacting with opioid receptors (B), all these other effects are pharmacological effects of ketamine and phencyclidine. However, NMDA antagonism is responsible for their analgesic and anesthetic effects.

MacDonald JF, et al. The PCP site of the NMDA receptor complex. *Adv Exp Med Biol*. 1990;268:27-34.

83.5. Answer: C. The characteristic findings associated with ketamine or phencyclidine use include hypertension, tachycardia, hyperthermia from psychomotor agitation, and nystagmus. Although rotatory and vertical nystagmus are commonly described as nearly pathognomonic, they are often absent. Both miosis and mydriasis are variably reported.

McCarron MM, et al. Acute phencyclidine intoxication: Clinical patterns, complications, and treatment. *Ann Emerg Med*. 1981;10:290-297.

Weiner AL, et al. Ketamine abusers presenting to the emergency department: A case series. *J Emerg Med*. 2000;18:447-451.

83.6. Answer: E. Phencyclidine and ketamine are adsorbed to activated charcoal. Because of ion trapping in the acidic environment of the stomach, continuous nasogastric suction will enhance elimination. However, most patients who present following a phencyclidine or ketamine overdose are either agitated or sedated. As such, the risks of activated charcoal administration outweigh the benefits, except in the rare event of a massive overdose requiring a protected airway. Similarly, nasogastric tubes are typically not recommended in agitated or sedated patients. The use of continuous nasogastric suction causes significant fluid and electrolyte imbalances. For most patients, supportive care is sufficient.

Picchioni AL, Consroe PF. Activated charcoal—a phencyclidine antidote, or hog in dogs. *N Engl J Med*. 1979;300:202.

83.7. Answer: E. Methoxetamine was promoted as a safer alternative to ketamine in that it produced less liver and kidney toxicity. Both clinical experience and animal studies proved otherwise. Both drugs are extensively metabolized by the same CYPs (3A4, 2B6, and 2C9) and have similar clinical effects.

Craig CL, Loeffler GH. The ketamine analog methoxetamine: A new designer drug to threaten military readiness. *Mil Med*. 2014;179: 1149-1157.

Hofer KE, et al. Ketamine-like effects after recreational use of methoxetamine. *Ann Emerg Med*. 2012;60:97-99.

Wood DM, et al. Acute toxicity associated with the recreational use of the ketamine derivative methoxetamine. *Eur J Clin Pharmacol*. 2012;68:853-856.

83.8. Answer: C. Emergence reactions are common with both therapeutic and recreational use of ketamine. In general, a benzodiazepine is preferred. While the choice of benzodiazepines is somewhat stylistic, in a severely agitated patient, choosing the drug with the most rapid effect is recommended as a delay to sedation poses a risk for the patient and staff. As this patient already has intravenous access, the use of intramuscular or oral medication is not recommended. Furthermore, the intramuscular absorption of diazepam is erratic, and this route should always be avoided. The time to peak effect of midazolam is significantly shorter than lorazepam, and therefore, midazolam is recommended for rapid control.

Cartwright PD, Pingel SM. Midazolam and diazepam in ketamine anaesthesia. *Anaesthesia*. 1984;39:439-442.

Chudnofsky CR, et al. A combination of midazolam and ketamine for procedural sedation and analgesia in adult emergency department patients. *Acad Emerg Med*. 2000;7:228-235.

83.9. Answer: A. Evidence for phencyclidine tolerance and withdrawal is well established in animals. Humans develop depression, anxiety, irritability, lack of energy, sleep disturbance, and disturbed thoughts after 1 day of abstinence from drug use. Neonates born to chronically using mothers also develop symptoms consistent with a withdrawal syndrome.

Balster RL, Woolverton WL. Continuous-access phencyclidine self-administration by rhesus monkeys leading to physical dependence. *Psychopharmacology*. 1980;70:5-10.

Rawson RA, et al. Characteristics of 68 chronic phencyclidine abusers who sought treatment. *Drug Alcohol Depend*. 1981;8:223-227.

Strauss AA, et al. Neonatal manifestations of maternal phencyclidine (PCP) abuse. *Pediatrics*. 1981;68:550-552.

83.10. Answer: D. The high lipid solubility of phencyclidine allows the drug to partition into the brain, where it becomes ion trapped in the relatively acidic environment, leading to prolonged clinical effects.

Misra AL, et al. Persistence of phencyclidine (PCP) and metabolites in brain and adipose tissue and implications for long-lasting behavioural effects. *Res Commun Chem Pathol Pharmacol*. 1979;24:431-445.

Aluminum

84

QUESTIONS

84.1. A 72-year-old man with a past medical history of stage III chronic kidney disease and radiation cystitis presents to the hospital with significant hematuria. The patient is taken to the operating room for persistent bleeding, and while there, a medication is applied directly into his bladder. Over the subsequent days, his mental status declines and his physical examination is remarkable for myoclonic jerking. What xenobiotic best explains this patient's presentation?
A. Potassium aluminum sulfate
B. Arsenic trioxide
C. Glycine
D. Hexavalent chromium
E. Mesna

84.2. Which of the following options is the chelator of choice in patients who present with acute aluminum toxicity?
A. Deferoxamine
B. Dimercaprol
C. Calcium disodium ethylenediaminetetraacetic acid
D. Penicillamine
E. Prussian blue

84.3. In patients with chronic aluminum toxicity, what organ system(s) are primarily affected?
A. Nervous, cardiac, and musculoskeletal
B. Cardiac, musculoskeletal, and hematopoietic
C. Dermatologic, cardiac, and hematopoietic
D. Hematopoietic, nervous, and musculoskeletal
E. Hematolopoietic alone

84.4. In 1947, 26% of potroom workers developed pulmonary fibrosis. Some of these patients went on to develop a progressive encephalopathy. What metal caused their symptoms?
A. Aluminum
B. Cobalt
C. Cadmium
D. Lead
E. Manganese

84.5. A 63-year-old man with a history of kidney disease is diagnosed with chronic aluminum toxicity. He is unaware of the exact names of the medications he is prescribed; however, he knows he has not changed his medication in at least 5 years. What class of medication most likely led to his toxicity?
A. Antacids
B. Migraine medication
C. Antidepressants
D. Antiepileptics
E. Antihypertensives

84.6. Which of the following options best explains how aluminum results in anemia?
A. Stimulation of hematopoietic cells
B. Inhibition of delta-aminolevulinic acid dehydrogenase
C. Vitamin D resistance
D. Oxidative stress
E. Impaired absorption of iron from the gastrointestinal tract

84.7. Which of the following options increases absorption of aluminum in the gastrointestinal tract?
A. Phosphorous
B. Silicone
C. Uremia
D. Hemochromatosis
E. Large organic acids

84.8. Which of the following options best explains how aluminum is metabolized in the body?
A. Acetyl-CoA oxidation
B. Sulfation
C. Glucuronidation
D. Cytochrome P450 2E1
E. Aluminum is not metabolized in the body

84.9. Which of the following options best explains the mechanism of action whereby aluminum causes osteomalacia?

A. Increased excretion of calcium
B. Decreased absorption of magnesium
C. Direct competition of aluminum with other cations in the bone
D. Increased aluminum concentration in the osteoclasts
E. Impaired excretion of phosphate

84.10. A 54-year-old man presents to the emergency department with shortness of breath. He is admitted to the hospital and is diagnosed with aluminosis. Which of the following pulmonary function tests is consistent with this diagnosis?
A. Normal pulmonary function test
B. Restrictive pattern
C. Reversible obstructive pattern
D. Irreversible obstructive pattern
E. Pure obstruction with air trapping

ANSWERS

84.1. Answer: A. Potassium aluminum sulfate (Alum) is used as a treatment for hemorrhagic cystitis. Patients who have kidney dysfunction and radiation cystitis are at a higher risk of developing neurotoxicity from absorbed aluminum. Acute neurotoxicity associated with aluminum includes encephalopathy, seizures, and myoclonus.

> Phelps KR, et al. Encephalopathy after bladder irrigation with alum: Case report and literature review. *Am J Med Sci.* 1999;318:181-185.

84.2. Answer: A. Deferoxamine chelates aluminum to form aluminoxamine. Aluminoxamine is excreted in the urine. In patients who have impaired kidney function, hemodialysis is indicated 6-8 hours following administration of the deferoxamine.

> Nakamura H, et al. Encephalopathy with seizures after use of aluminum-containing bone cement. *Lancet.* 1994;344:1647.

84.3. Answer: D. Patients with chronic aluminum toxicity develop a microcytic hypochromic anemia that does not improve with iron supplementation. Patients later develop encephalopathy and dementia. Aluminum toxicity also predisposes to osteomalacia and secondary fractures.

> Ward MK, et al. Osteomalacic dialysis osteodystrophy: Evidence for a water-borne aetiological agent, probably aluminium. *Lancet.* 1978;1: 841-845.

84.4. Answer: A. A pot is a large vessel in which aluminum is produced, and a potroom refers to the buildings where these pots are stored. Potroom asthma is an occupational asthma that occurred in workers who had chronic exposure to aluminum dust. Aluminum dust also predisposed patients to develop pulmonary fibrosis and an encephalopathy known as "potroom palsy."

> McLaughlin AI, et al. Pulmonary fibrosis and encephalopathy associated with the inhalation of aluminium dust. *Br J Ind Med.* 1962;19:253-263.

84.5. Answer: A. In patients with chronic kidney disease, ingestion of antacids that contain aluminum hydroxide leads to chronic aluminum toxicity. This occurs very rarely as patients with kidney disease are counseled to avoid aluminum-containing medications. Furthermore, toxicity typically only occurs months to years following ingestion of the aluminum-containing xenobiotics.

> Randall ME. Aluminium toxicity in an infant not on dialysis. *Lancet.* 1983;1:1327-1328.

84.6. Answer: B. Aluminum inhibits delta-aminolevulinic acid dehydrogenase in the heme synthesis pathway, leading to accumulation of erythrocyte protoporphyrins. Human hematopoietic cells are inhibited, not stimulated, in aluminum toxicity. Oxidative stress is a contributor to the pulmonary toxicity. Vitamin D resistance explains the osteomalacia caused by aluminum toxicity.

Abdulla M, et al. Antagonistic effects of zinc and aluminum on lead inhibition of delta-aminolevulinic acid dehydratase. *Arch Environ Health*. 1979;34:464-469.

84.7. Answer: C. Gastrointestinal absorption of aluminum occurs primarily in the small intestine. Gastrointestinal absorption is increased when uremia or iron deficiency anemia exist, or in the presence of citrate and other small organic acids. The presence of silicone and phosphorous decreases the absorption of aluminum.

Fernández Menéndez MJ, et al. Aluminium uptake by intestinal cells: Effect of iron status and precomplexation. *Nephrol Dial Transplant*. 1991;6:672-674.

84.8. Answer: E. Aluminum is not metabolized in the body. Approximately 95% gets excreted unchanged in the urine. In patients receiving dialysis, the elimination half-life is as long as 85 days.

Greger JL, Sutherland JE. Aluminum exposure and metabolism. *Crit Rev Clin Lab Sci*. 1997;34:439-474.

84.9. Answer: C. Aluminum toxicity leads to vitamin D–resistant osteomalacia. The osteopathy is primarily caused when aluminum competes with and replaces other cations in the bone. Aluminum concentrates in the mitochondria of osteoblasts not osteoclasts. Magnesium, calcium, and phosphate are not affected and do not appear to directly contribute to the osteomalacia.

Griswold WR, et al. Accumulation of aluminum in a nondialyzed uremic child receiving aluminum hydroxide. *Pediatrics*. 1983;71:56-58.

84.10. Answer: B. Aluminosis is a pneumoconiosis that occurs subsequent to chronic aluminum exposure. Pulmonary function tests performed on these patients demonstrate restrictive lung function. Potroom asthma is also associated with inhaled aluminum; patients present with cough, wheezing, and shortness of breath that often improve following cessation of exposure.

Riihimäki V, Aitio A. Occupational exposure to aluminum and its biomonitoring in perspective. *Crit Rev Toxicol*. 2012;42:827-853.

Antimony

QUESTIONS

85.1. A 22-year-old man is given a "traditional medication" that contains antimony potassium tartrate as a therapy for alcohol use disorder. Which of the following clinical effects is most likely to occur?
- A. Nausea and vomiting
- B. Prolongation of the QRS complex
- C. Prolongation of the PR interval
- D. Acute kidney injury
- E. Bone marrow suppression

85.2. Which of the following antimony compounds is most likely to cause pancreatitis?
- A. Stibine
- B. Antimony potassium tartrate
- C. Antimony trioxide
- D. Antimony pentoxide
- E. Meglumine antimoniate

85.3. Acute toxicity from ingestion of antimony salts most resembles toxicity from ingestion of which of the following metal salts?
- A. Aluminum
- B. Arsenic
- C. Bismuth
- D. Cadmium
- E. Chromium

85.4. Inhalation of which of the following antimony compounds is associated with metal fume fever?
- A. Stibine
- B. Antimony potassium tartrate
- C. Antimony trioxide
- D. Meglumine antimoniate
- E. Sodium stibogluconate

85.5. Which of the following statements best describes the role of oral activated charcoal in a patient who has ingested an antimony salt?
- A. There is no role for activated charcoal at all
- B. There is no role for delayed activated charcoal as antimony salts are rapidly absorbed
- C. There is a theoretical role for delayed activated charcoal because antimony undergoes enterohepatic circulation
- D. There is a demonstrated role for delayed activated charcoal because antimony undergoes enterohepatic circulation and activated charcoal increases survival in poisoned animals
- E. There is a demonstrated role for both early administration and repeat dose delayed administration of activated charcoal as each therapy improves survival in animals

85.6. Which of the following statements best describes the pattern of elimination of antimony salts?
- A. Both trivalent and pentavalent antimony are primarily eliminated in the bile
- B. Both trivalent and pentavalent antimony are primarily eliminated in the urine
- C. Trivalent antimony is primarily eliminated in the urine and pentavalent antimony is primarily eliminated in the bile
- D. Trivalent antimony is primarily eliminated in the bile and pentavalent antimony is primarily eliminated in the urine
- E. Trivalent antimony is primarily eliminated in the urine and pentavalent antimony is primarily eliminated in the breath and sweat

85.7. Which of the following antimony compounds is most likely to cause severe dermal injury on direct contact?

A. Antimony pentachloride
B. Antimony potassium tartrate
C. Antimony trioxide
D. Meglumine antimoniate
E. Sodium stibogluconate

85.8. A 20-year-old man is diagnosed with cutaneous leishmaniasis and started on a course of parenteral sodium stibogluconate. After 4 days of therapy, which of the following tests is most likely to be abnormal?

A. Chest radiograph
B. Complete blood count
C. Urinalysis
D. Kidney function tests
E. Prothrombin time

85.9. Which of the following therapies is most clinically indicated during the acute phase of severe antimony potassium tartrate poisoning?

A. Intramuscular dimercaprol
B. Intravenous calcium disodium EDTA
C. Intravenous N-acetylcysteine
D. Oral succimer
E. Oral D-penicillamine

85.10. A 53-year-old worker is trying to recharge lead storage batteries in a closed space. He notices an odd smell and leaves the area. Shortly thereafter, he develops nausea and abdominal pain and presents to the hospital. Which of the following diagnostic studies is most likely to be helpful?

A. A rapid glucose
B. Kidney function tests
C. A complete blood count
D. A chest radiograph
E. An electrocardiogram

ANSWERS

85.1. Answer: A. Antimony potassium tartrate, also known as "tartar emetic," causes severe gastrointestinal toxicity and was once used as a purgative. It has a sweet taste, and occasional reports document its use as an aversive therapy in patients with alcohol use disorder. Most complications result from the consequences of protracted vomiting, including fluid and electrolyte abnormalities and gastrointestinal irritation.

Tarabar AF, et al. Antimony toxicity from the use of tartar emetic for the treatment of alcohol abuse. *Vet Hum Toxicol.* 2004;46:331-333.

85.2. Answer: E. All the listed compounds are associated with nausea, vomiting, diarrhea, and abdominal pain. Only meglumine antimoniate and sodium stibogluconate are commonly associated with pancreatitis.

Delgado J, et al. High frequency of serious side effects from meglumine antimoniate given without an upper limit dose for the treatment of visceral leishmaniasis in human immunodeficiency virus type-1-infected patients. *Am J Trop Med Hyg.* 1999;61:766-769.

Gasser RA Jr, et al. Pancreatitis induced by pentavalent antimonial agents during treatment of leishmaniasis. *Clin Infect Dis.* 1994;18:83-90.

85.3. Answer: B. Antimony salts and arsenic salts have very similar acute toxicities, including gastrointestinal, bone marrow, and cardiovascular toxicities. Both metals also

occur together in nature so that whenever one is included in a differential diagnosis, it is reasonable to include the other.

Gerhardsson L, et al. Antimony in lung, liver and kidney tissue from deceased smelter workers. *Scand J Work Environ Health.* 1982;8:201-208.

Wu F, et al. Health risk associated with dietary co-exposure to high levels of antimony and arsenic in the world's largest antimony mine area. *Sci Total Environ.* 2011;409:3344-3351.

85.4. Answer: C. Antimony trioxide is used as a flame retardant. Inhalation is associated with signs and symptoms of metal fume fever. Metal fume fever is also reported with antimony pentoxide.

Anonymous. Metals and the lung. *Lancet.* 1984;2:903-904.

85.5. Answer: C. It is completely unknown whether antimony is adsorbed to the surface of pharmaceutical activated charcoal, but it is adsorbed to biochars used for environmental purposes. Based on demonstrated enterohepatic circulation in humans, delayed and/or repeat doses of activated charcoal are reasonable in patients with life-threating ingestions, as long as no contraindications exist.

Konstantopoulos MW, et al. Case records of the Massachusetts General Hospital. Case 22-2012. A 34-year-old man with intractable vomiting after ingestion of an unknown substance. *N Engl J Med.* 2012;367:259-268.

Bailly R, et al. Experimental and human studies on antimony metabolism: Their relevance for the biological monitoring of workers exposed to inorganic antimony. *Br J Ind Med.* 1991;48:93-97.

85.6. Answer: D. Trivalent and pentavalent forms of antimony are eliminated by different pathways. Trivalent antimony is glucuronidated in the liver, eliminated in the bile, and undergoes enterohepatic circulation, leading to prolonged elimination. The pentavalent forms are rapidly eliminated by the kidney.

Bailly R, et al. Experimental and human studies on antimony metabolism: Their relevance for the biological monitoring of workers exposed to inorganic antimony. *Br J Ind Med.* 1991;48:93-97.

Winship KA. Toxicity of antimony and its compounds. *Adverse Drug React Acute Poisoning Rev.* 1987;6:67-90.

85.7. Answer: A. Most antimony compounds are directly irritating to the skin and eyes, but antimony pentachloride forms hydrochloric acid on direct contact with water and is more likely to cause severe burns than the other forms.

Winship KA. Toxicity of antimony and its compounds. *Adverse Drug React Acute Poisoning Rev.* 1987;6:67-90.

Renes LE. Antimony poisoning in industry. *AMA Arch Ind Hyg Occup Med.* 1953;7:99-108.

85.8. Answer: B. Toxicity during treatment with parenteral sodium stibogluconate is common, as many patients develop myalgias, nausea, abdominal pain, and malaise. Furthermore, up to 50% of patients develop QT interval prolongation and >80% of patients develop transient elevations in hepatic aminotransferases. Virtually all patients develop some degree of bone marrow suppression that is most evident in lymphocyte and platelet counts. Most patients are able to continue therapy despite these adverse reactions.

Wise ES, et al. Monitoring toxicity associated with parenteral sodium stibogluconate in the day-case management of returned travellers with New World cutaneous leishmaniasis [corrected]. *PLoS Negl Trop Dis.* 2012;6:e1688.

85.9. Answer: A. In animal studies, dimercaprol, succimer, and dimercaptopropane sulfonic acid all improved survival, but the best human data are for dimercaprol. Although oral succimer is a reasonable alternative, acutely poisoned patients have severe nausea and vomiting, making oral administration challenging. There is a concern that oral chelation will enhance absorption.

Thompson RHS, Whittaker VP. Antidotal activity of British anti-Lewisite against compounds of antimony, gold and mercury. *Biochem J.* 1947;41:342-346.

Lauwers LF, et al. Oral antimony intoxications in man. *Crit Care Med.* 1990;18:324-326.

85.10. Answer: C. Stibine gas (SbH_3) is released while charging lead storage batteries. Clinical effects are similar to those of arsine gas (AsH_3). In addition to gastrointestinal effects, both produce massive hemolysis.

Winship KA. Toxicity of antimony and its compounds. *Adverse Drug React Acute Poisoning Rev.* 1987;6:67-90.

Arsenic

QUESTIONS

86.1. Which of the following findings is associated with chronic but not with acute arsenic poisoning?
   A. Nausea, vomiting, and diarrhea
   B. Peripheral neuropathy
   C. Elevated blood pressure
   D. Encephalopathy
   E. Dysrhythmias

86.2. Which of the following chelators is recommended for the initial management of acute arsenic poisoning?
   A. Deferoxamine
   B. Dimercaprol
   C. Succimer
   D. *N*-Acetylcysteine
   E. Penicillamine

86.3. More than 6,000 beer drinkers developed peripheral neuropathy in Staffordshire, England, in 1900. An investigation revealed that the sugar used to produce the beer was contaminated with which of the following options?
   A. Lead
   B. Arsenic
   C. Thallium
   D. *n*-Hexane
   E. Triorthocresyl phosphate (TOCP)

86.4. Which of the following options is the primary pathophysiologic lesion produced by trivalent arsenic?
   A. Pyruvate dehydrogenase complex inhibition
   B. Inhibition of gluconeogenesis
   C. Depletion of glutathione

   D. Inhibition of thiolase
   E. Uncoupling of oxidative phosphorylation

86.5. Which of the following diagnoses mimics arsenic toxicity?
   A. Aortic dissection
   B. Trigeminal neuralgia
   C. Tetanus
   D. Guillian-Barré syndrome
   E. Alcohol withdrawal

86.6. A 45-year-old woman presents to the hospital requesting toxicologic consultation because she is concerned that she has elevated arsenic concentrations. Which of the following species of arsenic is benign?
   A. Monomethylarsonic acid
   B. Arsenic^{3+}
   C. Arsenobetaine
   D. Arsenic^{5+}
   E. Dimethylarsinic acid

86.7. A medical alert is called on a patient who is being treated for acute promyelocytic leukemia (APML). The patient is found in cardiac arrest, and upon initial rhythm evaluation, torsade de pointes is seen on the monitor. What medication is the patient currently receiving as part of his chemotherapy regimen?
   A. Arsenic trioxide
   B. Cyclophosphamide
   C. Methotrexate
   D. 5-Fluorouracil
   E. Uridine triacetate

86.8. A 65-year-old man who immigrated to the United States from Bangladesh 10 years ago presents to the hospital seeking care for hyperkeratosis on his palms and soles. On examination, he also has squamous cell skin cancer. What else might this patient have?
A. Orthostatic hypotension
B. Rice water diarrhea
C. Restrictive lung disease
D. Acute respiratory distress syndrome
E. Fever

86.9. A 19-year-old man is being treated for the meningoencephalitic stage of African trypanosomiasis. He develops vomiting, abdominal pain, and peripheral neuropathy. He later develops seizures and becomes comatose. What medication was he being treated with?
A. Melarsoprol
B. Hydroxychloroquine
C. Abacavir
D. Cefepime
E. Acyclovir

86.10. Which of the following malignancies is associated with chronic arsenic exposure?
A. Leukemia
B. Lymphoma
C. Kaposi sarcoma
D. Breast
E. Bladder

ANSWERS

86.1. Answer: C. Chronic arsenic toxicity is associated with an increased risk of diabetes mellitus, peripheral vascular disease, hypertension, and several cancers, including skin, lung, bladder, kidney, and liver. Peripheral neuropathy is associated with both acute and chronic arsenic toxicity. While nausea and vomiting are reported in chronic arsenic toxicity, they occur much more commonly in acute toxicity. Dysrhythmias and encephalopathy occur much more commonly in acute toxicity as compared to chronic toxicity.

Cebrian ME, et al. Chronic arsenic poisoning in the north of Mexico. *Hum Toxicol.* 1983;2:121-133.

Das D, et al. Arsenic in ground water in six districts of West Bengal, India: The biggest arsenic calamity in the world. Part 2. Arsenic concentration in drinking water, hair, nails, urine, skin-scale and liver tissue (biopsy) of the affected people. *Analyst.* 1995;120:917-924.

Tay CH, Seah CS. Arsenic poisoning from anti-asthmatic herbal preparations. *Med J Aust.* 1975;2:424-428.

86.2. Answer: B. Dimercaprol is the standard therapy for arsenic toxicity and is the only chelator that is administered parenterally to critically ill patients. Succimer (DMSA) is not US Food and Drug Administration approved for arsenic chelation but was used successfully in a few reported cases. Its role in treating critically ill patients remains to be defined. The efficacy of penicillamine has never been proven, *N*-acetylcysteine remains an experimental therapy for arsenic toxicity, and deferoxamine is used to chelate iron.

Eagle H, Magnuson HJ. The systemic treatment of 227 cases of arsenic poisoning (encephalitis, dermatitis, blood dyscrasias, jaundice, fever) with 2,3-dimercaptopropanolol (BAL). *J Clin Invest.* 1946;25:420-441.

Lenz K, Hruby K, Drunl W, et al. 2,3-Dimercaptosuccinic acid in human arsenic poisoining. *Arch Toxicol.* 1981;47:241-243.

86.3. Answer: B. The use of arsenic-contaminated sugar in the production of beer in England in 1900 resulted in at least 6,000 cases of peripheral neuropathy and 70 deaths.

Final report of the Royal Commission on Arsenical Poisoning. *Lancet.* 1903;2:1674-1676.

86.4. Answer: A. Trivalent arsenic prevents the regeneration of lipoamide, a necessary cofactor in the conversion of pyruvate to acetyl coenzyme A (CoA). Pentavalent arsenic uncouples oxidative phosphorylation, while depletion of glutathione potentiates trivalent arsenic toxicity. The inhibition of gluconeogenesis and thiolase are less important toxic effects of trivalent arsenic.

Buchet JP, Lauwerys R. Role of thiols in the in-vitro methylation of inorganic arsenic by rate liver cytosol. *Biochem Parmacol.* 1988; 37:3149-3153.

Peters RA. I. Present state of knowledge of biochemical lesions induced trivalent arsenical poisoning. *Bull Johns Hopkins Hosp.* 1955;87:1-20.

Riechl F, et al. Effects of arsenic on carbohydrate metabolism after single or repeated injection in guinea pigs. *Arch Toxicol.* 1988;62:473-475.

86.5. Answer: D. Acute arsenic toxicity initially mimics cholera, patients present with loose, watery diarrhea, described as "rice water." This is followed by an ascending paralysis that resembles the Guillian-Barré syndrome (GBS). It is differentiated from GBS by the additional prolonged QT interval on the electrocardiogram (ECG) and the leukopenia that occurs with arsenic toxicity.

Heyman A, et al. Peripheral neuropathy caused by arsenical intoxication: A study of 41 cases with observations on the effects of BAL (2,3-dimercaptopropanol). *N Engl J Med.* 1956;254:401-409.

Le Quesne PM, McLeod J. Peripheral neuropathy following a single exposure arsenic: Clinical course in four patients with electrophysiological and histological studies. *J Neurol Sci.* 1977;32:437-451.

86.6. Answer: C. Arsenobetaine is the most common form of arsenic found in seafood. It is excreted unchanged in the urine, producing arsenic concentrations as high as 1,700 mcg/L (22.66 micromol/L), but does not cause toxicity.

Arbouine MW, Wilson HK. The effect of seafood consumption on the assessment of occupational exposure to arsenic by urinary arsenic speciation measurements. *J Trace Elem.* 1992;6:153-160.

86.7. Answer: A. Arsenic trioxide is currently used as a treatment for APML. A well-documented toxicity of arsenic trioxide is prolongation of the QT interval and increased risk of torsade de pointes. Other medications that prolong the QT should be avoided in these patients.

Kwong YL. Arsenic trioxide in the treatment of haematological malignancies. *Expert Opin Drug Saf.* 2004;3:589-597.

Soignet SL, et al. United States multicenter study of arsenic trioxide in relapsed acute promyelocytic leukemia. *J Clin Oncol.* 2001;19: 3852-3860.

86.8. Answer: C. In parts of Bangladesh, there is significant contamination of arsenic in the ground water. Chronic arsenic toxicity is endemic in these areas. Patients present with cutaneous manifestations (both malignant and non-malignant), hypertension, coronary vascular disease, restrictive lung disease, and cancers including lung, bladder, kidney, and liver. Characteristic skin changes include hyperkeratosis on the palms and soles. Rice-water diarrhea, orthostatic hypotension, acute respiratory distress syndrome, and fever are more characteristic of acute arsenic toxicity.

Das D, et al. Chronic low-level arsenic exposure reduces lung function in male population without skin lesions. *Int J Public Health.* 2014;59:655-663.

Yoshida T, et al. Chronic health effects in people exposed to arsenic via the drinking water: Dose–response relationships in review. *Toxicol Appl Pharmacol.* 2004;198:243-252.

Mostafa MG, Cherry N. Arsenic in drinking water and renal cancers in rural Bangladesh. *Occup Environ Med.* 2013;70:768-773.

86.9. Answer: A. Melarsoprol is an organoarsenical used to treat the meningoencephalitic stage of African trypanosomiasis. It is ineffective in the treatment of the American form. Toxic effects are similar to those of inorganic arsenic.

Bouteille B, et al. Treatment perspectives for human African trypanosomiasis. *Fundam Clin Pharmacol.* 2003;17:171-181.

86.10. Answer: E. Lung, liver, and bladder cancers are associated with arsenic toxicity. Bowen disease and squamous cell and basal cell carcinomas also occur. All of these malignancies occur following chronic arsenic exposure, due to medicinal preparations, industrial or mining processes, or from contaminated well water. Leukemia, lymphoma, Kaposi sarcoma, and breast cancer have not been associated with arsenic.

Chen C-J, et al. Malignant neoplasms among residents of a blackfoot disease-endemic area in Taiwan: High-arsenic artesian well water and cancers. *Cancer Res.* 1985;45:5895-5899.

Kasper ML, et al. Hepatic angiosarcoma and bronchioloalveolar carcinoma induced by Fowler's solution. *JAMA.* 1984;252:3407-3408.

Bismuth

QUESTIONS

87.1. In the early 20th century, children presented to the hospital with abdominal pain, oliguria, anuria, malaise, depressed mental status, and vomiting following administration of what medication used to treat teething?
A. Elemental bismuth
B. Bismuth thioglycollate
C. Diallylacetic acid
D. Bismuth subsalicylate
E. Benzyl alcohol

87.2. Which of the following statements about bismuth is most accurate?
A. Toxicity occurs typically as a result of acute exposure
B. Concomitant proton pump inhibitor (PPI) use decreases the risk of toxicity
C. Neurologic toxicity is the only feature of bismuth subsalicylate toxicity
D. Nephrotoxicity should be treated with chelation
E. Ceasing the exposure often leads to complete reversal of bismuth encephalopathy

87.3. A 34-year-old man has fractures in his scapula and two of his lumbar vertebral bodies on radiographs. Which toxin most likely contributed to these findings?
A. Arsenic
B. Bismuth
C. Cadmium
D. Copper
E. Chromium

87.4. A 29-year-old woman presents to the emergency department with encephalopathy and is ultimately diagnosed with bismuth toxicity. Her symptoms began as apathy and progressed to visual hallucinations. On examination, she has marked myoclonic jerking and tremors. Two days later, despite admission to the hospital and removal from all potential exposures, her severe encephalopathy persists. What chelation therapy would be reasonable?
A. Dimercaprol
B. D-Penicillamine
C. Calcium ethylenediaminetetraacetic acid
D. Deferoxamine
E. No chelation therapy is indicated

87.5. Which of the following options is a mimic of chronic bismuth toxicity?
A. Guillian-Barré syndrome
B. Creutzfeldt-Jakob disease
C. Myasthenia gravis
D. Multiple sclerosis
E. Botulism

87.6. Which of the following formulations of bismuth is most associated with neurologic toxicity?
A. Bismuth bicitropeptide
B. Dicitratobismuthate
C. Bismuth triglycollamate
D. Bismuth subnitrate
E. Bismuth subsalicylate

87.7. Which of the following formulations of bismuth is most associated with kidney toxicity?
  A. Bismuth bicitropeptide
  B. Dicitratobismuthate
  C. Bismuth subcarbonate
  D. Bismuth subnitrate
  E. Elemental bismuth

87.8. A 27-year-old woman presents to the emergency department 8 hours after an overdose of several bottles of a nonprescription bismuth antidiarrheal medication. Her vital signs are remarkable for a heart rate of 128 beats/min and a respiratory rate is 28 breaths/min. She is confused and diaphoretic. Which of the following diagnostic tests will confirm the patient's diagnosis?
  A. Brain computed tomography (CT)
  B. Electroencephalogram (EEG)
  C. Lumbar puncture
  D. Serum bismuth concentration
  E. Serum salicylate concentration

87.9. A 35-year-old man is admitted to the intensive care unit with a diagnosis of severe bismuth encephalopathy. On examination, he has pronounced myoclonic jerking. An electroencephalogram (EEG) is performed. Which of the following EEG patterns would be diagnostic?
  A. Nonspecific slow-wave changes
  B. Sharp-wave abnormalities
  C. Hypsarrhythmia
  D. Spike and wave pattern in the temporal lobes
  E. No corresponding EEG changes

87.10. A 19-year-old man presents to the emergency department concerned that his stool is black. A fecal occult blood test is performed and shows no blood. Which of the following choices best explains the black color of his stool?
  A. Ingestion of beets
  B. Supratherapeutic acetaminophen ingestion
  C. Frequent ibuprofen use
  D. Recent ingestion of bismuth subsalicylate
  E. Recent ingestion of lithium

ANSWERS

87.1. Answer: B. Bismuth thioglycollate, a medication available in the early 20th century, was administered intramuscularly to treatment gingivostomatitis. With as little as one dose, some children went on to develop kidney failure and altered mental status. Their symptoms improved with chelation and resolution of their uremia. Elemental bismuth is nontoxic. Bismuth subsalicylate is available without a prescription and is not used to treat teething. Diallylacetic acid led to hepatotoxicity. Benzyl alcohol led to "gasping baby syndrome."

McClendon SJ. Toxic effects with anuria from a single injection of a bismuth preparation. *Am J Dis Child.* 1941;61:339-341.

87.2. Answer: E. Toxicity typically occurs in the setting of chronic exposure. Concomitant PPI use increases the bioavailability of oral bismuth and increases the risk of toxicity. Toxicity from lipid-soluble organic formulations of bismuth subsalicylate and bismuth subgallate manifests as both kidney and central nervous system toxicity. The evidence for chelation is poor but therapy is typically reserved for neurotoxic presentations. Stopping the exposure and decontamination (whole bowel irrigation, removal of bismuth iodoform gauze) generally lead to complete reversal of bismuth encephalopathy within days to weeks.

Hasking GJ, Duggan JM. Encephalopathy from bismuth subsalicylate. *Med J Aust.* 1982;2:167.

Taylor EG, Klenerman P. Acute renal failure after bismuth subcitrate overdose. *Lancet.* 1990;335:670-671.

87.3. Answer: B. Patients who have bismuth encephalopathy develop very pronounced myoclonic jerks that are severe enough to lead to fractures. The fractures are not caused by a direct effect of the metal on the bone.

Emile J, et al. Osteoarticular complications in bismuth encephalopathy. *Clin Toxicol.* 1981;18:1285-1290.

87.4. Answer: A. Most patients have resolution of their bismuth toxicity with removal from the source and aggressive gastrointestinal decontamination alone. However, in patients who have severe, life-threatening encephalopathy that persists despite these measures, chelation with dimercaprol (BAL) is reasonable.

Molina JA, et al. Myoclonic encephalopathy due to bismuth salts: Treatment with dimercaprol and analysis of CSF transmitters. *Acta Neurol Scand.* 1989;79:200-203.

87.5. Answer: B. Chronic bismuth toxicity presents with a progressive encephalopathy that includes neurobehavioral findings and progresses to severe myoclonic jerking. Patients progress to seizures, eventually become comatose, and die.

Creutzfeldt-Jakob disease resembles chronic bismuth toxicity as it also leads to neurobehavioral findings, including hallucinations, and patients eventually develop severe myoclonic jerking.

Mendelowitz PC, et al. Bismuth absorption and myoclonic encephalopathy during bismuth subsalicylate therapy. *Ann Intern Med.* 1990; 112:140-141.

87.6. Answer: E. The more highly lipid soluble formulations of bismuth, such as bismuth subsalicylate and bismuth subgallate, are associated with neurotoxicity. The encephalopathy that results is due to neuronal sulfhydryl binding.

Liessens JL, et al. Bismuth encephalopathy. *Act Neurol Belg.* 1978; 78:301-309.

87.7. Answer: B. Acute kidney injury is due to exposure of the water-soluble bismuth salts, such as bismuth triglycollamate and dicitratobismuthate. Massive overdoses result in abdominal pain, vomiting, and oliguria followed by anuria. Bismuth causes degeneration of the proximal tubule.

Randall RE, et al. Bismuth nephrotoxicity. *Ann Intern Med.* 1972; 77:481-482.

87.8. Answer: E. Pepto-Bismol is a brand name product available in the United States without a prescription and contains bismuth subsalicylate. Many generic equivalents also exist. Up to 90% of the salicylate is absorbed. A serum salicylate concentration should be obtained in patients who present to health care after either an acute or chronic overdose of bismuth subsalicylate. The rapidity of the onset of toxicity, the tinnitus, and the bismuth formulation taken all are suggestive of salicylate toxicity.

Sainsbury SJ. Fatal salicylate toxicity from bismuth subsalicylate. *West J Med.* 1991;155:637-639.

87.9. Answer: E. In patients with severe bismuth toxicity, the myoclonic jerks exhibited by patients do not correspond to a particular EEG pattern. At low blood concentrations of bismuth (<5 mcg/dL), patients have diffuse slowing. At concentrations between 5 mcg/dL up to 150 mcg/dL, sharp-wave abnormalities are seen. As the concentration rises higher than 200 mcg/dL, the EEG no longer corresponds to the patient's neurologic examination. This occurs as a result of an inhibitory effect of bismuth at higher concentrations.

Buge A, et al. Epileptic phenomena in bismuth toxic encephalopathy. *J Neurol Neurosurg Psychiatry.* 1981;44:62-67.

87.10. Answer: D. Bismuth ingestion, even at therapeutic doses, causes black stool that will test negative for blood. The formation of bismuth sulfide in the gastrointestinal tract causes this discoloration. This same compound also leads to a dark discoloration of the gums. Both findings are benign.

Zala L, et al. Pigmentation following long-term bismuth therapy for pneumatosis cystoides intestinalis. *Dermatology.* 1993;187:288-289.

Cadmium

QUESTIONS

88.1. Itai-Itai disease resulted from cadmium contamination of local rice crops. What is the characteristic pathologic finding in patients with Itai-Itai disease?
A. Chronic kidney disease
B. Cardiomyopathy
C. Restrictive lung disease
D. Peripheral neuropathy
E. Osteomalacia

88.2. Where is most of the cadmium in the blood found?
A. Concentrated in the red blood cells
B. Free in the plasma
C. Bound to albumin and alpha$_2$ macroglobulin
D. Bound to transferrin
E. Bound to alpha-1-acid glycoprotein

88.3. In animal models of cadmium toxicity, which of the following organs ultimately has the highest concentration of cadmium?
A. Bone
B. Lung
C. Heart
D. Kidney
E. Central nervous system

88.4. A 54-year-old man presents to the occupational health clinic because he is concerned regarding his risk of developing cadmium-associated kidney injury. Which of the following options would be the best test to screen this patient?
A. Serum cadmium concentrations
B. Urine cadmium concentrations

C. Urine specific gravity
D. Urine nitrites
E. Urine protein

88.5. Which of the following choices is a cellular defense mechanism that is induced to protect against cadmium toxicity?
A. Metallothionein
B. Glutathione
C. Ceruloplasmin
D. Superoxide dismutase
E. Ferritin

88.6. A 37-year-old man presents to the emergency department with shortness of breath, cough, and chills that began approximately 8 hours after welding cadmium alloys. His initial chest radiograph is normal. While in the emergency department, he develops worsening shortness of breath, and his pulmonary examination is notable for crackles. What is the most likely etiology of his presentation?
A. Metal fume fever
B. Cadmium pneumonitis
C. Styrene sickness
D. Solderer's acute hypersensitivity pneumonitis
E. Hard metal disease

88.7. What chelation therapy is indicated for a patient who has chronic pulmonary toxicity secondary to occupational exposure to cadmium?
A. Succimer
B. Calcium disodium edetate
C. Dimercaprol
D. Penicillamine
E. None of the above

88.8. A 44-year-old woman with complaints of fatigue, weight gain, and trouble concentrating on work is evaluated by a holistic medicine doctor who orders a urine screen for metals. The patient is employed as a paralegal in a large law firm and enjoys hiking as her only hobby. Which of the following options best explains an elevated urinary cadmium concentration on the urine screening examination?
A. Excessive seafood diet
B. Multivitamin supplement use
C. Cigarette smoking
D. Drinking well water
E. Large chronic ingestion of Brazil nuts

88.9. A 16-year-old boy presents to the hospital with hypotension and facial edema after ingesting approximately 200 g of cadmium chloride that he obtained from the storeroom in his science class. His blood pressure responds to a fluid bolus, and his facial edema does not progress. Which of the following chelators would be most reasonable to administer?
A. Calcium disodium edetate
B. Dimercaprol
C. Succimer
D. Penicillamine
E. None of the above

88.10. Chronic exposure to cadmium is associated with cancer in which of the following organ systems in humans?
A. Pulmonary
B. Kidney
C. Bone
D. Hematopoietic
E. Gastrointestinal

ANSWERS

88.1. Answer: E. Contamination of the local water supply with the wastewater runoff from a zinc-lead-cadmium mine in Japan from 1939-1954 was believed to be responsible for Itai-Itai disease. Itai-Itai is translated to "ouch-ouch" and is an unusual chronic syndrome manifested by extreme bone pain and osteomalacia. Approximately 200 people who lived along the banks of the Jintsu River developed these symptoms, which were thought to be due to the cadmium.

Cadmium pollution and itai-itai disease. *Lancet.* 1971;2:382-383.

88.2. Answer: C. Following absorption, cadmium is transported in the blood by both albumin and alpha$_2$ macroglobulin before it is ultimately stored in tissues.

Watkins SR, et al. Cadmium-binding serum protein. *Biochem Biophys Res Commun.* 1977;74:1403-1410.

88.3. Answer: D. In a rat model of cadmium toxicity, cadmium is first transported to the liver, but ultimately cadmium is found in highest concentrations in the kidneys. This corelates well with findings in humans, in that kidney toxicity is a prominent manifestation of cadmium exposure.

Dudley RE, et al. Cadmium-induced hepatic and renal injury in chronically exposed rats: Likely role of hepatic cadmium-metallothionein in nephrotoxicity. *Toxicol Appl Pharmacol.* 1985;77:414-426.

88.4. Answer: E. Chronic exposure to cadmium leads to proximal tubular dysfunction, which eventually leads to both proteinuria and hypercalciuria. Routine urinalysis is indicated as part of an occupational health program in workers with known cadmium exposure.

Scott R, et al. Hypercalciuria related to cadmium exposure. *Urology.* 1978;11:462-465.

88.5. Answer: A. Metallothionein is a natural chelator with a strong affinity for cadmium. Binding is cytoprotective. The other choices are important cellular defense mechanisms against metals and oxidants but have little, if any, role in defense against cadmium toxicity. Because metallothionein-bound cadmium is delivered to the kidney, the complex is implicated in tubular toxicity.

Cherian MG, et al. Cadmium-metallothionein-induced nephropathy. *Toxicol Appl Pharmacol.* 1976;38:399-408.

Klaassen CD, et al. Metallothionein: An intracellular protein to protect against cadmium toxicity. *Annu Rev Pharmacol Toxicol.* 1999;39:267-294.

88.6. Answer: B. Cadmium pneumonitis is a potentially life-threatening illness that occurs because of exposure to cadmium, classically after soldering cadmium in an enclosed space. The initial presentation mimics metal fume fever, with an influenzalike illness and a normal chest radiograph. However, as opposed to metal fume fever, which is benign and self-limited, cadmium pneumonitis progresses to acute respiratory distress syndrome (ARDS) with respiratory failure and death in the most severe cases. Patients who survive are at risk of developing pulmonary fibrosis. Solderer's hypersensitivity pneumonitis is typically chronic in nature.

Hard metal disease is associated with exposures to tungsten and cobalt.

Barnhart S, Rosenstock L. Cadmium chemical pneumonitis. *Chest*. 1984; 86:791.

88.7. Answer: E. In patients with chronic cadmium toxicity, chelation therapy is not indicated. It does not improve the pulmonary or the kidney toxicity associated with chronic exposure. Dimercaprol potentially worsens toxicity as it removes cadmium from metallothionein and allows it to redistribute in the body.

Dalhamn T, Friberg L. Dimercaprol (2,3-dimercaptopropanol) in chronic cadmium poisoning. *Acta Pharmacol Toxicol*. 1955;11:68-71.

88.8. Answer: C. Cigarette smokers have higher cadmium concentrations than nonsmokers because of cadmium contamination of tobacco. The pulmonary effects of cadmium are believed to contribute to lung disease in smokers. Seafood is typically associated with mercury or arsenic exposure. As there is no biological role for cadmium, it is not included in vitamins and dietary supplements. Brazil nuts are high in selenium not cadmium. Well water is always a potential source of toxin exposure, but smoking is far more likely absent a known contamination.

Telisman S, et al. Cadmium in the blood and seminal fluid of nonoccupationally exposed adult male subjects with regard to smoking habits. *Int Arch Occup Environ Health*. 1997;70:243-248.

Mannino DM, et al. Urinary cadmium levels predict lower lung function in current and former smokers: Data from the Third National Health and Nutrition Examination Survey. *Thorax*. 2004;59:194-198.

88.9. Answer: C. The ingested dose is consistent with reported cases of lethal cadmium ingestion. There are no good data on chelation of acute cadmium poisoning in humans. Animal models are supportive of succimer as the primary chelator based largely on safety. Penicillamine, dimercaprol, and calcium disodium edetate are either ineffective or exacerbate toxicity. Diethylenetriaminepentaacetic acid (DTPA) and 2,3-dimercaptopropane sulfonate (DMPS), both reduce tissue burdens of cadmium and are reasonable alternatives to succimer.

Cantilena LR, Klaassen CD. Decreased effectiveness of chelation therapy with time after acute cadmium poisoning. *Toxicol Appl Pharmacol*. 1982;63:173-180.

Basinger MA, et al. Antagonists for acute oral cadmium chloride intoxication. *J Toxicol Environ Health*. 1988;23:77-89.

Jones MM, et al. The relative effectiveness of some chelating agents as antidotes in acute cadmium poisoning. *Res Commun Chem Pathol Pharmacol*. 1978;22:581-588.

88.10. Answer: A. In animal models, cadmium exposure is associated with tumors in multiple organ systems. Although the association is not as strong as for other carcinogens, the International Agency for Research on Cancer lists cadmium as a carcinogen with the primary target organ in humans being the lungs.

Park R, et al. Cadmium and lung cancer mortality accounting for simultaneous arsenic exposure. *Occup Environ Med*. 2012;69:303-309.

Cesium

QUESTIONS

89.1. A 41-year-old woman with end-stage ovarian cancer ingests cesium chloride to alkalinize and kill her cancer cells. Which of the following clinical manifestations is most likely to occur?
A. Acute liver injury
B. Acute kidney injury
C. Cardiac dysrhythmias
D. Aplastic anemia
E. Painful peripheral neuropathy

89.2. Which of the following options best describes the most important mechanism for the answer to Question 89.1?
A. Bone marrow supression
B. Potassium channel blockade
C. Sulfhydryl binding
D. Oxidant stress
E. Free radical formation

89.3. Which of the following electrolyte abnormalities is reported in patients who ingest cesium chloride?
A. Hypokalemia
B. Hyperkalemia
C. Hyponatremia
D. Hypernatremia
E. Hypocalcemia

89.4. Which of the following therapies would be safest in a 37-year-old man who has persistent nausea and vomiting after an intentional ingestion of cesium chloride?
A. Ondansetron
B. Diphenhydramine
C. Granisetron
D. Metoclopramide
E. Trimethobenzamide

89.5. A 32-year-old man presents to the emergency department shortly after an ingestion of 5 g of cesium chloride. Which of the following therapies is indicated to prevent the absorption of recently ingested cesium chloride?
A. Activated charcoal
B. Sorbitol
C. Whole bowel irrigation with polyethylene glycol electrolyte lavage solution
D. Sodium polystyrene sulfonate
E. None of the above

89.6. Which of the following factors increases the biological half-life of cesium in humans?
A. Younger age
B. Male sex
C. Pregnancy
D. Breastfeeding
E. High-fat diet

89.7. A 62-year-old man presents to the hospital 10 hours after an ingestion of cesium chloride and has serious clinical toxicity. Which of the following therapies is indicated to enhance the elimination of ingested cesium salts?
A. Forced diuresis
B. Hemodialysis
C. Dimercaprol
D. Prussian blue
E. Pentetate zinc trisodium (Zn-DTPA)

89.8. Which of the following factors contributes to the long biological half-life of ingested cesium salts?
  A. Prolonged gastrointestinal absorption phase
  B. Extensive enterohepatic recirculation
  C. Absence of urinary or fecal elimination
  D. Fixed intracellular binding
  E. Deposition into bone

89.9. Radioactive cesium (^{137}Cs) exposure raises concerns for which type of radiation?
  A. Alpha particles
  B. Beta particles
  C. Gamma rays
  D. Neutrons
  E. Both beta particles and gamma rays

89.10. A 27-year-old man unintentionally handles an unshielded radiocesium source (^{137}Cs) for a few seconds. What will be the first manifestation of his exposure?
  A. No findings
  B. Nausea and vomiting
  C. Cutaneous burns
  D. Lymphopenia
  E. Coagulopathy

ANSWERS

89.1. Answer: C. Acute toxicity from cesium salt ingestion is mostly likely to result in cardiotoxicity. Patients develop QT interval prolongation, torsade de pointes, and other ventricular dysrhythmias.

> Nayebpour M, Nattel S. Pharmacologic response of cesium-induced ventricular tachyarrhythmias in anesthetized dogs. *J Cardiovasc Pharmacol.* 1990;15:552-561.

> Senges JC, et al. Cesium chloride induced ventricular arrhythmias in dogs: Three-dimensional activation patterns and their relation to the cesium dose applied. *Basic Res Cardiol.* 2000;95:152-162.

89.2. Answer: B. Cesium mimics potassium to block potassium rectifier currents in the heart. The net result is prolongation of the QT interval and malignant ventricular dysrhythmias, including torsade de pointes. Sodium channel blockade plays a minor role.

> Zhang S, et al. Modulation of human ether-à-go-go-related K+ (HERG) channel inactivation by Cs+ and K+. *J Physiol.* 2003;548:691-702.

> Hanich RF, et al. Autonomic modulation of ventricular arrhythmia in cesium chloride-induced long QT syndrome. *Circulation.* 1988;77: 1149-1161.

89.3. Answer: A. Both hypokalemia and hypomagnesemia occur in patients with cesium-induced dysrhythmias. These abnormalities most likely result from gastrointestinal losses as nausea, vomiting, and diarrhea are common in patients who ingest cesium salts.

> Vyas H, et al. Acquired long QT syndrome secondary to cesium chloride supplement. *J Altern Complement Med.* 2006;12:1011-1014.

> Young F, Bolt J. Torsades de pointes—a report of a case induced by caesium taken as a complementary medicine, and the literature review. *J Clin Pharm Ther.* 2013;38:254-257.

89.4. Answer: E. Among the antiemetics listed, only trimethobenzamide is not associated with QT interval prolongation. The others should be specifically avoided in patients with known ingestions of cesium chloride as there is already a significant risk for ventricular dysrhythmias.

> https://crediblemeds.org/. Accessed on June 18, 2021.

89.5. Answer: E. Most patients with clinically significant ingestions of cesium will have nausea, vomiting, and diarrhea, making decontamination both challenging and less likely to be of benefit. Of note, adsorption to activated charcoal is poor and whole bowel irrigation is unlikely to be beneficial because of the rapid and complete absorption of cesium salts. Although polystyrene sulfonate is suggested by some authors in acute lithium poisoning, its role in cesium toxicity is unknown and therefore cannot be recommended. Cautious use of an antiemetic and Prussian blue are the most reasonable alternatives.

> Verzijl JM, et al. In vitro binding characteristics for cesium of two qualities of Prussian blue, activated charcoal, and Resonium-A. *Clin Toxicol.* 1992;30:215-222.

89.6. Answer: B. The elimination of cesium is prolonged in men and older patients. Women, including pregnant and breastfeeding women, and children eliminate cesium more rapidly. There is no evidence that dietary fat content has a significant impact on cesium elimination.

> Boni AL. Variations in the retention and excretion of 137Cs with age and sex. *Nature.* 1969;222:1188-1189.

89.7. Answer: D. The method of choice to enhance the elimination of either radioactive or nonradioactive cesium is Prussian blue. The crystal lattice of Prussian blue traps cesium in the gut to enhance elimination. In one human volunteer study, >90% of ingested cesium was eliminated after 14 days of Prussian blue therapy as compared to about 5% in controls. There is no evidence for either forced diuresis or hemodialysis. It is unlikely that Zn-DTAP or dimercaprol will have a significant effect.

Madshus K, Strömme A. Increased excretion of 137Cs in humans by Prussian Blue. *Z Naturforsch B*. 1968;23:391-392.

89.8. Answer: B. Cesium salts are rapidly and nearly completely absorbed in humans. Significant enterohepatic recirculation results in very limited fecal elimination with most of the absorbed cesium being eliminated from the kidneys. Unlike lead, there does not appear to be a large reservoir of cesium in bones, although cesium is extensively distributed into most organs.

Lipsztein JL, et al. Studies of Cs retention in the human body related to body parameters and Prussian blue administration. *Health Phys*. 1991;60:57-61.

Madshus K, Strömme A. Cesium behavior and distribution in man following a single dose of 137Cs. *Z Naturforsch B*. 1964;19:690-692.

Rääf CL, et al. Human metabolism of radiocesium revisited. *Radiat Prot Dosimetry*. 2004;112:395-404.

89.9. Answer: E. Radioactive cesium (^{137}Cs) emits beta particles as it decays to an unstable barium isotope, which subsequently emits gamma radiation. Exposure to ^{137}Cs should always lead to evaluation of both potential emissions.

Nakamura S, et al. Measurement of 90Sr radioactivity in cesium hot particles originating from the Fukushima Nuclear Power Plant Accident. *J Radiat Res*. 2018;59:677-684.

89.10. Answer: C. Beta emissions produce local burns that resemble thermal burns. No findings would be expected after a cutaneous exposure to an alpha emitter. All the other findings are manifestations of total-body irradiation that result from either incorporation events or total-body external exposure to a gamma source and are not likely from a transient exposure to the hand.

Oliveira AR, et al. Localized lesions induced by 137Cs during the Goiânia accident. *Health Phys*. 1991;60:25-29.

Oliveira AR, et al. Medical and related aspects of the Goiânia accident: An overview. *Health Phys*. 1991;60:17-24.

Chromium

QUESTIONS

90.1. Welding of which of the following metals is most likely to liberate chromium?
- A. Stainless steel
- B. Galvanized steel
- C. Wrought iron
- D. Brass
- E. Bronze

90.2. Which of the following options is true regarding the role of chromium in humans?
- A. There is no biological role for chromium
- B. Chromium is involved in glucose regulation
- C. Chromium is involved in skeletal mineralization
- D. Chromium is involved with hemoglobin synthesis
- E. Chromium is utilized in the electron transport chain

90.3. Which of the following malignancies is most associated with chronic chromium exposure?
- A. Brain
- B. Lung
- C. Liver
- D. Kidney
- E. Hematologic

90.4. Which of the following options is true once chromium enters the systemic circulation?
- A. It is tightly bound to transferrin
- B. It is tightly bound to albumin
- C. It is tightly bound to alpha-1-acid glycoprotein
- D. It is equally distributed between albumin and alpha-1-acid glycoprotein
- E. It is highly concentrated in red blood cells

90.5. After leaving the systemic circulation, most of the absorbed chromium is found in which of the following organs?
- A. Brain
- B. Lungs
- C. Muscles
- D. Kidneys
- E. Blood

90.6. Which of the following options is true regarding the biochemistry of chromium salt ingestion?
- A. Ingested hexavalent chromium is absorbed and rapidly converted to neutral chromium (Cr^0) in the circulation
- B. Ingested trivalent chromium is absorbed and rapidly converted to hexavalent chromium
- C. Ingested hexavalent chromium is absorbed and rapidly converted to trivalent chromium
- D. Ingested hexavalent chromium is rapidly converted to trivalent chromium in the stomach before it is absorbed
- E. Ingested trivalent chromium is rapidly converted to hexavalent chromium in the stomach before it is absorbed

90.7. Which of the following options best describes the dermatologic response that occurs in patients with occupational exposures to chromium compounds?
- A. Ulcers on exposed areas
- B. Chronic urticaria
- C. Allergic contact dermatitis
- D. Hyperkeratotic lesions
- E. Squamous cell carcinoma

90.8. Which of the following therapies would be best for a 26-year-old woman who presents to the hospital with nausea and vomiting 1 hour after ingestion of 40 chromium picolinate capsules?
A. An antiemetic followed by oral activated charcoal
B. *N*-Acetylcysteine (NAC)
C. Dimercaprol (BAL)
D. Hemodialysis
E. Supportive care

90.9. A 36-year-old man presents to the hospital with nausea and blood-tinged vomiting after an intentional ingestion of potassium dichromate. In addition to supportive care and an endoscopy to exclude significant gastrointestinal injury, which of the following therapies would best help lower his body burden of chromium?
A. Hemodialysis
B. Calcium edetate (CaEDTA)
C. Dimercaprol (BAL)
D. D-Penicillamine
E. *N*-Acetylcysteine (NAC)

90.10. Which of the following types of kidney toxicity would be expected to occur in a patient who had an acute, massive overdose of hexavalent chromium?
A. Acute tubular necrosis
B. Focal glomerulosclerosis
C. Obstructive uropathy
D. Acute interstitial nephritis
E. Eosinophiluria

ANSWERS

90.1. Answer: A. Steel is made from mixing iron and carbon. The addition of corrosion-resistant alloy metals, such as chromium or nickel, is what makes steel "stainless." Galvanized steel contains zinc; brass is made of copper and zinc; bronze is made of copper and tin. Welding stainless steel liberates chromium in respiratory particles.

> Stern RM, et al. In vitro toxicity of welding fumes and their constituents. *Environ Res.* 1988;46:168-180.

> Stern RM. In vitro assessment of equivalence of occupational health risk: Welders. *Environ Health Perspect.* 1983;51:217-222.

90.2. Answer: B. Chromium facilitates the effects of insulin in the regulation of glucose and lipid metabolism. Trivalent chromium, in the form of chromium picolinate, is sold as a supplement to support weight regulation and lean body mass, theoretically because of its biological role.

> Hua Y, et al. Molecular mechanisms of chromium in alleviating insulin resistance. *J Nutr Biochem.* 2012;23:313-319.

90.3. Answer: B. Epidemiologic studies demonstrate a significantly increased risk of lung cancer in individuals exposed to hexavalent chromium compounds, with small cell and poorly differentiated pulmonary carcinomas being the most common.

> Langard S, Vigander T. Occurrence of lung cancer in workers producing chromium pigments. *Br J Ind Med.* 1983;40:71-74.

> Satoh K, et al. Epidemiological study of workers engaged in the manufacture of chromium compounds. *J Occup Med.* 1981;23:835-838.

90.4. Answer: E. The red bloods cells serve as a protected reservoir for chromium in the systemic circulation. Release occurs on hemolysis or with red-cell senescence. As a result of this, plasma or serum concentrations do not adequately reflect the body burden of absorbed chromium.

> Iserson KV, et al. Failure of dialysis therapy in potassium dichromate poisoning. *J Emerg Med.* 1983;1:143-149.

> Costa M. Toxicity and carcinogenicity of Cr(VI) in animal models and humans. *Crit Rev Toxicol.* 1997;27:431-442.

90.5. Answer: D. After leaving the blood, most of the chromium is found in the liver and kidneys of experimentally exposed animals. It is unclear how this finding relates to either acute or chronic toxicity.

> Costa M. Toxicity and carcinogenicity of Cr(VI) in animal models and humans. *Crit Rev Toxicol.* 1997;27:431-442.

90.6. Answer: C. Hexavalent chromium has a greater bioavailability than trivalent chromium but is such a potent oxidizing agent that it is rapidly converted to trivalent chromium after absorption. This oxidation reaction is likely the cause of toxicity.

> Iserson KV, et al. Failure of dialysis therapy in potassium dichromate poisoning. *J Emerg Med.* 1983;1:143-149.

> Paustenbach DJ, et al. Observation of steady state in blood and urine following human ingestion of hexavalent chromium in drinking water. *J Toxicol Environ Health.* 1996;49:453-461.

90.7.   Answer: A. Occupational exposure to chromium compounds is associated with a variety of manifestations that most commonly include ulcerative disease of the skin and nasal perforation (chrome holes). The pathophysiology involves caustic injury from deposits that occur in microbreaks of the skin and nasal tissue. While some patients develop allergic contact dermatitis, they are often exposed to other metals, such as nickel, that are associated with allergic reactions. Hyperkeratosis and squamous cell carcinoma are associated with chronic arsenic toxicity.

Lee HS, Goh CL. Occupational dermatosis among chrome platers. *Contact Dermatitis.* 1988;18:89-93.

90.8.   Answer: E. Most acute ingestions of trivalent chromium compounds are relatively benign compared to hexavalent compounds. Chromium salts are not well adsorbed to activated charcoal. As such, the best therapy is general supportive care. There are rare cases of chronic excessive use of chromium picolinate associated with toxicity that resolves with discontinuation.

Cerulli J, et al. Chromium picolinate toxicity. *Ann Pharmacother.* 1998;32:428-431.

90.9.   Answer: E. Acute ingestions of hexavalent chromium compounds produce life-threating toxicity. Unfortunately, hemodialysis does not effectively remove chromium but is indicated based on standard criteria in patients who develop acute kidney injury. There is no reliable evidence that any of the traditional chelators substantially increase chromium elimination. Choices B-D have cost and safety concerns. In an animal model, NAC increased renal elimination of chromium and is generally safe and inexpensive.

Iserson KV, et al. Failure of dialysis therapy in potassium dichromate poisoning. *J Emerg Med.* 1983;1:143-149.

Nowak-Wiaderek W. Influence of various drugs on excretion and distribution of chromium-51 in acute poisoning in rats. *Mater Med Pol.* 1975;7:308-310.

Banner W Jr, et al. Experimental chelation therapy in chromium, lead, and boron intoxication with *N*-acetylcysteine and other compounds. *Toxicol Appl Pharmacol.* 1986;83:142-147.

90.10.   Answer: A. Following an acute overdose of hexavalent chromium, patients present with symptoms that are like other metal ingestions. This includes vomiting, gastrointestinal hemorrhage, and potentially bowel perforation. Patients also develop hemolysis because of the strong oxidative effects of hexavalent chromium. The primary kidney injury that occurs following an acute exposure is acute tubular necrosis.

Wedeen RP, Qian LF. Chromium-induced kidney disease. *Environ Health Perspect.* 1991;92:71-74.

QUESTIONS

91.1. In the 1960s, two outbreaks of disease were associated with beer drinking in the United States and Canada. Investigations revealed that cobalt sulfate was added to the beer as a foam stabilizer. Which organ system was primarily affected in these outbreaks?
A. Central nervous system
B. Ophthalmic
C. Pulmonary
D. Cardiac
E. Hepatic

91.2. Which of the following mechanisms best explains the effect of cobalt on red blood cells?
A. Cobalt produces intravascular hemolysis through an oxidation reaction
B. Cobalt increases iron absorption in the gut, improving hemoglobin synthesis
C. Cobalt produces an immune complex–mediated hemolytic anemia
D. Cobalt stimulates erythropoietin
E. Cobalt causes aplastic anemia

91.3. Which of the following mechanisms best describes the effect of cobalt on thyroid function?
A. Cobalt prevents peripheral conversion of tetraiodothyronine (T_4) to triiodothyronine (T_3)
B. Cobalt stimulates the peripheral conversion of T_4 to T_3
C. Cobalt inhibits iodine uptake in the thyroid gland
D. Cobalt stimulates iodine uptake in the thyroid gland
E. Cobalt stimulates thyroperoxidase

91.4. Workers in the tungsten carbide industry who are exposed to cobalt develop toxicity in which of the following organ systems?
A. Central nervous system
B. Pulmonary
C. Cardiac
D. Renal
E. Peripheral nervous system

91.5. Involvement of which organ systems is described in patients suffering from cobalt toxicity following failed arthroplasty but is not typically reported in other forms of cobalt poisoning?
A. Ophthalmic
B. Genitourinary
C. Pulmonary
D. Hepatic
E. Peripheral nervous system

91.6. A 75-year-old man has a metal-on-metal hip implant that has become acutely painful. Which imaging modality is advised for assessment of joint dysfunction?
A. Plain radiograph
B. Computed tomography (CT)
C. Contrast-enhanced CT
D. Magnetic resonance imaging (MRI) with contrast
E. Metal artifact reduction sequence (MARS) MRI

91.7. An 87-year-old woman presents to the emergency department with fatigue. Vital signs and basic laboratory studies, including a complete blood count, electrolytes, and kidney, liver, and thyroid function tests, are normal. Inflammatory markers and a urine analysis are also unremarkable. She asks whether her fatigue could be related to toxicity from a hip implant preformed many years earlier. She has no pain, swelling, or decreased range of motion of the hip, and her gait is unremarkable. Which of the following tests is indicated?
A. Plain radiograph of the hip
B. Blood for chromium and cobalt
C. 24-Hour urine collection for chromium and cobalt
D. Hip ultrasound
E. No testing is indicated

91.8. The pathophysiology of cobalt toxicity is related in part to an inhibitory effect on which of the following enzymes in the citric acid cycle?
A. Aconitase
B. Isocitrate dehydrogenase
C. Alpha-ketoglutarate dehydrogenase
D. Succinyl-CoA synthetase
E. Fumarase

91.9. Cobalt impairs neuromuscular transmission by competing for which of the following cations?
A. Sodium
B. Potassium
C. Calcium
D. Magnesium
E. Zinc

91.10. A 79-year-old man with a history of a metal-on-metal hip implant develops pain and swelling around his surgical scar, trouble hearing, and severe fatigue over many months. Testing indicates abnormal wear at the joint, and his blood cobalt concentrations are significantly elevated. Prior to hip revision, treatment with which of the following chelators is reasonable?
A. *N*-Acetylcysteine
B. Calcium disodium edetate
C. Dimercaprol
D. Succimer
E. Penicillamine

ANSWERS

91.1. Answer: D. The disorder that became known as "beer drinker's cardiomyopathy" required both cobalt excess and the presence of high concentrations of NADH that resulted from metabolism of large quantities of ethanol. In experimental models, neither cobalt alone nor ethanol that was free of cobalt was able to reproduce the disease.

Morin Y, Daniel P. Quebec beer-drinkers' cardiomyopathy: Etiological considerations. *Can Med Assoc J.* 1967;97:926-928.

McDermott PH, et al. Myocardosis and cardiac failure in men. *JAMA.* 1966;198:253-256.

91.2. Answer: D. One of the first uses for cobalt was as a hematinic as it was felt to be less toxic than iron. Cobalt increases erythropoietin production by upregulating the production of hypoxia-inducible factor 1 (HIF-1).

Samelko L, et al. Cobalt-alloy implant debris induce HIF-1alpha hypoxia associated responses: A mechanism for metal-specific orthopedic implant failure. *PLoS One.* 2013;8:e67127.

91.3. Answer: C. Cobalt induces hypothyroidism by a complex mechanism that includes inhibition of iodine uptake, inhibition of thyroperoxidase, and inhibition of iodine oxidation, all of which are required for incorporation into thyroxine.

Kriss JP, et al. Hypothyroidism and thyroid hyperplasia in patients treated with cobalt. *JAMA.* 1955;157:117-121.

Prescott E, et al. Effect of occupational exposure to cobalt blue dyes on the thyroid volume and function of female plate painters. *Scand J Work Environ Health.* 1992;18:101-104.

91.4. Answer: B. "Hard-metal disease" was first described in workers in the tungsten carbide industry, which uses very high temperatures to combine cobalt and tungsten. Workers develop upper respiratory tract irritation, exertional dyspnea, severe dry cough, wheezing, and interstitial lung disease ranging from alveolitis to progressive fibrosis. A characteristic finding of this disease is multinucleated giant cells in bronchoalveolar lavage specimens. This suggests an immune-mediated response to cobalt.

Cugell DW, et al. The respiratory effects of cobalt. *Arch Intern Med.* 1990;150:177-183.

Fairhall LT, et al. Cobalt and dust environment of the cemented tungsten carbide industry. *Public Health Rep.* 1949;64:485-490.

Harding HE. Notes on the toxicology of cobalt metal. *Br J Ind Med.* 1950;7:76-78.

91.5. **Answer: A.** When hip prostheses that contain metal-on-metal surfaces fail, they liberate both cobalt and chromium into the systemic circulation. In addition to the other manifestations of systemic cobalt toxicity, several case reports demonstrate an association with loss of visual function.

Rizzetti MC, et al. Loss of sight and sound. Could it be the hip? *Lancet.* 2009;373:1052.

Steens W, et al. Severe cobalt poisoning with loss of sight after ceramic-metal pairing in a hip—a case report. *Acta Orthop.* 2006;77:830-832.

91.6. **Answer: E.** Diagnostic imaging is indicated in patients with symptoms that are potentially related to dysfunction of metal-on-metal hip implants. The preferred methods of evaluation of the implant include ultrasound and metal artifact reduction sequence (MARS) MRI.

Kwon YM, et al. Risk stratification algorithm for management of patients with metal-on-metal hip arthroplasty: Consensus statement of the American Association of Hip and Knee Surgeons, the American Academy of Orthopaedic Surgeons, and the Hip Society. *J Bone Joint Surg Am.* 2014;96:e4.

91.7. **Answer: E.** There is extensive debate as to what to do with the few remaining patients who have metal-on-metal hip implants and have no clinical evidence of joint dysfunction or an increase in pain. Societies differ in recommendations due to lack of data. While some societies recommend routine testing, there is no evidence-based threshold for action in asymptomatic patients. The philosophy of the US Food and Drug Administration (FDA) is essentially to leave asymptomatic patients alone.

Australian Government-Department of Health Therapeutic Goods Administration. Metal-on-metal hip replacement implants—information for general practitioners, orthopaedic surgeons and other health professionals, 2012. https://www.tga.gov.au/metal-metal-hip-replacement-implants

US Food and Drug Administration. Concerns about metal-on-metal hip implants. https://www.fda.gov/MedicalDevices/ProductsandMedicalProcedures/ImplantsandProsthetics/MetalonMetalHipImplants/ucm241604.htm. Accessed March 18, 2017.

Medicines and Healthcare Products Regulatory Agency. Management recommendations for patients with metal-on-metal hip replacement implants 2012. https://www.gov.uk/drug-device-alerts/all-metal-on-metal-mom-hip-replacements-updated-advice-for-follow-up-of-patients

91.8. **Answer: C.** Like other divalent cations, cobalt has an inhibitory effect on alpha-ketoglutarate dehydrogenase. While this effect is weak by comparison, it is greatly enhanced in the presence of NADH. This mechanism likely explains the similarity between beer drinker's cardiomyopathy and beriberi, as alpha-ketoglutarate dehydrogenase is a thiamine-dependent enzyme.

Daniel M, et al. The biological action of cobalt and other metals. I. The effect of cobalt on the morphology and metabolism of rat fibroblasts in vitro. *Br J Exp Pathol.* 1963;44:163-176.

Wiberg GS. The effect of cobalt ions on energy metabolism in the rat. *Can J Biochem.* 1968;46:549-554.

91.9. **Answer: C.** Weakness is a common complaint in patients with elevated cobalt concentrations. Although the etiology for weakness is likely multifactorial, at least one animal model demonstrates that cobalt competes for calcium at the neuromuscular junction and that this effect is largely inhibitory.

Weakly JN. The action of cobalt ions on neuromuscular transmission in the frog. *J Physiol.* 1973;234:597-612.

91.10. **Answer: A.** Controlled trials of chelation therapy for cobalt toxicity in humans have not been performed. Based on animal models and human case reports, *N*-acetylcysteine is preferred based on both safety and efficacy endpoints.

Giampreti A, et al. Chelation in suspected prosthetic hip-associated cobalt toxicity. *Can J Cardiol.* 2014;30:465.e13.

Domingo JL, et al. *N*-acetyl-l-cysteine in acute cobalt poisoning. *Arch Farmacol Toxicolw.* 1985;11:55-62.

Copper

QUESTIONS

92.1. Which of the following statements is true regarding absorption of small amounts of dietary oral copper salts?
A. Absorption is largely from passive diffusion in the stomach
B. Absorption is largely from passive diffusion in the small bowel
C. Absorption is largely from active transport in the stomach
D. Absorption is largely from active transport in the small bowel
E. Absorption is by passive diffusion throughout the stomach and small bowel

92.2. A 24-year-old man presents to the emergency department after an acute overdose of a septic tank cleaning product. On his emergency department assessment, he is found to have blue-colored vomitus and abdominal pain. Within 24 hours, his hemoglobin falls from normal to 4 g/dL (2.5 mmol/L) and a methemoglobin of 18% develops. Subsequently, he develops hypotension to 70/30 mmHg, scleral icterus, and diffuse abdominal tenderness. Which of the following therapies is indicated at this time?
A. Activated charcoal
B. D-Penicillamine
C. Methylene blue
D. Dimercaptopropane sulfonate
E. Zinc

92.3. A 5-month-old boy who just immigrated to the United States from India presents to the hospital with new cirrhosis. A diagnosis of idiopathic copper toxicosis is suspected. What laboratory results would confirm this diagnosis?
A. Low serum copper and low serum ceruloplasmin
B. Low serum copper and high serum ceruloplasmin
C. High serum copper and normal serum ceruloplasmin
D. High serum copper and high serum ceruloplasmin
E. Normal serum copper and high serum ceruloplasmin

92.4. A 70-year-old Portuguese man who previously worked in a vineyard is found to have interstitial pulmonary fibrosis and histiocytic granulomas. What occupational exposure contributed to the development of these findings?
A. Asbestos
B. Lead
C. Silicosis
D. Bordeaux solution
E. Lye

92.5. Which of the following mechanisms best describes the efficacy of zinc supplementation in copper poisoning?
A. Zinc induces ceruloplasmin synthesis
B. Zinc induces metallothionine synthesis
C. Zinc stabilizes red blood cells to prevent hemolysis
D. Zinc prevents copper absorption into the hepatocytes
E. Zinc competes for copper absorption in the gut

92.6. Which of the following tests is most useful in assessing acute copper poisoning?
A. Whole blood copper concentration
B. Serum copper concentration
C. 24-hour copper concentration following oral succimer challenge
D. 24-hour urine copper concentration
E. Ceruloplasmin concentration

92.7. Central nervous system manifestations of copper poisoning result from abnormalities in which of the following structures?
A. Corpus collosum
B. Periaqueductal gray
C. Globus pallidus
D. Lenticular nucleus
E. Cerebellum

92.8. Which of the following statements is true about the use of extracorporeal techniques in a patient with severe acute copper poisoning?
A. Intermittent hemodialysis is preferred
B. Peritoneal dialysis is useful
C. Exchange transfusion removes a clinically significant amount of copper
D. Therapeutic plasma exchange is the modality of choice
E. Extracorporeal removal is not indicated

92.9. Which of the following choices is the most common adverse effect of D-penicillamine therapy when used for short-term chelation of acute copper poisoning?
A. Worsening neurologic toxicity
B. Agranulocytosis
C. Toxic epidermal necrolysis (TEN)
D. Hypersensitivity
E. Acute kidney injury

92.10. Diethyldithiocarbamate chelates copper lead, and thallium. Which of the following metals is also chelated by diethyldithiocarbamate?
A. Cobalt
B. Iron
C. Nickel
D. Arsenic
E. Magnesium

ANSWERS

92.1. Answer: D. As an essential trace metal, an active transport mechanism known as Menkes ATPase is present in the small bowel. Under normal conditions, only about 12% of an ingested dose of copper is absorbed. In overdose, however, absorption increases and becomes passive through damaged mucosa. Menkes syndrome is a severe congenital disorder of this transporter that results in copper deficiency.

Goodman VL, et al. Copper deficiency as an anti-cancer strategy. *Endocr Relat Cancer*. 2004;11:255-263.

Harvey LJ, et al. Copper absorption from foods labelled intrinsically and extrinsically with Cu-65 stable isotope. *Eur J Clin Nutr*. 2005;59:363-368.

Kaler SG. Diagnosis and therapy of Menkes syndrome, a genetic form of copper deficiency. *Am J Clin Nutr*. 1998;67(5 Suppl):1029S-1034S.

92.2. Answer: B. This patient ingested copper sulfate, which is commonly used to clean septic systems and is associated with blue-green emesis. D-Penicillamine is used as a treatment in the management of Wilson disease and, is helpful in preventing copper-induced hemolysis. An acute overdose of copper salts is often caustic; therefore, activated charcoal should be avoided as it will interfere with adequate visualization on endoscopy. Although copper causes methemoglobinemia, which is associated with a high incidence of hemolysis, the methemoglobin is released in the plasma and methylene blue will not reliably reduce the ferric ion. Dimercaptopropane sulfonate worsens copper-induced hemolysis in vitro and should be avoided. While zinc is used in the management of patients who have Wilson disease, it should be avoided in the acute setting because it leads to gastrointestinal irritation.

Vieira J, et al. Urinary copper excretion before and after oral intake of D-penicillamine in parents of patients with Wilson's disease. *Dig Liver Dis*. 2012;44:323-327.

Aaseth J, et al. The interaction of copper (Cu++) with the erythrocyte membrane and 2,3-dimercaptopropanesulphonate in vitro: A source of activated oxygen species. *Pharmacol Toxicol*. 1987;61:250-253.

Yang CC, et al. Prolonged hemolysis and methemoglobinemia following organic copper fungicide ingestion. *Vet Hum Toxicol*. 2004;46:321-323.

92.3. Answer: D. Idiopathic copper toxicosis is associated with excessive dietary intake of copper. This usually occurs because of copper leaching out of brass storage containers into milk and water. The elevation of both the serum copper and the serum ceruloplasmin distinguishes this from Wilson disease, which is notable for an inability of the liver to eliminate excess copper and low ceruloplasmin concentration.

Normal ceruloplasmin is not expected since ceruloplasmin concentrations rise in patients with copper poisoning.

Nayak NC, Chitale AR. Indian childhood cirrhosis (ICC) & ICC-like diseases: The changing scenario of facts versus notions. *Indian J Med Res*. 2013;137:1029-1042.

Johncilla M, Mitchell KA. Pathology of the liver in copper overload. *Semin Liver Dis*. 2011;31:239-244.

92.4. Answer: D. "Vineyard sprayer's lung" is an occupational disease that was described in Portuguese vineyard workers who used Bordeaux solution, which contains 1-2% copper sulfate, lime, and calcium sulfate.

Pimentel JC, Marques F. "Vineyard sprayer's lung": A new occupational disease. *Thorax*. 1969;24:678-688.

92.5. Answer: B. Zinc is used in patients with chronic copper overload because it increases the synthesis of metallothionine, which serves as a binding protein for free copper. It is unclear what, if any, role zinc serves in patients with acute copper poisoning because the induction takes time. Large ingestions of zinc do limit copper absorption from the gut, but this would not be a reasonable therapeutic approach.

Santiago R, et al. Zinc therapy for Wilson disease in children in French pediatric centers. *J Pediatr Gastroenterol Nutr*. 2015;61:613-618.

92.6. Answer: B. Because copper is sequestered in red blood cells, the whole blood copper concentration correlates better with tissue stores and prognosis than either serum or 24-hour urine concentrations. There is never a role for provocative testing. Ceruloplasmin is useful in assessing patients for Wilson disease.

Adelstein SJ, Vallee BL. Copper metabolism in man. *N Engl J Med*. 1961;265:892-897.

Wahal PK, et al. Study of whole blood, red cell and plasma copper levels in acute copper sulphate poisoning and their relationship with complications and prognosis. *J Assoc Physicians India*. 1976;24:153-158.

92.7. Answer: D. Wilson disease is also known as hepatolenticular degeneration. For unclear reasons, copper targets the lenticular nucleus of the basal ganglia to produce tremor, ataxia, dysphagia, dysphonia, and parkinsonism.

Lorincz MT. Neurologic Wilson's disease. *Ann N Y Acad Sci*. 2010;1184: 173-187.

Oder W, et al. Wilson's disease: Evidence of subgroups derived from clinical findings and brain lesions. *Neurology*. 1993;43:120-124.

92.8. Answer: E. Although copper ions are small enough to fit through a hemodialysis filter, the large volume of distribution and high protein binding almost certainly make all extracorporeal attempts to remove copper futile. The is supported by quantification in a variety of case reports. While some techniques are used as bridging therapy in patients with severe Wilson disease, it is unclear if the limited benefits reported are related to copper removal.

Agarwal BN, et al. Ineffectiveness of hemodialysis in copper sulphate poisoning. *Nephron*. 1975;15:74-77.

Oldenquist G, Salem M. Parenteral copper sulfate poisoning causing acute renal failure. *Nephrol Dial Transplant*. 1999;14:441-443.

Kiss JE, et al. Effective removal of copper by plasma exchange in fulminant Wilson's disease. *Transfusion*. 1998;38:327-331.

Kreymann B, et al. Albumin dialysis: Effective removal of copper in a patient with fulminant Wilson disease and successful bridging to liver transplantation: A new possibility for the elimination of protein-bound toxins. *J Hepatol*. 1999;31:1080-1085.

Kuno T, et al. Severely decompensated abdominal Wilson disease treated with peritoneal dialysis: A case report. *Acta Paediatr Jpn*. 1998;40:85-87.

92.9. Answer: D. Chronic use of D-penicillamine in patients with Wilson disease is associated with worsening neurologic toxicity, TEN, agranulocytosis, and nephrotic syndrome. But with short-term use, the only common serious adverse event is a hypersensitivity reaction, which occurs in 25% of people who are penicillin allergic. This likely occurs from contamination rather than a true allergy.

Herbst D. Detection of penicillin G and ampicillin as contaminants in tetracyclines and penicillamine. *J Pharm Sci*. 1977;66:1646-1648.

Juhlin L, et al. Antibody reactivity in penicillin-sensitive patients determinated with different penicillin derivatives. *Int Arch Allergy Appl Immunol*. 1977;54:19-28.

92.10. Answer: C. Diethyldithiocarbamate chelates copper, which is essential to the activity of dopamine beta-hydroxylase, resulting in less norepinephrine synthesis. Other metals chelated experimentally include nickel, cadmium, thallium, copper, and mercury.

Goldstein M, et al. Inhibition of dopamine beta hydroxylase by disulfiram. *Life Sci*. 1964;3:763-767.

Sunderman FW Sr. Therapeutic properties of sodium diethyldithiocarbamate: its role as an inhibitor in the progression of AIDS. *Ann Clin Lab Sci*. 1991;21:70-81.

Lead

QUESTIONS

93.1. What is the most common adverse health effect observed in adults with chronic lead toxicity?
A. Hypertension
B. Cognitive decline
C. Anemia
D. Peripheral neuropathy
E. Glaucoma

93.2. Which of the following mechanisms best explains how lead toxicity leads to saturnine gout?
A. Binding with oxalate to form crystals
B. Increasing uric acid production
C. Inhibiting protein degradation
D. Decreasing uric acid excretion in the distal renal tubule
E. Increasing cellular destruction

93.3. A 3-year-old child presents to the emergency department after an outpatient screening venous lead concentration returned at 55 mcg/dL (2.65 micromol/L). The child is entirely asymptomatic with a normal examination. Which of the following interventions is indicated in this patient?
A. Succimer
B. Sodium edetate (sodium EDTA)
C. Dimercaprol (BAL) and calcium disodium edetate (Ca Na$_2$EDTA)
D. Penicillamine
E. Routine chelation is not indicated

93.4. Which of the following choices is a manifestation of severe lead toxicity?
A. Metabolic acidosis
B. Hypokalemia
C. Cerebral edema
D. Hypotension
E. Liver failure

93.5. Through which of the following routes is inorganic and metallic lead most efficiently absorbed in adults?
A. Cutaneous
B. Gastrointestinal
C. Pulmonary
D. Ophthalmic
E. Rectal

93.6. A 15-month-old boy presents to the emergency department with vomiting, lethargy, and irritability. He was recently diagnosed with developmental delay. On further history, the mother reveals that they recently remodeled her childhood home. While waiting for blood lead concentrations, what test will strengthen the diagnosis of childhood lead toxicity?
A. Lumbar puncture
B. Liver function tests
C. Computed tomography (CT) scan of the brain
D. Long-bone radiograph
E. Serum creatinine

93.7. Lead interferes with the conversion of which of the following steps in the synthesis of hemoglobin?
   A. Delta-aminolevulinic acid to porphobilinogen
   B. Porphobilinogen to uroporphyrinogen III
   C. Uroporphyrinogen III to delta-aminolevulinic acid
   D. Coproporphyrinogen to delta-aminolevulinic acid
   E. Delta-aminolevulinic acid to coproporphyrinogen

93.8. Dimercaprol (BAL) should be used with caution in patients with which of the following characteristics?
   A. Lead encephalopathy
   B. Hypertension
   C. A urine pH of 8.0
   D. Peanut allergy
   E. Age younger than 1 year

93.9. Which of the following processes will cause a significant rise in blood lead concentrations in patients who have a chronic lead exposure?

   A. Hypothyroidism
   B. Pregnancy
   C. New gunshot wound with a bullet lodged in the soft tissue
   D. Sepsis
   E. Constipation

93.10. A 4-year-old boy presents to the emergency department for further evaluation of an elevated lead concentration. An abdominal radiograph reveals several paint chips in his gastrointestinal tract. Which of the following therapies would be most reasonable to perform next?
   A. Orogastric lavage
   B. Endoscopic removal
   C. Surgical removal
   D. Activated charcoal
   E. Whole bowel irrigation

ANSWERS

93.1. Answer: A. Hypertension is the most prevalent adverse health effect in adults with chronic lead toxicity. The association between elevation in blood pressure and blood lead concentrations is demonstrated in epidemiological and experimental models and follows a dose-response relationship. A systematic review showed an estimated increase of 0.6-1.25 mmHg in systolic blood pressure associated with a two-fold increase in blood lead concentrations.

> Navas-Acien A, et al. Lead exposure and cardiovascular disease—a systematic review. *Environ Health Perspect* 2007;115:472-482.

93.2. Answer: D. Lead competitively decreases uric acid excretion in the distal renal tubule. This results in elevations in blood urate concentrations and in articular urate crystal deposition. In contrast to gouty arthritis not associated with lead, there is a more equal gender ratio and an increased tendency for polyarticular involvement, particularly in the knee. Saturnine gout is also associated with chronic kidney disease.

> Dalvi SR, Pillinger MH. Saturnine gout, redux: A review. *Am J Med.* 2013;126:450.e451-450.e458.

93.3. Answer: A. In addition to source remediation and nutritional support, chelation therapy is recommended for asymptomatic children with blood lead concentrations >45 mcg/dL (2.17 micromol/L). For children without overt symptoms and a concentration up to 69 mcg/dL (3.33 micromol/L), we recommend treatment with succimer

alone. CaNa$_2$EDTA is another reasonable chelator to administer alone but is expensive, requires parenteral administration, and is less well tolerated. Sodium EDTA, however, should not be administered as there is a significant risk of life-threatening hypocalcemia and death. Penicillamine is reserved for patients who have adverse reactions to either succimer or CaNa$_2$EDTA.

> Centers for Disease Control and Prevention. Managing elevated blood lead levels among young children: Recommendations from the Advisory Committee on Childhood Lead Poisoning Prevention. Atlanta, GA: Centers for Disease Control and Prevention; 2002.

> American Academy of Pediatrics Committee on Drugs. Treatment guidelines for lead exposure in children. *Pediatrics.* 1995;96:155-160.

93.4. Answer: C. Patients are at risk of developing encephalopathy from lead poisoning, which leads to intractable seizures, cerebral edema, and coma with resultant herniation.

> Hagelmeyer CD, et al. Fatal lead encephalopathy following foreign body ingestion: Case report. *J Emerg Med.* 1988;6:397-400.

93.5. Answer: C. Pulmonary absorption of lead (mostly in the occupational setting) is about 30-40% of exposed lead, while gastrointestinal (GI) absorption is 10-15% in nonfasting adults. GI absorption in children is 4-5 times as much as in adults. Respiratory absorption occurs quickly and is dependent on both minute ventilation and the concentration of airborne lead. Thus, an individual engaging in vigorous physical activity will absorb considerably more then when at rest. Ophthalmic, rectal, and cutaneous absorption are limited.

Agency for Toxic Substances and Disease Registry. *The Nature and Extent of Lead Poisoning in Children in the United States: A Report to Congress.* Atlanta, GA: Agency for Toxic Substances and Disease Registry; 1988.

93.6. Answer: D. The presence of "lead lines" on radiographs of long bones is suggestive of lead toxicity while waiting for concentrations. The bands of increased metaphyseal density represent increased calcium deposition and not lead deposition. Lead inhibits osteoclastic remodeling but does not affect osteoblastic action. Lumbar puncture should be avoided due to concern of increased intracranial pressure from cerebral edema in lead encephalopathy. Significant liver toxicity does not typically occur in patients with lead toxicity. A CT scan of the head occasionally shows signs of encephalopathy, but this is not specific for lead. An elevated creatinine occasionally occurs, but it is also a nonspecific finding.

Gandi D, et al. Lead lines. *Lancet.* 2003;362:197.

93.7. Answer: A. Lead prevents the conversion of delta-aminolevulinic acid (ALA) to porphobilinogen and the conversion of coproporphyrinogen III to protoporphyrin IX by blocking the action of ALA dehydratase and coproporphyrinogen decarboxylase. This in turn causes ALA and coproporphyrin to accumulate in the urine where they serve as "markers" for lead poisoning. Lead also blocks ferrochelatase from incorporating iron into protoporphyrin to form heme, which causes protoporphyrin to accumulate in the red blood cells. Lead also inhibits the transport of iron across mitochondrial membranes in maturing normoblasts in the bone marrow, contributing to the accumulation of protoporphyrin.

Schwartz BS, Hu H. Adult lead exposure: Time for change. *Environ Health Perspect.* 2007;115:451-454.

93.8. Answer: D. Dimercaprol (BAL) is formulated in peanut oil; therefore, patients should be asked about a known peanut allergy, and a risk-benefit analysis is indicated. Severe lead toxicity is an indication to treat with BAL. BAL should precede the first dose of CaNa$_2$EDTA by 4 hours to prevent redistribution of lead to the central nervous system. Age and hypertension are not contraindications to administer BAL. Alkalinization of the urine with parenteral sodium bicarbonate is recommended to prevent liberation of the metal from the chelated complex.

Committee on Drugs. Treatment guidelines for lead exposure in children. *Pediatrics.* 1995;96:155-160.

BAL in oil ampules (dimercaprol injection USP) [package insert]. Decatur, IL: Taylor Pharmaceuticals; 2006.

93.9. Answer: B. Bone lead is mobilized and contributes to as much as 50% of the blood lead content at times when rapid bone turnover occurs, such as pregnancy, lactation, in patients with osteoporosis, and in children with immobilization.

Silbergeld EK, et al. Lead and osteoporosis: Mobilization of lead from bone in post-menopausal women. *Environ Res.* 1988;47:79-94.

Markowitz ME, Weinberger HL. Immobilization-related lead toxicity in previously lead-poisoned children. *Pediatrics.* 1990;86:455-457.

93.10. Answer: E. We recommend prompt institution of whole bowel irrigation for patients who have a large burden of paint chips on abdominal imaging. If the lead foreign body is a fish sinker, bullet, or curtain weight, patients are at risk of developing significantly elevated blood lead concentrations within 24 hours of ingestion. These patients should have prompt endoscopic removal of any gastric foreign bodies. If the foreign body is past the stomach and in the small bowel, a trial of whole bowel irrigation or a bulk laxative is reasonable. If there is delayed passage or rapidly rising blood lead concentrations, then endoscopic or surgical removal is recommended. There is no indication to administer activated charcoal if the ingestion is solely paint chips.

Fergusson L, et al. Lead foreign body ingestion in children. *J Paediatr Child Health.* 1997;33:542-544.

McKinney PE. Acute elevation of blood lead levels within hours of ingestion of large quantities of lead shot. *J Toxicol Clin Toxicol.* 2000;38:435-440.

Manganese

QUESTIONS

94.1. Welders chronically exposed to ferromanganese metals develop which of the following disorders?
A. Cardiomyopathy
B. Chronic kidney disease
C. Aplastic anemia
D. Chronic obstructive pulmonary disease
E. Parkinsonism

94.2. Which of the following disorders increases the risk of manganese toxicity?
A. Kidney disease
B. Liver disease
C. Asthma
D. Congestive heart failure
E. Psoriasis

94.3. Manganese accumulates in which area of the central nervous system?
A. Frontal cortex
B. Temporal lobes
C. Cerebellum
D. Basal ganglia
E. Brain stem

94.4. Manganese exposure in the central nervous system is best assessed using which of the following diagnostic modalities?
A. Noncontrast computed tomography
B. Contrast computed tomography
C. T1-weighted magnetic resonance imaging
D. T2-weighted magnetic resonance imaging
E. Electroencephalogram

94.5. Dietary deficiency of which of the following nutrients increases manganese absorption?
A. Iron
B. Copper
C. Zinc
D. Calcium
E. Magnesium

94.6. Which of the following laboratory tests is recommended to confirm an acute manganese exposure?
A. Hair manganese concentration
B. Serum or plasma manganese concentration
C. Whole blood manganese concentration
D. 24-hour urine manganese concentration
E. 24-hour fecal manganese concentration

94.7. Which of the following genetic abnormalities increases the risk of manganese toxicity?
A. Alpha-1-antitrypsin deficiency
B. SLC30A10 transporter mutation
C. Glucose-6-phosphate dehydrogenase (G6PD) deficiency
D. SLC19A3 genetic deficiency
E. SCN1A mutation

94.8. A 37-year-old man presents to the hospital following an intentional ingestion of potassium permanganate. Which of the following clinical effects is expected first?
A. Stridor
B. Aplastic anemia
C. Dilated cardiomyopathy
D. Parkinsonian tremor
E. Alopecia

94.9. A 22-year-old woman visits a naturopathic office and is given an injection of manganese chloride instead of magnesium chloride. Which of the following therapies would be reasonable to use to enhance manganese elimination?

   A. Hemodialysis
   B. Cholestyramine
   C. Succimer
   D. Calcium disodium edetate (Ca_2Na_2EDTA)
   E. *N*-Acetylcysteine

94.10. A 52-year-old-man develops symptoms consistent with a chronic occupational exposure to manganese. Which of the following therapies is demonstrated to improve the outcome in patients with manganese toxicity?

   A. Levodopa/carbidopa
   B. Cholestyramine
   C. Succimer
   D. Selegiline
   E. None of the above

ANSWERS

94.1. Answer: E. Welders with chronic occupational exposure to manganese develop neurologic manifestations consistent with parkinsonism. The association between manganese and parkinsonism was first described in the 1800s and is well documented in miners and other occupations with poor industrial hygiene.

> Josephs KA, et al. Neurologic manifestations in welders with pallidal MRI T1 hyperintensity. *Neurology.* 2005;64:2033-2039.

> Couper J. On the effects of black oxide of manganese when inhaled into the lungs. *Br Ann Med Pharmacol.* 1837;1:41-42.

> Schuler P, et al. Manganese poisoning; environmental and medical study at a Chilean mine. *Ind Med Surg.* 1957;26:167-173.

94.2. Answer: B. Manganese accumulates in patients with liver dysfunction who are undergoing total parenteral nutrition. This is also described in patients with severe liver disease and normal dietary manganese intake.

> Fell JME, et al. Manganese toxicity in children receiving long-term parenteral nutrition. *Lancet.* 1996;347:1218-1221.

> Masumoto K, et al. Manganese intoxication during intermittent parenteral nutrition: Report of two cases. *JPEN J Parenter Enteral Nutr.* 2016;25:95-99.

> Nagatomo S, et al. Manganese intoxication during total parenteral nutrition: Report of two cases and review of the literature. *J Neurol Sci.* 1999;162:102-105.

> Rose C, et al. Manganese deposition in basal ganglia structures results from both portal-systemic shunting and liver dysfunction. *Gastroenterology.* 1999;117:640-644.

94.3. Answer: D. Manganese accumulates in the basal ganglia and, more specifically, at the level of the globus pallidus.

> Josephs KA, et al. Neurologic manifestations in welders with pallidal MRI T1 hyperintensity. *Neurology.* 2005;64:2033-2039.

> Arjona A, et al. Diagnosis of chronic manganese intoxication by magnetic resonance imaging. *N Engl J Med.* 1997;336:964-965.

94.4. Answer: C. T1-weighted magnetic resonance imaging (MRI) characteristically shows hyperintensity in the basal ganglia at the level of the globus pallidus, representing manganese accumulation. These findings are, unfortunately, not well correlated with clinical manifestations of toxicity. The substantia nigra findings in patients with Parkinson disease are best demonstrated with T2-weighted MRI.

> Arjona A, et al. Diagnosis of chronic manganese intoxication by magnetic resonance imaging. *N Engl J Med.* 1997;336:964-965.

> Nagatomo S, et al. Manganese intoxication during total parenteral nutrition: Report of two cases and review of the literature. *J Neurol Sci.* 1999;162:102-105.

94.5. Answer: A. Iron deficiency is associated with an increase in manganese absorption from the gastrointestinal tract. Iron defficiency also increases lead absorption.

> Finley JW. Manganese absorption and retention by young women is associated with serum ferritin concentration. *Am J Clin Nutr.* 1999;70:37-43.

94.6. Answer: C. The best test to confirm an exposure to manganese is a whole blood concentration, although concentrations do not correlate with symptoms. Unfortunately, following an acute exposure, manganese rapidly leaves the blood and distributes into other compartments. There is no role for the routine use of the other diagnostic modalities listed here. Although urine manganese elimination will increase with provocative testing, this does not correlate with body burden.

Spencer A. Whole blood manganese levels in pregnancy and the neonate. *Nutrition.* 1999;15:731-734.

Bader M, et al. Biomonitoring of manganese in blood, urine and axillary hair following low-dose exposure during the manufacture of dry cell batteries. *Int Arch Occup Environ Health.* 1999;72:521-527.

Laohaudomchok W, et al. Toenail, blood and urine as biomarkers of occupational exposure to manganese. *Epidemiology.* 2011;22:S93-S94.

94.7. Answer: B. A defect in the SLC30A10 transporter allows manganese to accumulate in the central nervous system and predisposes individuals to clinical toxicity despite relatively low-level exposures. Alpha-1-antitrypsin deficiency is associated with early pulmonary disease and is not related to manganese. G6PD deficiency is responsible for hemolysis on exposure to oxidant stress. An SLC19A3 genetic deficiency impairs thiamine transport and is associated with Wernicke encephalopathy despite normal dietary intake. The SCN1A mutation is responsible for congenital epilepsy.

Peres TV, et al. Manganese-induced neurotoxicity: A review of its behavioral consequences and neuroprotective strategies. *BMC Pharmacol Toxicol.* 2016;17:57.

94.8. Answer: A. Potassium permanganate is a potent oxidizer that is often fatal following a small ingestion of either crystals or solution. Immediate effects include stridor and gastrointestinal burns. Subsequently, cardiovascular collapse, liver and kidney failure, and central nervous system toxicity are all reported.

Young RJ, et al. Fatal acute hepatorenal failure following potassium permanganate ingestion. *Hum Exp Toxicol.* 2016;15:259-261.

94.9. Answer: D. Unfortunately, the ability to enhance the elimination of manganese is limited. Despite hepatic clearance, there is no good support for either *N*-acetylcysteine or bile salt binding therapies such as cholestyramine. Data suggest that hemodialysis and succimer are both futile. There is support for the use of calcium disodium edetate but its effect on clinical symptoms is unclear at best.

Angle CR. Dimercaptosuccinic acid (DMSA): Negligible effect on manganese in urine and blood. *Occup Environ Med.* 1995;52:846.

Herrero Hernandez E, et al. Follow-up of patients affected by manganese-induced Parkinsonism after treatment with CaNa2EDTA. *Neurotoxicology.* 2006;27:333-339.

Hines EQ, et al. Massive intravenous manganese overdose due to compounding error: minimal role for hemodialysis. *Clin Toxicol (Phila).* 2016;54:523-525.

Stepens A, et al. A Parkinsonian syndrome in methcathinone users and the role of manganese. *N Engl J Med.* 2008;358:1009-1017.

94.10. Answer: E. While there is support for the use of Ca_2Na_2EDTA to enhance elimination, there is no controlled evidence to suggest that any therapy improves survival. Experience with antiparkinsonian therapies suggests limited, if any, benefit. It is reasonable to supplement iron in patients with iron deficiency and to terminate exposure, when possible, but the overall prognosis for recovery is poor once neurotoxicity manifests.

Stepens A, et al. A Parkinsonian syndrome in methcathinone users and the role of manganese. *N Engl J Med.* 2008;358:1009-1017.

95

Mercury

QUESTIONS

95.1. The Minamata Bay disaster was caused by water contamination from a vinyl chloride plant. What compound was implicated in this mass poisoning?
A. Mercuric sulfide
B. Mercuric chloride
C. Phosgene
D. Hydrogen chloride
E. Methylmercury

95.2. A 22-year-old man calls the poison control center because he broke a mercury thermometer purchased at an antique store. What is the best way to clean up the spill?
A. Call the local HAZMAT team
B. Vacuum the spill
C. Dry with paper towels and then flush the paper towels down the toilet
D. Pour sand onto the mercury and sweep it into a tightly sealed container
E. Dilute the spill with water and then mop up the spill

95.3. In the early 1900s, children who received a teething powder developed an erythematous, edematous, hyperkeratotic, pink papular rash. The rash was associated with irritability, insomnia, and decreased deep tendon reflexes. Which of the following substances led to the development of these symptoms?
A. Calamine
B. Methylene chloride
C. Mercuric sulfide
D. Mercurous chloride
E. Sucrose and water

95.4. Organic mercury poisoning from methylmercury and dimethylmercury affects which part of the brain?
A. Basal ganglia
B. Cerebellum
C. Mammillary bodies
D. Frontal lobe
E. Pituitary gland

95.5. A 26-year-old woman presents to the emergency department with 1 week of lower extremity swelling. She recently traveled to the United States from China. Her urinalysis demonstrates 4+ protein. On further history, the patient states that she has been using a skin-whitening cream for the past 8 months. What metal is likely found in this cream?
A. Lead
B. Chromium
C. Lithium
D. Mercury
E. Fluoride

95.6. Hematemesis is most closely associated with which of the following forms of mercury poisoning?
A. Elemental mercury
B. Methylmercury
C. Mercuric chloride
D. Mercurous chloride
E. Phenylmercury

95.7. Which of the following clinical presentations is most characteristic of chronic inorganic mercury intoxication?
  A. Irritability, tremor, ataxia
  B. Irritability, morbilliform rash, respiratory distress
  C. Anorexia, tunnel vision, kidney failure
  D. Anorexia, respiratory distress, ataxia
  E. Irritability, anorexia, hematochezia

95.8. Which of the following statements is true regarding the pharmacokinetic properties of mercury?
  A. Methylmercury is poorly absorbed in the gastrointestinal tract
  B. Inhalation is the most common route of mercuric chloride intoxication
  C. Absorbed elemental mercury is methylated to form methylmercury in the central nervous system
  D. Methoxyethylmercury is cleaved shortly following absorption to release the inorganic mercury ion
  E. The excretion of mercuric ions is predominantly fecal, with a total-body half-life of 30-60 days

95.9. Which of the following chelators is recommended in the treatment of methylmercury toxicity?
  A. Dimercaprol (BAL)
  B. Dimercaptosuccinic acid (DMSA)
  C. D-Penicillamine
  D. Calcium disodium edetate
  E. Deferoxamine

95.10. Which of the following options is correct regarding mercury analysis?
  A. Acceptable maximum blood and urine concentrations of mercury compounds are well established
  B. Toxic blood and urine concentrations of mercury compounds are well established
  C. Analysis of hair for mercury provides an accurate predictor of total-body inorganic mercury load
  D. Urine mercury concentrations are useful in confirming exposure and monitoring efficacy of therapy
  E. Stool analysis provides an accurate estimate of total-body methylmercury load

ANSWERS

95.1. Answer: E. In the 1940s, an epidemic of mercury poisoning occurred in Minamata Bay, Japan. Methylmercury accumulated in the marine life and poisoned the local fishing community along with surrounding wildlife. Thousands were poisoned; as a result, the disease is now renamed Minamata disease. Polyvinyl chloride, when thermally degraded, produces hydrogen chloride and phosgene; however, neither causes Minamata disease.

Powell P. Minamata disease: A story of mercury's malevolence. *South Med J.* 1991;84:1352-1358.

Stefanidou M, et al. Health impacts of fire smoke inhalation. *Inhal Toxicol.* 2008;20:761-766.

Borak J, Diller WF. Phosgene exposure: Mechanisms of injury and treatment strategies. *J Occup Environ Med.* 2001;43:110-119.

95.2. Answer: D. Elemental mercury should be removed from hard surfaces by pouring sand onto the spill and then sweeping it into a tightly sealed container. Vacuuming should be avoided as it aerosolizes the mercury. HAZMAT does not need to be contacted for simple elemental mercury spills.

Caldwell KL, et al. Total blood mercury concentrations in the U.S. population: 1999–2006. *Int J Hyg Environ Health.* 2009;212:588-598.

95.3. Answer: D. Children who were exposed to mercurous chloride–containing teething powder in the early 1900s developed an idiosyncratic hypersensitivity to mercury ions, resulting in acrodynia (pink, dusky appearance to the hands and feet that is painful) and neurologic symptoms. The children had a complete recovery once the exposure was removed. Acrodynia is still rarely reported today following other mercury exposures.

Warkany J, Hubbard DM. Adverse mercurial reactions in the form of acrodynia and related conditions. *AMA Am J Dis Child.* 1951;81:335-373.

Black J. The puzzle of pink disease. *J R Soc Med.* 1999;92:478-481.

Ahmed AE, et al. Halogenated methanes: Metabolism and toxicity. *Fed Proc.* 1980;39:3150-3155.

95.4. Answer: B. While methylmercury and dimethylmercury cause diffuse brain atrophy, the cerebellum is affected the most. The characteristic pathologic findings in methylmercury poisoning manifest clinically as visual constriction and ataxia.

Korogi Y, et al. MR findings in seven patients with organic mercury poisoning (Minamata disease). *AJNR Am J Neuroradiol.* 1994;15:1575-1578.

Siegler RW, et al. Fatal poisoning from liquid dimethylmercury: A neuropathologic study. *Hum Pathol.* 1999;30:720-723.

95.5. Answer: D. Chronic toxicity from inorganic mercury results in nephrotic syndrome and lower extremity swelling. Mercury-containing skin-whitening creams are not legal in the United States but are available internationally.

Sin KW, Tsang HS. Large-scale mercury exposure due to a cream cosmetic: Community-wide case series. *Hong Kong Med J.* 2003;9:329-334.

95.6. Answer: C. Caustic gastroenteritis is characteristic of the inorganic salts of mercury, in particular, mercuric chloride. Mercurous chloride is less soluble and therefore less well absorbed than mercuric chloride.

Troen P, et al. Mercuric bichloride poisoning. *N Engl J Med.* 1951; 244:459-463.

95.7. Answer: A. This triad is characteristic of chronic or subacute inorganic mercury poisoning. While anorexia, visual field constriction ("tunnel vision"), and acrodynia (morbilliform rash) are also findings in chronic inorganic mercury poisoning, respiratory distress, kidney failure, and hematochezia are not.

Mortensen ME, et al. Elemental mercury poisoning in a household. *MMWR.* 1990;39:424-425.

Taueg C, et al. Acute and chronic poisoning from residential exposures to elemental mercury—Michigan, 1989–1990. *J Toxicol Clin Toxicol.* 1992;30:63-67.

95.8. Answer: D. Methoxyethylmercury, a long chain alkyl organic compound, undergoes cleavage shortly following absorption to release the inorganic mercuric ion. Therefore, after absorption, this compound has clinical manifestations like the inorganic mercury compounds. Methylmercury is well absorbed from the gut (approximately 90%). The excretion of inorganic mercury is predominantly renal.

Klaassen C. Heavy metals and heavy-metal antagonists. In: Gilman AG, et al, eds. *Goodman & Gilman's The Pharmacological Basis of Therapeutics.* 8th ed. New York, NY: Pergamon Press; 1990:1592-1614.

Magos L. Mercury. In: Seiler HG, Sigel H, eds. *Handbook on Toxicity of Inorganic Compounds.* New York, NY: Marcel Dekker; 1988:419-436.

95.9. Answer: B. The neurotoxicity of methylmercury is relatively resistant to treatment. Dimercaptosuccinic acid was superior to penicillamine and dimercaptopropanesulfonic acid (DMPS) in reducing brain mercury in mice poisoned with methylmercury.

Aaseth J, Friedheim EAH. Treatment of methyl mercury poisoning in mice with 2,3-dimercaptosuccinic acid and other complexing thiols. *Acta Pharmacol Toxicol.* 1978;42:248-252.

95.10. Answer: D. Urine and blood mercury concentrations are not well established to confirm or exclude toxicity. However, they are useful in confirming exposure and monitoring treatment efficacy. Hair analysis is similarly useful for analyzing exposure to organic mercury.

Rosenman KD, et al. Sensitive indicators of inorganic mercury toxicity. *Arch Environ Health.* 1986;41:208-215.

Suzuki T, et al. The hair–organ relationship in mercury concentration in contemporary Japanese. *Arch Environ Health.* 1993;48:221-229.

Nickel

QUESTIONS

96.1. Nickel carbonyl is formed by the reaction of nickel with which of the following options?
A. Water
B. Carbon dioxide
C. Carbon monoxide
D. Benzene
E. Phenol

96.2. A 23-year-old woman presents to the emergency department with a rash around her ear lobes that corresponds to nickel earrings she was wearing. What type of hypersensitivity did she develop?
A. Type I
B. Type II
C. Type III
D. Type IV
E. Type V

96.3. In the patient in Question 96.2 who presents with dermatitis, which of the following therapies is recommended?
A. Epinephrine
B. Oral corticosteroids
C. Topical corticosteroids
D. Icatibant
E. Transexemic acid

96.4. A 34-year-old man is brought into the emergency department directly from his work site, a petroleum processing plant, because he developed severe shortness of breath. A radiograph performed demonstrates findings consistent with acute respiratory distress syndrome (ARDS). During his evaluation, he has a generalized tonic-clonic seizure and has a decline in his mental status. Which of the following xenobiotics would be the best chelator to add to his management?
A. Diethyldithiocarbamate
B. Calcium disodium edetate
C. Dimercaprol
D. D-Penicillamine
E. Succimer

96.5. In patients receiving chelation therapy for nickel carbonyl toxicity, which of the following should they avoid?
A. Metoclopramide
B. Rocuronium
C. Propofol
D. Aged chese
E. Ethanol

96.6. Which of the following symptoms occurs most commonly in nickel carbonyl poisoning?
A. Chest pain
B. Abdominal pain
C. Somnolence
D. Fever
E. Dyspnea

96.7. In patients who survive nickel carbonyl poisoning, which of the following options is the most common sequela?
A. Parkinsonism
B. Neurasthenic syndrome
C. Trigeminal neuralgia
D. Bilateral facial nerve palsy
E. Alopecia

96.8. Which of the following options is the primary route of elimination of absorbed nickel?
A. Pulmonary
B. Gastrointestinal
C. Kidney
D. Skin
E. Hepatic

96.9. A 67-year-old man presented to the emergency department following an acute parenteral exposure to nickel. This occurred at his dialysis center where water was heated through a nickel-plated tank. Which of the following symptoms would you expect him to develop?
A. Headache
B. Cough
C. Shortness of breath
D. Hemoptysis
E. Dermatitis

96.10. An 18-year-old woman presents to the emergency department with a widespread, systemic dermatitis. Ingestion of which of the following metals led to this rash?
A. Aluminum
B. Nickel
C. Iron
D. Lead
E. Barium

ANSWERS

96.1. Answer: C. Nickel carbonyl is a highly volatile and dangerous nickel compound that occurs when nickel reacts with carbon monoxide. It is used as a chemical reagent in nickel refining and petroleum processing.

Sunderman FW. A pilgrimage into the archives of nickel toxicology. *Ann Clin Lab Sci.* 1989;19:1–16.

96.2. Answer: D. By far, the most common toxicity associated with nickel is dermatitis. The allergic reaction caused by nickel is a type IV delayed hypersensitivity reaction. Nickel allergies are the most frequent positive results on allergen skin-patch testing.

Lu LK, et al. Prevention of nickel allergy: The case for regulation? *Dermatol Clin.* 2009;27:155-161.

96.3. Answer: C. In patients who present with a contact dermatitis caused by nickel, the mainstay of therapy is to avoid future exposure. Topical corticosteroids and oral antihistamines are used in the acute management.

Saito M, et al. Molecular mechanisms of nickel allergy. *Int J Mol Sci.* 2016;17:202.

96.4. Answer: A. Diethyldithiocarbamate (DDC) is the chelator that is recommended in the treatment of patients poisoned by nickel carbonyl. Calcium disodium edetate has no protective effect. While dimercaprol and D-penicillamine demonstrated some benefit in rats, they are not currently the chelators of choice.

Bradberry SM, Vale JA. Therapeutic review: Do diethyldithiocarbamate and disulfiram have a role in acute nickel carbonyl poisoning? *J Toxicol Clin Toxicol.* 1999;37:259-264.

96.5. Answer: E. Diethyldithiocarbamate (DDC) is the current chelator of choice in the treatment of nickel carbonyl. Diethyldithiocarbamate leads to a disulfiram reaction, and therefore, patients should be counseled to avoid drinking ethanol while receiving this therapy.

Sunderman FW Sr. The treatment of acute nickel carbonyl poisoning with sodium diethyldithiocarbamate. *Ann Clin Res.* 1971;3:182-185.

96.6. Answer: A. While all the listed findings occur in nickel carbonyl poisoning, chest pain is the most common symptom, occurring in 67% of patients. Abdominal pain occurs in 1.7%, somnolence in 5.1%, fever in 6.7%, and dyspnea in 8.9% of patients.

Shi ZC. Acute nickel carbonyl poisoning: A report of 179 cases. *Br J Ind Med.* 1986;43:422-424.

96.7. Answer: B. Neurasthenic syndrome resembles chronic fatigue syndrome and consists of symptoms that include fatigue, headache, anxiety, and depressed mood. While most survivors of nickel carbonyl poisoning recover completely, some patients develop this syndrome.

> Shi ZC. Acute nickel carbonyl poisoning: A report of 179 cases. *Br J Ind Med.* 1986;43:422-424.

96.8. Answer: C. While most nickel is excreted through the gastrointestinal tract, this reflects unabsorbed nickel. When the nickel is absorbed, it is excreted primarily through the kidneys.

> Sunderman FW Jr, et al. Nickel absorption and kinetics in human volunteers. *Proc Soc Exp Biol Med.* 1989;191:5-11.

96.9. Answer: A. Patients exposed to parenteral nickel develop symptoms similar to nickel carbonyl toxicity. The main difference, however, is that patients exposed to isolated nickel do not develop any respiratory complaints.

> Webster JD, et al. Acute nickel intoxication by dialysis. *Ann Intern Med.* 1980;92:631-633.

96.10. Answer: B. While nickel is one of the most common causes of a local dermatitis, the secondary form involves a more widespread dermatitis. This degree of dermatitis occurs when nickel is either ingested or inhaled.

> Rahilly G, Price N. Nickel allergy and orthodontics. *J Orthod.* 2003; 30:171-174.

Selenium

97.1. Selenium is an essential trace element in the human diet. It serves as an important cofactor for which enzyme?
A. Glutathione peroxidase
B. Alcohol dehydrogenase
C. Aconitase
D. Succinate dehydrogenase
E. ATP synthase

97.2. In 1979, Keshan disease was first described in China in an area where selenium deficiency was endemic. Which of the following clinical presentations is associated with Keshan disease?
A. Sensory neuropathy
B. Kidney toxicity
C. Liver toxicity
D. Cardiomyopathy
E. Aplastic anemia

97.3. A 6-year-old girl is given a nutritional supplement containing selenium. Although intended to contain 7 mcg/mL, this unregulated supplement contains 800 mcg/mL. What finding would you expect to see on this child's nails?
A. Photoonycholysis
B. Mees lines
C. Clubbing
D. Black discoloration
E. Subungual hematoma

97.4. Which of the following options best compares the toxicity of acute elemental selenium exposure to that of selenium ion?
A. Greater risk of cardiotoxicity
B. Greater risk of hemorrhagic gastritis
C. Greater risk of hemolysis
D. Greater risk of death
E. Acute exposure to elemental selenium is nontoxic

97.5. A 2-year-old boy presents to the emergency department 1 hour after ingesting gun bluing solution. He appears critically ill and immediately vomits on arrival. What odor would you expect?
A. Rotting fish
B. Pears
C. Garlic
D. Chloroformlike
E. Freshly mown hay

97.6. You are in the emergency department taking care of the patient in Question 97.5, who ingested gun bluing solution. The patient is hypotensive with a metabolic acidosis, hemolysis, and an elevated creatine phosphokinase. Which of the following therapies would be reasonable to be performed next?
A. Chelation with dimercaprol
B. Nasogastric lavage
C. *N*-Acetylcysteine
D. Chelation with succimer
E. Chelation with calcium disodium edetate

97.7. A 34-year-old woman with a history of schizophrenia presents to an outpatient clinic for further evaluation of brittle hair and nails. She ate a diet primarily consisting of brazil nuts for 3 months. You suspect chronic selenium toxicity. Which of the following sources would be the most appropriate to use to test for confirmation?
A. Urine
B. Hair
C. Serum
D. Whole blood
E. Skin biopsy

97.8. Although not currently recommended for the treatment of selenium toxicity in humans, which other metal increases the biliary excretion of selenium?
A. Bismuth
B. Copper
C. Thallium
D. Cesium
E. Arsenic

97.9. A 32-year-old man presents to the emergency department following exposure to hydrogen selenide gas at his workplace. He has a cough and shortness of breath. A chest radiograph is performed and is normal. Which of the following outcomes is to be expected in this patient?
A. Progression to acute respiratory distress syndrome (ARDS)
B. Cerebral edema and death
C. Mesothelioma
D. Long-term reactive airway disease
E. No long-term toxicity

97.10. Selenium is generated through electrolytic copper refining and is also used in the rubber, paper, waste, and fossil fuel industries. Workers chronically exposed to selenium develop which of the following symptoms?
A. Eyelid dermatitis
B. Changes to iris color
C. Blackened tongue
D. Angioedema
E. Dysphagia

ANSWERS

97.1. Answer: A. In patients who are selenium deficient, glutathione peroxidase activity in whole blood is decreased. Glutathione peroxidase catalyzes the conversion of hydrogen peroxide to water. Both glutathione and selenium are essential for this conversion.

> Barceloux DG. Selenium. *J Toxicol Clin Toxicol*. 1999;37:146-172.

97.2. Answer: D. Keshan disease is an endemic cardiomyopathy in China that affects patients in rural areas who ingest a selenium-poor diet. Patients with Keshan disease develop cardiogenic shock, dysrhythmias, and pulmonary edema.

> Ge K, et al. Keshan disease—an endemic cardiomyopathy in China. *Virchows Arch*. 1983;401:1-15.

97.3. Answer: B. Although selenium is a nonmetal, its toxicity resembles heavy metal toxicity. While Mees lines typically occur in heavy metal toxicity, they also occur with selenosis as selenium is substituted for sulfur in keratin proteins. Selenosis also produces brittleness and yellow nail discoloration.

> Webb A, Kerns W. What is the origin of these nail changes in an otherwise healthy young patient? *J Med Toxicol*. 2009;5:39-40.

97.4. Answer: E. Elemental selenium following an acute exposure does not produce toxicity. Chronic exposure to elemental selenium, however, produces toxicity. In comparison, acute overdoses of selenite and selenious acid both cause severe toxicity.

> Nantel AJ, et al. Acute poisoning by selenious acid. *Vet Hum Toxicol*. 1985;27:531-533.

97.5. Answer: C. Gun bluing solution contains primarily selenious acid and, occasionally, nitric acid and copper nitrate. Selenious acid is caustic and results in vomiting, abdominal pain, and burns of the esophagus and stomach. Vomit that contains selenious acid has a garlic odor.

> Nantel AJ, et al. Acute poisoning by selenious acid. *Vet Hum Toxicol*. 1985;27:531-533.

97.6. Answer: B. Gun bluing solution contains selenious acid and leads to severe toxicity within 1 hour, which rapidly progresses to death. While there are limited data to support gastrointestinal decontamination following a gun bluing solution overdose, given the lack of antidotal therapy, gastrointestinal decontamination should be emphasized to reduce exposure. As selenious acid is caustic in nature, judicious use of a small nasogastric lavage would be reasonable and is preferred over larger orogastric tubes. Chelation with dimercaprol, calcium disodium edetate, or succimer is not advised because they form nephrotoxic complexes with selenium and exacerbate toxicity. There is no indication for *N*-acetylcysteine in the treatment of selenious acid at this time.

Kise Y, et al. Acute oral selenium intoxication with ten times the lethal dose resulting in deep gastric ulcer. *J Emerg Med*. 2004;26:183-187.

97.7. Answer: D. In chronic selenium exposure, selenium is incorporated into red blood cells and other proteins. Therefore, whole blood is the most appropriate method of testing. This is in comparison to acute exposures, which are best evaluated with serum. Selenium is found in the urine within the first 4 hours of exposure, but its concentration is affected by hydration.

Nuttall KL. Evaluating selenium poisoning. *Ann Clin Lab Sci*. 2006; 36:406-420.

97.8. Answer: E. Arsenical compounds, such as arsenite, increase the biliary elimination of selenium 10-fold. However, given the toxicity of arsenic, addition of arsenical compounds for the purpose of treatment of selenium toxicity is not recommended.

Levander OA. Metabolic interrelationships and adaptations in selenium toxicity. *Ann N Y Acad Sci*. 1972;192:181-192.

97.9. Answer: D. Hydrogen selenide gas causes respiratory irritation. Like hydrogen sulfide, hydrogen selenide produces olfactory fatigue, which poses a risk of a higher dose of exposure. Respiratory symptoms that occur after exposure to hydrogen selenide last several days, with some patients progressing to long-term reactive airway disease.

Schecter A, et al. Acute hydrogen selenide inhalation. *Chest*. 1980; 77:554-555.

97.10. Answer: A. Patients chronically exposed to dermal selenium develop erythematous eyelid edema and inflammation. This is coined "rose eye." Patients also develop conjunctivitis, dental decay, yellow skin discoloration, and nail abnormalities. Direct ocular exposure to selenium causes a conjunctival burn.

Holness DL, et al. Health status of copper refinery workers with specific reference to selenium exposure. *Arch Environ Health*. 1989;44:291-297.

QUESTIONS

98.1. Which of the following statements is consistent with the US Food and Drug Administration (FDA)'s final rule on the use of nonprescription drugs that contain colloidal silver or silver salts?
A. They are not recognized as safe and effective and are therefore misbranded
B. There is limited evidence of benefit and no evidence of harm
C. More data are necessary to define appropriate therapeutic indications
D. Because of some evidence of harm, they should be restricted to very narrow therapeutic indications
E. They are overtly harmful and therefore prohibited

98.2. Which of the following options is the most common complication of chronic silver ingestion in humans?
A. Kidney injury
B. Liver injury
C. Cardiac injury
D. Bone marrow toxicity
E. Skin pigmentation

98.3. Which of the following options best describes the pathophysiology of argyria?
A. An acute and chronic inflammatory reaction
B. Increased melanin production
C. Direct deposition of silver in the tissue
D. Silver-induced selenium deficiency
E. Increased melanin production and direct deposition of silver in the tissue

98.4. Which of the following treatments is currently recommended in patients with argyria?
A. Oral selenium supplementation
B. Chelation with succimer
C. Topical hydroquinone and sunscreens
D. Oral vitamin E
E. Oral sulfur supplementation

98.5. Following cessation of exposure, how long will serum concentrations of silver remain elevated in patients with argyria?
A. 3 days
B. 3 weeks
C. 3 months
D. 3 years
E. >30 years

98.6. Which of the following abnormalities occurs following large chronic exposures to silver?
A. Abnormal taste
B. Abnormal smell
C. Abnormal balance
D. Abnormal gait
E. All of the above

98.7. Which of the following complaints is the most common in workers exposed to greater than acceptable silver oxide concentrations for prolonged periods of time?
A. Abdominal pain
B. Impaired hearing
C. Upper respiratory tract irritation
D. Lower respiratory tract irritation
E. Impaired taste

98.8. In addition to silver, which of the following xenobiotics causes a slate-gray skin discoloration?
   A. Furosemide
   B. Amiodarone
   C. Tetracycline
   D. Procainamide
   E. Disulfiram

98.9. The use of silver in cement for hip arthroplasty is associated with which of the following adverse effects?
   A. Disseminated argyria
   B. Peripheral neuropathy
   C. Acute kidney injury
   D. Myocarditis
   E. Systemic embolization

98.10. Kidney injury from silver is rarely reported. Which of the following kidney lesions is documented in humans?
   A. Interstitial nephritis
   B. Minimal change disease
   C. Membranoproliferative glomerulonephritis
   D. Acute tubular necrosis
   E. Renal papillary necrosis

ANSWERS

98.1. Answer: A. In 1999, the US FDA issued its final rule on nonprescription drugs containing colloidal silver or silver salts using this exact wording: "They are not recognized as safe and effective and are therefore misbranded." Silver is still available in devices as an antibacterial, topically in burn creams, and in the dietary supplement market, which has protections against FDA regulations.

Food and Drug Administration. *FDA Issues Final Rule on OTC Drug Products Containing Colloidal Silver*. Rockville, MD: US Department of Health and Human Services, Food and Drug Administration; August 17, 1999.

98.2. Answer: E. Argyria causes a blue-gray discoloration of the skin, which is the most common manifestation of silver ingestion in humans. Although other organ toxicities are reported, they are distinctly uncommon.

Gettler AO, et al. A contribution to the pathology of generalized argyria with a discussion of the fate of silver in the human body. *Am J Pathol*. 1927;3:631-652.

98.3. Answer: E. The pathophysiology of argyria is complex. Although increased melanocyte activity is noted, there is an additional effect of direct deposition of silver ions in the skin. The subsequent reduction by sunlight occurs in the presence of selenium and sulfur, which leads to the abnormal coloration.

Liu J, et al. Chemical transformations of nanosilver in biological environments. *ACS Nano*. 2012;6:9887-9899.

98.4. Answer: C. At the present time, there is no definitive cure for argyria. Sunscreens and hydroquinone reduce the silver burden and limit the ability of sunlight to further the pigmentation process. Other therapies such as laser treatment, selenium, and vitamin E have some experimental support but are too preliminary to be routinely recommended.

Browning JC, Levy ML. Argyria attributed to silvadene application in a patient with dystrophic epidermolysis bullosa. *Dermatol Online J*. 2008;14:9.

98.5. Answer: D. Silver that is deposited in the skin and elsewhere slowly leaches out of tissues back into the serum. In one report, this persisted for at least 3 years. As serum silver concentrations have no relationship to the clinical findings, it is not recommended that they be used to either confirm exposure or follow therapy.

White JM, et al. Severe generalized argyria secondary to ingestion of colloidal silver protein. *Clin Exp Dermatol*. 2003;28:254-256.

98.6. Answer: E. At least one report describes weakness and all these other findings in a patient with silver toxicity in which no other cause was identified. While uncommon, these finding are consistent with animal experiments and are rarely reported in large cohorts of silver workers.

Westhofen M, Schäfer H. Generalized argyrosis in man: Neurotological, ultrastructural and X-ray microanalytical findings. *Arch Otorhinolaryngol*. 1986;243:260-264.

98.7. Answer: C. In one study that evaluated 30 silver workers, 25 (83.3%) complained of upper respiratory tract irritation, defined as itchy, red, and watery eyes or sneezing, stuffiness and running nose, or sore throat. Sixty percent had nose bleeds. Cutaneous burns were common on direct contact with silver nitrate, and many reported that their skin color had changed.

Rosenman KD, et al. Argyria: Clinical implications of exposure to silver nitrate and silver oxide. *J Occup Med*. 1979;21:430-435.

98.8. **Answer: B.** Chronic use of amiodarone is associated with a slate-gray discoloration of the skin that resembles argyria. Microscopic findings suggest that this is related to an accumulation of iodine in the skin, which is believed to represent deposition of the drug itself or a metabolite. Gold, some antimalarials, and some antipsychotics are also associated with a similar color change. While xenobiotics that induce methemoglobin or sulfhemoglobin should also be included in the differential diagnosis, they do not change the skin color per se.

Trimble JW, et al. Cutaneous pigmentation secondary to amiodarone therapy. *Arch Dermatol* 1983;119:914-918.

98.9. **Answer: B.** Rare cases of peripheral neuropathy are reported after both cutaneous application of sliver sulfadiazine and the use of silver in cement for hip arthroplasty. Some improvement is noted on cessation of exposure.

Vik H, et al. Neuropathy caused by silver absorption from arthroplasty cement. *Lancet.* 1985;1:872.

Payne CM, et al. Argyria from excessive use of topical silver sulphadiazine. *Lancet.* 1992;340:126.

98.10. **Answer: A.** In one severely burned patient, the application of silver sulfadiazine was associated with interstitial nephritis. Since this is uncommon, the authors speculate whether this represents an adverse reaction to silver or the sulfonamide. Kidney injury is also reported in some animal experiments.

Owens CJ, Yarbrough DR 3rd, Brackett NC Jr. Nephrotic syndrome following topically applied sulfadiazine silver therapy. *Arch Intern Med.* 1974;134:332-335.

Thallium

QUESTIONS

99.1. Because of its ionic radius, which of the following options is correct regarding thallium?
   A. It is poorly absorbed through the gastrointestinal tract
   B. It accumulates in areas of high potassium concentration
   C. It accumulates in bone
   D. It is similar to sodium
   E. It undergoes renal elimination similar to chlorine

99.2. Which of the following options describes the role of activated charcoal in the management of thallium poisoning?
   A. It has no role in treating exposures as small ions are not adsorbed to activated charcoal
   B. It should only be given to prevent absorption of potential co-ingestants
   C. It has demonstrated limited adsorption binding in vitro but no clinical utility
   D. It is indicated only as a single dose to prevent absorption of thallium
   E. It should be given in multiple doses both to prevent absorption and to enhance elimination

99.3. The role of potassium administration in thallium poisoning is best described by which of the following statements?
   A. Potassium administration enhances thallium elimination by competing for renal elimination
   B. Potassium administration enhances thallium elimination by liberating tissue stores of thallium
   C. Potassium administration enhances lethality of thallium in some animal models
   D. Potassium administration is associated with an exacerbation of neurologic symptoms in humans with thallium poisoning
   E. All of the above

99.4. Which of the following symptoms is characteristic of an acute thallium overdose?
   A. Alopecia
   B. Painful descending neuropathy
   C. Macrocytic anemia
   D. Voluminous diarrhea
   E. Torsade de pointes

99.5. Which of the following statements is most correct regarding the role of extracorporeal removal in thallium poisoning?
   A. Combined hemoperfusion and hemodialysis produce a clinically useful clearance rate
   B. Peritoneal dialysis is an acceptable choice, especially if the patient has kidney failure
   C. A standard 4-hour session of hemodialysis will effectively remove a significant amount of thallium
   D. Continuous arteriovenous hemofiltration (CAVH) improves survival in animal models
   E. There is no role for extracorporeal removal in thallium poisoning

STUDY GUIDE FOR GOLDFRANK'S TOXICOLOGIC EMERGENCIES

99.6. A 27-year-old woman is being evaluated in the intensive care unit for a presumed diagnosis of thallium toxicity. Which of the following tests is necessary to establish a definitive diagnosis?
A. A urine qualitative test
B. Potassium mobilization test
C. Calcium disodium edetate mobilization test
D. 24-hour urine sample for atomic absorption spectroscopy
E. No definitive test is available

99.7. Which of the following chelators improves survival or significantly enhances elimination in experimental models of thallium poisoning?
A. British anti-Lewisite (BAL)
B. Calcium disodium edetate
C. *N*-Acetylcysteine
D. D-Penicillamine
E. 2,3-Dimercaptosuccinic acid

99.8. Which of the following statements about Prussian blue is correct?
A. Oral Prussian blue is rapidly absorbed and binds thallium to enhance renal elimination
B. Prussian blue binds thallium in the gastrointestinal tract to enhance fecal elimination of thallium
C. Oral Prussian blue enhances both renal and fecal elimination of thallium

D. The major adverse effect of Prussian blue therapy is constipation, so it should be given with mannitol
E. Prussian blue should be dosed with caution in patients with kidney failure because it liberates cyanide

99.9. Most modern cases of thallium poisoning in the United States resulted from which of the following options?
A. Intentional adulteration of a cocaine supply
B. Intentional adulteration of an MDMA (XTC) supply
C. Unintentional exposure to thallium-containing rodenticides
D. Unintentional overdose with radiolabeled thallium for cardiac imaging
E. Attempted or successful homicide

99.10. Which of following statements about thallium poisoning in pregnancy is true?
A. Thallium is not teratogenic in animal models
B. Breastfeeding is recommended after delivery since thallium is not eliminated in breast milk
C. Thallium exposure has resulted in normal fetal outcomes despite severe maternal poisoning
D. Prussian blue is teratogenic and should not be used in pregnant patients with thallium toxicity
E. Absence of fetal movements in utero is indicative of impending fetal demise

ANSWERS

99.1. Answer: B. Thallium and potassium have similar ionic radii: 1.33 Å for potassium and 1.47 Å for thallium. As such, thallium distributes into tissues similarly to potassium. While this has significant relevance to toxicity, it also serves as the basis for the use of radiolabeled thallium for cardiac stress tests.

Mulkey JP, Oehme FW. A review of thallium toxicity. *Vet Hum Toxicol.* 1993;35:445-453.

99.2. Answer: E. Activated charcoal adsorbs thallium in vitro and should be used to prevent thallium absorption. Since thallium is enterohepatically recirculated, multiple-dose activated charcoal (MDAC) is reasonable to enhance thallium elimination, especially if Prussian blue is unavailable. In an animal model, MDAC proved efficacious against thallium poisoning.

Lund A. The effect of various substances on the excretion and the toxicity of thallium in the rat. *Acta Pharmacol Toxicol.* 1956;12:260-268.

99.3. Answer: E. All of the answers are true. Although potassium administration enhances thallium elimination by at least the two mechanisms described (choices A and B), it redistributes thallium to the central nervous system. Because this is associated with an exacerbation of neurologic symptoms in humans and enhanced lethality in animal models we recommend against using potassium in thallium poisoned patients.

Meggs WJ, et al. Effects of potassium in a murine model of thallium poisoning. *J Toxicol Clin Toxicol.* 1995;33:559.

Papp JP, et al. Potassium chloride treatment in thallotoxicosis. *Ann Intern Med.* 1969;71:119-123.

99.4. Answer: A. Alopecia and a painful ascending peripheral neuropathy are classic findings associated with thallium toxicity. Unlike most other metal salts, the gastrointestinal symptoms associated with thallium poisoning are mild and include both limited diarrhea and constipation. Effects on hematopoiesis are not described. Torsade de pointes is characteristic of arsenic or cesium poisonings, not thallium poisoning.

Chamberlain PH, et al. Thallium poisoning. *Pediatrics.* 1958;12: 1170-1182.

Moeschlin S. Thallium poisoning. *Clin Toxicol.* 1980;17:133-146.

99.5. Answer: A. Combined hemodialysis and hemoperfusion removed as much as 93 mg of thallium during a 3-hour session. This is at least 3-4 times more effective than hemodialysis alone and far superior to peritoneal dialysis. Although unstudied, it is expected that modern hemodialysis could be sufficient and is recommended by the Extracorporeal Treatments in Poisoning Workgroup. The use of CAVH and continuous arteriovenous hemofiltration with dialysis have not been studied.

Aoyama H, et al. Acute poisoning by intentional ingestion of thallous malonate. *Hum Toxicol.* 1986; 5:389-392.

De Backer W, et al. Thallium intoxication treated with combined hemoperfusion-hemodialysis. *Clin Toxicol.* 1982;19:259-264.

Ghannoum M, et al. Extracorporeal treatment for thallium poisoning: Recommendations from the EXTRIP Workgroup. *Clin J Am Soc Nephrol.* 2012;7:1682-1690.

99.6. Answer: D. The standard testing method to confirm a diagnosis of thallium toxicity is to obtain a 24-hour urine sample and to assay the urine using atomic absorption spectroscopy. Urine qualitative tests should not be performed as there is a high rate of false-negative results. Both potassium mobilization and calcium disodium edetate mobilization tests should not be performed. These mobilization tests exacerbate neurologic toxicity.

Saddique A, Peterson CD. Thallium poisoning: A review. *Vet Hum Toxicol.* 1983;25:16-22.

Wakid NW, Cortas NK. Chemical and atomic absorption methods for thallium in urine compared. *Clin Chem.* 1984;30:587-588.

99.7. Answer: D. Of all the chelators listed, only D-penicillamine enhances the elimination of thallium in poisoned animals. Unfortunately, like diethyldithiocarbamate (dithiocarb), D-penicillamine also redistributes thallium into vital organs. It should not be used alone, but it potentially has some role when combined with Prussian blue.

Rios C, Monroy-Noyola A. D-Penicillamine and Prussian blue as antidotes against thallium intoxication in rats. *Toxicology.* 1992;74:69-76.

99.8. Answer: B. Prussian blue is poorly absorbed from the gastrointestinal tract. It functions as an exchange resin forming a tight bond with thallium to enhance fecal elimination. No data support the assertion that the potassium liberated by Prussian blue contributes to thallium elimination by enhancing renal clearance. Prussian blue does not cause constipation or diarrhea. Mannitol is added to the therapeutic regimen because of the constipation often associated with thallium poisoning not Prussian blue. Although Prussian blue contains a cyanide group, there is good evidence that liberation is of no consequence.

Heydlauf H. Ferric-cyanoferrate(II): An effective antidote in thallium poisoning. *Eur J Pharmacol.* 1969;6:340-344.

Krazov J, et al. Relationship between physiochemical properties of Prussian blue and its efficacy as antidote against thallium poisoning. *J Appl Toxicol.* 1993;13: 213-216.

99.9. Answer: E. Although three cases of thallium poisoning from adulterated cocaine were reported in 1986, this seems to be an isolated event. No cases of adulterated MDMA have been reported. Unintentional exposure to rodenticides is no longer a significant concern in the United States because thallium-containing rodenticides have been banned for many years. This is not the case in other countries. The amount of thallium used for radiolabeled studies is so small that even a massive overdose would be unlikely to produce clinical signs or symptoms of toxicity. Unfortunately, attempted and successful homicide cases of thallium poisoning still exist.

Insley BM, et al. Thallium poisoning in cocaine users. *Am J Emerg Med.* 1986;4:545-548.

Meggs WJ, et al. Thallium poisoning from maliciously contaminated food. *J Toxicol Clin Toxicol.* 1994;32:723-730.

99.10. Answer: C. Animal evidence supports the teratogenicity of thallium. Although some authors report normal births following thallium poisoning during pregnancy, both fetal demise and neonatal toxicity are also reported. One author reported absent fetal movements and the subsequent birth of a normal child. Although not well studied, no evidence exists to support teratogenicity of Prussian blue. Therefore, Prussian blue should be administered to pregnant women with thallium poisoning, if indicated. After delivery, breastfeeding is discouraged because of significant thallium elimination in breast milk.

English JC. A case of thallium poisoning complicating pregnancy. *Med J Aust*. 1954;1:780-782.

Moeschlin S. Thallium poisoning. *Clin Toxicol*. 1980;17:133-146.

Hoffman RS. Thallium poisoning during pregnancy: A case report and comprehensive literature review. *J Toxicol Clin Toxicol*. 2000;38:767-775.

Zinc

QUESTIONS

100.1. Following absorption from the gut, which of the following proteins is important for the intracellular storage and regulation of zinc?
A. Albumin
B. Alpha-1-acid glycoprotein
C. Transferrin
D. Metallothionein
E. Protoporphyrin

100.2. Which of the following organs has the highest concentration of zinc?
A. Prostate
B. Liver
C. Kidneys
D. Heart
E. Brain

100.3. Zinc supplementation is approved by the US Food and Drug Administration (FDA) to treat which of the following diseases?
A. Addison
B. Cushing
C. Ménière
D. Parkinson
E. Wilson

100.4. A 37-year-old healthy man was using a torch all day to cut up galvanized steel on a construction site. The next day, he develops fever, chills, cough, myalgias, muscle cramping, chest pain, dyspnea, dry throat, and a metallic taste in his mouth. At the hospital, he has a normal chest radiograph, complete blood count, and procalcitonin. Which of the following therapies is most reasonable?
A. Reassurance that this is a benign self-limited disease
B. Discharge on antibiotics for likely community-acquired pneumonia
C. Discharge with a pulse oximeter to return if his saturation falls below 92%
D. Admit and prepare for transfusion if hemolysis occurs
E. Admit as this will likely progress to acute respiratory distress syndrome (ARDS)

100.5. A 24 year old man ingests zinc chloride in a suicide attempt. He presents with multiple episodes of vomiting and abdominal pain. In addition to supportive care, which of the follow interventions is most likely to be helpful?
A. Calcium disodium edetate (CaNa$_2$EDTA)
B. Dimercaprol
C. Endoscopy
D. Systemic corticosteroids
E. Succimer

100.6. A 19-year-old healthy military recruit is exposed to a zinc chloride smoke bomb in a closed space. He immediately develops lacrimation, rhinitis, dyspnea, and chest pain. Which of the following therapies is most reasonable?
- A. Reassurance that this is a benign self-limited disease
- B. Discharge on antibiotics for likely community-acquired pneumonia
- C. Discharge with a pulse oximeter to return if his saturation falls below 92%
- D. Admit and prepare for transfusion if hemolysis occurs
- E. Admit as this will likely progress to acute respiratory distress syndrome (ARDS)

100.7. An 85-year-old woman presents to the hospital complaining of progressive numbness and weakness of her arms and legs, incontinence, and cognitive decline. Neuroimaging is normal. She is found to be copper deficient. Which of the following is the likely source of her toxicity?
- A. Toothpaste
- B. Denture cream
- C. Dental rinse
- D. Drinking water
- E. Ingested coins

100.8. A 33-year-old man presents to the emergency department with vomiting after a large intentional ingestion of zinc sulfate. An abdominal radiograph demonstrates >20 round foreign bodies in the patient's stomach. Which of the following decontamination strategies would be most reasonable?
- A. Orogastric lavage
- B. Activated charcoal
- C. Whole bowel irrigation
- D. Endoscopy
- E. No therapy is needed

100.9. A 44-year-old-man with poorly controlled schizophrenia chronically ingests US pennies. An abdominal radiograph is obtained, and the radiologist estimates that hundreds are present. The patient refuses any attempts at removal. He is lost to follow-up and returns 1 year later. Many coins are still present and there is no mechanical obstruction. Which of the following findings is most likely to be present on his evaluation?
- A. None; the coins are inert
- B. Hepatic dysfunction and an abnormal magnetic resonance imaging (MRI)
- C. Kayser-Fleischer rings
- D. Sideroblastic anemia
- E. Hemolytic anemia

100.10. Which of the following therapies is **NOT** advisable in a patient with severe acute zinc toxicity?
- A. Dimercaprol
- B. Calcium disodium edetate (CaNa$_2$EDTA)
- C. Deferiprone
- D. Diethylenetriaminepentaacetic acid (DTPA)
- E. N-Acetylcysteine

ANSWERS

100.1. Answer: D. Metallothionein is an inducible family of low-molecular-weight proteins that are rich in thiol groups and thus useful for binding and regulating many essential and nonessential metals. Albumin binds about two-thirds of intravascular zinc.

Fosmire GJ. Zinc toxicity. *Am J Clin Nutr.* 1990;51:225-227.

Roney N, et al. ATSDR evaluation of potential for human exposure to zinc. *Toxicol Ind Health.* 2007;23:247-308.

100.2. Answer: A. The high concentration of zinc in the prostate is attributed to the presence of acid phosphatase, which is a zinc-containing enzyme.

Barceloux D. Zinc. *J Toxicol Clin Toxicol.* 1999;37:279-292.

100.3. Answer: E. Zinc effectively treats the copper excess in Wilson disease by inducing metallothionine, which serves as an alternative copper storage protein to ceruloplasmin.

Babula P, et al. Mammalian metallothioneins: Properties and functions. *Metallomics.* 2012;4:739-750.

Leitzmann MF, et al. Zinc supplement use and risk of prostate cancer. *J Natl Cancer Inst.* 2003;95:1004-1007.

100.4. Answer: A. Galvanization is a process of coating metals with zinc to prevent corrosion and rust. Cutting it with a torch liberates zinc oxide, which leads to metal fume fever as illustrated by this patient's symptoms. Hemolysis would occur from arsine or stibine gas, which is not possible in this scenario. Typically, cadmium pneumonitis progresses to ARDS. Most patients with metal fume fever are managed as outpatients with reassurance and supportive care alone. Antibiotics are not necessary.

El Safty A, et al. Zinc toxicity among galvanization workers in the iron and steel industry. *Ann N Y Acad Sci.* 2008;1140:256-262.

100.5. Answer: C. Zinc chloride, which is used in soldering flux, is highly caustic, with even small ingestions capable of producing devastating esophageal and gastric injuries. Although systemic toxicity is possible and would be an indication for chelation, the caustic injury should be addressed first.

Yamataka A, et al. A case of zinc chloride ingestion. *J Pediatr Surg.* 1998;33:660-662.

Knapp JF, et al. Case 01-1994: A toddler with caustic ingestion. *Pediatr Emerg Care.* 1994;10:54-58.

100.6. Answer: E. Zinc chloride is highly water soluble and liberates hydrochloric acid on contact. There are many cases of progression to ARDS and death following exposures in a closed space. This occurs without other manifestations of zinc toxicity and should be treated much like exposures to other pulmonary irritants.

Hjortso E, et al. ARDS after accidental inhalation of zinc chloride smoke. *Intensive Care Med.* 1988;14:17-24.

Homma S, et al. Pulmonary vascular lesions in the adult respiratory distress syndrome caused by inhalation of zinc chloride smoke: A morphometric study. *Hum Pathol.* 1992;23:45-50.

Matarese SL, Matthews JI. Zinc chloride (smoke bomb) inhalational lung injury. *Chest.* 1986;89:308-309.

100.7. Answer: B. Multiple reports link a syndrome of progressive myeloneuropathy to hypocupremia that is induced by excessive use of denture creams that are high in zinc. Risk factors include large-volume use of cream, poor-fitting dentures, and wearing the dentures during sleep. These patients typically improve with cessation of exposure and copper supplementation.

Nations SP, et al. Denture cream: An unusual source of excess zinc, leading to hypocupremia and neurologic disease. *Neurology.* 2008;71:639-643.

100.8. Answer: C. Given the number of tablets and their likely size, neither orogastric lavage nor endoscopy is likely to be successful. Most metals are not well adsorbed to activated charcoal. In at least one reported case, whole bowel irrigation seemed to rapidly propel zinc sulfate tablets through the gastrointestinal tract.

Burkhart KK, et al. Whole bowel irrigation as treatment for zinc sulfate overdose. *Ann Emerg Med.* 1990;19:1167-1170.

100.9. Answer: D. For nearly 40 years, the US penny is >97% zinc with the rest being copper. As such, absorption of the metal contents is more likely to produces zinc excess and resulting copper deficiency, making the findings of Wilson disease (choices B and C) unlikely. In one such case, the patient presented with pancytopenia with sideroblasts on peripheral smear. A high zinc concentration and a low copper concentration were measured. Hemolytic anemia is characteristic of acute copper salt overdose.

Kumar A, Jazieh AR. Case report of sideroblastic anemia caused by ingestion of coins. *Am J Hematol.* 2001;66:126-129.

100.10. Answer: A. All the listed therapies are associated with increased zinc elimination and have some support in either experimental models or human case reports. However, because dimercaprol also increases copper elimination and copper deficiency is expected with zinc toxicity, this choice is not optimal.

Cantilena LR Jr, Klaassen CD. The effect of chelating agents on the excretion of endogenous metals. *Toxicol Appl Pharmacol.* 1982;63:344-50.

Cao Y, et al. Chelation therapy in intoxications with mercury, lead and copper. *J Trace Elem Med Biol.* 2015;31:188-192.

Lusky LM, et al. The protective action of BAL on experimental poisoning by lead, tungsten, copper and Paris green. *Fed Proc.* 1948;7:242.

Antiseptics, Disinfectants, and Sterilants

101

QUESTIONS

101.1. A 40-year-old man presents to the emergency department with cyanosis and is diagnosed with methemoglobinemia. One hour prior to presentation, he intentionally ingested 0.5% chlorhexidine in a 70% ethanol solution. What degradation product led to his methemoglobinemia?
   A. Hexachlorophene
   B. *p*-Chloroaniline
   C. Hexachlorobenzene
   D. Methylene dianiline
   E. Paraphenylenediamine

101.2. A 72-year-old woman with a history of pancreatic cancer purchases a solution to use as an alternative cancer therapy. Three hours after ingestion, she experiences severe abdominal pain, hemiparesis, and aphasia. Which xenobiotic best explains her symptoms?
   A. Phenol
   B. Potassium permanganate
   C. Hydrogen peroxide
   D. Iodine
   E. Sodium hypochlorite

101.3. Which of the following antiseptics is associated with hypothyroidism in neonates and infants?
   A. Hexachlorophene
   B. Benzyl alcohol
   C. Hexachlorobenzene
   D. Iodine
   E. Chlorhexidine

101.4. A 67-year-old woman presents to the hospital for evaluation of a resting tremor and gait abnormality. Nine months prior to presentation, she ingested a medication that was intended to be applied topically to treat eczema. Which of the following xenobiotics best explains her symptoms?
   A. Potassium permanganate
   B. Ammonium lactate
   C. Sodium perborate
   D. Lugol solution
   E. Merbromin

101.5. A 2-year-old boy is brought into the emergency department after drinking household bleach. What is the expected toxicity following this ingestion?
   A. Methemoglobinemia
   B. Esophageal burn
   C. Multiorgan failure
   D. Aspiration pneumonitis
   E. No toxicity expected

101.6. A 45-year-old medical school professor is found at work with altered mental status, emesis, and a high anion gap metabolic acidosis. An overdose of which of the following xenobiotics led to his presentation?
   A. Povidine
   B. Ethylene oxide
   C. Isopropanol
   D. Formaldehyde
   E. Hydrogen peroxide

101.7. Dermal exposure to which of the following antiseptics is associated with the development of vacuolar encephalopathy?
  A. Chloroxylenol
  B. Cresol
  C. Hexachlorophene
  D. Phenol
  E. Sodium octylphenoxyethoxyethyl ether sulfonate

101.8. A 26-year-old man has an episode of loss of consciousness followed by a tonic-clonic seizure while at work in the hospital. On physical examination, his conjunctiva are injected and he has blistering of his mucus membranes. His symptoms began after a vial of sterilant was dropped in the colonoscopy recovery room. What is the likely sterilant that led to his presentation?
  A. Glutaraldehyde
  B. Chloroform
  C. Sodium chlorate

D. Benzalkonium chloride
E. Ethylene oxide

101.9. Which of the following xenobiotics induces a colitis that is similar to inflammatory bowel disease?
  A. Formaldehyde
  B. Ethylene oxide
  C. Glutaraldehyde
  D. Mercuric bichloride
  E. Lanolin

101.10. If an ingestion is not identified, boric acid toxicity is often misdiagnosed as which of the following illnesses?
  A. Toxic shock syndrome
  B. Botulism
  C. Smallpox
  D. Toxic alimentary aleukia
  E. Tularemia

ANSWERS

101.1. Answer: B. When ingested, chlorhexidine produces acute respiratory distress syndrome, caustic injury, and methemoglobinemia. Chlorhexidine is degraded to *p*-chloroaniline, which is a strong oxidant and is responsible for the production of methemoglobinemia.

Kuypers MI, et al. A case of methemoglobinemia after ingestion of a chlorhexidine in alcohol solution in an alcohol-dependent patient. *Clin Toxicol (Phila)*. 2016;54:604.

101.2. Answer: C. Dilute over-the-counter 3% hydrogen peroxide is generally well tolerated. Concentrated solutions >30%, however, produce substantial toxicity. One milliliter of 35% hydrogen peroxide liberates >100 mL of oxygen. Rare cases of arterial gas embolism presenting as portal venous gas, respiratory distress, and acute stroke are reported. Hyperbaric oxygen therapy is recommended in patients with a life-threatening toxicity following a hydrogen peroxide ingestion.

Rider SP, et al. Cerebral air gas embolism from concentrated hydrogen peroxide ingestion. *Clin Toxicol (Phila)*. 2008;46:9,815-818.

101.3. Answer: D. A controlled trial in 1997 compared iodine and chlorhexidine use as disinfectants in infants. When used on umbilical stumps, iodine was associated with subclinical hypothyroidism and an elevated thyroid-stimulating hormone (TSH).

Linder N, et al. Topical iodine-containing antiseptics and subclinical hypothyroidism in preterm infants. *J Pediatr*. 1997;131:434-439.

101.4. Answer: A. Manganese causes a Parkinsonism characterized by autonomic symptoms, behavioral changes, and movement disorders. In this case, potassium iodate, used as an expectorant, was unintentionally mistaken for potassium permanganate, which is used topically for eczema and as a dermal disinfectant.

Holzgraefe M, et al. Chronic enteral poisoning caused by potassium permanganate: A case report. *J Toxicol Clin Toxicol*. 1986;24:235-244.

101.5. Answer: E. Household bleach usually contains approximately 5% sodium hypochlorite. If large quantities are ingested, this dilute sodium hypochlorite solution causes caustic injury. However, in the majority of exposures in children, acute caustic injury is so uncommon that patients do not need further evaluation if they are otherwise well appearing.

Pike DG, et al. A re-evaluation of the dangers of Clorox ingestion. *J Pediatr*. 1963;63:303-305.

101.6. Answer: D. Formaldehyde is used as a tissue fixative and embalming agent. Formaldehyde is rapidly metabolized to formic acid and causes an anion gap metabolic acidosis. When ingested, formaldehyde also causes severe caustic injury.

Eells JT, et al. Formaldehyde poisoning. Rapid metabolism to formic acid. *JAMA*. 1981;246:1237-1238.

101.7. Answer: C. The bathing of premature infants with hexachlorophene (pHisoHex) was associated with significant neurologic abnormalities, including the development of vacuolar encephalopathy.

Martinez AJ, et al. Acute hexachlorophene encephalopathy: Cliniconeuropathological correlation. *Acta Neuropathol.* 1974;28:93-103.

101.8. Answer: E. Typically used as a sterilant for high-risk medical equipment, ethylene oxide causes severe toxicity manifesting as mucus membrane irritation, gastrointestinal symptoms, loss of consciousness, and recurrent seizures. Toxicity from acute exposures lasts hours to days. Chronic exposure is associated with an increased incidence of several cancers, including breast, lymphatic, and hematopoietic. Chronic exposure leads to an increased risk of spontaneous abortions as well as mild cognitive impairment and neuropathy. The treatment is primarily supportive.

Salinas E, et al. Acute ethylene oxide intoxication. *Drug Intell Clin Pharm.* 1981;15:384-386.

101.9. Answer: C. Glutaraldehyde is a sterilant used to disinfect colonoscopes. Care must be taken to ensure that all of the glutaraldehyde is removed from the colonoscope prior to use as it causes colitis. Glutaraldehyde-induced colitis typically presents within 48 hours of exposure with severe abdominal pain, fever, and bloody diarrhea.

Sheibani S, Gerson LB. Chemical colitis. *J Clin Gastroenterol.* 2008; 42:115-121.

101.10. Answer: A. Boric acid toxicity is characterized by altered mental status, gastrointestinal symptoms, kidney injury, and a classic "boiled-lobster" rash consisting of erythroderma and exfoliative dermatitis. The clinical manifestations are very similar to toxic shock syndrome, toxic epidermal necrolysis, and staphylococcal scalded skin syndrome.

Mukaigawara M, et al. A curve ball. *N Engl J Med.* 2020;838:970-975.

Camphor and Moth Repellents

QUESTIONS

102.1. Which of the following disorders is most reported following chronic exposure to paradichlorobenzene?
  A. Hemolytic anemia
  B. Leukoencephalopathy
  C. Myocarditis
  D. Chronic kidney disease
  E. Osteomalacia

102.2. Which of the following statements about radiographs of moth repellents is correct?
  A. Camphor is more radiopaque than paradichlorobenzene
  B. Naphthalene is more radiopaque than paradichlorobenzene
  C. Paradichlorobenzene is more radiopaque than naphthalene
  D. Camphor is more radiopaque than naphthalene
  E. Camphor and naphthalene have similar radiographic appearances

102.3. The onset of seizures after an ingestion of a toxic dose of camphor most commonly occurs in which of the following time frames?
  A. Within 5 minutes
  B. 15-20 minutes
  C. 1-2 hours
  D. 4-6 hours
  E. 12-24 hours

102.4. Which of the following statements is true regarding the differentiation between naphthalene and paradichlorobenzene mothballs?
  A. Naphthalene will float in water, whereas paradichlorobenzene sinks
  B. Paradichlorobenzene will float in water, whereas naphthalene sinks
  C. Both sink in water but paradichlorobenzene will float if salt is added
  D. Both sink in water but naphthalene will float if salt is added
  E. Both float in water but paradichlorobenzene will sink if ethanol or isopropanol is added

102.5. A healthy, 15-kg, 2-year-old boy is found playing with a naphthalene mothball. The parent removes it from the child's mouth and thinks about half of the mothball is missing. Which of the following management strategies is most appropriate?
  A. Send the child to the hospital for oral activated charcoal and discharge
  B. Send the child to the hospital for oral activated charcoal followed by discharge and referral for daily blood work for 5 days
  C. Send the child to the hospital for oral activated charcoal and admission for observation
  D. Send the child to the hospital for whole bowel irrigation and admission for observation
  E. No therapy needed

102.6. A 4-year-old boy is brought to the hospital 4 days after ingesting one or two mothballs. Originally, the parents thought that it was of no consequence, but over the last few days, he has become irritable and pale, and his urine has turned dark. Laboratory testing reveals a hemoglobin of 7 g/dL, with an elevated reticulocyte count, an elevated indirect bilirubin, and a low haptoglobin. The child has no acid–base abnormalities and a normal mental status. Which of the following therapies is most indicated?
   A. Admission for observation alone
   B. Methylene blue
   C. Exchange transfusion
   D. Hemodialysis
   E. Ascorbic acid

102.7. Which of the following statements about naphthalene-induced hemolysis is correct?
   A. Hemolysis occurs only in patients with a glucose-6-phosphate dehydrogenase (G6PD) deficiency
   B. Following ingestion of naphthalene, signs and symptoms are usually delayed for several days
   C. Methylene blue prevents hemolysis
   D. Methemoglobinemia usually precedes hemolysis
   E. *N*-Acetylcysteine (NAC) helps limit hemolysis

102.8. A 3-year-old boy is brought to the hospital with pallor, jaundice, tachycardia, and irritability. Which of the following findings on peripheral blood smear is supportive of a diagnosis of naphthalene toxicity?
   A. Howell-Jolly bodies
   B. Poikilocytoses
   C. Ovalocytosis
   D. Heinz bodies
   E. Basophilic stippling

102.9. Which of the following statements is true when trying to confirm the ingestion of paradichlorobenzene in a patient with presumed chronic toxicity?
   A. Finding paradichlorobenzene in the urine confirms an acute ingestion
   B. Finding paradichlorobenzene in the blood confirms an acute ingestion
   C. Finding 2,5-dicholorphenol in the urine confirms an acute ingestion
   D. Finding 2,5-dicholorphenol in the blood confirms an acute ingestion
   E. There is no good test to confirm ingestion

102.10. Which of the following events was responsible for the US Food and Drug Administration's (FDA) ban on concentrated camphor oil products?
   A. Confusion over castor oil and cod liver oil
   B. A recognition that lower concentrations were equally efficacious
   C. A lack of proven efficacy
   D. Higher toxicity of more concentrated products
   E. Illegal use as an abortifacient

ANSWERS

102.1. Answer: B. Paradichlorobenzene is less acutely toxic than camphor and naphthalene, but in no way benign. Rare cases of hepatic, renal, and hematologic toxicity are reported. However, the most well-reported disorder following chronic exposure or massive acute ingestion is leukoencephalopathy. The mechanism is unknown. Most patients improve or completely recover once the exposure is terminated.

Avila E, et al. Pica with paradichlorobenzene mothball ingestion associated with toxic leukoencephalopathy. *J Neuroimaging.* 2006;16:78-81.

Dubey D, et al. *Para*-Dichlorobenzene toxicity—a review of potential neurotoxic manifestations. *Ther Adv Neurol Disord.* 2014;7:177-187.

102.2. Answer: C. Paradichlorobenzene is more radiopaque than naphthalene, which is more radiopaque than camphor. Radiopacity relates to the atomic number in relation to surrounding tissues. The chlorine content of paradichlorobenzene renders it more radiopaque that the other two. If samples of all three are available, then an unknown is identified by comparison.

Woolf AD, et al. Radiopacity of household deodorizers, air fresheners, and moth repellents. *J Toxicol Clin Toxicol.* 1993;31:415-428.

102.3. Answer: C. Most seizures occur between 1-2 hours after an ingestion of camphor. An onset as quick as 5 minutes is occasionally reported and might be related to liquid versus solid products. The mechanism for seizures is unknown. Most seizures are self-limited or respond to a benzodiazepine.

Kressel JJ. Camphor. *Clin Toxicol Rev.* 1982;4:1-4.

Benz RW. Camphorated oil poisoning with no mortality: Report of twenty cases. *JAMA.* 1919;72:1217-1218.

Khine H, et al. A cluster of children with seizures caused by camphor poisoning. *Pediatrics.* 2009;123:1269-1272.

102.4. **Answer: C.** There are many techniques to differentiate moth repellents that are complex and involve melting, burning, or utilizing reagents that are not readily available. One of the easiest techniques is to differentiate the mothballs based on density. If camphor, naphthalene, and paradichlorobenzene are placed in water, only the camphor will float and the other two will sink. If salt is added to the water, the naphthalene will float and the paradichlorobenzene will remain submerged.

Ambre J, et al. Mothball composition: Three simple tests for distinguishing paradichlorobenzene from naphthalene. *Ann Emerg Med.* 1986;15:724-726.

Winkler JV, et al. Mothball differentiation: Naphthalene from paradichlorobenzene. *Ann Emerg Med.* 1985;14:30-32.

102.5. **Answer: E.** Although ingestions of a single naphthalene mothball cause hemolytic anemia, ingestions of smaller amounts in healthy children are rarely of consequence. Regardless, the onset of symptoms is not for at least 24-48 hours after ingestion, and it is unclear if activated charcoal or any other therapy is preventative. Healthy children with small ingestions are managed at home. For children brought to the hospital, activated charcoal and discharge are reasonable even for high-risk children, as long as follow-up is assured.

Zuelzer WW, Apt L. Acute hemolytic anemia due to naphthalene poisoning; a clinical and experimental study. *JAMA.* 1949;141:185-190.

102.6. **Answer: A.** Naphthalene-induced hemolytic anemia is usually a self-limited process. Since the etiology is oxidant-mediated stress, older cells are more susceptible and hemolyze first. Since all new cells are resistant to oxidation, if the bone marrow is functioning, most children recover quickly. Indications for transfusion should be based on clinical grounds, remembering that stored blood is relatively deficient in glucose-6-phosphate dehydrogenase and therefore susceptible to hemolysis. Methylene blue and ascorbic acid treat methemoglobinemia, which is not present. Hemodialysis treats kidney injury only and will not remove the toxin. There is little, if any, role for formal exchange transfusion.

Pannu AK, Singla V. Naphthalene toxicity in clinical practice. *Curr Drug Metab.* 2020;21:63-66.

102.7. **Answer: B.** Following ingestion of naphthalene, signs and symptoms of hemolysis are delayed for several days because time is required for the liver to metabolize naphthalene to 1-naphthol (alpha-naphthol), which is responsible for the hemolysis. Patients do not have to be deficient in G6PD activity for hemolysis to occur, although those with G6PD deficiency are more susceptible. While methemoglobinemia, hemolysis, or both occur, neither is a prerequisite for the other. There is no demonstrable role for NAC therapy. Methylene blue does not prevent or treat hemolysis.

Chusid E, Fried CT. Acute hemolytic anemia due to naphthalene ingestion. *Am J Dis Child.* 1955;87:612-614.

Gidron E, Leuren J. Naphthalene poisoning. *Lancet.* 1956;1:228-230.

Mackell JV, et al. Acute hemolytic anemia due to ingestion of naphthalene mothballs: I: Clinical aspects. *Pediatrics.* 1951;7:722-725.

102.8. **Answer D.** The characteristic findings in naphthalene-induced anemia are Heinz bodies. Heinz bodies are inclusions in red blood cells that result from denatured hemoglobin. These abnormalities impair the ability of the cells to deform as they go through the reticuloendothelial system and serve as lead points for hemolysis.

Zuelzer WW, Apt L. Acute hemolytic anemia due to naphthalene poisoning; a clinical and experimental study. *JAMA.* 1949;141:185-190.

102.9. **Answer: E.** Paradichlorobenzene is so ubiquitous in the modern environment that >90% of Americans tested had the metabolite 2,5-dichlorophenol found. Presumably most of these result from casual exposure. Since finding the metabolite should be expected in everyone, a positive result is not considered confirmatory.

Hill RH Jr, et al. *p*-Dichlorobenzene exposure among 1,000 adults in the United States. *Arch Environ Health.* 1995;50:277-280.

Hill RH, et al. Residues of chlorinated phenols and phenoxy acid herbicides in the urine of Arkansas children. *Arch Envrion Contam Toxicol.* 1989;18:469-474.

Ye X, et al. Urinary concentrations of 2,4-dichlorophenol and 2,5-dichlorophenol in the U.S. population (National Health Nutrition Examination Survey, 2003-2010): Trends and predictors. *Environ Health Perspect.* 2014;122:351-355.

102.10. **Answer: A.** There is no proven benefit of concentrated camphorated oil, and higher concentrations are more likely to be toxic. Bottles were labeled in such a fashion that they were confused for castor oil and cod liver oil, resulting in them being used for the treatment of children. Strong lobbying efforts by the pharmacy community resulted in the US FDA's final decision.

Trestrail JH 3rd, Spartz ME. Camphorated and castor oil confusion and its toxic results. *Clin Toxicol.* 1977;11:151-158.

QUESTIONS

103.1. Which of the following options best describes the epidemiology of caustic ingestions?
   A. Most ingestions requiring admission are in children, and children comprise most of the cases requiring operative repair
   B. Most ingestions requiring admission are in adults, and children comprise most of the cases requiring operative repair
   C. Most ingestions requiring admission are in children, and adults comprise most of the cases requiring operative repair
   D. Most ingestions requiring admission are in adults, and adults comprise most of the cases requiring operative repair
   E. The total number of cases requiring admission and those requiring operative repair are essentially equally split between adults and children

103.2. A 20-year-old man complains of eye pain after someone threw a hydrochloric acid–containing toilet bowl cleaner in his face as a means of retribution. Which statement about caustics in the eye is most accurate?
   A. Acid injuries penetrate deeply and often require prolonged irrigation
   B. Alkali injuries only injure superficial structures and should be irrigated for a short period of time
   C. Acid injuries only injure superficial structures and should be irrigated for a short period of time
   D. Alkali injuries penetrate deeply and often require prolonged irrigation
   E. The pathophysiologies of acid and alkali injuries are similar, and they should be treated in a similar fashion

103.3. When is the ideal time to perform an endoscopy for patients who present following a caustic ingestion?
   A. No sooner than 24 hours after exposure to fully appreciate the degree of injury
   B. Within 12 hours of the exposure
   C. Only after water-soluble contrast studies are negative
   D. Between days 1 and 5 after the exposure
   E. Between weeks 1 and 2 after the exposure

103.4. A 15-year-old boy took a bite of a liquid laundry detergent pod as part of a dare. Which of the following is most likely to occur?
   A. Vomiting
   B. Coughing
   C. Lethargy
   D. Rash
   E. Seizure

103.5. A 5-year-old boy has an unwitnessed ingestion of a sodium hydroxide–containing drain opener. He vomited once at home and now presents with drooling and an oropharyngeal burn. When is therapy with corticosteroids indicated?
- A. Immediately
- B. Only when an endoscopy demonstrates that his maximal esophageal injury is graded as a 2A lesion
- C. Only when an endoscopy demonstrates that his maximal esophageal injury is graded as a 2B lesion
- D. Only when an endoscopy demonstrates that his maximal esophageal injury is graded as a 3A lesion
- E. Never

103.6. When is antibiotic therapy indicated in children with alkaline esophageal injuries?
- A. Always as prophylactic therapy
- B. Only when there is an obvious infection
- C. In combination with corticosteroids
- D. For all grade 1 injuries on endoscopy
- E. For all grade 4 injuries on endocopy

103.7. Which of the following options most accurately describes the variability of caustic injuries?
- A. Alkalis causes coagulation necrosis
- B. Acids causes liquefication necrosis
- C. Alkalis tend to preferentially injure the stomach
- D. Acids tend to preferentially injure the esophagus
- E. The anatomical location of the injury is more dependent on formulation than pH

103.8. A 2-year-old boy takes a sip of a household bleach that contains sodium hypochlorite and vomits once at home. What is the most appropriate next step?
- A. The child should go to the pediatrician within a few days
- B. Reassure the caregiver that serious injury is extremely unlikely and inform them that the child can remain at home if he is able to drink liquids
- C. The child should go to the hospital immediately for observation
- D. The child should go to the hospital immediately for endoscopy
- E. The child should be given a dilute sodium bicarbonate solution for neutralization

103.9. A 2-year-old girl has an unsupervised ingestion of an alkaline hair care product. Which of the following should prompt a consult for endoscopy?
- A. One or two episodes of vomiting
- B. Drooling
- C. An obvious burn on the lip
- D. Both vomiting and drooling
- E. No additional criteria are needed beyond history; all children with alkaline ingestions should undergo endoscopy

103.10. Which of the following options best describes the role of computed tomography imaging (CT scan) in patients with caustic injuries?
- A. It is a second choice best used when endoscopy is unavailable or unsafe
- B. It is superior to endoscopy and will likely make endoscopy obsolete
- C. It produces results equivalent to endoscopy
- D. It is best used as an adjunct to endoscopy
- E. Data are inconclusive to define a clear role

ANSWERS

103.1. Answer: C. Children are more frequently involved in caustic ingestions as products are commonly available and there is a lack of sound poison prevention. Fortunately, these unsupervised ingestions tend to be smaller in volume. Adult ingestions, however, are often suicidal. In one study, children comprised 39% of all admissions, whereas adults comprised 81% of cases needing operative repair.

Hawkins DB, et al. Caustic ingestion: Controversies in management. A review of 214 cases. *Laryngoscope*. 1980;90:98-109.

103.2. Answer: D. Caustic injuries to the eye can be devastating and should prompt an emergent consultation with an ophthalmologist. Acids tend to have limited penetration, whereas alkalis often penetrate deeply and damage posterior structures. Both require immediate irrigation with the first available fluid. Water is a perfectly acceptable irrigation solution and is readily available. The duration of irrigation should be expected to be longer with alkali injuries, but for both acids and alkalis, irrigation should continue until the pH of the eye is normal. One exception is hydrofluoric acid which should not be irrigated with more than 1L routinely.

Hirst LW, et al. Controlled trial of hyperbaric oxygen treatment for alkali corneal burn in the rabbit. *Clin Experiment Ophthalmol*. 2004;32:67-70.

Burns FR, Paterson CA. Prompt irrigation of chemical eye injuries may avert severe damage. *Occup Health Saf*. 1989;58:33-36.

Wagoner MD. Chemical injuries of the eye: Current concepts in pathophysiology and therapy. *Surv Ophthalmol*. 1997;41:275-312.

103.3. Answer: B. Endoscopy is ideally performed within 12 hours of the exposure. No contrast studies are required prior to endoscopy. As wound healing occurs, the tissues soften; therefore, the risk of perforation from endoscopy is highest between 3 and 14 days.

Zargar SA, et al. The role of fiberoptic endoscopy in the management of corrosive ingestion and modified endoscopic classification of burns. *Gastrointest Endosc*. 1991;37:165-169.

103.4. Answer A. Brightly colored laundry pods are attractive to children who bite them because they look like candy. Biting into laundry pods also became popular among teenagers as a result of a social media fad. Vomiting is the most common symptom, occurring in 55% of patients. One unique finding is lethargy (found in 7% of cases), which often leads to airway compromise.

Centers for Disease Control and Prevention. Health hazards associated with laundry detergent pods — United States, May–June 2012. *MMWR Morbid Mortal Wkly Rep*. 2012;61:825-829.

103.5. Answer: C. The goal of corticosteroid therapy is to prevent stricture formation, which is associated with lifelong pain, nutritional disorders, and need for invasive procedures. Prolonged courses of corticosteroids are associated with immunosuppression and infection. The current recommended 3-day corticosteroid protocol reduces the incidence and severity of strictures but was only studied in grade 2B injuries.

Usta M, et al. High doses of methylprednisolone in the management of caustic esophageal burns. *Pediatrics*. 2014;133:E1518-1524.

103.6. Answer: C. It is generally accepted that there is no role for prophylactic antibiotics as they have no proven benefit and are likely to select for resistant organisms. However, when patients with alkaline esophageal injuries have grade 2B lesions and are placed on corticosteroid therapy, the full protocol should be followed, which includes H_2 antagonists and antibiotics.

Usta M, et al. High doses of methylprednisolone in the management of caustic esophageal burns. *Pediatrics*. 2014;133:E1518-1524.

103.7. Answer: E. Acid injuries produce coagulation necrosis and alkali injuries produce liquification necrosis. While it was commonly said that alkalis preferentially injury the esophagus and acids preferentially injure the stomach, this is not accurate. This finding is the result of most acids being low-viscosity liquids that pool in the stomach, and many alkalis are solids and viscous fluids that adhere to the esophagus. In many large series of acid ingestions, esophageal injuries are common.

Ashcraft KW, Padula RT. The effect of dilute corrosives on the esophagus. *Pediatrics*. 1974;53:226-232.

Dilawari JB, et al. Corrosive acid ingestion in man—a clinical and endoscopic study. *Gut*. 1984;25:183-187.

Zargar SA, et al. Ingestion of corrosive acids. Spectrum of injury to upper gastrointestinal tract and natural history. *Gastroenterology*. 1989;97:702-707.

103.8. Answer: B. Household bleach (sodium hypochlorite) rarely causes significant injury in unintentional exposures. Rare cases of large intentional ingestions are reported to cause clinically significant burns. Most children with unsupervised ingestions are managed at home if they are able to tolerate liquids. There is no role for neutralization therapy which may actually be harmful.

Landau GD, Saunders WH. The effect of chlorine bleach on the esophagus. *Arch Otolaryngol*. 1964;80:174-176.

103.9. Answer: D. Following alkaline caustic ingestion in children, endoscopy is not routinely indicated as there are costs and risks and, in many settings, a transfer is required. Signs and symptoms are predictive of the need for urgent endoscopy. Children with stridor or the combination of both vomiting and drooling have a high likelihood of a clinically significant finding on endoscopy. The presence or absence of obvious burns is poorly predictive. The goal of endoscopy is to identify patients with low-risk injuries that are discharged or observed as their diet is advanced, severe injuries that require computed tomography (CT) scan and surgical consultation, and grade 2B injuries that are amenable to corticosteroid therapy.

Crain EF, et al. Caustic ingestions. Symptoms as predictors of esophageal injury. *Am J Dis Child*. 1984;138:863-865.

Previtera C, et al. Predictive value of visible lesions (cheeks, lips, oropharynx) in suspected caustic ingestion: May endoscopy reasonably be omitted in completely negative pediatric patients? *Pediatr Emerg Care*. 1990;6:176-178.

103.10. Answer: D. Endoscopy has several significant limitations, including the need for specialized equipment and personnel, and often requires endotracheal intubation or an operating room to be performed safely in children. Endoscopy is also limited by technique and the inability to pass the scope beyond the first significant lesion. CT scanning has an advantage of characterizing the serosal surface of the gastrointestinal tract as well as identifying small perforations. However, CT scanning does not adequately identify grade 2B injuries that should receive corticosteroids. As such, these modalities are best viewed as complementary techniques.

Ryu HH, et al. Caustic injury: Can CT grading system enable prediction of esophageal stricture? *Clin Toxicol (Phila)*. 2010;48:137-142.

Hydrofluoric Acid and Fluorides

QUESTIONS

104.1. A 21-year-old construction worker is assigned to clean grease and dirt from the tire wheel rims of his supervisor's personal vehicle. He was wearing gloves but noted that the tip of his index finger was wet when he removed his gloves. He immediately washed his hands. He presented to the hospital 8 hours later with severe throbbing pain to his finger. His finger appeared normal on examination. Which of the following xenobiotics was present in the cleaning product?
A. Ammonium bifluoride
B. Nitric acid
C. Sodium hydroxide
D. Oxalic acid
E. Ethylene glycol butyl ether

104.2. Which of the following properties makes hydrofluoric acid (HF) a uniquely toxic xenobiotic?
A. It liberates more hydrogen ions in solution than equimolar hydrochloric acid
B. The fluoride anion is a highly toxic
C. It is more commonly available in highly concentrated solutions than other acids
D. It has a very high heat of solution
E. It has high volatility, adding inhalational injury to many dermal exposures

104.3. A 43-year-old man tried to remove a metal water stain from an antique porcelain sink with a 40% hydrofluoric acid (HF) solution. Shortly after he removed his glove, he noted severe pain on his thumb and index fingers and irrigated them with tap water for 20 minutes. By the time he arrives to the emergency department, his two fingertips are blistered and painful. Which of the following options is the best next step?
A. Arrange transfer to a burn center
B. Deliver intravenous calcium gluconate
C. Deliver intravenous magnesium sulfate
D. Irrigate for an additional 20 minutes with cold water
E. Deliver intraarterial calcium gluconate to the affected hand

104.4. A 35-year-old woman ingests a bottle of household rust remover in a suicide attempt. She is vomiting and complaining of abdominal pain. Which diagnostic test is most likely to alter her therapy?
A. A complete blood count
B. Kidney function tests
C. Liver function tests
D. An electrocardiogram (ECG)
E. An abdominal radiograph

104.5. Following an ingestion of hydrofluoric acid (HF), a 29-year-old man has several episodes of ventricular tachycardia, despite intravenous calcium and magnesium supplementation. Which of the following antidysrhythmics is most likely to be of benefit?
A. Lidocaine
B. Procainamide
C. Quinidine
D. Phenytoin
E. Adenosine

104.6. A 5-year-old (25-kg) boy is found in his parent's bathroom with an open tube of fluoride-containing toothpaste. The child has one episode of vomiting 30 minutes after the ingestion, so he is brought to the hospital. The child is well appearing with unremarkable vital signs. Which of the following courses of action is most indicated?

A. Administer 1 g/kg of oral activated charcoal
B. Admit the child for overnight observation
C. Consult gastroenterology for endoscopy
D. Have the patient drink a glass of milk and observe for a few hours
E. Insert an intravenous catheter and administer calcium gluconate and magnesium sulfate

104.7. A 56-year-old man presents to the hospital complaining of thigh pain. Approximately 12 hours earlier, he was cleaning a rusted hand saw with a dilute solution of hydrofluoric acid (HF). A small amount of the liquid spilled on his thigh. He now complains of anterior thigh pain over an area about the size of his palm. His vital signs and physical examination are completely normal. Which of the following courses of action would be the next best step?

A. Obtain an electrocardiogram and serum electrolytes
B. Insert an intravenous line and administer calcium gluconate and magnesium sulfate
C. Insert a femoral arterial line on the affected side and infuse dilute calcium gluconate
D. Apply topical calcium gel, administer an analgesic, and reassess 1 hour later
E. Reassure him that the pain will resolve, treat with acetaminophen, and discharge

104.8. A 47-year-old man develops a cough and shortness of breath after an industrial release of hydrogen fluoride gas. After evacuation, his eyes and skin are irrigated. He has no dermal pain or visual complaints. An electrocardiogram and electrolytes are normal. What is the most important next step in his management?

A. Insert an intravenous catheter and administer calcium gluconate and magnesium sulfate
B. Administer inhaled racemic epinephrine
C. Administer inhaled calcium gluconate
D. Intubate for emergent bronchioalveolar lavage
E. Administer intravenous corticosteroids

104.9. Which of the following statements about irrigation solutions for ocular hydrofluoric acid (HF) exposure is true?

A. A proprietary amphoteric solution outperforms other irrigating solutions
B. A 10% calcium gluconate irrigation will rapidly bind fluorides and improves symptoms and outcome
C. A 10% magnesium sulfate irrigation will rapidly bind fluoride and improves symptoms and outcome
D. Topical calcium gel is applied following irrigation to reduce injury
E. Immediate irrigation with 0.9% saline, lactated Ringer solution, or tap water is recommended

104.10. In the setting of hydrofluoric acid (HF) exposure, which of the following statements best describes the fate of fluoride ions that reach the systemic circulation?

A. They bind with hydroxyapatite to form fluorapatite
B. They precipitate as calcium fluoride
C. They precipitate as magnesium fluoride
D. They are freely filtered by the kidney and eliminated in the urine
E. They are selectively concentrated in red blood cells

ANSWERS

104.1. Answer: A. While all the xenobiotics listed are cleaning products, the delayed pain with an unremarkable examination is characteristic of hydrofluoric acid. Ammonium bifluoride is a similar xenobiotic, commonly available in the United States as an automobile wheel cleaner. This product is highly toxic and has injured a number of children following unsupervised ingestions.

Maddry JK, et al. Prolonged hypocalcemia refractory to calcium gluconate after ammonium bifluoride ingestion in a pediatric patient. *Am J Emerg Med.* 2017;35:378.e371-378.e372.

104.2. Answer: B. Hydrofluoric acid (HF) is uniquely toxic because of the fluoride anion. The high electronegativity of fluoride limits dissociation, which allows tissue penetration. Fluoride is released and is toxic to most enzyme systems. Massive HF exposures are lethal.

Boink AB, et al. The mechanism of fluoride-induced hypocalcaemia. *Hum Exp Toxicol.* 1994;13:149-155.

Lepke S, Passow H. Effects of fluoride on potassium and sodium permeability of the erythrocyte membrane. *J Gen Physiol.* 1968;51:365-372.

McClure F. A review of fluorine and its physiologic effects. *Physiol Rev.* 1933;13:277-300.

104.3.   Answer: E. The immediate pain and tissue injury are consistent with a dermal exposure to concentrated hydrofluoric acid (HF). While this patient could ultimately benefit from transfer to a burn center, delayed care will almost certainly exacerbate tissue loss. Intravenous calcium and magnesium are indicated for systemic toxicity, which is unlikely given the small burn area. No further irrigation is needed. Once tissue injury is evident, definitive therapy is provided with intraarterial calcium.

Vance MV, et al. Digital hydrofluoric acid burns: Treatment with intraarterial calcium infusion. *Ann Emerg Med.* 1986;15:890-896.

104.4.   Answer: D. Systemic toxicity following ingestion of hydrofluoric acid (HF) produces hyperkalemia and hypocalcemia. The ECG provides one of the earliest clues to these electrolyte abnormalities. Although the other tests are important, unless bedside electrolytes are available, the ECG will be the most rapid guide to therapy. If perforation is a concern, then an upright chest radiograph has greater sensitivity and specificity compared to an abdominal radiograph.

Holstege C, et al. The electrocardiographic toxidrome: The ECG presentation of hydrofluoric acid ingestion. *Am J Emerg Med.* 2005;23:171-176.

104.5.   Answer: C. Although hypocalcemia, hypomagnesemia, and hyperkalemia all contribute to ventricular dysrhythmias in patients with HF toxicity, correction of these electrolyte abnormalities is not necessarily adequate. Part of the pathophysiology of HF poisoning involves the unregulated efflux of potassium from the cells, which results from the blockade of Na^+,K^+-ATPase. In experimental models, potassium efflux blockers, such as quinidine and amiodarone, protect against ventricular dysrhythmias caused by this mechanism.

Dalamaga M, et al. Hypocalcemia, hypomagnesemia, and hypokalemia following hydrofluoric acid chemical injury. *J Burn Care Res.* 2008;29:541-543.

Su M, et al. Amiodarone attenuates fluoride-induced hyperkalemia in vitro. *Acad Emerg Med.* 2003;10:105-109.

104.6.   Answer: D. Most children tolerate oral fluoride doses of <5 mg/kg with either no symptoms or transient gastrointestinal distress. The American Dentistry Association recommends that no fluoride-containing dental product be dispensed with a fluoride content >120 mg. Since this child weighs 25 kg, it would be expected that he could tolerate an entire tube of toothpaste, a quantity that would be unlikely

to be consumed. Milk is a reasonable fluid to offer, as it has some calcium available to bond to residual fluoride in the gastrointestinal tract.

Shulman JD, Wells LM. Acute fluoride toxicity from ingesting home-use dental products in children, birth to 6 years of age. *J Public Health Dent.* 1997;57:150-158.

104.7.   Answer: D. Patients who have a topical exposure to dilute HF present with delayed pain, and it almost never results in either systemic toxicity or tissue loss. For these cases, application of a topical calcium gel and analgesia with either acetaminophen or a nonsteroidal antiinflammatory drug are usually sufficient. Patients can be discharged with a small supply of gel for repeated topical administration and should be referred to follow-up for a wound check in 24-48 hours. In patients with topical, dilute HF exposures, it is usually unnecessary to obtain serum electrolytes. Patients with dilute HF exposures do not typically require intravenous or intraarterial therapies.

Burkhart KK, et al. Comparison of topical magnesium and calcium treatment for dermal hydrofluoric acid burns. *Ann Emerg Med.* 1994;24:9-13.

Kirkpatrick JJ, Burd DA. An algorithmic approach to the treatment of hydrofluoric acid burns. *Burns.* 1995;21:495-499.

104.8.   Answer: C. Gaseous hydrogen fluoride exposures have the potential to simultaneously cause dermal, ocular, pulmonary, and systemic toxicity. For the pulmonary toxicity, administration of nebulized calcium gluconate is associated with symptomatic relief.

Wing JS, et al. Acute health effects in a community after a release of hydrofluoric acid. *Arch Environ Health.* 1991;46:155-160.

Lee DC, et al. Treatment of inhalational exposure to hydrofluoric acid with nebulized calcium gluconate. *J Occup Med.* 1993;35:470.

Kirkpatrick JJ, Burd DA. An algorithmic approach to the treatment of hydrofluoric acid burns. *Burns.* 1995;21:495-499.

104.9.   Answer: E. Most patients with ocular exposures to hydrofluoric acid will require an ophthalmology consultation. However, immediate therapy helps preserve vision. While there is some evidence for dilute (1%) calcium gluconate administration following irrigation, more concentrated salts are very irritating and are not recommended. Proprietary solutions claim benefit without the support of rigorous controlled data. They are also costly and not universally available. The most important therapy is immediate irrigation with either a sterile isotonic solution or tap water.

Sterile isotonic solutions are preferred, but tap water will suffice in the prehospital setting. It is recommended to limit the irrigation to 1 L in each eye and larger volumes are detrimental.

Beiran I, et al. The efficacy of calcium gluconate in ocular hydrofluoric acid burns. *Hum Exp Toxicol.* 1997;16:223-228.

McCulley JP, et al. Hydrofluoric acid burns of the eye. *J Occup Med.* 1983;25:447-450.

104.10. Answer: A. While the exact fate of excess fluoride is still in debate, the prevailing thought is that, in the presence of phosphate and hydroxyapatite, fluoride forms fluoroapatite and is deposited in bone.

Boink AB, et al. The mechanism of fluoride-induced hypocalcaemia. *Hum Exp Toxicol.* 1994;13:149-155.

Hydrocarbons

QUESTIONS

105.1. Following a hydrocarbon ingestion, which of the characteristics predisposes patients to pulmonary toxicity?
A. High viscosity
B. High surface tension
C. High volatility
D. High boiling point
E. High freezing point

105.2. A 2-year-old boy presents to the emergency department 30 minutes following an ingestion of kerosene. The ingestion was witnessed by his parents who describe an immediate episode of vomiting as well as coughing. The patient appears well upon presentation to the emergency department and a radiograph of his chest performed 1 hour after the ingestion is read as "normal." What is the best next management step?
A. Observation for 6 hours followed by a repeat chest radiograph
B. Consultation with an ear, nose, and throat (ENT) specialist for evaluation of vocal cord edema
C. Consultation with a gastroenterologist for an urgent upper endoscopy
D. If patient is able to tolerate food, then discharge home with close outpatient follow-up
E. Prophylactic intubation and transfer to a center with extracorporeal membrane oxygenation (ECMO) capabilities

105.3. Which of the following treatments is useful for hydrocarbon-induced pulmonary toxicity?
A. Prophylactic antibiotics
B. Mineral oil lavage
C. Corticosteroids
D. Positive end-expiratory pressure ventilation
E. Olive oil lavage

105.4. A 16-year-old boy became unresponsive in the bathroom when his mother walked in and startled him. Emergency medical services (EMS) found him pulseless and initiated chest compressions. In the emergency department, his electrocardiogram (ECG) rhythm is ventricular tachycardia that is unresponsive to defibrillation. What medication should be administered next to the patient?
A. Naloxone
B. Epinephrine
C. Albuterol
D. Esmolol
E. Atropine

105.5. A 64-year-old shoemaker presents with numbness that began in his distal extremities and progressed proximally. What occupational exposure best explains this finding?
A. Benzene
B. *n*-Hexane
C. Hexavalent chromium
D. Lead
E. Trichloroethylene

105.6. A 45-year-old woman presents with severe, episodic facial pain that is triggered by talking and brushing her teeth. The pain has been persistent and debilitating for several days. What exposure most likely caused this disorder?
- A. Carbamazepine
- B. Amitriptyline
- C. Trichloroethylene
- D. Methyl-*n*-butyl ketone
- E. 2,5-Hexanedione

105.7. A 32-year-old man presents to the emergency department because he is no longer able to walk. On examination, he has severe muscle weakness and gold paint around his nose and mouth. What is the most likely etiology for the weakness in this patient?
- A. Rhabdomyolysis
- B. Metabolic acidosis
- C. Hippuric acid accumulation
- D. Hypokalemia
- E. Dehydration

105.8. A 26-year-old woman presents after a phenol exposure to her skin. What is the best intervention?
- A. Irrigation with polyethylene glycol electrolyte lavage solution
- B. Irrigation with polyethylene glycol 400

- C. Irrigation with soap and water
- D. Irrigation with water alone
- E. Irrigation with olive oil

105.9. In patients who present following a kerosene ingestion, what type of gastrointestinal decontamination is indicated?
- A. Activated charcoal
- B. Gastric lavage
- C. Induced emesis
- D. Whole bowel irrigation
- E. No gastrointestinal decontamination

105.10. A 42-year-old man presents to the emergency department after being found unresponsive in his garage. An initial chest radiograph, electrocardiogram, and co-oximetry panel are within normal limits. His mental status improves, and he is admitted to the hospital for observation. A venous blood gas with a co-oximetry panel performed 12 hours later shows a rising carbon monoxide level to 17%. Which of the following substances explains his presentation?
- A. Toluene
- B. Carbon tetrachloride
- C. Benzene
- D. Terpene
- E. Methylene chloride

ANSWERS

105.1. Answer: C. The greatest concern with hydrocarbon ingestion is the risk of aspiration and the secondary development of pulmonary toxicity. Viscosity is the tendency of a substance to resist flow. Surface tension is a cohesive force generated between molecules. Volatility is the tendency for a liquid to change to a gas. Hydrocarbons with a low viscosity, low surface tension, and high volatility have a higher propensity for aspiration.

Gerard HW. Toxicological studies on hydrocarbons: V. Kerosone. *Toxic Appl Pharmacol.* 1959;1:462-469.

Gerard HW. Toxicological studies on hydrocarbons: IX. The aspiration hazard and toxicity of hydrocarbons and hydrocarbon mixtures. *Arch Environ Health.* 1963;6:329-341.

105.2. Answer: A. Kerosene, also known as paraffin, is a hydrocarbon that is associated with significant pulmonary injury when aspirated. Vomiting and coughing are common immediately following ingestion; however, there is a delay to the development of abnormal radiographic findings. The correct management following an exposure to a hydrocarbon is

observation for at least 6 hours followed by a chest radiograph. This child did not have drooling or stridor; therefore, the likelihood of a significant caustic injury is low, and an endoscopy is not indicated. He does not have any symptoms of airway edema or injury at this time, so a consultation with an ENT specialist is not necessary.

Anas N, et al. Criteria for hospitalizing children who have ingested products containing hydrocarbons. *JAMA.* 1981;246:840-843.

105.3. Answer: D. Prophylactic antibiotics and steroids have not proven to be useful in both animal and human studies. Olive oil and mineral oil lavage were used in the past as a means of increasing the viscosity of the resultant hydrocarbon mixture. There is no evidence that either of these is useful, and there are reports of toxicity from ingestion of these oils. Jet ventilation and positive end-expiratory pressure are useful in patients who have severe pulmonary injury.

Balme KH, et al. The efficacy of prophylactic antibiotics in the management of children with kerosene-associated pneumonitis: A double-blind randomised controlled trial. *Clin toxicol (Phil).* 2015;53:789-796.

Beamon RF, et al. Hydrocarbon ingestion in children: A six-year retrospective study. *JACEP*. 1976;5:771-775.

Bysani GK, et al. Treatment of hydrocarbon pneumonitis. High frequency jet ventilation as an alternative to extracorporeal membrane oxygenation. *Chest*. 1994;106:300-303.

Marks MI, et al. Adrenocorticosteroid treatment of hydrocarbon pneumonia in children—a cooperative study. *J Pediatr*. 1972;81:366-369.

105.4. Answer: D. This patient was abusing inhalants while in the bathroom, which are associated with myocardial sensitization. When his mother startled him, he had a catecholamine response that precipitated the cardiac dysrhythmia. This phenomenon is known as "sudden sniffing death syndrome." Beta adrenergic antagonists treat the ventricular tachycardias that occur because of myocardial sensitization; as esmolol is short acting, it would be an ideal therapy. Beta adrenergic agonists, such as epinephrine and albuterol, exacerbate the underlying condition and should be avoided if cardiac arrest follows hydrocarbon exposure. This patient's presentation is atypical for an opioid overdose; while naloxone is not contraindicated, it would not help.

Mortiz F, et al. Esmolol in the treatment of severe arrhythmia after acute trichloroethylene poisoning. *Intensive Care Med*. 2000;26:256.

105.5. Answer: B. Shoemaker's polyneuropathy is associated with occupational exposure to *n*-hexane. The metabolite of *n*-hexane, 2,5-hexanedione, causes a peripheral neuropathy that begins distally and progresses more proximally, also known as a dying-back neuropathy. 2,5-Hexanedione is also a metabolic intermediate of methyl-*n*-butyl ketone (MBK). While benezene is also an occupational exposure in shoemaking, it does not cause a polyneuropathy. Hexavalent chromium causes painless ulcers and a perforated nasal septum, known as "chrome holes," but is not typically associated with a neuropathy. Lead causes bilateral wrist drop but does not typically cause a dying-back neuropathy. Trichloroethylene is associated with trigeminal neuralgia.

Bos PM, et al. Critical review of the toxicity of methyl n-butyl ketone: Risk from occupational exposure. *Am J Ind Med*. 1991;20:175-194.

105.6. Answer: C. The patient is presenting with symptoms consistent with trigeminal neuralgia. Trichloroethylene exposure is associated with the development of trigeminal neuralgia, which occurs within 12 hours of exposure and persists for years. Carbamazepine and amitriptyline are often used as treatments for trigeminal neuralgia. Both methyl-*n*-butyl ketone and 2,5-hexanedione cause a peripheral neuropathy that classically begins distally and progresses proximally.

Leandri M, et al. Electrophysiological evidence of trigeminal root damage after trichloroethylene exposure. *Muscle Nerve*. 1995;18:467-468.

105.7. Answer: D. Toluene is available in many commercial products, including spray paint. Toluene abuse leads to renal potassium loss and subsequent symptomatic hypokalemia. The degree of muscle weakness is associated with the extent of the potassium deficit, and the symptoms resolve with replacement of potassium.

Cohr KH, Stolkholm J. Toluene, a toxicologic review. *Sand J Work Environ Health*. 1979;5:71-90.

Echeverria D, et al. Acute neurobehavioral effects of toluene. *Br J Ind Med*. 1989;46:483-495.

Fischman C, Oster VR. Toxic effects of toluene. *JAMA*. 1979;242:1491.

105.8. Answer: B. In patients who have a dermal exposure to hydrocarbons, local decontamination should be a priority. While for most hydrocarbons irrigation with soap and water is adequate, that is not the case with phenol. The ideal solution for irrigation following phenol exposure is polyethylene glycol 400 (PEG 400). Polyethylene glycol with electrolytes (PEG ELS) is the formulation routinely used for whole bowel irrigation and is not effective in phenol exposures. If PEG 400 is not immediately available, then irrigation with water should be used.

Monteiro-Riviere NA, et al. Efficacy of topical phenol decontamination strategies on severity of acute phenol chemical burns and dermal absorption: In vitro and in vivo studies in pig skin. *Toxicol Ind Health*. 2001;17:95-104.

105.9. Answer: E. Following hydrocarbon ingestion, the largest concern is for aspiration and subsequent development of a pneumonitis. In this exposure, the risks of induced emesis, activated charcoal, and gastric lavage outweigh the benefits and should be avoided. However, if the hydrocarbon was used as a vehicle for other toxins (such as a pesticide) or was inherently highly toxic (such as benzene) then some form of gastrointestinal decontamination is reasonable.

Laass W. Therapy of acute oral poisoning by organic solvents: Treatment by activated charcoal in combination with laxatives. *Arch Toxicol Suppl*. 1980;4:406-409.

Press E, et al. Cooperative kerosene poisoning study: Evaluation of gastric lavage and other factors in the treatment of accidental ingestion of petroleum distillate products. *Pediatrics*. 1962;29:648-674.

105.10. Answer: E. In 2019, the US Environmental Protection Agency (EPA) banned methylene chloride from products available for general consumer use. Prior to that, methylene chloride was found commonly in paint removers and degreasers. When it is inhaled or ingested it directly produces central nervous system depression. Methylene chloride is a one-carbon halomethane and is degraded by CYP2E1 to form carbon monoxide. Methylene chloride and other one-carbon halomethanes, such as methylene dibromide, should be suspected in patients who present to the hospital with a delayed elevation in carbon monoxide levels.

Ahmed AE, et al. Halogenated methanes: Metabolism and toxicity. *Fed Proc.* 1980;39:3150-3155.

QUESTIONS

106.1. The retinal toxicity caused by methanol poisoning is due to which of the following options?
A. Hyperosmolarity
B. Elevated lactic acid concentrations
C. Accumulation of formaldehyde
D. Accumulation of formic acid
E. Destruction of the retinal phospholipid membrane

106.2. A 26-year-old man has an elevated anion gap on his laboratory investigations. Which of the following options suggests an overdose of ethylene glycol?
A. Ketonuria
B. Lactate gap
C. Hypokalemia
D. Radiopaque density in the stomach
E. Hyperemic optic disks

106.3. Which of the following enzymes is involved in the metabolism of ethylene glycol to glycolic acid?
A. Cytochrome P450 isozyme CYP3A4
B. Glutamic acid decarboxylase
C. Aldehyde dehydrogenase
D. Pyruvic acid dehydrogenase
E. Reduced nicotinic acid dehydrogenase

106.4. A 16-year-old girl presents to the hospital after an intentional overdose of a bottle of rubbing alcohol. Which of the following would be characteristic of isopropanol (isopropyl alcohol) toxicity?
A. Crystaluria
B. A high anion gap

C. Ocular toxicity
D. Ketonuria
E. Metabolic acidosis

106.5. Which of the following alcohols causes central nervous system toxicity, respiratory distress, hypotension, and kidney and liver failure in neonates?
A. Benzyl alcohol
B. Propylene glycol
C. Isopropyl alcohol
D. Diethylene glycol
E. Methanol

106.6. A 15-year-old boy presents to the emergency department with an altered mental status. His laboratory results demonstrate an elevated creatinine to 2.2 mg/dL (194.5 micromol/L), an anion gap of 10 mEq/L, an osmol gap of 52 mOsm/L, and an undetectable ethanol concentration. His urinalysis reveals large ketones. Which of the following should be performed as part of his medical management?
A. Administration of oral ethanol
B. Administration of intravenous fomepizole
C. Emergent hemodialysis
D. Intravenous hydration with dextrose supplementation
E. Intravenous sodium bicarbonate infusion

106.7. A 45-year-old man presents to the hospital following an intentional overdose of methanol. His serum pH is 6.89, his serum bicarbonate is undetectably low, and his anion gap is 36 mEq/L. An osmol gap is calculated and it is 8 mOsm/L. Which of the following options should be performed next in this patient?
   A. Intravenous (IV) hydration and thiamine alone
   B. Oral ethanol alone
   C. Immediate IV hypertonic sodium bicarbonate
   D. IV fomepizole alone
   E. Continuous veno-venous hemofiltration

106.8. A 63-year-old man presents to the hospital 1.5 hours after an intentional ingestion of ethylene glycol. His laboratory findings demonstrate an osmol gap of 55 mOsm/L, an anion gap of 12 mEq/L, an undetectable ethanol concentration, and a serum creatinine of 0.8 mg/dL (70.7 micromol/L). Which of the following options would be the best initial therapy for this patient?
   A. Intravenous (IV) hydration and thiamine alone
   B. Oral ethanol alone
   C. Immediate hemodialysis
   D. IV fomepizole alone
   E. Continuous veno-venous hemofiltration

106.9. A toxicologist is working in a country that does not have fomepizole readily available and only has ethanol as an antidote for toxic alcohols. Which of the following statements is correct about ethanol therapy for methanol overdoses?
   A. Ethanol has no more adverse effects than fomepizole
   B. Patients receiving ethanol therapy are routinely managed in a lower acuity setting
   C. Ethanol is as effective as fomepizole
   D. Ethanol is easier to use than fomepizole
   E. Ethanol therapy should target a blood ethanol level of 50 mg/dL (10.8 mmol/L)

106.10. A 28-year-old man presents to the hospital with vague gastrointestinal complaints after an unknown ingestion. His laboratory investigations reveal an acute kidney injury. Several days later, he develops bilateral facial nerve paralysis and peripheral extremity weakness. What ingestion explains his presentation?
   A. Ethylene glycol
   B. Isopropyl alcohol
   C. Diethylene glycol
   D. Methanol
   E. Benzyl alcohol

ANSWERS

106.1. Answer: D. The retinal toxicity from methanol is the direct result of the accumulation of the metabolite formic acid. Formate inhibits the cytochrome oxidase chain, increasing lactate production and metabolic acidosis at the cellular level.

Sejersted OM. Formate concentrations in plasma from patients poisoned with methanol. *Acta Med Scand.* 1983;213:105-110.

106.2. Answer: B. Many hospitals do not have ready access to a laboratory that provides ethylene glycol, methanol, and isopropyl alcohol concentrations in a time that would assist in medical decision making. Clinicians must, therefore, use surrogate findings that suggest a toxic alcohol ingestion. A lactate gap points towards an ingestion of ethylene glycol. Glycolate, one of the metabolites of ethylene glycol, only differs structurally from lactate by one carbon, which leads to a false-positive lactate elevation in certain analyzers. When two blood lactate concentrations are requested simultaneously and run on two different analyzers with a large discrepancy in results, a "lactate gap" is present. This finding suggests an ethylene glycol ingestion.

Tintu A, et al. Interference of ethylene glycol with (L)-lactate measurement is assay-dependent. *Ann Clin Biochem.* 2013;50:70-72.

106.3. Answer: C. Ethylene glycol is metabolized by alcohol dehydrogenase to glycoaldehyde and then by aldehyde dehydrogenase to glycolic acid, which is then slowly metabolized to glyoxylic acid and then to oxalic acid. Fomepizole inhibits alcohol dehydrogenase, thereby preventing metabolism and the subsequent accumulation of glycolic acid and ultimately oxalic acid.

Jacobsen D, et al. Ethylene glycol intoxication: Evaluation of kinetics and crystalluria. *Am J Med.* 1988;84:145-152.

106.4. Answer: D. The finding of ketones in the blood and urine in the absence of a metabolic acidosis, crystalluria, or an elevated anion gap is consistent with an isopropyl alcohol ingestion.

Daniel DR, et al. Isopropyl alcohol metabolism after acute intoxication in humans. *J Anal Toxicol.* 1981;5:110-112.

Rich J, et al. Isopropyl alcohol intoxication. *Arch Neurol.* 1990;47:322-324.

106.5. Answer A. The administration of bacteriostatic sodium chloride or bacteriostatic water, which contained benzyl alcohol, was responsible for central nervous system toxicity, respiratory distress, hypotension, metabolic acidosis, and kidney and liver failure in neonates. This syndrome is also known as the gasping baby syndrome. Benzyl alcohol is metabolized to benzoic acid and conjugated with glycine and excreted as hippuric acid. Neonates have an immature conjugation pathway and limited glycine reserves, generating a high anion gap metabolic acidosis caused by the accumulation of benzoic acid.

Gershank JJ, et al. The gasping syndrome and benzyl alcohol poisoning. *N Engl J Med.* 1982;307:1384-1388.

Vest, et al. Conjugation reactions in the newborn infant. *Arch Dis Child.* 1965;40:97-105.

106.6. Answer: D. Although isopropanol is usually categorized as a toxic alcohol, it is relatively benign compared to ethylene glycol and methanol. Isopropanol is associated with inebriation, which is usually more prolonged than ethanol. Isopropanol is metabolized by alcohol dehydrogenase to form acetone and both lead to an elevated osmolar gap with a normal anion gap. An elevated creatinine often occurs; however, this is secondary to a laboratory interference from the acetone and not a true acute kidney injury. While hemodialysis will remove both the isopropyl alcohol and the acetone, it is rarely indicated as the risks of hemodialysis usually outweigh the benefits. Ingestion of isopropanol rarely leads to end-organ injury, and usually supportive care is adequate.

Dyer S, et al. Hemorrhagic gastritis from topical isopropanol exposure. *Ann Pharmacother.* 2002;36:1733-1735.

Killeen C, et al. Pseudorenal insufficiency with isopropyl alcohol ingestion. *Am J Ther.* 2011;18:e113-e116.

106.7. Answer: C. In patients who present early following an ingestion of a toxic alcohol, the osmol gap is elevated. However, as the alcohol is metabolized to its toxic metabolites, the osmol gap will drop as the anion gap becomes elevated. A normal osmol gap ranges from −14 to +10 mOsm/L. For these two reasons, an elevated osmol gap should not be used to exclude a toxic alcohol. However, if the osmol gap is >40 mOsm/L, then a toxic alcohol ingestion becomes more likely. In this patient, immediate administration of IV hypertonic sodium bicarbonate to correct the metabolic acidosis and to alter the distribution of the formate metabolite from the eye and into the urine is critical. Since it is unknown if there is still any parent compound present, following this with IV fomepizole is appropriate. Furthermore, as this patient already has a severe metabolic acidosis, emergent hemodialysis is warranted to correct the acid–base disorder and to remove any remaining formic acid and methanol. Continuous veno-venous hemofiltration is not ideal, and

intermittent hemodialysis is the more appropriate extracorporeal removal technique.

Hoffman RS, et al. Osmol gaps revisited: Normal values and limitations. *J Toxicol Clin Toxicol.* 1993;31:81-93.

Roberts DM, et al. Recommendations for the role of extracorporeal treatments in the management of acute methanol poisoning: A systematic review and consensus statement. *Crit Care Med.* 2015;43:461-472.

106.8. Answer: D. Given this patient's elevated osmol gap, normal anion gap, normal creatinine, and reported history of ingestion 1.5 hours ago, it is likely that this patient is presenting early enough that the ethylene glycol has not been metabolized to toxic metabolites. Administration of IV fomepizole is indicated to prevent the metabolism of the ethylene glycol. While ethanol would also prevent the metabolism of ethylene glycol, the disadvantages that come with administering it are many, and it should not be given when fomepizole is available. Intravenous ethanol is not commercially available in the US and would have to be compounded, likely delaying administration. Oral ethanol is a reasonable temporizing method if a patient presents to a critical access hospital with no fomepizole available or in an epidemic situation when there is a shortage of fomepizole. If possible, this patient would be better cared for in a tertiary hospital where definitive care, such as hemodialysis and fomepizole, would be available. Ethylene glycol is rapidly eliminated by the kidney if kidney function is preserved. If IV fomepizole is given and the patient has adequate kidney function, that will be adequate treatment. Hemodialysis could be needed if this patient's creatinine begins to rise. In contrast, methanol is primarily cleared through the lungs, and it takes as long 7-10 days to be fully eliminated from the body; therefore, if a patient presents following a methanol overdose, administration of IV fomepizole followed by hemodialysis is the correct option. Hemodialysis alone is not adequate in someone who likely has significant parent compound as the ethylene glycol continues to be metabolized.

Cheng JT, et al. Clearance of ethylene glycol by kidneys and hemodialysis. *J Toxicol Clin Toxicol.* 1987;25:95-108.

106.9. Answer: C. Although never directly compared in a randomized trial, outbreak data suggest that ethanol therapy is as effective as fomepizole therapy in preventing death from methanol. The goal of ethanol therapy is to achieve a blood ethanol concentration of 100-150 mg/dL (21.7-32.5 mmol/L). This is most often achieved with oral ethanol since intravenous (IV) ethanol is no longer commercially available in the US and would need to be compounded, delaying the time to administration. Ethanol is associated with significantly more complications than IV fomepizole, including hypotension, central nervous system depression, hypoglycemia, pancreatitis, and gastritis. Patients receiving ethanol therapy require frequent evaluation of their serum ethanol concentration to ensure that they remain within the appropriate therapeutic window. Furthermore, given the high incidence of adverse events, these patients frequently require an intensive care unit for appropriate monitoring.

> Noker PE, et al. Methanol toxicity: Treatment with folic acid and 5-formyltetrahydrofolic acid. *Alcohol: Clin Exp Res.* 1980;4:378-383.

> Zakharov S, et al. Fomepizole versus ethanol in the treatment of acute methanol poisoning: Comparison of clinical effectiveness in a mass poisoning outbreak. *Clin Toxicol.* 2015;53:797-806.

106.10. Answer: C. Diethylene glycol (DEG) is used as an antifreeze; however it is sweet tasting and was used as a diluent. There have been numerous mass poisonings associated with the use of DEG in liquid medicines. The first outbreak was elixir of sulfanilamide in 1937 that played a large role in the development of the modern-day Food and Drug Administration in the United States. A more recent outbreak of DEG toxicity was in 2006 in Panama, where DEG was found in cough syrup. DEG is a potent neurotoxin as well as a nephrotoxin. Patients initially present with vague gastrointestinal or respiratory complaints but then progress to develop severe kidney injury necessitating dialysis and neurologic injury that progresses to coma. DEG causes both unilateral and bilateral seventh cranial nerve paralysis. Fomepizole and hemodialysis are recommended as soon as possible in patients in whom DEG toxicity is suspected.

> Alfred S, et al. Delayed neurologic sequelae resulting from epidemic diethylene glycol poisoning. *Clin Toxicol.* 2005;43:155-159.

> Sosa NR, et al. Clinical, laboratory, diagnostic, and histopathologic features of diethylene glycol poisoning—Panama, 2006. *Ann Emerg Med.* 2014;64:38-47.

QUESTIONS

107.1. A 24-year-old man ingests a depilatory sold for patients with folliculitis barbae. He presents with nausea and vomiting. Which of the following electrolyte abnormalities are most likely to occur?
A. Hyperkalemia, hypermagnesemia
B. Hypokalemia, hyperphosphatemia
C. Hypokalemia, hypophosphatemia
D. Hyperkalemia, hyperphosphatemia
E. Hyperkalemia, hypophosphatemia

107.2. A 4-year-old girl is brought to the hospital 30 minutes after an ingestion of a barium carbonate rodenticide. Which of the following methods of gastrointestinal decontamination is reasonable?
A. Oral activated charcoal
B. Oral sodium or magnesium sulfate
C. Oral sorbitol
D. Whole bowel irrigation with polyethylene glycol electrolyte lavage solution
E. No gastrointestinal decontamination is recommended

107.3. Which of the following mechanisms bests explains toxicity from barium salt ingestion?
A. Inhibition of calcium-activated potassium rectifier channels
B. Blockade of Na^+,K^+-ATPase
C. Potassium wasting in the renal tubules
D. Binding of potassium in the gastrointestinal tract
E. Glucose-mediated intracellular potassium shift

107.4. Weakness in the setting of barium toxicity is best correlated with which of the following findings?
A. Hypokalemia
B. Hyperkalemia
C. Hypermagnesemia
D. Hypophosphatemia
E. Barium concentration

107.5. Which of the following statements is true regarding the toxicokinetics of barium salts?
A. As water solubility increases, absorption decreases
B. As water solubility increases, absorption increases
C. Water solubility has little effect on absorption
D. Most absorbed barium is renally eliminated
E. Because of deep compartmental stores, the terminal elimination half-life of barium is about 30 days

107.6. Which analyte is preferred to confirm acute barium poisoning?
A. Serum
B. Urine
C. Hair
D. Stool
E. Whole blood

107.7. Which of the following extracorporeal modalities would be reasonable in a patient with barium poisoning who is not responsive to standard therapies?
A. Peritoneal dialysis
B. Hemodialysis
C. Hemoperfusion
D. Therapeutic plasma exchange
E. Continuous veno-venous hemodialysis

107.8. During a barium enema contrast study in a 23-year-old man, contrast is noted in the portal vein. Which of the following clinical effects is expected?
- A. Hypokalemia
- B. Weakness
- C. Cardiovascular collapse
- D. Hepatotoxicity
- E. Acute kidney injury

107.9. What radiologic findings are expected on chest imaging after occupational exposure to inhaled particulate insoluble barium?
- A. Ground-glass opacities
- B. Hilar lymphadenopathy resembling sarcoidosis
- C. Egg shell calcifications
- D. Very fine punctate and annular lesions and some slightly larger nodules
- E. Calcified pleural plaques

107.10. A 40-year-old factory worker is exposed to barium styphnate. Which of the following manifestations is unique to barium styphnate?
- A. Electrolyte abnormalities
- B. Cardiac dysrhythmias
- C. Weakness
- D. Nausea and vomiting
- E. Cutaneous burns

ANSWERS

107.1. Answer: C. Barium sulfide is sold as a depilatory. Severe hypokalemia is a cardinal feature of barium toxicity and is exacerbated by blood transfusions. Patients are subject to many complications of hypokalemia, such as ventricular dysrhythmias, hypotension, muscular weakness, and respiratory failure. Hypophosphatemia is another less commonly associated electrolyte abnormality that occurs in patients with barium toxicity.

Johnson CH, VanTassell VJ. Acute barium poisoning with respiratory failure and rhabdomyolysis. *Ann Emerg Med.* 1991;20:1138-1142.

Bhoelan BS, et al. Barium toxicity and the role of the potassium inward rectifier current. *Clin Toxicol (Phila)* 2014;52:584-593.

107.2. Answer: B. It is unlikely that barium is adsorbed to activated charcoal. Soluble oral barium is rapidly absorbed so that attempts at catharsis are unlikely to be beneficial. However, the administration of oral sodium or magnesium sulfate converts barium carbonate or barium chloride to the less soluble sulfate form, thereby limiting absorption.

Payen C, et al. Intoxication by large amounts of barium nitrate overcome by early massive K supplementation and oral administration of magnesium sulphate. *Hum Exp Toxicol.* 2011;30:34-37.

Mills K, Kunkel D. Prevention of severe barium carbonate toxicity with oral magnesium sulfate. *Vet Human Toxicol.* 1993;35:342.

107.3. Answer: A. Barium inhibits calcium-activated potassium rectifier channels, reducing outward flow of potassium. There is also a persistent Na^+,K^+-ATPase pump electrogenesis, which leads to a shift of extracellular potassium into the cell. The net effect is hypokalemia.

Bhoelan BS, et al. Barium toxicity and the role of the potassium inward rectifier current. *Clin Toxicol (Phila)* 2014;52:584-593.

107.4. Answer: E. Although hypokalemia is often severe enough to account for weakness and paralysis, the fact that weakness correlates better with the barium concentration than with the potassium concentration suggests that there is an additional direct effect of barium on skeletal muscle.

Phelan DM, et al. Is hypokalaemia the cause of paralysis in barium poisoning? *BMJ (Clin Res Ed).* 1984;289:882.

Thomas M, et al. Acute barium intoxication following ingestion of ceramic glaze. *Postgrad Med J.* 1998;74:545-546.

107.5. Answer: B. Absorption of barium salts is directly correlated with water solubility. Compounds such as barium sulfate (used for enteral contrast) are essentially not absorbed. Barium chloride, on the other hand, is rapidly absorbed. Fecal elimination is the primary mode of excretion. Unlike lead, there is no deep compartmental reservoir for barium.

Johnson CH, VanTassell VJ. Acute barium poisoning with respiratory failure and rhabdomyolysis. *Ann Emerg Med.* 1991;20:1138-1142.

Schorn TF, et al. Barium carbonate intoxication. *Intensive Care Med.* 1991;17:60-62.

107.6. Answer: A. Although barium is measured in a variety of analytes, it is important to remember that the results will rarely be available in a time frame to assist with clinical decision making. Standards and normal concentrations are best described for serum, and therefore, it is the preferred analyte.

Phelan DM, et al. Is hypokalaemia the cause of paralysis in barium poisoning? *BMJ (Clin Res Ed).* 1984;289:882.

Thomas M, et al. Acute barium intoxication following ingestion of ceramic glaze. *Postgrad Med J.* 1998;74:545-546.

Łukasik-Głębocka M, et al. Barium determination in gastric contents, blood and urine by inductively coupled plasma mass spectrometry in the case of oral barium chloride poisoning. *J Anal Toxicol.* 2014;38:380-382.

107.7. Answer: B. In this instance, the goal of extracorporeal therapy is to rapidly restore and maintain a normal serum potassium (any elimination of barium would be secondary). This is best achieved with the high blood flow rates of hemodialysis with a relatively high potassium concentration in the dialysate. Continuous veno-venous hemodialysis would be the next best choice.

Bahlmann H, et al. Acute barium nitrate intoxication treated by hemodialysis. *Acta Anaesthesiol Scand.* 2005;49:110-112.

Wells JA, Wood KE. Acute barium poisoning treated with hemodialysis. *Am J Emerg Med.* 2001;19:175-177.

107.8. Answer: C. When barium contrast is instilled under pressure, intravasation (leakage into the circulation) is rarely reported. Patients are at risk for both air and contrast embolism with sudden cardiovascular collapse. Intraabdominal sepsis also occurs. The typical manifestations of barium toxicity (hypokalemia) are not usually expected.

O'Hara DE, et al. Barium intravasation during an upper gastrointestinal examination: A case report and literature review. *Am Surg.* 1995;61:330-333.

Takahashi M, et al. Nonfatal barium intravasation into the portal venous system during barium enema examination. *Intern Med.* 2004;43: 1145-1150.

107.9. Answer: D. Pulmonary baritosis is a benign pneumoconiosis that is described in workers exposed to ground insoluble barium salts. Radiographic findings consist of very fine punctate and annular lesions and some slightly larger nodular lesions. Ground-glass opacities (A) are typically seen with viral diseases and were reported as a complication of vaping (E-cigarette or vaping use-associated lung injury). Berylliosis resembles sarcoidosis (B). Egg-shell calcifications are seen in silicosis (C). Calcified pleural plaques (E) are observed after chronic asbestos exposure and are typical of mesothelioma.

Doig AT. Baritosis: A benign pneumoconiosis. *Thorax.* 1976;31:30-39.

107.10. Answer: E. Barium styphnate is a highly explosive compound. Exposure resulting from the explosion produces cutaneous burns and trauma followed by classic signs and symptoms of barium toxicity. Although this patient's potassium concentration was 3.5 mEq/L on presentation, an hour later, his hypokalemia worsened to 2.9 mEq/L.

Jacobs IA, et al. Poisoning as a result of barium styphnate explosion. *Am J Ind Med.* 2002;41:285-288.

Fumigants

QUESTIONS

108.1. In 1987, the Montreal Protocol was created as an international agreement to reduce the environmental impact of fumigants. Reduction of which of the following options was the main target of this agreement?
A. Deforestation
B. Water contamination
C. Fossil fuel use
D. Carbon emissions
E. Ozone depletion

108.2. A 3-year-old boy unintentionally ingests zinc phosphide after it was added to a cookie meant to attract and eliminate rodents in the home. The child presents in cardiovascular collapse. What odor might be present on the child's breath?
A. Rotting fish
B. Freshly mown hay
C. Pears
D. Apple blossoms
E. Bitter almonds

108.3. What is the underlying mechanism of toxicity from metal phosphides?
A. Reaction with sulfhydryl groups
B. Suicide inhibition of aconitase
C. Induction of P-glycoprotein
D. Inhibition of cytochrome c oxidase
E. Glutathione depletion

108.4. Phosphine is metabolized to phosphite and hypophosphite rapidly in the blood, and therefore, serum testing for diagnostic purposes is limited. What other test is easily used at the bedside to aid with diagnosis?
A. Sodium periodate
B. Alcohol oxidase
C. Urine fluorescence
D. Ferric chloride
E. Silver nitrate

108.5. A 4-year-old boy presents to the emergency department following an unintentional ingestion of aluminum phosphide. Which antidote is reasonable to administer?
A. *N*-Acetylcysteine
B. Octreotide
C. Fomepizole
D. Physostigmine
E. Flumazenil

108.6. A family vacationing in the US Virgin Islands all develop varying degrees of neurologic effects. The two teenage sons both present to the emergency department with generalized tonic-clonic seizures. The father presents with tremor and difficulty walking. On further investigation, it is discovered that the villa below theirs was being fumigated. Which fumigant is responsible for their neurologic effects?
A. Dichloropropene
B. Methyl bromide
C. Aluminum phosphide
D. Zinc phosphide
E. Sulfuryl fluoride

108.7. A magnetitic resonance imaging (MRI) is performed on the two teenage boys from Question 108.6. The findings seen on their MRI mimics which pathology?
  A. Intrathecal methotrexate toxicity
  B. Multiple sclerosis
  C. Parkinson disease
  D. Herpes simplex encephalitis
  E. Wernicke encephalopathy

108.8. A 62-year-old man with a chronic occupational exposure to 1,3-dichloropropene should be screened for which malignancy?
  A. Hepatocellular carcinoma
  B. Pancreatic malignancy
  C. Lymphoma and leukemia
  D. Small cell adenocarcinoma
  E. Urothelial tumors

108.9. A 46-year-old-man presents to the emergency department after being found unresponsive at work. His electrocardiogram (ECG) demonstrates both QRS complex widening and QT interval prolongation. His colleague said that they were working with sulfuryl fluoride gas. Which medication should be administered?
  A. Isoproterenol
  B. Lidocaine
  C. Calcium gluconate
  D. Esmolol
  E. Sodium bicarbonate

108.10. A 27-year-old agricultural worker presents to clinic with cognitive and neurobehavioral changes. He has a history of a severe burn from a chemical used at work. Which fumigant is associated with late neuropsychiatric sequelae?
  A. Methyl iodide
  B. 1,3-Dibromochloropropane
  C. Sulfuryl fluoride
  D. Zinc phosphide
  E. Glyphosate

ANSWERS

108.1. Answer: E. The Montreal Protocol was established to protect the environment through reduction of production and consumption of products that deplete ozone. This includes chlorofluorocarbons and halons, such as methyl bromide. Unfortunately, many corporations have exceptions and are still able to produce these chemicals.

US Department of State. The Montreal Protocol on Substances That Deplete the Ozone Layer. https://www.state.gov/key-topics-office-of-environmental-quality-and-transboundary-issues/the-montreal-protocol-on-substances-that-deplete-the-ozone-layer/. Accessed April 2, 2021.

108.2. Answer: A. Exposure to metal phosphides results in the production of phosphine gas when combined with moisture in the mouth and hydrochloric acid in the stomach. Pure phosphine gas is odorless; it is the substituted phosphines and diphosphines that are associated with this characteristic smell. Phosphines are described to have a fishy or garlic odor, even at small amounts of 0.2 to 3 parts per million.

Popp W, et al. Phosphine gas poisoning in a German office. *Lancet.* 2002;359:1574.

108.3. Answer: D. Metal phosphides, such as zinc and aluminum phosphide, react with water or acid to produce phosphine gas. Phosphine gas is a noncompetitive inhibitor of oxidative phosphorylation and interferes with mitochondrial complexes I through IV, in addition to inhibition of catalase.

Singh S, et al. Cytochrome-c oxidase inhibition in 26 aluminum phosphide poisoned patients. *Clin Toxicol.* 2006;44:155-158.

108.4. Answer: E. Phosphine, when exhaled, will cause silver nitrate to turn black, with a detection limit of 0.05 ppm. Ammonium molybdate produces canary yellow precipitates when combined with phosphides in stomach acid; however, this test is more appropriately used post-mortem.

Koreti S, et al. Aluminum phosphide poisoning in children—challenges in diagnosis and management. *Sch Acad J Biosci.* 2014;2:505-509.

108.5. Answer: A. In a small, randomized, controlled trial, the addition of *N*-acetylcysteine (NAC) to supportive care, compared to supportive care alone, resulted in decreased mortality, decreased intubation rates, and decreased length of stay. NAC also reduced blood thiobarbituric acid reactive substances, which are a marker of lipid peroxidation. Given the low cost and ease of use, NAC is recommended.

Tehrani H, et al. Protective effects of N-acetylcysteine on aluminum phosphide-induced oxidative stress in acute human poisoning. *Clin Toxicol.* 2013;51:23-28.

108.6 Answer: B. Methyl bromide inhalation leads to seizures, coma, dysrhythmias, acute respiratory distress syndrome, and death. At lower concentrations, neurotoxicity such as tremor, diplopia, dysmetria, and dysarthria occurs.

The mainstay of therapy is to remove patients from the exposure. The seizures are very difficult to control, and multiple antiepileptics, such as propofol, thiopental, and pentobarbital, are often needed.

Lifshitz M, Gavrilov V. Central nervous system toxicity and early peripheral neuropathy following dermal exposure to methyl bromide. *Clin Toxicol*. 2000;38:799-801.

Hustinx WNM, et al. Systemic effects of inhalational methyl bromide poisoning: A study of nine cases occupationally exposed due to inadvertent spread during fumigation. *Br J Ind Med*. 1993;50:155-159.

108.7. Answer: E. After poisoning with methyl bromide, classic MRI findings include symmetric T2 signal abnormalities in the inferior colliculi. Other areas involved include the subthalamic nuclei, periaqueductal gray matter, and basal ganglia. These findings are reversible and reflect an overall energy-depleted state. Thiamine deficiency and resultant Wernicke encephalopathy lead to a similar distribution of findings as methyl bromide. Wernicke encephalopathy is associated with damage to the mammillary bodies and also causes symmetric changes in the periventricular areas of the thalamus, hypothalamus, brainstem, periaqueductal midbrain, and cerebellar cortex.

Geyer HL, et al. Methyl bromide intoxication causes reversible symmetric brainstem and cerebellar MRI lesions. *Neurology*. 2005;64:1279-1281.

Koguchi K, et al. Wernicke's encephalopathy after glucose infusion. *Neurology* 2004;62:512.

108.8. Answer: C. 1,3-Dichloropropene was introduced in 1945 as a nematicide to decrease exposure to dibromochloropropane. It has structural similarity to vinyl chloride, which is a known carcinogen. Case reports suggest that patients exposed to 1,3-dichloropropene are at increased risk for developing hematologic malignancies, such as leukemia and lymphoma.

Markovitz A, Crosby WH. Chemical carcinogenesis: A soil fumigant, 1,3-dichloropropene, as possible cause of hematologic malignancies. *Arch Intern Med*. 1984;144:1409-1411.

108.9. Answer: C. ECG changes secondary to sulfuryl fluoride toxicity are mediated via fluoride toxicity, which results in hypocalcemia. Hypocalcemia causes both QRS complex widening and QT interval prolongation, leading to dysrhythmias. Calcium gluconate or calcium chloride should be administered in this setting. Other potential electrolyte abnormalities include hyperkalemia and hypomagnesemia.

Nuckolls JG, et al. Fatalities resulting from sulfuryl fluoride exposure after home fumigation—Virginia. *JAMA*. 1987;258:2041-2042.

Scheuerman EH. Case report: Suicide by exposure to sulfuryl fluoride. *J Forensic Sci*. 1986;31:1154-1158.

108.10. Answer: A. After massive methyl iodide exposure, patients demonstrate personality changes and cognitive impairment, often as late effects. Specifically, deficits related to attention, recent memory, information processing, and visual memory occur. The exact mechanism is unclear, but neurotoxicity is believed to be a result of glutathione depletion and metabolism, similar to what occurs with methyl bromide toxicity.

Schwartz MD, et al. Acute methyl iodide exposure with delayed neuropsychiatric sequelae: Report of a case. *Am J Ind Med*. 2005;47:550-556.

QUESTIONS

109.1. Which of the following xenobiotics is an appropriate treatment for a patient with acute 2,4-dichlorophenoxyacetic acid toxicity?
A. *N*-Acetylcysteine (NAC)
B. Methylene blue
C. Cyclophosphamide
D. Fomepizole
E. Sodium bicarbonate

109.2. A 45-year-old man presents to the hospital with influenzalike symptoms, shortness of breath, and an acute kidney injury. Approximately 36 hours prior to arrival, he ate mushrooms brought from Poland. The toxin in this mushroom resembles which of the following herbicides?
A. Dinitrophenol
B. Glyphosate
C. Bromoxynil
D. Diquat
E. Atrazine

109.3. Which of the following statements about the pulmonary toxicity of paraquat is correct?
A. The superoxide radical consumes electrons and depletes cells of NADH
B. An acute alveolitis occurs with the loss of only type II cells
C. The pulmonary toxicity of diquat is almost identical to the toxicity of paraquat
D. A proliferation of fibroblasts and extensive deposition of collagen in the interstitium and alveolar spaces cause a loss of alveolar integrity
E. Paraquat acts as an antiinflammatory in the lungs

109.4. Which of the following antidotes is beneficial in the treatment of paraquat poisoning?
A. Deferoxamine
B. Ascorbic acid
C. Vitamin E
D. *N*-Acetylcysteine
E. None of the above

109.5. Which of the following standard therapies is harmful in patients with paraquat toxicity?
A. 50% dextrose
B. 100% oxygen
C. Naloxone
D. Thiamine
E. *N*-Acetylcysteine

109.6. Which of the following tests is used to confirm ingestion of paraquat or diquat?
A. Urinary dithionate
B. Urinary ferric chloride
C. Expose venous blood to air and observe for color change
D. Serum butyrylcholinesterase
E. Negative inspiratory force (NIF)

109.7. A 32-year-old man presents to the emergency department following an intentional ingestion of the herbicide dinitrophenol. Which of the following treatments is most important in the management of this patient?
A. Sodium bicarbonate
B. *N*-Acetylcysteine
C. Fuller's earth
D. Hemodialysis
E. Ice water immersion

109.8. A 26-year-old woman presents to the emergency department following an intentional ingestion of the herbicide propanil. Which of the following tests will be helpful in guiding the management of this patient?
A. Urinary dithionate
B. Urinary ferric chloride
C. Expose venous blood to air and observe for color change
D. Serum butyrylcholinesterase
E. Negative inspiratory force (NIF)

109.9. A 62-year-old woman presents to the emergency department following an intentional ingestion of an herbicide. She has initial vomiting and is admitted to the hospital for observation. Twenty-four hour later, she has altered mental status and a seizure. She then develops an elevated temperature and respiratory failure requiring mechanical ventilation. Her laboratory analysis demonstrates an elevated ammonia concentration. Which of the following herbicides did she ingest?
A. Paraquat
B. Diquat
C. Glufosinate
D. Glyphosate
E. Atrazine

109.10. A 27-year-old man presents to the hospital following an intentional ingestion of glyphosate. He eventually develops severe toxicity, requiring mechanical ventilation. Which of the following therapies will this patient most likely require?
A. Calcium gluconate
B. Ice water immersion
C. Methylene blue
D. Fomepizole
E. *N*-Acetylcysteine

ANSWERS

109.1. Answer: E. Patients who present following an ingestion of 2,4-dichlorophenoxyacetic acid (2,4-D) need to be observed for 24-48 hours. Urinary alkalinization increases the urinary excretion of 2,4-D. In patients who are symptomatic urine alkalinization (with a goal urine pH of >7.50) helps to limit the distribution of phenoxy compounds from the central circulation. In patients who have severe toxicity, hemodialysis is reasonable, given 2,4-D is small and water-soluble, with saturable protein binding. None of the other answers play a specific role in the management of acute phenoxy herbicide toxicity.

Prescott LF, et al. Treatment of severe 2,4-D and mecoprop intoxication with alkaline diuresis. *Br J Clin Pharmacol.* 1979;7:111-116.

109.2. Answer: D. The patient in this case ate a *Cortinarius orellanus* mushroom which contain orellanine. Orellanine is a bipyridyl compound with a chemical structure that resembles paraquat and diquat. Although it creates reactive oxygen species, it does not concentrate in the lungs to the same extent as paraquat, so severe pulmonary toxicity does not occur.

Richard JM, et al. Nephrotoxicity of orellanine, a toxin from the mushroom *Cortinarius orellanus. Arch Toxicol.* 1988;62:242-245.

109.3. Answer: D. The effects in the lungs following a paraquat ingestion result from proliferation of fibroblasts and extensive deposition of collagen in the interstitium and alveolar spaces, causing a loss of alveolar integrity.

Barbás K, et al. Inhibition of lung damage caused by paraquat with lymphokines or cytokines. *Exp Pathol.* 1990;38:189-195.

109.4. Answer: E. There is no effective antidote for paraquat poisoning. Therapy is directed at preventing absorption, enhancing elimination, and providing supportive care. Death occurs following ingestions of as little as 10 to 20 mL of a 20% wt/vol solution. As outcomes from an overdose of this herbicide are so devastating, the only real solution is to ban this herbicide.

Bismuth C, et al. Prognosis and treatment of paraquat poisoning: A review of 28 cases. *J Toxicol Clin Toxicol.* 1982;19:461-474.

109.5. Answer: B. The spontaneous reaction of paraquat with molecular oxygen in the lungs yields a superoxide radical and reforms a paraquat cation, which again takes part in a redox reaction. Supplemental oxygen increases the generation of reactive oxygen species.

Smith LL. The toxicity of paraquat. *Adverse Drug React Acute Poisoning Rev.* 1988;1:1-17.

109.6. Answer: A. The urinary dithionate test is used to confirm exposure to either paraquat or diquat. The urine will turn blue if paraquat is present and green if diquat is present. The darker the color, the higher the concentration.

Koo JR, et al. Rapid analysis of plasma paraquat using sodium dithionite as a predictor of outcome in acute paraquat poisoning. *Am J Med Sci.* 2009;338:373-377.

109.7. Answer: E. Dinitrophenol is an herbicide that causes uncoupling of oxidative phosphorylation in the mitochondria. Dinitrophenol is also used as a weight loss supplement. Patients who overdose on dinitrophenol develop severe, life-threatening hyperthermia. Management of these patients must include rapid cooling.

Grundlingh J, et al. 2,4-dinitrophenol (DNP): A weight loss agent with significant acute toxicity and risk of death. *J Med Toxicol.* 2011;7:205-212.

109.8. Answer: C. Propanil gets metabolized to 3,4-dichloroaniline and causes methemoglobinemia. Because concentrations of 3,4-dichloroaniline remain elevated in the body for prolonged periods of time, patients are at risk for protracted production of methemoglobin. Patients should be treated with methylene blue. Patients are also at risk of developing rebound methemobloginemia; this is prevented by the administration of methylene blue as a constant infusion.

Roberts DM, et al. Clinical outcomes and kinetics of propanil following acute self-poisoning: A prospective case series. *BMC Clin Pharmacol.* 2009;9:3.

109.9. Answer: C. Glufosinate is an herbicide that primarily causes neurologic toxicity and respiratory impairment. Patients who ingest glufosinate need to be admitted and observed for 48 hours as clinical symptoms are often delayed. Ammonia concentrations are elevated following an ingestion of glufosinate; the concentration peaks at 24 to 48 hours after ingestion, and increasing concentrations suggest an increased risk of neurotoxicity. There are no specific antidotes available to treat this overdose. The mainstay of therapy is supportive care, management of the seizures, and early intubation in patients who demonstrate signs of respiratory impairment.

Mao YC, et al. Acute human glufosinate-containing herbicide poisoning. *Clin Toxicol (Phila).* 2012;50:396-402.

Mao YC, et al. Hyperammonemia following glufosinate-containing herbicide poisoning: A potential marker of severe neurotoxicity. *Clin Toxicol (Phila).* 2011;49:48-52.

109.10. Answer: A. Glyphosate causes nausea and vomiting, gastrointestinal burns and necrosis, multisystem organ dysfunction, pancreatitis, acute respiratory distress syndrome, and pneumonitis. Electrolytes need to be monitored closely, as several formulations of glyphosate contain glyphosate as a potassium salt and overdoses often lead to severe hyperkalemia with electrocardiographic changes.

Garlich FM, et al. Hemodialysis clearance of glyphosate following a life-threatening ingestion of glyphosate-surfactant herbicide. *Clin Toxicol.* 2014;52:66-71.

Insecticides: Organic Phosphorus Compounds and Carbamates

QUESTIONS

110.1. A 32-year-old man ingests an unknown insecticide in a suicide attempt. He presents with bronchorrhea, bradycardia, miosis, diaphoresis, and vomiting. When administering atropine, which of the following is an appropriate endpoint of therapy?
A. Tachycardia
B. Mydriasis
C. Dry skin
D. Dry pulmonary secretions
E. Cessation of vomiting

110.2. Which of the following options is the most efficient way to reduce the fatality rate from organic phosphorus insecticide?
A. Child-resistant closures on bottles
B. Limiting bottle size
C. Limiting the concentration of active ingredients
D. Providing families with locked boxes
E. Prohibiting importation and sale of the most toxic insecticides

110.3. A 28-year-old man presents to the hospital with cholinergic symptoms after an intentional ingestion of parathion. Which of the following intravenous atropine dosing strategies is preferred to appropriately manage this patient?
A. 1 mg repeated every 15 minutes as needed
B. 5 mg repeated every 30 minutes as needed

C. 1-5 mg repeated every 2-20 minutes as needed
D. An initial dose of 1 mg doubled every 15 minutes as needed
E. An initial dose of 1-3 mg doubled every 5 minutes as needed

110.4. Which of the following options best distinguishes dimethoxy versus diethoxy organic phosphorus insecticides?
A. Diethoxy insecticides age faster than dimethoxy insecticides
B. Diethoxy and dimethoxy insecticides age at similar rates
C. Acetylcholinesterase spontaneous reactivates faster for dimethoxy insecticides than for diethoxy insecticides
D. Acetylcholinesterase spontaneous acetylcholinesterase faster for diethoxy insecticides than for dimethoxy insecticides
E. Acetylcholinesterase spontaneous acetylcholinesterase at about the same rate for dimethoxy and diethoxy insecticides

110.5. Which of the following symptoms would likely respond to pralidoxime therapy in a 47-year-old woman with a known malathion ingestion?
A. Bronchorrhea that failed to respond to 3 mg of atropine
B. Repeated episodes of vomiting
C. Muscle weakness with hypoventilation
D. A seizure that did not respond to a standard dose of intravenous lorazepam
E. A QT interval that is >500 msec with a heart rate of 40 beats/min

110.6. What is the difference between organic phosphorus and carbamate insecticides?
  A. Carbamate poisoning is always mild by comparison
  B. Carbamate poisoning resolves quicker than organic phosphorus poisoning
  C. Pralidoxime makes carbamate poisoning worse
  D. Intermediate syndrome occurs more commonly in carbamate poisoning
  E. Delayed neuropathy occurs more commonly in carbamate poisoning

110.7. Which of the following options is most characteristic of the intermediate syndrome in patients with organic phosphorus insecticide poisoning?
  A. Neuromuscular paralysis that follows only mild cholinergic crisis
  B. Clinical effects that occur at a time between spontaneous acetylcholinesterase reactivation and aging
  C. Clinical effects that result from select organic phosphorus insecticides that behave more like carbamate insecticides
  D. Proximal muscle weakness that occurs 1-3 days after poisoning and after cholinergic symptoms have resolved
  E. Recurrent cholinergic symptoms that occur after both weakness and cholinergic symptoms initially resolved

110.8. Which of the following options best describes the delayed neuropathy associated with organic phosphorus insecticide poisoning?

  A. Severe cholinergic crisis was initially present in most patients
  B. It is a demyelinating disease of large distal neurons
  C. Symptoms typically present 1 to 2 years following poisoning
  D. A similar syndrome is commonly reported following carbamate poisoning
  E. It characteristically presents with weakness of the neck flexors

110.9. Which of the following statements is true regarding cholinesterase testing in patients with organic phosphorus insecticide poisoning?
  A. Red cell cholinesterase is more reflective of synaptic inhibition than butyrylcholinesterase
  B. Oxime therapy improves both red cell and butyrylcholinesterase activity
  C. Without oxime treatment, butyrylcholinesterase activity returns to normal more rapidly than red cell cholinesterase activity
  D. Red cell cholinesterase activity is easier to assay than butyrylcholinesterase activity
  E. Pregnancy falsely increases butyrylcholinesterase activity

110.10. Which of the following paralytics will have its metabolism altered by organic phosphorous insecticide poisoning?
  A. Rocuronium
  B. Vecuronium
  C. Cisatracurium
  D. Atracurium
  E. Mivacurium

ANSWERS

110.1. Answer: D. The muscarinic manifestations of the cholinergic syndrome include salivation, lacrimation, urination, defecation, bradycardia, bronchorrhea, and emesis. Although atropine will correct all these findings, some will respond to lower doses than the others. It is important to remember that the only commonly life-threatening manifestation of muscarinic excess is bronchorrhea. Atropine should be dosed until pulmonary secretions dry, regardless of pupillary size, heart rate, or gastrointestinal symptoms.

Eddleston M, et al. Management of acute organophosphorus pesticide poisoning. *Lancet.* 2008;371:597-607.

110.2. Answer: E. In theory, all these choices might help reduce fatality from organic phosphorus insecticides, but only removing access to the most lethal members of this class of insecticides has demonstrable efficacy.

Buckley NA, et al. Case fatality of agricultural pesticides after self-poisoning in Sri Lanka: A prospective cohort study. *Lancet Glob Health.* 2021;23:S2214-109X(21)00086-3.

Pearson M, et al. Effectiveness of household lockable pesticide storage to reduce pesticide self-poisoning in rural Asia: A community-based, cluster-randomised controlled trial. *Lancet.* 2017;390:1863-1872.

110.3. Answer: E. The goal of therapy with atropine is to rapidly control secretions. Although many regimens are recommended, strong evidence-based guidance is lacking. However, based on clinical experience, this rapid doubling strategy allows for the most efficient use of time and resources and will typically control patients in the shortest amount of time.

> Eddleston M, et al. Speed of initial atropinisation in significant organophosphorus pesticide poisoning—a systematic comparison of recommended regimens. *J Toxicol Clin Toxicol.* 2004;42:865-875.

110.4. Answer: C. Acetylcholinesterase exposed to dimethoxy organic phosphorus insecticides spontaneously reactivates faster than if exposed to diethoxy organic phosphorus insecticides, which is important with mild or moderate overdoses. When the dose is increased such that there is an excess of insecticide present, regenerated enzyme becomes inactivated again. In contrast, dimethoxy organic phosphorus insecticides age quicker, making them more resistant to reactivation by oximes as time goes on.

> Eyer P. The role of oximes in the management of organophosphorus pesticide poisoning. *Toxicol Rev.* 2003;22:165-190.

110.5. Answer: C. All of the listed events occur in patients with organic phosphorus insecticide poisoning. Oximes only directly improve nicotinic effects that include muscle weakness and fasciculations as well as paralysis. Muscarinic effects (A and B), QT interval prolongation, and seizures are not likely to respond to oximes.

> Merrill DG, Mihm FG. Prolonged toxicity of organophosphate poisoning. *Crit Care Med.* 1982;10:550-551.

> Namba T, Hiraki K. PAM (pyridine-2-aldoxime methiodide) therapy of alkylphosphate poisoning. *JAMA.* 1958;166:1834-1839.

110.6. Answer: B. Carbamates and organic phosphorus insecticides both inhibit cholinesterase to produce muscarinic and nicotinic symptoms that are indistinguishable on clinical presentation and are equally severe. However, because carbamates do not age, symptoms tend to resolve more quickly than organic phosphorus insecticides. Because of rapid resolution, both the intermediate syndrome and delayed neuropathy are distinctly uncommon with carbamate poisoning. Although often unnecessary, oximes do not make carbamate poisoning worse as was once thought.

> Lamb T, et al. High lethality and minimal variation after acute self-poisoning with carbamate insecticides in Sri Lanka–implications for global suicide prevention. *Clin Toxicol (Phila).* 2016;54:624-631.

> Mercurio-Zappala M, et al. Pralidoxime in carbaryl poisoning: An animal model. *Hum Exp Toxicol.* 2007;26:125-129.

110.7. Answer: D. The intermediate syndrome occurs 24 to 96 hours after acute organic phosphorus insecticide poisoning and following resolution of the cholinergic crisis. Patients develop proximal muscle weakness, especially of the neck flexors, and cranial nerve palsies and progress to respiratory failure that lasts up to several weeks.

> Wadia RS, et al. Neurological manifestations of organophosphate insecticide poisoning. *J Neurol Neurosurg Psychiatry.* 1974;37:841-847.

> Senanayake N, Karalliedde L. Neurotoxic effects of organophosphate insecticides: An intermediate syndrome. *N Engl J Med.* 1987;316:761-763.

110.8. Answer: B. Peripheral neuropathies occur days to weeks following acute organic phosphorous insecticide poisoning. These neuropathies also result from exposures to organic phosphorus compounds that do not inhibit red blood cell cholinesterase or produce clinical cholinergic toxicity. Pathologic findings demonstrate effects primarily on large distal neurons, with axonal degeneration preceding demyelination.

> Cavanagh JB, et al. Comparison of the functional effects of dyflos, tri-o-cresyl phosphate and tri-pethylphenyl phosphate in chickens. *Br J Pharmacol.* 1961;17:21-27.

> Johnson MK. The delayed neurotoxic effect of some organophosphorus compounds. Identification of the phosphorylation site as an esterase. *Biochem J.* 1969;114:711-717.

> Glynn P. A mechanism for organophosphate-induced delayed neuropathy. *Toxicol Lett.* 2006;162:94-97.

110.9. Answer: A. Most patients with organic phosphorus insecticide poisoning are treated based on clinical grounds as laboratory testing is frequently unavailable or unable to be resulted in a clinically useful time frame. However, for workplace monitoring, assessing the response to treatment, and experimental evaluation, testing is sometimes used. Red cell cholinesterase activity is more reflective of synaptic activity but more difficulty to assay and must be adjusted for abnormal hemoglobin concentrations. Depending on the timing of oxime therapy, no response, partial, or complete reversal of red cell cholinesterase activity is possible. In the absence of therapy, however, activity only returns to normal as red cells regenerate, which is a slow process.

> Namba T, et al. Poisoning due to organophosphate insecticides. *Am J Med.* 1971;50:475-492.

> Eddleston M, et al. Management of acute organophosphorus pesticide poisoning. *Lancet.* 2008;371:597-607.

110.10. Answer: E. Among the listed non depolarizing neuromuscular blockers, only mivacurium is metabolized by butyrylcholinesterase (plasma cholinesterase) and is, therefore, subject to alteration in the setting of organic phosphorus poisoning. It should be expected that the normal duration of effect of mivacurium is substantially prolonged in this clinical setting. While this is not a contraindication per se, prolonged paralysis can be confused for worsening organic phosphorus-induced neuromuscular dysfunction. A similarly prolonged effect is expected with succinylcholine.

Sener EB, et al. Prolonged apnea following succinylcholine administration in undiagnosed acute organophosphate poisoning. *Acta Anaesthesiol Scand.* 2002;46:1046-1048.

QUESTIONS

111.1. A 3-year-old boy with a history of eczema has a topical medication applied as a treatment for scabies. He presents to the emergency department 2 hours following the exposure for evaluation of a generalized tonic-clonic seizure. This medication leads to seizures by binding to which of the following receptor sites in the brain?
A. Serotonergic A_3 binding site
B. Central dopaminergic receptors
C. Glycinergic binding sites
D. Ivermectin binding site on the chloride channel
E. Picrotoxin binding site on the GABA receptor

111.2. Dichlorodiphenyltrichloroethane (DDT) causes toxicity by binding to which of the following sites?
A. Serotonergic A_3 binding site
B. Sodium channel
C. Glycinergic binding sites
D. Ivermectin binding site on the chloride channel
E. Picrotoxin binding site on the GABA receptor

111.3. A 62-year-old man presents to the emergency department with a very prominent tremor that is attributed to chlordecone exposure. Which of the following medications will exacerbate his tremor?
A. Digoxin
B. Ibuprofen
C. Phenytoin
D. Acetaminophen
E. Cyproheptadine

111.4. A 74-year-old woman is being evaluated in the emergency department for multiple neurologic symptoms, including ataxia and opsoclonus. On examination, she has an exaggerated startle response. She is a housewife and her husband was a factory worker in the 1970s. Which of the following xenobiotics could explain her presentation?
A. Asbestos
B. Benzene
C. Acrylamide
D. Chlordecone
E. Dichlorodiphenyltrichloroethane (DDT)

111.5. Which of the following organochlorine pesticides is poorly absorbed dermally?
A. Dichorodiphenyltrichloroethane (DDT)
B. Aldrin
C. Dieldrin
D. Endosulfan
E. Endrin

111.6. Which of the following options is the primary route of excretion of organic chlorine?
A. Bile
B. Pulmonary
C. Kidney
D. Dermal
E. Hair

111.7. Which of the following signs or symptoms is the most common cause of morbidity in patients who overdose on endosulfan?
A. Esophageal strictures
B. Delayed neuropsychiatric symptoms
C. Gastrointestinal hemorrhage
D. Status epilepticus
E. Acute respiratory distress syndrome (ARDS)

111.8. A 27-year-old woman presents to the emergency department 1 hour after an intentional ingestion of an organic chlorine pesticide. Which of the following diagnostic tests is most likely to be abnormal?
A. Computed tomography (CT) scan of the brain
B. Chest radiograph
C. Abdominal radiograph
D. Co-oximetry
E. Complete blood cell count

111.9. Which of the following odors is associated with a toxaphene ingestion?
A. Rotten egg
B. Garlic
C. Pears
D. Bitter almonds
E. Turpentine

111.10. A 52-year-old man presents to the emergency department following an intentional overdose of an organic chlorine pesticide. Which of the following interventions is recommended as part of the management of this patient?
A. Activated charcoal
B. *N*-Acetylcysteine
C. Sodium bicarbonate
D. Cholestyramine
E. Oil-based cathartic

ANSWERS

111.1. Answer: E. This patient had lindane applied as a topical treatment for scabies; eczema, broken skin, and hot baths increase its absorption. Lindane acts as a GABA antagonist by binding to the picrotoxin receptor on the GABA$_A$ receptor–chloride ionophore complex in the central nervous system. GABA agonists, such as benzodiazepines and phenobarbital, are usually efficacious in the treatment of the seizures and neurotoxicity of lindane.

> Narahashi T. Neuronal ion channels as the target sites of insecticides. *Pharmacol Toxicol.* 1996;79:1-14.

111.2. Answer: B. DDT causes toxicity by binding to sodium channels. It lengthens the period of time in which this channel remains in its open configuration. Chronic DDT exposure leads to a tremor. Following large ingestions of DDT, nausea, vomiting, hyperesthesia of the mouth and face, headache, dizziness, myoclonus, leg weakness, agitation, and seizures occur.

> Tilson HA, et al. Effects of 5,5-diphenylhydantoin (phenytoin) on neurobehavioral toxicity of organochlorine pesticides and permethrin. *J Pharmacol Exp Ther.* 1985;233:285-289.

111.3. Answer: C. Phenytoin and serotonin agonists exacerbate the prominent tremor that occurs with chlordecone. This is in contradistinction to dichlorodiphenyltrichloroethane (DDT), in that the tremor induced by DDT is improved with phenytoin.

> Herr DW, et al. Pharmacological modification of tremor and enhanced acoustic startle by chlordecone and *p,p'*-DDT. *Psychopharmacology (Berl).* 1987;91:320–325.

111.4. Answer: D. In Hopewell, Virginia, between 1973 and 1974, factory workers heavily exposed to chlordecone developed insidious, chronic toxicity. Their symptoms included a prominent tremor of the hands and head, known as the "Kepone shakes," weakness, opsoclonus, ataxia, weight loss, and elevated liver enzymes. Some workers had exaggerated startle responses. Several of the workers' wives developed chlordecone toxicity as well, likely because of laundering their husband's work clothes.

> Faroon O, et al. ATSDR evaluation of health effects of chemicals. II. Mirex and chlordecone: Health effects, toxicokinetics, human exposure, and environmental fate. *Toxicol Ind Health.* 1995;11:1-203.

111.5. Answer: A. DDT and its analogues methoxychlor, dicofol, and chlorobenzilate are very poorly absorbed transdermally, unless the pesticide is dissolved in a suitable hydrocarbon solvent. All of the other options listed are very well absorbed through both an intact or a broken dermal barrier.

> Reigart JR, Roberts JR. *Recognition and Management of Pesticide Poisonings.* EPA Document No. EPA 735-R-98-003. Washington, DC: Environmental Protection Agency; 1999.

111.6. Answer: A. The primary route of excretion of the organic chlorines is in the bile. Most organic chlorines also produce detectable urinary metabolites. Due to their excretion in the bile, most organic chlorines have significant enterohepatic recirculation.

Cohn WJ, et al. Treatment of chlordecone (Kepone) toxicity with cholestyramine. Results of a controlled clinical trial. *N Engl J Med.* 1978;298:243-248.

Faroon O, et al. ATSDR evaluation of health effects of chemicals. II. Mirex and chlordecone: Health effects, toxicokinetics, human exposure, and environmental fate. *Toxicol Ind Health.* 1995;11:1-203.

111.7. Answer: D. Status epilepticus occurs frequently in patients who have an intentional (suicidal) endosulfan ingestion. In a Nepalese study more than half of patients developed refractory status epilepticus and 32% died.

Lohani S, et al. Abstract 146: Status epilepticus after acute endosulfan poisoning: A study of 25 cases. *Clin Toxicol.* 2012;50:574-720.

111.8. Answer: C. Following an ingestion of an organic chlorine pesticide, an abdominal radiograph will often reveal the presence of a radiopaque substance in the stomach. This is due to the chlorine, which increases the radiopacity of xenobiotics.

Choi SH, et al. Diagnostic radiopacity and hepatotoxicity following chloroform ingestion: A case report. *Emerg Med J.* 2006;23:394-395.

111.9. Answer: E. Toxaphene, a chlorinated pinene, has a turpentinelike odor. Endosulfan has a rotten egg odor due to its sulfur moiety. The odor of violets in the urine is associated with a turpentine overdose. Chloral hydrate toxicity is associated with the smell of pears. Cyanide is associated with a bitter almond–like odor. Many organic phosphorus compounds smell like garlic.

Goldfrank LR, et al. Teaching the recognition of odors. *Ann Emerg Med.* 1982;11:684-686.

111.10. Answer: D. Cholestyramine is recommended in the management of all patients who overdose on chlordecone or other organic chlorine pesticides. Cholestyramine, a nonabsorbable bile acid–binding anion exchange resin, decreases the incidence of seizures and morality. Oil-based cathartics should be avoided because they increase absorption of organic chlorine pesticides. Most organic chlorine pesticides contain petroleum distillates as part of their mixture, so the role of activated charcoal is limited. Sodium bicarbonate and *N*-acetylcysteine are not used in the management of organic chlorine overdoses.

Kassner JT, et al. Cholestyramine as an adsorbent in acute lindane poisoning: A murine model. *Ann Emerg Med.* 1993;22:1392-1397.

QUESTIONS

112.1. Which of the following findings occurs in workers chronically exposed to white phosphorus?
A. Osteonecrosis of the mandible
B. Cardiac atrophy
C. Splenic enlargement
D. Ascending neuropathy
E. Punctate keratitis

112.2. Which of the following forms of phosphorus is known for its luminescent appearance and its ability to spontaneously combust in air?
A. Red phosphorus
B. White phosphorus
C. Black phosphorus
D. Blue phosphorus
E. Green phosphorus

112.3. Following ingestion, the greatest concentration of white phosphorus is found in which organ?
A. Brain
B. Heart
C. Kidney
D. Liver
E. Spleen

112.4. Which of the following forms of phosphorus is used to make methamphetamine and leads to the production of phosphine gas?
A. Red phosphorus
B. White phosphorus
C. Black phosphorus
D. Blue phosphorus
E. Green phosphorus

112.5. A 50-year-old man presents to the emergency department after ingesting an unknown substance. His vital signs are: blood pressure, 154/93 mmHg; heart rate, 119 beats/min; respiratory rate, 18 breaths/min; temperature, 98.7 °F (37.1 °C), and oxygen saturation, 100%. He has abdominal pain, vomiting, and diarrhea. Which of the following signs or symptoms would suggest that the patient ingested white phosphorus?
A. Blue vomitus
B. Red meat allergy
C. Tardieu spots
D. Alopecia
E. Smoking stools

112.6. A 17-year-old girl presents to the emergency department after ingesting white phosphorus. Despite appropriate management, she dies and is taken to the medical examiner. The patient's autopsy will most likely demonstrate which of the following changes in the liver?
A. Zone 1 injury
B. Zone 2 injury
C. Zone 3 injury
D. Zone 4 injury
E. Zone 5 injury

112.7. A 47-year-old man presents to the emergency department after ingesting white phosphorus in a suicide attempt. Which of the following electrolyte abnormalities is most likely to occur?
A. Hypophosphatemia
B. Hypernatremia
C. Hyperkalemia
D. Hypermagnesemia
E. Hyperchloremia

112.8. A 34-year-old man presents to the emergency department following a cutaneous exposure to white phosphorus munitions. Which of the following choices helps to safely identify areas that need decontamination?

    A. Wood's lamp

    B. Prussian blue applied to the skin

    C. Concentrated copper sulfate applied to the skin

    D. Ice packs applied to suspected exposure sites

    E. Subcutaneous methylene blue administration

112.9. Which of the following methods is the best way to halt continuing injury from dermal white phosphorus?

    A. Applying a gauze that is soaked in water directly on the skin and removing it 3-5 minutes later

    B. Irrigating the exposed area with copious water

    C. Applying a concentrated copper sulfate solution over the area

    D. Neutralizing the area by applying sodium bicarbonate directly onto the affected skin

    E. Gently fanning the exposed area

112.10. A 34-year-old man presents to the emergency department after ingesting white phosphorus 4 hours prior to presentation. Which of the following findings is a poor prognostic sign in white phosphorus exposure?

    A. Cherry red skin

    B. Altered mental status

    C. Metabolic alkalosis

    D. Hypokalemia

    E. Hyperglycemia

ANSWERS

112.1. Answer: A. Workers chronically exposed to white phosphorus are at risk of developing "phossy jaw." This illness is characterized by osteonecrosis of the mandible and presents with abscesses and bony loss. Historically, this occurred in workers making "strike anywhere" matches.

Hughes JP, et al. Phosphorus necrosis of the jaw: A present-day study. *Br J Ind Med*. 1962;19:83-99.

112.2. Answer: B. White phosphorus is known for its luminescent appearance; it spontaneously combusts in air and is the phosphorus of most toxicologic significance. Red phosphorus is a red powdery compound that is found in current-day matches. Yellow phosphorus is white phosphorus that takes on a waxy appearance when exposed to light and has basically the same toxicologic manifestations. There is no such thing as black, blue, or green phosphorus.

Witkowski W, et al. Experimental comparison of efficiency of first aid dressings in burning white phosphorus on bacon model. *Med Sci Monit*. 2015;21:2361-2366.

112.3. Answer: D. Following an ingestion, the greatest concentration of phosphorus is found in the liver. White phosphorus is well absorbed from the gastrointestinal tract. Coingestion with fats, alcohols, and liquids increases the toxicity of white phosphorus.

Cameron J, Patrick RS. Acute phosphorus poisoning—the distribution of toxic doses of yellow phosphorus in the tissues of experimental animals. *Med Sci Law*. 1966;6:209-214.

Ghoshal AK, et al. Isotopic studies on the absorption and tissue distribution of white phosphorus in rats. *Exp Mol Pathol*. 1971;14:212-219.

112.4. Answer: A. Red phosphorus is used with elemental iodine to produce hydroiodic acid, which is a reducing agent required to convert ephedrine to methamphetamine. During heating, red phosphorus and iodine generate phosphine (PH_3) gas, which leads to pulmonary symptoms and death. Black, blue, and green phosphorus do not exist.

Willers-Russo LJ. Three fatalities involving phosphine gas, produced as a result of methamphetamine manufacturing. *J Forensic Sci*. 1999;44:647-652.

112.5. Answer: E. Ingested white phosphorus that is not absorbed is excreted in the stool. The combustion of the phosphorus upon its exposure to air is responsible for the "smoking stool syndrome" that occurs with white phosphorus ingestion.

Simon FA, Pickering LK. Acute yellow phosphorus poisoning: "Smoking stool syndrome." *JAMA*. 1976;235:1343-1344.

112.6. Answer: A. Unlike acetaminophen and carbon tetrachloride, which cause a zone 3, or centrilobular, pattern of liver injury, white phosphorus causes a zone 1, or periportal, pattern of hepatic injury.

Fletcher GF, Galambos JT. Phosphorus poisoning in humans. *Arch Intern Med*. 1963;112:846-852.

112.7. Answer: C. In a rat model of dermal burns from phosphorus, an initial diuresis occurs followed by acute kidney injury manifested by hyperkalemia, hyponatremia, and hyperphosphatemia. Both hypo- and hypercalcemia are also reported.

BenHur N, et al. Phosphorus burns—a pathophysiological study. *Br J Plast Surg*. 1972;25:238-244.

Brewer E, Haggerty R. Toxic hazards rat poisons II—phosphorus. *N Engl J Med*. 1958;258:147-148.

Konjoyan T. White phosphorus burns: Case report and literature review. *Mil Med*. 1983;148:881-884.

112.8. Answer: A. A Wood's lamp helps to identify areas that need decontamination by taking advantage of the phosphorescent characteristic of white phosphorus. Although there are articles suggesting the use of a copper sulfate solution, *concentrated* copper sulfate puts the patient at risk of systemic toxicity and oxidant injury.

Conner J, Bebarta V. White phosphorus dermal burns. *N Engl J Med*. 2007;357:1530.

Aviv U, et al. The burning issue of white phosphorus: A case report and review of the literature. *Disaster Mil Med*. 2017;3:6.

112.9. Answer: A. Because white phosphorus reacts with atmospheric oxygen, taking a gauze soaked in water and limiting the amount of contact the white phosphorus has with oxygen is important. Pouring water over the area is dangerous as burning phosphorus splashes unpredictably and health care workers risk being exposed and injured. *Concentrated* copper sulfate places the patient at risk for systemic toxicity. Fanning the exposed area increases the exposure to oxygen. Applying sodium bicarbonate directly to the exposed area is not indicated.

Witkowski W, et al. Experimental comparison of efficiency of first aid dressings in burning white phosphorus on bacon model. *Med Sci Monit*. 2015;21:2361-2366.

112.10. Answer: B. Cyanosis, hypotension, metabolic acidosis, altered sensorium, an elevated prothrombin time (PT), and hypoglycemia occurring in the first 6 hours following an exposure to white phosphorus are all poor prognostic signs.

Diaz-Rivera R, et al. Acute phosphorus poisoning in man: A study of 56 cases. *Medicine*. 1950;29:269-298.

Sodium Monofluoroacetate and Fluoroacetamide

QUESTIONS

113.1. Which of the following options is a modern-day use of sodium monofluoroacetate (SMFA) in the United States?
A. Foam stabilizer in beer
B. Embedded in collars of livestock
C. Protection against cisplatin-induced kidney failure
D. Preservative in cosmetics, foods, and pharmaceuticals
E. Sweetener, moistening agent, and a diluent

113.2. Fluorocitrate prevents which of the following enzymes from further metabolic activity?
A. Alpha-ketoglutarate
B. Pyruvate dehydrogenase
C. CYP2E1
D. Aconitase
E. CYP3A4

113.3. A 54-year-old man presents to the emergency department after an overdose of sodium monofluoroacetate (SMFA). Which of the following findings is most likely to develop first?
A. Vomiting
B. Agitation
C. Abdominal pain
D. Chest pain
E. Altered mental status

113.4. A 77-year-old woman presents to the emergency department after an intentional ingestion of sodium monofluoroacetate (SMFA). She develops polymorphic ventricular tachycardia. Which of the following options best explains this event?
A. Myocardial sensitization
B. Catecholamine surge
C. Cardiac ischemia
D. Hypomagnesemia
E. Hypocalcemia

113.5. An 18-year-old man ingests sodium monofluoroacetate (SMFA) in a suicide attempt. He presents to the emergency department 2 hours later with abdominal pain and tachycardia. He is awake and following commands. Which of the following therapies is the best next step in his management?
A. High-dose insulin
B. Activated charcoal
C. Magnesium bolus
D. Flumazenil
E. Naloxone

113.6. You are working in a very remote clinic when a 20-year-old man presents after ingesting sodium monofluoroacetate (SMFA). Due to weather conditions, transport to a nearby hospital is impossible. Your clinic is very poorly stocked. Which of the following therapies limits toxicity?
A. Acetic acid
B. Ethanol
C. Mineral oil
D. N-Acetylcysteine
E. Sodium bicarbonate

113.7. What is the mechanism of action of glycerol mono-acetate when used to treat sodium monofluoroac-etate (SMFA) toxicity?
A. Glycerol monoacetate acts as an acetate donor
B. Glycerol monoacetate acts as an electron acceptor
C. Glycerol monoacetate has antimicrobial prop-erties that prevent infection
D. Glycerol monoacetate becomes directly con-verted to alpha-ketoglutarate
E. Glycerol monoacetate regenerates pyruvate dehydrogenase

113.8. Which of the following plants is a natural source of sodium monofluoroacetate (SMFA)?
A. *Dichapetalum braunii*
B. *Colchicum autumnale*
C. *Areca catechu*
D. *Citrus aurantium*
E. *Angelica polymorpha*

113.9. A 26-year-old man presents to the emergency department with an altered mental status following a sodium monofluoroacetate (SMFA) overdose. He has an elevated ammonia to 100 micromol/L. What is the best explanation for this abnormality?
A. Glutamate depletion
B. Increased ammonia absorption from gastroin-testinal tract
C. Carnitine depletion
D. Oxaloacetate depletion
E. SMFA preparations often contain ammonia

113.10. Which of the following options is associated with poor prognosis following sodium monofluoroac-etate (SMFA) ingestion?
A. Hypertension
B. Premature ventricular contractions
C. Poor capillary refill
D. Early emesis
E. Seizures

ANSWERS

113.1. Answer: B. Sodium monofluoroacetate (SMFA) is restricted in the United States to placement in collars of sheep and cattle to protect against coyotes. Cobalt was added as a foam stabilizer to beer in the 1960s and led to an outbreak of cardiomyopathy. Amifostine is used to protect against cisplatin-induced kidney failure. Parabens, also known as parahydroxybenzoic acids, are a group of com-pounds widely employed as preservatives in cosmetics, foods, and pharmaceuticals. Sorbitol is used as a sweetener, moistening agent, and a diluent.

Burns RJ, Connolly GE. Toxicity of Compound 1080 livestock protection collars to sheep. *Arch Environ Contam Toxicol.* 1995;28:141-144.

Robinson RF, et al. Intoxication with sodium monofluoroacetate (compound 1080). *Vet Hum Toxicol.* 2002;44:93-95.

113.2. Answer: D. Sodium monofluoroacetate (SMFA) is an irreversible inhibitor of the citric acid cycle. It enters the mitochondria as monofluoroacetic acid and is converted to monofluoroacetyl-coenzyme A (CoA) by acetate thiokinase. This compound then joins with mitochondrial citrate syn-thase and oxaloacetate to form fluorocitrate. Fluorocitrate then covalently binds aconitase, preventing the enzyme from any further metabolic activity in the citric acid cycle.

Liébecq C, Peters RA. The toxicity of fluoroacetate and the tricarboxylic acid cycle. 1949. *Biochim Biophys Acta.* 1989;1000:254-269.

113.3. Answer: A. In a large case series of patients who ingested SMFA, the most common findings were nausea and vomiting (74%), followed by diarrhea (29%), and agitation (29%).

Chi CH, et al. Clinical presentation and prognostic factors in sodium monofluoroacetate intoxication. *J Toxicol Clin Toxicol.* 1996;34:707-712.

113.4. Answer: E. The most predominant electrolyte abnor-mality after an SMFA ingestion is hypocalcemia. This is due to the elevated citrate concentrations. Hypocalcemia leads to a prolonged QT interval and subsequent torsade de pointes, a type of polymorphic ventricular tachycardia. SMFA also causes hypokalemia and atrial fibrillation. Myocardial sensiti-zation occurs in "sudden sniffing death syndrome" following hydrocarbon exposure.

Proudfoot AT, et al. Sodium fluoroacetate poisoning. *Toxicol Rev.* 2006;25:213-219.

113.5. Answer: B. The immediate management of an SMFA overdose includes removal of clothes and the cleaning of skin with soap and water. Activated charcoal (1 g/kg) binds to SMFA and should be administered. Although colestipol is more effective at binding SMFA than activated charcoal, activated charcoal is more readily accessible.

Norris W, et al. Sorption of fluoroacetate (compound 1080) by colesti-pol, activated charcoal and anion-exchange in resins in vitro and gastro-intestinal decontamination in rats. *Vet Hum Toxicol.* 2000;42:269-275.

113.6. Answer: B. Although the appropriate dose is unknown, ethanol decreases the toxicity of SMFA. Ethanol accomplishes this by providing a source of acetyl-CoA that competes with monofluoroacetyl-CoA for binding of citrate synthase. A reasonable serum ethanol concentration goal is 100 mg/dL (21.7 mmol/L).

Chi CH, et al. Clinical presentation and prognostic factors in sodium monofluoroacetate intoxication. *J Toxicol Clin Toxicol*. 1996;34:707-712.

Chi CH, et al. Hemodynamic abnormalities in sodium monofluoroacetate intoxication. *Hum Exp Toxicol*. 1999;18:351-353.

Ramirez M. Inebriation with pyridoxine and fluoroacetate: A case report. *Vet Hum Toxicol*. 1986;28:154.

Hutchens JO, et al. The effect of ethanol and various metabolites on fluoroacetate poisoning. *J Pharmacol Exp Ther*. 1949;95:62-70.

113.7. Answer: A. Glycerol monoacetate has two mechanisms of action when used to treat SMFA poisoning. First, it is converted to acetyl-CoA and is able to compete with monofluoroacetyl-CoA for binding of citrate synthase. Second, glycerol monoacetate donates an acetate that will compete with monofluoroacetate for incorporation into citrate in place of fluoroacetate.

Taitelman U, et al. The effect of monoacetin and calcium chloride on acid-base balance and survival in experimental sodium fluoroacetate poisoning. *Arch Toxicol Suppl*. 1983;6:222-227.

113.8. Answer: A. *Dichapetalum braunii* is a naturally occurring plant that contains up to 8.0 mg/g of SMFA in its seeds. *Colchicum autmnale* (autumn crocus) contains colchicine. *Areca catechu* (Betel nut) contains arecoline. *Citrus aurantium* (bitter orange) contains synephrine. *Angelica polymorpha* (Dong Quai) contains coumarin.

Eason CT. Sodium monofluoroacetate (1080) risk assessment and risk communication. *Toxicology*. 2002;181-182:523-530.

113.9. Answer: A. Because SMFA leads to the inhibition of aconitase, a biochemical "dead end" occurs within the citric acid cycle. Depletion of alpha-ketoglutarate leads to glutamate depletion, which disrupts the urea cycle disruption and causes ammonia accumulation. Carnitine depletion describes one of the mechanisms of action of valproate toxicity. Increased ammonia absorption and oxaloacetate depletion are not mechanisms associated with SMFA. SMFA preparations do not contain ammonia.

Proudfoot AT, Bradberry SM, Vale JA. Sodium fluoroacetate poisoning. *Toxicol Rev*. 2006;25:213-219.

Tsuji H, et al. Effects of sodium monofluoroacetate on glucose, amino-acid, and fatty-acid metabolism and risk assessment of glucose supplementation. *Drug Chem Toxicol*. 2009;32:353-361.

113.10. Answer. E. In a Taiwanese case series all deaths following SMFA ingestions occurred within 72 hours of admission to the hospital. The presence of respiratory distress or seizures was a poor prognostic sign.

Chi CH, et al. Clinical presentation and prognostic factors in sodium monofluoroacetate intoxication. *J Toxicol Clin Toxicol*. 1996;34:707-712.

Strychnine

114.1. Which of the following neurotransmitters is antagonized by strychnine?
A. Glycine
B. Gamma aminobutyric acid (GABA)
C. Glutamate
D. Acetylcholine
E. Adenosine

114.2. Which of the following disorders most closely mimics strychnine poisoning?
A. Myasthenia gravis
B. Tetanus
C. Guillain-Barré
D. Lambert-Eaton
E. Botulism

114.3. A 50-year-old man presents to the emergency department with involuntary, generalized muscle contractions. A family member brings over a bag of supplements that the patient takes for his rheumatoid arthritis. Which of the following supplements explains his presentation?
A. Chan Su
B. Vitamin B_{17}
C. Black cohosh
D. Maqianzi
E. Pokeweed

114.4. Early in the course of strychnine poisoning, mortality is mainly a result of which of the following causes?
A. Multiorgan failure
B. Rhabdomyolysis

C. Hypoventilation
D. Aspiration pneumonitis
E. Compartment syndrome

114.5. Which of the following xenobiotics could potentially *harm* a patient who is strychnine poisoned?
A. Midazolam
B. Propofol
C. Phenobarbital
D. Rocuronium
E. Succinylcholine

114.6. Symptoms of strychnine toxicity tend to occur within what time frame following an ingestion?
A. 5-10 minutes
B. 15-60 minutes
C. 70-120 minutes
D. 4-6 hours
E. 12-24 hours

114.7. Which of the following gastrointestinal decontamination techniques would be best in strychnine poisoning?
A. Sodium polystyrene sulfonate
B. Induction of vomiting
C. Whole bowel irrigation
D. Activated charcoal
E. Any form of gastrointestinal decontamination is contraindicated

114.8. Which of the following options is true regarding the toxicokinetics of strychnine?

A. It is poorly absorbed from the gastrointestinal (GI) tract and mucous membranes

B. It has a low volume of distribution

C. It is largely bound to protein

D. It is metabolized primarily by CYP3A4

E. Its metabolite, strychnine-*N*-oxide, is 50% as toxic as strychnine

114.9. Which of the following options best describes the muscle contractions in strychnine poisoning?

A. They are triggered by trivial stimuli, such as turning on a light

B. Episodes last for at least 15 minutes at a time

C. Patients are unresponsive during these episodes

D. Episodes recur and last for 7-10 days

E. The muscle contractions are unilateral

114.10. A 36-year-old physician presents to the emergency department 2 hours after ingesting strychnine from an antique medication kit. She is awake and speaking to you; however, she is having involuntary contractions and is hyperreflexic. Her vital signs are: blood pressure 148/90 mmHg; heart rate 158 beats/min; respiratory rate 28 breaths/min; oxygen saturation 92% on room air; temperature 109.2 °F (42.9 °C). Which of the following is best be performed next?

A. Orogastric lavage

B. Administer dantrolene

C. Ice water immersion

D. Electrical cardioversion

E. Urinary alkalinization

ANSWERS

114.1. Answer: A. Strychnine competitively inhibits the binding of glycine to the postsynaptic receptor in the spinal cord. Specifically, it inhibits the binding of glycine to the alpha-subunit of the glycinergic chloride channel. It does not directly antagonize GABA, glutamate, adenosine, or acetylcholine.

Boyd RE, et al. Strychnine poisoning. Recovery from profound lactic acidosis, hyperthermia, and rhabdomyolysis. *Am J Med.* 1983;74:507-512.

Curtis DR, et al. The specificity of strychnine as a glycine antagonist in the mammalian spinal cord. *Exp Brain Res.* 1971;12:547-565.

Woodbury DM. Convulsant drugs: Mechanism of action. *Adv Neurol.* 1980;27:249-303.

114.2 Answer: B. Tetanus toxin causes a syndrome of muscular contractions that is almost indistinguishable from strychnine poisoning. However, it does so by preventing the release of presynaptic glycine. Myasthenia gravis is a neuromuscular disease caused by autoantibodies to the postsynaptic nicotinic acetylcholine receptor at the neuromuscular junction. Guillain-Barré syndrome is an acute immune-mediated polyneuropathy leading to nerve demyelination and progressive, ascending muscle weakness. Lambert-Eaton is a syndrome caused by antibodies to voltage-gated calcium channels and leads to limb weakness, usually in the context of a neoplasm such as small cell lung cancer. Botulinum toxin binds to neurons containing acetylcholine and prevents release, leading to weakness.

Hassel B. Tetanus: Pathophysiology, treatment, and the possibility of using botulinum toxin against tetanus-induced rigidity and spasms. *Toxins (Basel).* 2013;5:73-83.

114.3 Answer: D. Maqianzi, a Chinese herbal medicine used to treat limb paralysis, rheumatism, inflammatory disease, and skeletal fluorosis, contains strychnine. Chan Su is an herbal supplement used as an aphrodisiac and contains bufadienolides. Black cohosh is a plant that contains triterpene glycosides and is used as an abortifacient. Amygdalin, sometimes referred to inappropriately as the non existent "vitamin B_{17}," is a cyanogenic glycoside found in apricot pits, cherry pits, and peach pits. Pokeweed (phytolacca americana) is a plant that causes gastrointestinal symptoms and leukocytosis.

Chan TY. Herbal medicine causing likely strychnine poisoning. *Hum Exp Toxicol.* 2002;21:467-468.

Kong HY, et al. Safety of individual medication of Ma Qian Zi (semen strychni) based upon assessment of therapeutic effects of Guo's therapy against moderate fluorosis of bone. *J Tradit Chin Med.* 2011;31:297-302.

114.4. Answer: C. Early in the course of strychnine poisoning, mortality is mainly due to hypoventilation and hypoxia secondary to muscular contractions. Later, life-threatening complications, such as rhabdomyolysis, kidney injury, hyperthermia-induced organ failure, and aspiration develop.

Flood RG. Strychnine poisoning. *Pediatr Emerg Care.* 1999;15:286-287.

114.5. Answer: E. The judicious use of benzodiazepines is the first-line therapy for strychnine poisoning. When benzodiazepines fail to achieve control of convulsions, propofol and barbiturates are added. A last-line agent to control muscular hyperactivity in strychnine poisoning is a neuromuscular blocker. However, depolarizing neuromuscular blockers, such as succinylcholine, will induce muscle contractions and cause hyperkalemia, worsening the clinical picture. If using a neuromuscular blocker, it is recommended to use nondepolarizing neuromuscular blockers, such as rocuronium. Succinylcholine is contraindicated.

Maron BJ, et al. Strychnine poisoning successfully treated with diazepam. *J Pediatr.* 1971;78:697-699.

Haggard H, Greenberg L. Antidotes for strychnine poisoning. *JAMA.* 1983;98:1133-1136.

O'Callaghan WG, et al. Unusual strychnine poisoning and its treatment: Report of eight cases. *BMJ (Clin Res Ed).* 1982;285:478.

Sgaragli GP, Mannaioni PF. Pharmacokinetic observations on a case of massive strychnine poisoning. *Clin Toxicol.* 1973;6:533-540.

114.6. Answer: B. Oral strychnine poisoning is characterized by a rapid onset of toxicity beginning within 15-60 minutes of ingestion. A delayed onset of clinical effects is uncommon.

Gordon AM, Richards DW. Strychnine intoxication. *JACEP.* 1979;8:520-522.

114.7. Answer: D. Induction of vomiting is absolutely contraindicated in a patient with strychnine poisoning. The risk of aspiration in a patient who already has muscular contractions impeding respirations potentially leads to death. Activated charcoal (AC) binds strychnine effectively (1 g AC binds 950 mg strychnine) and is recommended when there is little concern for aspiration, such as when the airway is protected or if the patient is not vomiting. Orogastric lavage is reasonable to perform in patients who present early following a large strychnine overdose. There is no evidence for whole bowel irrigation or sodium polystyrene sulfonate in strychnine poisoning.

Anderson AH. Experimental studies on the pharmacology of activated charcoal. *Acta Pharmacol.* 1946;2:69-78.

Teitelbaum DT, Ott JE. Acute strychnine intoxication. *Clin Toxicol.* 1970;3:267-273.

American Academy of Clinical Toxicology, European Association of Poisons Centres and Clinical Toxicologists. Position statement: Gastric lavage. *J Toxicol Clin Toxicol.* 2004;42:933-943.

114.8. Answer: D. Strychnine is rapidly absorbed from the GI tract and mucous membranes. Although protein binding is minimal, strychnine has a large volume of distribution, making it a poor candidate for extracorporeal drug removal. Strychnine is metabolized by cytochrome P450 enzymes, mostly CYP3A4, that forms a metabolite called strychnine-*N*-oxide which is one-tenth as toxic as the original alkaloid.

Adamson RH, Fouts JR. Enzymatic metabolism of strychnine. *J Pharmacol Exp Ther.* 1959;127:87-91.

Heiser JM, et al. Massive strychnine intoxication: Serial blood levels in a fatal case. *J Toxicol Clin Toxicol.* 1992;30:269-283.

114.9. Answer: A. Typical findings of strychnine poisoning include involuntary, generalized muscular contractions, usually occurring in the back, neck, and limbs. The contractions affect both sides of the body. These contractions are easily triggered by trivial stimuli such as turning on a light, and each episode lasts from 30-120 seconds. The episodes recur for as long as 12-24 hours. Because the spinal cord is more affected than the brain, the mental status is usually preserved during these episodes.

Smith BA. Strychnine poisoning. *J Emerg Med.* 1990;8:321-325.

114.10. Answer: C. This patient is hyperthermic, and the single most important next step is rapid cooling. The morbidity and mortality rise dramatically when patients remain hyperthemic for longer than 30 minutes. Ice water immersion is the most effective technique to rapidly cool patients. Cooling should take precedence over other therapies; in patients who require intubation, cooling should occur concurrently. Dantrolene is not indicated as this patient does not have malignant hyperthermia.

Casa DJ, et al. Cold water immersion: the gold standard for exertional heatstroke treatment. *Exerc Sport Sci Rev.* 2007;35:141-149.

Arthropods

115.1. Which of the following statements about *Latrodectus mactans* envenomations is correct?
  A. Only the male spider is capable of envenomating humans
  B. There is usually a severe local reaction
  C. Muscle cramps, nausea, weakness, and tremor develop within several hours
  D. Whole immunoglobulin antivenon is recommended for patients with at least mild symptoms
  E. The spider is identified by the violin markings on the its black abdomen

115.2. Which of the following statements about the Loxosceles reclusa spider is correct?
  A. Only the male spider is capable of envenomating humans
  B. The location of the bite is initially very painful
  C. Within 1 hour, the bite blisters and becomes necrotic
  D. Antivenom should be administered at the first sign of tissue necrosis
  E. Rare victims develop fever, arthralgias, hemolysis, and disseminated intravascular coagulation (DIC)

115.3. Which of the following statements about a sting from a *Centruroides* scorpion in North America is correct?
  A. Stings occur predominantly in the Northwestern United States
  B. Mortality is approximately 25% in children
  C. Mannitol relieves muscle cramps
  D. Adults develop muscle fasciculations and cramps, seizures, kidney failure, and cardiovascular collapse
  E. Antivenom significantly reduces the need for large doses of sedatives in children

115.4. Which of the following statements about tick paralysis is correct?
  A. Improvement occurs after the entire tick is removed from the skin
  B. The tick must be on the skin for 2-3 hours before symptoms develop
  C. Absent deep tendon reflexes at 6 hours following the bite is expected
  D. Calcium gluconate will effectively reverse muscle weakness
  E. Boys get tick paralysis more commonly than girls

115.5. Which of the following statements about *Hymenoptera* stings is correct?
  A. The venom produced by wasps, hornets, and yellow jackets is almost identical
  B. Direct venom toxicity is more common than anaphylaxis
  C. A delayed reaction of fever, malaise, headache, polyarthritis, and lymphadenopathy rarely occurs 1-2 days after a sting
  D. The venom of Africanized honeybees is more toxic than common honeybees
  E. Apamin, one of the toxic components of venom, binds to glycine receptors in the spinal cord

115.6. Which of the following statements about *Atrax robustus* spider bites is correct?
- A. Atracotoxin is a sodium channel blocker
- B. Female spiders cause more severe injuries in humans than male spiders
- C. Initial local pain progresses to muscle spasms and cardiovascular collapse
- D. Pressure immobilization is not indicated
- E. Antivenom administration is associated with severe allergic reactions

115.7. Which of the following options is found in the venom of fire ants?
- A. Phospholipase
- B. Hyaluronidase
- C. *N*-Acetyl-beta-glucosamidase
- D. Piperidine
- E. All of the above

115.8. Which of the following North American spiders causes a necrotic lesion?
- A. *Eratigena* spp
- B. *Drassodes* spp
- C. *Ummidia* spp
- D. *Latrodectus* spp
- E. *Heteropoda* spp

115.9. Which of the following reactions would be most common after a tarantula bite in the United States (US)?
- A. A large necrotic lesion
- B. Hypotension
- C. Bronchospasm
- D. Localized pain and irritation
- E. Myoglobinuric acute kidney injury

115.10. Which of the following therapies is most indicated following ocular exposure to the urticarial hairs of a tarantula?
- A. A topical antibiotic
- B. A topical cycloplegic
- C. A topical corticosteroid
- D. A systemic corticosteroid
- E. Ophthalmology consultation

ANSWERS

115.1. Answer: C. Severe muscle cramps, nausea, weakness, and tremor develop within several hours of a black widow spider envenomation. Although both the male and female spiders are venomous, only the female spider has a jaw apparatus that is sufficiently large to penetrate human skin. Significant local reactions are rare. The spider is identified by a red to orange hourglass on the abdomen. Different *Latrodectus* spp have different shapes and colors to their markings. The whole immunoglobulin antivenon is reserved for patients with severe pain refractory to other therapy as it is an equine antivenin with a risk of anaphylaxis. A newer F(ab')$_2$ antivenom shows promise.

Clark RF, et al. Clinical presentation and treatment of black widow spider envenomation: A review of 163 cases. *Ann Emerg Med.* 1992;21:782-787.

Dart RC, et al. A randomized, double-blind, placebo-controlled trial of a highly purified equine F(ab)2 antibody black widow spider antivenom. *Ann Emerg Med.* 2013;61:458-467.

115.2. Answer: E. While the most common description of a brown recluse spider bite is a purple papule that develops hours after a painless bite, rare victims develop fever, arthralgias, hemolysis, and DIC. Both male and female spiders are capable of envenomating victims.

Gendron BP. *Loxosceles reclusa* envenomation. *Am J Emerg Med.* 1990;8: 51-54.

Franca FO, et al. Rhabdomyolysis in presumed viscero-cutaneous loxoscelism: Report of two cases. *Trans R Soc Trop Med Hyg.* 2002;96:287-290.

Williams ST, et al. Severe intravascular hemolysis associated with brown recluse spider envenomation. A report of two cases and review of the literature. *Am J Clin Pathol.* 1995;104:463-467.

115.3. Answer: E. Victims develop muscle fasciculations and cramps, seizures, kidney failure, and, rarely, cardiovascular collapse after a *Centruroides* scorpion sting. This presentation occurs in children, but is rarely reported in adults. The *Centruroides* scorpion is found predominantly in the Southwestern states and Mexico. Mortality is rare. Mannitol is used to treat ciguatera poisoning but not scorpion stings. A newer, safer antivenom is now available and significantly reduces the need for large doses of sedatives.

Boyer LV, et al. Antivenom for critically ill children with neurotoxicity from scorpion stings. *N Engl J Med.* 2009;360:2090-2098.

Boyer LV, et al. Effectiveness of Centruroides scorpion antivenom compared to historical controls. *Toxicon.* 2013;76:377-385.

115.4. Answer: A. Improvement in paralysis occurs rapidly after the entire tick is removed from the skin. The tick must remain on the person for 5-6 days before symptoms occur.

Absent or decreased deep tendon reflexes is often the earliest sign of toxicity. Girls develop tick paralysis more commonly than boys, as the tick often hides in the scalp under long hair.

Needham GR. Evaluation of five popular methods for tick removal. *Pediatrics*. 1985;75:997-1002.

115.5. Answer: A. Because the venom produced by wasps, hornets, and yellow jackets is almost identical, immunotherapy was developed from a common venom. Although direct toxicity occurs, it usually follows massive, multiple envenomations. As such, IgE-mediated anaphylaxis is far more common as it occurs following a single sting. Delayed reactions occur 1-2 weeks after the sting. Africanized honeybees do not have more toxic venom, but are a greater risk because they tend to be aggressive and attack together, leading to multiple stings. Apamin binds to spinal Ca^{2+}-triggered K^+ channels.

Abramowicz M, ed. Insect venoms. *Med Lett Drug Ther*. 1983;25:53-54.

Bresolin NL, et al. Acute renal failure following massive attack by Africanized bee stings. *Pediatr Nephrol*. 2002;17:625-627.

Habermann E. Apamin. *Pharmacol Ther*. 1984;25:255-270.

115.6. Answer: C. The funnel web spider is found in Queensland, New South Wales, Tasmania, and Victoria. The male is the more dangerous, containing high concentrations of a neurotoxin, atracotoxin, that fixes the sodium channel in an open configuration. Fatalities are more commonly reported in children. Pressure immobilization is recommended to slow venom movement in the lymphatic space. Funnel web spider antivenom is generally considered safe, effective, and of very low acute allergenicity.

Gray RR. Getting to known funnel-webs. *Aust Nat Hist*. 1981;20: 256-258.

Isbister GK, et al. Funnel-web spider bite: A systematic review of recorded clinical cases. *Med J Aust*. 2005;182:407-411.

115.7. Answer: E. All substances listed are found in the venom of fire ants.

Stafford CT, et al. Allergy to imported fire ants. *South Med J*. 1989;82:1520-1527.

115.8. Answer: A. Outside of envenomations from *Loxosceles* spp, confirmed dermatonecrotic spider bites in North America are distinctly uncommon. There is at least one confirmed necrotic lesion produced by the bite of the hobo spider, *Eratigena agrestis* (formerly known as *Tegenaria agrestis*).

Centers for Disease Control and Prevention. Necrotic arachnidism— Pacific Northwest, 1988-1996. *MMWR Morb Mortal Wkly Rep*. 1996;45:433-436.

115.9. Answer: D. Tarantula bites, which are rare in the US, usually cause minor localized histamine-related effects, including localized pruritis, erythema, and swelling.

Schanbacher FL, et al. Composition and properties of tarantula *Dugsiella henzi* (Girard) venom. *Toxicon*. 1979;11:21-29.

115.10. Answer: E. The urticarial hairs of a tarantula become imbedded in the cornea of exposed individuals and, if not removed and properly treated, lead to a debilitating chronic reaction called ophthalmia nodosa. Specialty consultation is always recommended following these exposures.

Belyea DA, et al. The red eye revisited: Ophthalmia nodosa due to tarantula hairs. *South Med J*. 1998;91:565-567.

Bernardino CR, Rapuano C. Ophthalmia nodosa caused by casual handling of a tarantula. *CLAO J*. 2000;26:111-112.

QUESTIONS

116.1. A 4-year-old girl is found on the beach in Australia with flaccid paralysis and is immediately transported to the emergency department. Envenomation from which animal best explains this presentation?
A. *Carukia barnesi*
B. *Conus geographus*
C. *Physalia physalis*
D. *Synanceia horrida*
E. *Chironex fleckeri*

116.2. A 27-year-old man presents to the emergency department with a rash confined to the genital area 1 day after swimming in the ocean. Which of the following exposures best explains his presentation?
A. Hydroids
B. Sea anemones
C. Box jellyfish
D. Corals
E. *Linuche unguiculata*

116.3. A 22-year-old woman presents to an emergency department in Australia with extreme hypertension, tachycardia, and diaphoresis. Which of the following exposures best explains her presentation?
A. *Carukia barnesi*
B. *Hapalochlaena maculosa*
C. *Chironex fleckeri*
D. *Conus geographus*
E. *Enhydrina schistosa*

116.4. Which of the following options best explains the mechanism of action of the toxin found in blue-ringed octopi?
A. It is an agonist of the nicotinic acetylcholine (ACh) receptor
B. It is an antagonist of the nicotinic ACh receptor
C. It is an antagonist of the voltage-gated sodium channel
D. It is an antagonist of the muscarinic ACh receptor
E. It is an antagonist of the N-methyl-D-aspartate (NMDA) receptor

116.5. A 37-year-old man presents to the emergency department for evaluation of an injury he sustained to his left foot while working on the beach. The injury occured in shallow water despite wearing leather boots. Which of the following fish have dorsal spines that are powerful enough to penetrate a leather boot?
A. Stingray
B. Weeverfish
C. Lionfish
D. Starfish
E. Tigerfish

116.6. Which of the following Scorpaenidae envenomations has the greatest mortality?
A. Lionfish
B. Stonefish
C. Turkeyfish
D. Zebrafish
E. Tigerfish

116.7. Which of the following statements about the tentacles of the Portuguese man-of-war is correct?
  A. They are several hundred feet long
  B. Each man-of-war has several hundred tentacles
  C. Once detached, tentacles are no longer capable of stinging
  D. The tentacles contain nematocysts that deliver a neurotoxic venom
  E. Envenomation is best treated with ice packs

116.8. Which of the following statements about the venom isolated from the sea snake is correct?
  A. It inhibits the reuptake of calcium into the sarcoplasmic reticulum
  B. It interferes with Na^+,K^+-ATPase activity
  C. It inhibits the slow calcium channels
  D. It causes direct stimulation of postsynaptic glycine receptors
  E. It alters both sodium and chloride permeability at peripheral nerve endings

116.9. A 42-year-old man presents to the emergency department after stepping on a stonefish. In addition to other therapies, which of the following antibiotics would be appropriate to administer to this patient?
  A. Amoxicillin
  B. Nitrofurantoin
  C. Levofloxacin
  D. Trimethoprim/sulfamethoxazole
  E. Penicillin G

116.10. Which of the following statements about Cnidaria envenomations is most accurate?
  A. Most people who are envenomated do not present to health care facilities
  B. All patients with *Chironex fleckeri* envenomation should be admitted for cardiovascular monitoring
  C. Cnidaria antivenom administration is a lifesaving intervention
  D. 15-20% of *C. fleckeri* envenomations are fatal
  E. Stinger nets are very effective in preventing human envenomation

ANSWERS

116.1. Answer: B. Cone snail venom contains multiple peptide toxins ("conotoxins") that cause flaccid paralysis through different mechanisms, including nicotinic acetylcholine receptor inhibition and voltage-dependent sodium channel inhibition.

Norton RS, Olivera BM. Conotoxins down under *Toxicon*. 2006;48:780-798.

116.2. Answer: E. *Linuche unguiculata*, the larvae of the jellyfish, cause a dermatitis by attaching to the fibers of bathing suits (seabathers, eruption). The inflammatory reaction is treated with a topical corticosteroid.

Tomchik RS, et al. Clinical perspectives on seabather's eruption, also known as sea lice. *JAMA*. 1993;269:1669-1672.

116.3. Answer: A. The symptoms are consistent with Irukandji syndrome following *Carukia barnesi* envenomation. The condition is characterized by hyperactivation of the sympathetic nervous system caused by the painful discharge of toxin from the nematocysts. Other members of the phylum Cnidaria also cause this condition. Treatment of the hypertension with phentolamine is recommended.

Underwood AH, Seymour JE. Venom ontogeny, diet and morphology in *Carukia barnesi*, a species of Australian box jellyfish that causes Irukandji syndrome. *Toxicon*. 2007;49:1073-1082.

116.4. Answer: C. Tetrodotoxin is found in both blue-ringed octopi and puffer fish. It is a heat-stable antagonist of the voltage-gated sodium channel and leads to flaccid paralysis when it is ingested or injected.

Ahasan HA, et al. Paralytic complications of puffer fish (tetrodotoxin) poisoning. *Singapore Med J*. 2004;45:73-74.

116.5. Answer: B. The weeverfish has dorsal spines that are sharp and powerful enough to penetrate a leather boot. Following envenomation, the victim will experience a burning or crushing pain that increases in intensity as it spreads through the affected limb.

Halstead BW, Modglin FR. Weeverfish stings and venom apparatus of weever (*Trachinus*). *Z Tropenmed Parasitol*. 1958;9:129.

116.6. Answer: B. The stonefish is the most dangerous of the Scorpaenidae family. It is an aggressive fish and will not swim away from humans. It is a bottom dweller; therefore, most injuries occur when divers step on the fish in deep water. The stonefish causes immediate muscle spasm and excruciating pain. This sometimes prevents the diver from surfacing and getting help.

Wiener S. Observations on the venom of the stonefish (*Synanceja trachynis*). *Med J Aust*. 1959;2:260-265.

116.7. Answer: D. The Portuguese man-of-war contains a neurotoxic venom capable of causing excruciating pain. The tentacles are usually about 10 feet long, number about 40, and remain active for many hours after they are detached. Most Portuguese man-of-war are found in the southern Atlantic Ocean and in the Caribbean Sea. The initial management of Cnidaria envenomation should be focused on stabilization of any cardiopulmonary abnormalities. This is followed by other measures to prevent further discharge of nematocysts to limit pain and toxicity. Topical application of either vinegar or stingose, an aqueous solution of 20% aluminum sulfate and 1.1% surfactant is recommended.

Stein MR, et al. Fatal Portuguese man-of-war (*Physalia physalis*) envenomation. *Ann Emerg Med.* 1989;18:312-315.

116.8. Answer: E. The venom isolated from the toxic sea snakes alters both sodium and chloride permeability at peripheral nerve endings without affecting the Na^+,K^+-ATPase pump.

Gerencser GA, Loo SY. Effect of *Laticauda semifasciata* (sea snake) venom on sodium transport across frog skin. *Comp Biochem Physiol.* 1982;72A:727.

116.9. Answer: C. Prophylactic antibiotics decrease the rates of wound infection. The current recommended therapy following stone fish envenomation is either a quinolone or cefazolin. In patients who are undergoing hot water immersion, early antibiotic administration decreases the rate of growth of *Vibrio vulnificus* and the risk of developing necrotizing fasciitis.

Tang WM, et al. Rapidly progressive necrotising fasciitis following a stonefish sting: A report of two cases. *J Orthop Surg (Hong Kong).* 2006;14:67-70.

Clark RF, et al. Stingray envenomation: A retrospective review of clinical presentation and treatment in 119 cases. *J Emerg Med.* 2007;33:33-37.

116.10. Answer: A. Most jellyfish envenomations are mild to moderate and an injured person can be treated as an outpatient. Estimates on the rate of cardiovascular toxicity and mortality in the literature are skewed higher due to referral bias. Small jellyfish pass through the stinger nets; one Australian study found that the majority of stings occurred in netted waters.

Rosson CL, Tolle SW. Management of marine stings and scrapes. *West J Med.* 1989;150:97.

Little M, Mulcahy RF. A year's experience of Irukandji envenomation in far north Queensland. *Med J Aust.* 1998;169:638-641.

Mushrooms

QUESTIONS

117.1. A 22-year-old man with lethargy presents to the hospital following an ingestion of an *Amanita muscaria* mushroom. His presentation is explained by direct activity at which receptor site?
A. Kainate receptor
B. *N*-Methyl-D-aspartate (NMDA) receptor
C. Dopamine A_1 receptor
D. Gamma-aminobutyric acid $(GABA)_A$ receptor
E. Glycine receptor

117.2. A 27-year-old man is found seizing after eating mushrooms he foraged while on vacation. Lorazepam 4 mg is administered intravenously with no resolution of his seizures. Ingestion of which of the following mushrooms would explain his presentation?
A. *Amanita gemmata*
B. *Clitocybe nebularis*
C. *Gyromitra esculenta*
D. *Cortinarius orellanus*
E. *Paxillus involutus*

117.3. An otherwise healthy 33-year-old woman develops a headache, flushing, nausea, and vomiting while drinking mojitos with her friends. During her history, she states that she had eaten a salad containing foraged mushrooms the day prior to presentation. Which mushroom is likely responsible?
A. *Amanita muscaria*
B. *Clitocybe nebularis*
C. *Gyromitra esculenta*
D. *Cortinarius orellanus*
E. *Coprinus atramentarius*

117.4. A 3-year-old girl is brought into the emergency department by her mother because she developed vomiting, diarrhea, and difficulty breathing. On examination, the child is bradycardic, diaphoretic, and has significant wheezing. Ingestion of which of the following mushrooms would explain her presentation?
A. *Amanita gemmata*
B. *Clitocybe dealbata*
C. *Gyromitra esculenta*
D. *Cortinarius orellanus*
E. *Psilocybe cubensis*

117.5. A 65-year-old woman is brought to the emergency department confused and jaundiced. Her laboratory data demonstrate fulminant liver failure. Her family reveals that the patient ate a mushroom stew 3 days prior to presentation. The physician suspects *Amanita phalloides* as the culprit. Alpha-amanitin causes toxicity by interfering with which of the following options?
A. DNA transcriptase II
B. RNA polymerase II
C. RNA synthetase I
D. DNA synthetase II
E. DNA transcriptase I

117.6. A 68-year-old man develops nausea and vomiting 2 hours after eating a mushroom while on vacation in Washington State in the United States. Four days later, he notes fatigue and decreased urine output and presents to the hospital. There he is found to be in acute kidney failure. What toxin explains his symptoms?
A. Allenic norleucine
B. Ibotenic acid
C. Gyrometrin
D. 1-Aminocyclopropanol
E. Phallotoxin

117.7. A 29-year-old man presents with myalgias and tea-colored urine after a recent mushroom ingestion. On blood work, he has an elevated CPK >100,000 U/L (>1,666,666 nkat/L). Which mushroom did he eat?
A. *Amanita smithiana*
B. *Lycoperdon perlatum*
C. *Amanita muscaria*
D. *Tricholoma equestre*
E. *Cortinarius orellanus*

117.8. A 7-year-old boy is brought to the emergency department for shortness of breath and wheezing. Several hours earlier, he and his brothers were running around their backyard and jumping on giant mushrooms. What mushroom would explain the symptoms?
A. *Amanita smithiana*
B. *Lycoperdon perlatum*
C. *Amanita muscaria*
D. *Tricholoma equestre*
E. *Cortinarius orellanus*

117.9. A 17-year-old boy presents with ataxia and hallucinations following an intentional ingestion of *Psilocybe caerulipes*. The toxin in this mushroom resembles which neurotransmitter?
A. Gamma-aminobutyric acid (GABA)
B. Glutamate
C. Serotonin
D. Acetylcholine
E. Glycine

117.10. A 34-year-old-man presents to the emergency department for evaluation of painful paresthesias to his distal extremities. He has a history of foraging for mushrooms. His extremities are edematous and erythematous. What mushroom would explain his presentation?
A. *Clitocybe amoenolens*
B. *Amanita smithiana*
C. *Tricholoma equestre*
D. *Hapalopilus rutilans*
E. *Gymnopilus spectabilis*

ANSWERS

117.1. Answer: D. *Amanita muscaria* mushrooms contain both muscimol and ibotenic acid. The muscimol binds directly to the GABA$_A$ receptor and the ibotenic acid binds to the NMDA receptor. The structure of muscimol resembles GABA and the structure of ibotenic acid resembles glutamate. Ibotenic acid is decarboxylated to muscimol by the same process that glutamate is decarboxylated to GABA. Children are more prone to the effects of the ibotenic acid, while adults are more likely to experience effects of the muscimol.

Olsen RW. The GABA postsynaptic membrane receptor-ionophore complex. *Mol Cell Biochem.* 1981;39:261-279.

117.2. Answer: C. *Gyromitra esculenta* contains a toxin, gyromitrin, which on hydrolysis yields monomethylhydrazine. The hydrazine reacts with pyridoxine, inhibiting gamma-aminobutyric acid (GABA) formation. This causes seizures by a mechanism identical to isoniazid toxicity. Treatment with pyridoxine is indicated for seizures that do not respond to a standard dose of a benzodiazepine.

Sotaniemi E, et al. Hydrazine toxicity in the human: Report of fatal cases. *Ann Clin Res.* 1971;3:30-33.

117.3. Answer: E. *Coprinus atramentarius* contains 1-aminocyclopropanol, which inhibits aldehyde dehydrogenase. While the mushroom alone is benign, when ethanol is ingested within 48-72 hours following eating the mushroom, patients often present with a disulfiramlike reaction due to the accumulation of acetaldehyde.

Carlson A, et al. On the disulfiram-like effect of coprine, the pharmacologically active principle of *Coprinus atramentarius*. *Acta Pharmacol Toxicol.* 1978;42:292-297.

117.4. Answer: B. *Clitocybe dealbata* contains muscarine, which when ingested, leads to muscarinic symptoms. Patients present with diaphoresis, miosis, bradycardia, hypersalivation, lacrimation, urination, and defecation. These symptoms are reversed with the administration of atropine. As muscarine does not contain an ester bond and the toxicity is not due to an inhibition of acetylcholinesterase, there is no utility in the administration of pralidoxime. Furthermore, as muscarine does not cross the blood–brain barrier, patients do not manifest central nervous system toxicity.

Carder CA, et al. Management of mushroom poisoning. *Clin Toxicol Consult.* 1983;5:103-118.

117.5 Answer: B. Alpha-amanitin causes toxicity by interfering with RNA polymerase II. This inhibits protein synthesis and eventually causes fulminant liver failure. Alpha-amanitin is heat stable and is therefore still present and active, even if a mushroom is cooked. Alpha-amanitin is detected in the body several days after ingestion. Cyclopeptides also alter the regulation of glucose, calcium, and thyroid hormones. It is, therefore, important to monitor for hypoglycemia, which often precedes the hepatotoxicity.

Sperti S, et al. Dissociation constants of the complexes between RNA polymerase II and amanitins. *Experientia*. 1973;29:33-34.

117.6. Answer: A. Allenic norleucine, the toxin in *Amanita smithiana*, is considered a "rule breaker," as patients present with early vomiting (within 5 hours) following ingestion and then develop significant kidney toxicity. Most other mushrooms that produce symptoms this early are benign. Currently, this mushroom is only found in the Pacific Northwest region of North America.

Tulloss RE, et al. *Amanita smithiana* – taxonomy, distribution and poisonings. *Mycotaxon*. 1992;45:373-387.

117.7. Answer: D. *Tricholoma equestre*, a mushroom found primarily in Europe, causes atraumatic rhabdomyolysis. It has a 25% mortality, presumably due to cardiac rhabdomyolysis.

Bedry R, et al. Wild-mushroom intoxication as a cause of rhabdomyolysis. *N Engl J Med*. 2001;345:798-802.

117.8. Answer: B. *Lycoperdon perlatum* is commonly known as a puffball mushroom. They are edible and nontoxic when ingested. However, when they are mature and stomped on, they cause a massive inhalational exposure to spores. This leads to lycoperdonosis, which is an allergic bronchoalveolitis. The pneumonitis develops within hours of exposure, and patients present with cough, shortness of breath, fatigue, myalgias, and fever. The management of lycoperdonosis includes corticosteroids and antifungals, such as amphotericin B.

Strand RD, et al. Lycoperdonosis. *N Engl J Med*. 1967;277:89-91.

117.9. Answer: C. The structure of psilocybin resembles that of serotonin, which explains many of the symptoms noted. It is rare for patients who ingest this mushroom to seek care in the emergency department, as the mushroom is intentionally ingested for its hallucinogenic effect. However, if a patient does present to the hospital, they respond well to supportive care and benzodiazepines.

Curry SC, et al. Intravenous mushroom poisoning. *Ann Emerg Med*. 1985;14:900-902.

117.10. Answer: A. This patient's presentation is consistent with erythromelalgia, which is reported in Japan and France. It is attributed to the ingestion of *Clitocybe acromelaga* and *Clitocybe amoenolens*. The toxic substances within this mushroom are acromelic acids A to E. The management is largely supportive, and patients usually have resolution of their symptoms within several months.

Nakajima N, et al. Erythromelalgia associated with *Clitocybe acromelalga* intoxication. *Clin Toxicol (Phila)*. 2013;51:451-454.

118

Plants

118.1. A 27-year-old woman presents to the emergency department with seizurelike activity. The team is concerned that she is having "pseudoseizures" as she is awake and talking during the tonic-clonic movements. The movements are made worse when she is startled. Ingestion of what plant explains these movements?
A. *Conium maculatum*
B. *Cicuta maculata*
C. *Strychnos nux vomica*
D. *Aconitum napellus*
E. *Rhododendron ferrugineum*

118.2. A 35-year-old man is brought into the emergency department after spending a day working outdoors in the summer heat. His examination is notable for tachycardia, vomiting, diarrhea, agitation, and convulsions. What plant was he harvesting?
A. *Lathyrus sativus*
B. *Nicotiana tabacum*
C. *Catha edulis*
D. *Artemisia absinthium*
E. *Convallaria majalis*

118.3. A 61-year-old man presents to the emergency department with severe diarrhea after eating berries he found on the side of the road. He has profound lymphocytosis. What plant led to this presentation.
A. American pokeweed (*Phytolacca americana*)
B. American pennyroyal (*Hedeoma pulegioides*)
C. Chickling pea (*Lathyrus sativus*)
D. Water hemlock (*Cicuta maculata*)
E. Ackee fruit (*Bligha sapida*)

118.4. A 39-year-old man is brought into the emergency department while on vacation in the Caribbean. His family found him confused and diaphoretic. His point-of-care blood glucose is 15 mg/dL (0.8 mmol/L). Which plant could have led to this?
A. Ackee fruit
B. Jimsonweed
C. Lily of the valley
D. Pennyroyal
E. Blue cohosh

118.5. A 62-year-old man presents with generalized tonic-clonic seizures after an ingestion of a plant. Which of the following plants is the most likely cause?
A. Poison hemlock
B. Water hemlock
C. Foxglove
D. Dumb cane
E. Mistletoe

118.6. A 13-year-old boy is admitted to the hospital for further evaluation of his hypertension. He is also hypokalemic with a metabolic alkalosis. Further history reveals he had eaten an after-dinner treat every day for weeks that contains a toxin that comes from which plant?
A. *Manihot esculenta*
B. *Glycyrrhiza glabra*
C. *Taxus baccata*
D. *Abrus precatorius*
E. *Blighia sapida*

118.7. A 61-year-old woman presents with diarrhea and dehydration. She is admitted to the hospital, where she is found to have bone marrow suppression. During her hospital course, she develops a peripheral neuropathy. This toxicity is explained by the ingestion of what plant?
A. Birthwort (*Aristolochia* spp)
B. Dumb cane (*Dieffenbachia* spp)
C. Blue cohosh (*Caulophyllum thalictroides*)
D. St. John's wort (*Hypericum perforatum*)
E. Mayapple (*Podophyllum peltatum*)

118.8. A 54-year-old woman presents to the emergency department with right upper quadrant pain and new jaundice. She is diagnosed with hepatic veno-occlusive syndrome. Which plant did she ingest?
A. *Aristolochia* spp
B. *Abrus precatorius*
C. *Heliotropium amplexicaule*
D. *Catha edulis*
E. *Digitalis lanata*

118.9. A 16-year-old boy presents to the emergency department after ingesting a tea made from *Datura stramonium* seeds. What antidote would be reasonable to use as part of his management?
A. Atropine
B. Digoxin-specific FAb fragments
C. Pyridoxine
D. *N*-Acetylcysteine
E. Physostigmine

118.10. A 2-year-old boy is brought into the emergency department due to painful and swollen lips. The remainder of his examination is within normal. Which plant explains his symptoms?
A. *Dieffenbachia* spp
B. *Phytolacca americana*
C. *Colchicum autumnale*
D. *Rhododendron ferrugineum*
E. *Lathyrus sativus*

ANSWERS

118.1. Answer: C. *Strychnos nux vomica* contains strychnine, which antagonizes the postsynaptic glycine receptor. As glycine is an inhibitory neurotransmitter primarily in the spinal cord and not in the brain, patients present with "awake seizures." Poison hemlock contains conine, which acts as a nicotinic agonist. Water hemlock leads to seizures due to cicutoxin, which antagonizes $GABA_A$; however, these patients will not be awake. Monkshood contains aconite, which is a sodium channel opener that leads to cardiac toxicity. Rhododendron contains grayanotoxin, which acts in a similar mechanism to aconite.

Smith BA. Strychnine poisoning. *J Emerg Med*. 1990;8:321-325.

118.2. Answer: B. Green tobacco sickness occurs in workers who are out picking tobacco on hot days. The nicotine from *Nicotiana tabacum* is absorbed through the skin, causing nicotine toxicity. The chickling pea (*Lathyrus sativus*) contains beta-*N*-oxalylamino-L-alanine (BOAA) and causes neurolathyrism. Khat (*Catha edulis*) contains cathinones, leading to a sympathomimetic toxidrome. Wormwood (*Artemisia absinthium*) contains absinthe and causes hallucinations. Lily of the valley (*Convallaria majalis*) contains convallotoxin, a cardiac glycoside, and causes toxicity that resembles digoxin toxicity.

Bartholomay P, et al. Epidemiologic investigation of an occupational illness of tobacco harvesters in southern Brazil, a worldwide leader in tobacco production. *Occup Environ Med*. 2012;69:514-518.

118.3. Answer: A. *Phytolacca americana*, also known as American pokeweed, produces profound gastrointestinal distress and significant leukocytosis. If the pokeweed is parboiled much of the toxin is removed, and it is edible. Poke salad is eaten commonly in many parts of the United States.

Roberge R, et al. The root of evil—pokeweed intoxication. *Ann Emerg Med*. 1986;15:470-473.

118.4. Answer: A. When *Blighia sapida*, or ackee fruit, is unripe, it contains the toxin hypoglycin A, which leads to severe hypoglycemia. Jimsonweed produces an anticholinergic toxidrome. Lily of the valley produces cardiac toxicity. Pennyroyal leads to liver toxicity. Blue cohosh leads to nicotinic toxicity.

Bressler R, et al. Hypoglycin and hypoglycin-like compounds. *Pharmacol Rev*. 1969;21:105-130.

Jelliffe DB, Stuart KL. Acute toxic hypoglycemia in the vomiting sickness of Jamaica. *Br Med J*. 1954;1:75.

118.5. Answer: B. *Cicuta maculata*, or water hemlock, contains cicutoxin. Cicutoxin binds and antagonizes $GABA_A$ receptors. People ingest this plant due to its similar appearance to wild carrots and a fennellike odor. Poison hemlock contains coniine, which causes nicotinelike toxicity. Foxglove contains digitalis, a cardioactive steroid. Dumb cane causes local toxicity due to calcium oxalate crystals. Mistletoe causes hepatitis and gastrointestinal (GI) side effects.

Gompertz LM. Poisoning with water hemlock (*cicuta maculate*). A report of 17 cases. *JAMA*. 1926;87:1277-1278.

Knutsen OH, Paszkowshi P. New aspects in the treatment of water hemlock poisoning. *J Toxicol Clin Toxicol*. 1984;22:157-166.

118.6.   Answer: B. This child ate his father's European licorice. Real licorice that comes from licorice root contains glycyrrhizin. This causes inhibition of 11-beta-hydroxysteroid dehydrogenase and leads to hypermineralocorticoid syndrome. Linamarin is a cyanogenic glycoside that comes from cassava. Yew berry, from the *Taxus* species, contains taxine, which leads to sodium channel blockade and dysrhythmias. *Abrus precatorius* (also known as the rosary pea or the jequirity bean) contains abrin, a toxin similar to ricin that binds to the 60S ribosomal subunit and inhibits RNA polymerase and protein synthesis. *Blighia sapida*, also known as ackee fruit, contains the toxin hypoglycin A and leads to hypoglycemia and hepatotoxicity.

Farese RV, et al. Licorice-induced hypermineralocorticoidism. *N Engl J Med*. 1991;325:1223-1227.

118.7.   Answer: E. The toxicity of mayapple, or *Podophyllum peltatum*, resembles colchicine toxicity. Patients initially develop gastrointestinal effects, which are followed by bone marrow suppression and peripheral neuropathy. *Aristolochia* spp were used as uterine stimulants and were found in weight loss supplements, causing renal fibrosis and an increased risk of urothelial cancer. Blue cohosh is used as an abortifacient and has nicotinic effects from *N*-methylcysteine. St. John's wort is used to treat depression; it leads to serotonin toxicity when taken in conjunction with another serotonergic xenobiotic. It has important drug interactions with numerous other medications, such as digoxin, oral contraceptives, and warfarin. *Dieffenbachia* spp cause oropharyngeal toxicity due to calcium oxalate crystals.

Ng TH, et al. Encephalopathy and neuropathy following ingestion of a Chinese herbal broth containing podophyllin. *J Neurol Sci*. 1991;101:107-113.

118.8.   Answer: C. *Heliotropium* contains pyrrolizidine alkaloids. These alkaloids produce a veno-occlusive syndrome that results from proliferation of the intimal tissue of hepatic vasculature. In large, acute overdoses, centrilobular hepatic necrosis develops following metabolism by the cytochrome P450 system. Hepatic congestion, ascites, and edema result from vascular occlusion. Patients either die, develop cirrhosis or hepatic carcinomas, or recover completely.

Fu PP, et al. Pyrrolizidine alkaloids—genotoxicity, metabolism enzymes, metabolic activation, and mechanisms. *Drug Metab Rev*. 2004;36:1-55.

118.9.   Answer: E. *Datura stramonium,* commonly known as jimson weed, contains belladonna alkaloids, such as atropine and scopolamine, and leads to antimuscarinic symptoms when ingested. It is used recreationally by adolescents and young adults to achieve a hallucinatory effect. Physostigmine reverses the antimuscarinic toxicity that these patients develop.

Centers for Disease Control and Prevention (CDC). Anticholinergic poisoning associated with an herbal tea—New York City, 1994. *MMWR Morb Mortal Wkly Rep*. 1995;44:193-195.

118.10.   Answer: A. *Dieffenbachia* spp, also known as dumb cane, are very common house plants. Their leaves contain tiny needlelike calcium oxalate crystals called raphides. When the leaves are chewed, these crystals cause pain and swelling to the oropharynx. The treatment is largely supportive; however, in very rare cases, the swelling is severe enough that airway protection is indicated.

Altin G, et al. Severe destruction of the upper respiratory structures after brief exposure to a dieffenbachia plant. *J Craniofac Surg*. 2013;24: e245-e247.

QUESTIONS

119.1. A 22-year-old man presents to the emergency department after he was bitten by a Gila monster (*Heloderma suspectum*). Which of the following statements is true regarding Gila bites?
A. Best treated with antivenin
B. Associated with kidney failure
C. Cause severe pain and moderate edema
D. Are commonly fatal
E. Often associated with a coagulopathy

119.2. A 45-year-old man presents to the emergency department after he was bitten by his pet coral snake. Which of the following symptoms is consistent with an envenomation by this snake?
A. Significant local swelling and pain
B. Early coagulopathy
C. Metallic taste and tongue edema
D. Diplopia
E. Chest pain

119.3. An 18-year-old man presents to the emergency department for evaluation of a crotaline envenomation. On physical examination, he has obvious fang marks. Eight hours later, he has minor, nonprogressing, local swelling and discomfort. He has no systemic manifestations or hematologic abnormalities. Which of the following therapies is indicated in this patient?
A. Intravenous fluids
B. Cardiac monitoring
C. Antivenom administration
D. Oxygen therapy
E. Tetanus prophylaxis

119.4. Which of the following characteristics of pit vipers differentiates them from native nonvenomous species?
A. Rounded head
B. Vertically elliptical pupils
C. Double row of plates on the undersurface
D. Lack of a rattling sound
E. Hidden fangs

119.5. A 22-year-old man presents to the emergency department after he was bitten by a rattlesnake. Which of the following antibiotics should be administered prophylactically to this patient?
A. Ciprofloxacin
B. Amoxicillin/clavulanic acid
C. Doxycycline
D. Cefalexin
E. No antibiotic is indicated at this time

119.6. Crotalidae polyvalent immune Fab (Crofab) antivenom is developed from commonly encountered North American pit vipers. Which of the following snakes is used in the development of this antivenom?
A. *Cerastes cerastes*
B. *Crotalus lepidus*
C. *Crotalus viridis*
D. *Agkistrodon piscivorus*
E. *Agkistrodon contortrix*

119.7. A 21-year-old man presents to the emergency department after he was bitten by an eastern coral snake. He is entirely asymptomatic at presentation but his arm was wrapped by a friend who is a paramedic. His hand is warm and well perfused. Which of the following management strategies is indicated in this patient?
   A. Observe in the emergency department for 6 hours
   B. Empiric administration of crotaline antivenom
   C. Empiric administration of North American Coral Snake Antivenom
   D. Immediate removal of the pressure immobilization bandage (PIB)
   E. Admit to an intensive care unit for at least 24 hours for airway monitoring

119.8. A 24-year-old, 27-week pregnant woman presents to the emergency department after she was bitten on the foot by a pit viper in Texas. Her examination is remarkable for markedly progressive swelling around the bite, and her blood work reveals thrombocytopenia. Which of the following management strategies is indicated in this patient?
   A. Observe in the emergency department for 6 hours
   B. Administration of crotaline antivenom

   C. Administration of North American coral snake antivenom
   D. Immediate delivery of fetus
   E. Immediate fasciotomy of the foot and leg

119.9. A 27-year-old man presents to the emergency department with diplopia and ptosis after he was bitten by the Mojave rattlesnake *Crotalus scutulatus*. Which of the following options best explains the mechanism of his symptoms?
   A. Impaired metabolism of acetylcholine
   B. Presynaptic inhibition of acetylcholine release
   C. Postsynaptic inhibition at the acetylcholine receptor
   D. Presynaptic inhibition of the glycine receptor
   E. Postsynaptic inhibition of the glycine receptor

119.10. A 5-year-old boy presents to a hospital in Colorado with a snake bite to his left index finger. The finger is cyanotic and lacks sensation. Which of the following interventions is reasonable in this patient?
   A. Topical nitroglycerin paste
   B. Topical nifedipine
   C. Local infiltration with calcium gluconate
   D. Dermotomy
   E. Antivenom alone

ANSWERS

119.1. Answer: C. Gila monster bites are extremely uncommon and almost always occur in captive animals. They have very forceful bites and will hang on and chew for as long as 15 minutes. The most common symptoms are pain and edema. As these bites are very rare and there are no reported fatalities, there is no antivenin available. Coagulopathy is an extremely rare finding following Gila monster bites. Kidney failure does not occur following Gila monster bites.

French RN, et al. Gila monster bite. *Clin Toxicol*. 2012;50:151-152.

Hooker KR, et al. Gila monster envenomation. *Ann Emerg Med*. 1994; 24:731-735.

119.2. Answer: D. Only about 40% of coral snake bites are associated with envenomation. Because coral snake fangs are small and nonmobile they do not always produce easily identifiable wounds. Symptoms are often delayed for several hours and are neurologic, including diplopia, ptosis, dysphagia, muscle weakness, fasciculations, and, eventually, paralysis.

Kitchens CS, Van Mierop LH. Envenomation by the Eastern coral snake (*Micrurus fulvius*). A study of 39 victims. *JAMA*. 1987;258:1615-1618.

119.3. Answer: E. This patient has minimal toxicity from a crotaline envenomation and does not need to be treated with antivenom, intravenous fluids, or oxygen. He also does not need to be admitted for cardiac or serial laboratory monitoring. Tetanus prophylaxis is the only reasonable therapy following this bite. Bites that have progression of swelling beyond the area of the bite (with or without local tissue destruction), hematologic abnormalities, or non-life-threatening systemic effects are considered moderate envenomations. These patients should be admitted to an intensive care unit, receive antivenom therapy, have cardiac monitoring, and have their laboratory parameters monitored. Intravenous fluids and analgesics will likely also be needed. Severe envenomations have marked progressive swelling, pain (with or without local tissue destruction), and systemic effects such as diarrhea, weakness, shock, or angioedema. They also develop pronounced thrombocytopenia or coagulopathy. These patients also need vasopressor support in addition to the other interventions listed for moderate envenomations.

Dart RC, et al. Validation of a severity score for the assessment of crotalid snakebite. *Ann Emerg Med*. 1996;27:321-326.

119.4. Answer: B. Pit vipers are distinguished from native nonvenomous species of snakes by a triangle-shaped head, vertically elliptical pupils, a single row of plates on the under-surface, and easily identifiable fangs. Depending on their maturity, rattlesnakes do not always have a rattle.

Russell FE. Identification and distribution of North American venomous snakes. In: Russell FE, ed. *Snake Venom Poisoning*. Philadelphia, PA: Lippincott; 1980:45-86.

119.5. Answer: E. Prophylactic antibiotics should not be given to patients who present to the hospital following a rattlesnake envenomation as studies demonstrate a <3% rate of wound infection.

LoVecchio F, et al. Antibiotics after rattlesnake envenomation. *J Emerg Med*. 2002;23:327-328.

119.6. Answer: D. Crotalidae polyvalent immune Fab (Cro-fab) is an ovine-derived Fab fragment antivenom developed from commonly encountered North American pit vipers. The four snakes included in this antivenom are *Crotalus atrox* (western diamondback rattlesnake), *Crotalus adamanteus* (eastern diamondback), *Crotalus scutulatus* (Mojave rattle-snake), and *Agkistrodon piscivorus* (cottonmouth).

BTG. CroFab. https://crofab.com/about-crofab/Manufacturing. Accessed July 3, 2021.

119.7. Answer: E. Patients with a history concerning for a bite by either a Texas or eastern coral snake should be admitted for at least 24 hours in a setting capable of close airway monitoring and endotracheal intubation. There is no indication to administer crotaline antivenom in this patient as he was bitten by a coral snake. The package insert of the North American coral snake antivenom lists administration to asymptomatic patients as a contraindication. Pressure immobilization bandages (PIBs) delay the systemic absorption of snake venom; patients who present to health care with a PIB dressing in place should have the dressing left in place until resuscitative equipment and personnel are available.

Pfizer. North American Coral Snake Antivenin. 2016. http://labeling.pfizer.com/showlabeling.aspx?id=441. Accessed July 3, 2021.

119.8. Answer: B. While crotalidae polyvalent immune Fab (Crofab) is listed as pregnancy category C, it is used safely during pregnancy. As there is a potential for fetal demise after envenomation, there should be a low threshold for treatment with antivenom. Emergent delivery is only indicated for fetal distress as venom is unlikely to cross the placenta.

LaMonica GE, et al. Rattlesnake bites in pregnant women. *J Reprod Med*. 2010;55:520-522.

Langley RL. Snakebite during pregnancy: A literature review. *Wilderness Environ Med*. 2010;21:54-60.

119.9. Answer: B. The Mojave rattlesnake *C. scutulatus* possesses a neurotoxin, Mojave toxin, which is phospholipase A_2 (PLA_2). This toxin acts at the presynaptic terminal of the neuromuscular junction to inhibit acetylcholine release.

Glenn JL, et al. Geographical variation in *Crotalus scutulatus* (Mojave rattlesnake) venom properties. *Toxicon*. 1983;21:119-130.

Wooldridge BJ, et al. Mojave rattlesnakes (*Crotalus scutulatus*) lacking the acidic subunit DNA sequence lack Mojave toxin in their venom. *Comp Biochem Physiol B Biochem Mol Biol*. 2001;130:169-179.

119.10. Answer: D. As the diameter of fingers is small, there is limited ability of the skin to expand. This patient is presenting with evidence of ischemia. It is recommended in cases such as this to perform a digital dermotomy, in which a longitudinal incision is made through the skin at the medial or lateral aspect of the digit to decompress the neurovascular structures. In addition to performing a dermotomy, antivenom should also be administered. Prophylactic dermotomy should not be performed in cases of digital envenomation with no signs of ischemia. When compartment syndrome is suspected in other parts of the body that have larger diameters, such as an arm or leg, it is reasonable to start with antivenom alone and monitor compartment pressures closely.

Hall EL. Role of surgical intervention in the management of crotaline snake envenomation. *Ann Emerg Med*. 2001;37:175-180.

Cumpston KL. Is there a role for fasciotomy in Crotalinae envenomations in North America? *Clin Toxicol*. 2011;49:351-365.

Smoke Inhalation

120.1. What percentage of fire-related deaths are due to smoke inhalation?
A. <10%
B. 10-30%
C. 50-80%
D. 85-90%
E. >90%

120.2. Which of the following toxic gases is produced by combustion of plastics?
A. Sulfur dioxide
B. Styrene
C. Hydrogen fluoride
D. Cyanide
E. Phosphine

120.3. Which of the following toxic gases is produced by the combustion of polyvinyl chloride?
A. Phosgene
B. Arsine
C. Stibine
D. Phosphine
E. Cyanide

120.4. Which of the following physical properties of a toxin is most important in determining the location of lung injury?
A. pH
B. Particle size
C. Water solubility
D. Molecular weight
E. Fat solubility

120.5. Which of the following gases is a chemical asphyxiant found in fire or smoke?
A. Carbon monoxide
B. Phosgene
C. Carbon dioxide
D. Stibine
E. Nitric oxide

120.6. Which of the following statements best explains why acrolein causes toxicity at the alveoli and the terminal bronchioles?
A. It has low water solubility
B. It is carried to deep lung areas by soot particles
C. It has a low molecular weight that allows it to bypass the upper respiratory system
D. It has high lipid solubility and is readily absorbed by the cells of the lower respiratory system
E. It has a high molecular weight

120.7. Which of the following thermal degradation products will primarily cause pulmonary parenchymal injury?
A. Ammonia
B. Hydrogen chloride
C. Sulfur dioxide
D. Isocyanates
E. Oxides of nitrogen

120.8. A 40-year-old man is removed from a house fire. Which of the following biomarkers is the best indication to administer hydroxocobalamin?
A. A blood lactate of 10 mmol/L
B. A carbon monoxide of 45%
C. A methemoglobin of 30%
D. A blood cyanide of 40 micromol/L (1 mg/L)
E. Soot visualized in the airway with associated singed nasal hairs

120.9. Which of the following xenobiotics would be reasonable to use in the management of a patient who was a victim of a fire with suspected cyanide toxicity?

A. Amyl nitrite
B. Sodium nitrite
C. Sodium thiosulfate
D. Hyperbaric oxygen therapy
E. Sodium azide

120.10. Which of the following thermal degradation products is produced from the burning of melamine?
A. Styrene
B. Acrolein
C. Hydrogen sulfide
D. Ammonia
E. Sulfur dioxide

ANSWERS

120.1. Answer: C. Disastrous fires are frequent reminders of the role of inhalation injuries in fire deaths. From 1955 to 1972, a threefold increase in death from inhalational injury was reported and was attributed to abundant use of newer synthetic materials for building and furnishings. An estimated 50-80% of fire deaths are due to inhalation injuries rather than burns or trauma. Deaths from smoke inhalation occur more often in an enclosed-space environment.

Bowes PC. Casualties attributed to toxic gas and smoke at fires: A survey of statistics. *Med Sci Law.* 1976;16:104-110.

Harwood B, Hall JR. What kills in fires: Smoke inhalation or burns? *Fire J.* 1989;84:29-34.

120.2. Answer: D. Cyanide is produced from combustion of many nitrogen-containing products such as plastics, melamine resins, polyurethanes, wool, silk, nylon, nitrocellulose, polyacrylonitriles, synthetic rubber, and paper. High concentrations of cyanide are measured in air samples from fires, and elevated blood cyanide concentrations are reported in both fire survivors and fire fatalities. In addition to cyanide, combustion of plastics produces hydrogen chloride (HCl), aldehydes, ammonia, nitrogen oxides, phosgene, and chlorine.

Baud FJ, et al. Elevated blood cyanide concentrations in victims of smoke inhalation. *N Engl J Med.* 1991;325:1761-1766.

Stoll S, et al. Concentrations of cyanide in blood samples of corpses after smoke inhalation of varying origin. *Int J Legal Med.* 2017;131:123-129.

Grabowska T, et al. Prevalence of hydrogen cyanide and carboxyhaemoglobin in victims of smoke inhalation during enclosed-space fires: A combined toxicological risk. *Clin Toxicol (Phila).* 2012;50:759-763.

120.3. Answer: A. Polyvinyl chloride (PVC) is widely used in home and office furnishings, floor coverings, and electrical insulation. Therefore, high concentrations of its combustion products such as phosgene, carbon monoxide, hydrogen chloride, and chlorine are present in many fires. Phosgene toxicity leads to acute respiratory distress syndrome (ARDS).

Dyer RF, Esch VH. Polyvinyl chloride toxicity in fires: Hydrogen chloride toxicity in fire fighters. *JAMA.* 1976;235:393-397.

Markowitz JS, et al. Acute health effects among firefighters exposed to a polyvinyl chloride (PVC) fire. *Am J Epidemiol.* 1989;129:1023-1031.

120.4. Answer: C. Many irritant chemicals generated during combustion injure the upper airway, tracheobronchial tree, or pulmonary parenchyma. Water solubility is the most important chemical characteristic in determining the level of the respiratory tract injury. Highly water-soluble gases react with the upper airway mucosa to produce intense upper mucosal injury and inflammatory reaction. Unless toxic gas concentrations are extremely high or the duration of exposure is prolonged, injury is limited to the mucosa of the upper respiratory tract. Conversely, chemicals with low water solubility do not react with the upper airway mucosa and reach the lung parenchyma, where they react slowly to create a delayed toxic effect. In addition to water solubility, concentration of the substance inhaled, duration of exposure, particle size, respiratory rate, absence of protective reflexes, and preexisting disease influence the level of the respiratory tract injury.

Prien T. Toxic smoke compounds and inhalation injury: A review. *Burns.* 1988;14:451-460.

120.5. Answer: A. Carbon monoxide and cyanide are the two primary chemical asphyxiants that are formed in fires. Other chemical asphyxiants that are toxic thermal degradation products include hydrogen sulfide and oxides of nitrogen. Chemical asphyxiants impair aerobic respiration without any direct pulmonary toxicity.

Norris JC, et al. Synergistic lethality induced by the combination of carbon monoxide and cyanide. *Toxicology*. 1986;40:121-129.

120.6. Answer: B. Inhalation of soot particles and aerosols enhances the exposure to toxins in a fire environment. Soot adheres to the mucosa of the airways, allowing adsorbed irritant chemicals to react with the mucosal surface moisture. The deposition of these particles in the respiratory tract depends on their size, with those of 1-3 microm reaching the alveoli. Experimental animals have markedly decreased lung injury when exposed to smoke filtered to remove particulates. Also, irritant gases "piggyback" on aerosol droplets and alter the site of deposition of the gas.

Morgan WK. The respiratory effects of particles, vapours, and fumes. *Am Ind Hyg Assoc J*. 1986;47:670-673.

120.7. Answer: E. Oxides of nitrogen have a low water solubility and will therefore cause pulmonary parenchymal injury. Phosgene is another thermal degradation product that has a low water solubility. Ammonia, hydrogen chloride, and sulfur dioxide are highly water soluble and will affect the upper airway. Chlorine and isocyanates have intermediate water solubility and will injure both the upper and lower respiratory tracts.

Orzel RA. Toxicological aspects of firesmoke: Polymer pyrolysis and combustion. *Occup Med*. 1993;8:414-429.

120.8. Answer: A. A patient's hemodynamic status as well as their blood pH and lactate are the most useful tools in accurately assessing for cyanide toxicity. A blood lactate concentration of 10 mmol/L or greater in the setting of smoke inhalation suggests cyanide poisoning. While a blood cyanide concentration of 40 micromol/L (1 mg/L) is consistent with life-threatening cyanide toxicity, blood cyanide analysis is currently of limited value because the results are typically not available for hours to days.

Baud FJ, et al. Elevated blood cyanide concentrations in victims of smoke inhalation. *N Engl J Med*. 1991;325:1761-1766.

120.9. Answer: C. The gold standard for the management of patients who have suspected cyanide toxicity is hydroxocobalamin. However, not all hospitals have access to this antidote. The alternative cyanide antidote in the United States contains sodium nitrite and sodium thiosulfate. The amyl nitrite was removed because of its misuse potential. Sodium nitrite has a more detrimental side effect profile, including causing methemoglobinemia. In patients who already have carbon monoxide toxicity it should be avoided. Administering sodium thiosulfate alone is reasonable if that is the only option available. When sodium thiosulfate and hydroxocobalamin were compared, hydroxocobalamin was found to be a superior antidote.

Bebarta VS, et al. Hydroxocobalamin versus sodium thiosulfate for the treatment of acute cyanide toxicity in a swine (sus scrofa) model. *Ann Emerg Med*. 2012;59:532-539.

120.10. Answer: D. Melamine is a nitrogen-containing product that is used in adhesives and plastics. When it is burned, it produces both ammonia and cyanide. Ammonia, which is highly water soluble, causes injury to the upper airways by rapidly combining with mucosal water.

Prien T, Traber DL. Toxic smoke compounds and inhalation injury—a review. *Burns Incl Therm Inj*. 1988;14:451-460.

Orzel RA. Toxicologic aspects of firesmoke: Polymer pyrolysis and combustion. *Occup Med*. 1993;8:414-429.

Simple Asphyxiants and Pulmonary Irritants

QUESTIONS

121.1. Which of the following statements is correct about simple asphyxiant gases?
A. Simple asphyxiant gases never produce measurable laboratory abnormalities
B. Certain simple asphyxiant gases mediate physiologic changes in addition to causing hypoxia
C. Simple asphyxiant gases vary in their ability to produce hypoxia
D. Symptoms of simple asphyxia include shortness of breath and frothy, blood-tinged sputum
E. It is impossible to succumb to simple asphyxiant gases outdoors

121.2. Which of the following statements best describes phosgene toxicity?
A. Phosgene toxicity no longer occurs since its use as a war gas was banned by the Geneva Convention
B. Prolonged exposure is unlikely due to its foul odor
C. Dissolution in mucosal water is rapid, but the onset of toxicity is delayed
D. Once dissolved, the acidic products generate an influx of inflammatory cells
E. Pulmonary toxicity is completely averted with N-acetylcysteine (NAC)

121.3. Nebulized 2% sodium bicarbonate is recommended in patients exposed to which of the following pulmonary irritants?
A. Nitrogen dioxide
B. Chloroacetophenone
C. Chlorine
D. Ammonia
E. Ozone

121.4. Which of the following statements best describes metal fume fever?
A. Direct pulmonary toxicity occurs in conjunction with elevated serum metal concentrations
B. It is a recurrent influenzalike syndrome that develops shortly after exposure to metal oxide fumes
C. Exacerbation of symptoms during the workweek is typical
D. British anti-Lewisite (BAL) is the therapy of choice
E. Chest radiography usually reveals patchy pulmonary infiltrates

121.5. In the early 1930s, as many as 1,000 people died in the creation of Gauley Bridge Tunnel at Hawks Nest, West Virginia. Patients presented to health care with dyspnea, fever, fatigue, and weight loss. Which of the following was responsible for this disaster?
A. Asbestos
B. Sulfur dioxide
C. Nitrogen dioxide
D. Silica
E. Cadmium

121.6. A 22-year-old man presents to the hospital with shortness of breath. Earlier that morning, he was cleaning a toilet. While doing that, he mixed ammonia and bleach. Which of the following gases explains his symptoms?
A. Chloramine gas
B. Chlorine gas
C. Sulfur dioxide
D. Nitrogen dioxide
E. Phosgene gas

121.7. A scientist is found dead in an enclosed space. Further history revealed that he was in the process of transporting his specimens from one freezer to another and the door appeared to have locked behind him. What is the likely cause of his death?
A. Hydrogen cyanide
B. Carbon monoxide
C. Carbon dioxide
D. Methyl isocyanate
E. Zinc phosphide

121.8. In the 1952 London Fog disaster, approximately 4,000 people died, primarily due to respiratory causes. What toxin in the fog was the likely cause?
A. Carbon monoxide
B. Carbon dioxide
C. Sulfur dioxide
D. Phosgene
E. Chlorine

121.9. A member of the janitorial staff is found dead next to a sink in the hospital. The sink is in a room primarily used by orthopedic surgeons for the application of plaster casts. What toxicologic exposure could explanation his death?
A. Carbon monoxide
B. Hydrogen sulfide
C. Phosgene
D. Nitrogen dioxide
E. Carbon dioxide

121.10. A 34-year-old man presents to the emergency department with severe shortness of breath. He relates that approximately 5 hours prior to presentation he was working at his farm checking on the grain storage in his silo. What toxin likely contributed to his shortness of breath?
A. Nitrogen dioxide
B. Carbon dioxide
C. Carbon monoxide
D. Hydrogen sulfide
E. *Claviceps purpurea* fungus

ANSWERS

121.1. Answer: B. Simple asphyxiants produce their clinical toxicity by limiting the supply of available oxygen. Therefore, toxicity is directly related to the concentration of gas present and is independent of which gas it is. By definition, they produce hypoxia (and a low PO_2 and O_2 saturation). A few asphyxiant gases produce clinical toxicity even in the absence of hypoxia. For example, carbon dioxide produces a respiratory acidosis and nitrogen produces "nitrogen narcosis." Asphyxiant gases do not produce dyspnea or acute respiratory distress syndrome (ARDS) since gas exchange (PCO_2) is initially normal and there is no pulmonary irritation. The finding of blood-tinged sputum should suggest ARDS. Although uncommon, simple asphyxiation occurs outdoors, as in Lake Nyos in 1986.

Suruda A, Agnew J. Deaths from asphyxiation and poisoning at work in the United States, 1984-1986. *Br J Ind Med.* 1989;46:541-546.

121.2. Answer: D. Phosgene poisoning occurs as a result of fires and industrial use. It is suggested that sarin gas, chlorine, and possibly phosgene were used in some civil wars. Phosgene has a pleasant odor ("freshly cut hay"), which accounts in part for its success as a war gas. Its dissolution in lung water is slow, but once dissolved, it generates acid products that incite an inflammatory response. Treatments such as *N*-acetylcysteine are used to limit the inflammatory influx, most without dramatic success.

Ghio AJ, et al. Reduction of neutrophil influx diminishes lung injury and mortality following phosgene inhalation. *J Appl Physiol.* 1991; 71:657-665.

121.3. Answer: C. Nebulized sodium bicarbonate provides relief from pain and coughing in patients exposed to chlorine gas. This probably results from neutralization of the hydrochloric acid that forms when chlorine gas dissolves in the respiratory tract water. Although not studied, it is reasonable to treat patients exposed to hydrogen chloride, sulfur dioxide, or other acid-forming gases with dilute (2%) nebulized sodium bicarbonate.

Chisholm CD, et al. Inhaled sodium bicarbonate therapy for chlorine inhalational injuries. *Ann Emerg Med.* 1989;18;466.

121.4. Answer: B. A recurrent influenzalike illness (dyspnea, myalgia, and headache) associated with fever in patients exposed to metal fumes defines metal fume fever. The etiology is likely to be immunologic, and direct pulmonary toxicity does not occur. Patients have normal chest radiographs, and serum metal concentrations are not elevated. Acute tolerance develops so that repeat daily exposure produces milder symptoms, but after a short work hiatus, such as a weekend, the tolerance is lost. Galvanized steel, which contains zinc, is most frequently implicated. The management of patients with metal fume fever is supportive and includes analgesics and antipyretics. There is no specific antidote, and chelation is unnecessary.

Blanc P, et al. An experimental human model of metal fume fever. *Ann Intern Med*. 1991;114:930-936.

Blount BW. Two types of metal fume fever: Mild vs. serious. *Milit Med*. 1990;155:372-377.

121.5. Answer: D. Silicosis is caused by the inhalation of silica dust. Chronic silicosis takes as long as 45 years to develop, and patients present with exertional dyspnea. Acute silicosis, by contrast, develops in a few weeks and leads to dyspnea, fatigue, weight loss, and pleuritic chest pain. The prognosis is poor in acute silicosis and patients progress to rapid respiratory failure. It is believed that acute silicosis contributed to many of the deaths in the Hawks Nest disaster.

Leung CC, et al. Silicosis. *Lancet*. 2012;379:2008-2018.

121.6. Answer: A. When ammonia is added to hypochlorous acid (bleach), chloramine gas is formed ($NH_4^+ + HOCl \rightarrow H^+ + H_2O + NH_2Cl$). Chlorine gas is formed when bleach is combined with any strong acid, such as hydrochloric or sulfuric acid. Sulfur dioxide is formed when sulfurous acid is added to water. Silo filler's disease is caused by the formation of nitrogen dioxide due to silage decay. Combustion of certain plastics liberates phosgene gas.

Hattis RP, et al. Chlorine gas toxicity from mixture of bleach with other cleaning products—California. *MMWR*. 1991;40;619-629.

Manahan SE. *Toxicologic Chemistry*. 2nd ed. Boca Raton, FL: Lewis Publishers; 1992.

Ryrfeldt A, et al. Free radicals and lung disease. *Br Med Bull*. 1993;49:588-603.

121.7. Answer: C. Scientists frequently use dry ice to transport specimens. Dry ice is a solid form of carbon dioxide. It necessitates respectful care since it is potentially fatal if improperly handled or if a person is in an enclosed space with a large amount of dry ice. Not only does carbon dioxide act as a simple asphyxiant, it also acts on the respiratory center to increase the respiratory drive, causing a victim to die faster than would be expected if exposed to a simple asphyxiant.

Gill JR, et al. Environmental gas displacement: Three accidental deaths in the workplace. *Am J Forensic Med Pathol*. 2002;23:26-30.

Halpern P, et al. Exposure to extremely high concentrations of carbon dioxide: A clinical description of a mass casualty incident. *Ann Emerg Med*. 2004;43:196-199.

121.8 Answer: C. Smog, which is a portmanteau of smoke and fog, led to several disasters around the globe. The photochemical components of smog primarily include sulfur dioxide and oxides of nitrogen. Smog leads to exacerbations of underlying respiratory illnesses. Deaths attributed to bronchitis rose 10-fold during the London fog. Mortality from tuberculosis and lung cancer also increased. Deaths attributed to cardiac illness were three times as high as in prior years. A considerable number of animals also needed to be slaughtered as they also experienced respiratory distress.

Scott JA. Fog and deaths in London, December 1952. *Public Health Rep*. 1953;68:474-479.

121.9 Answer: B. Hydrogen sulfide has a rotten egg odor; however, at high concentrations, olfactory fatigue develops. Hydrogen sulfide toxicity occurs in hospital workers when acid cleaners are used to unclog drains that are clogged due to plaster of Paris sludge. While carbon monoxide leads to cardiac arrest, it would be unusual to just have a single person be ill and for the hospital carbon monoxide detectors to not alarm. Phosgene smells like freshly mown hay, and symptoms of toxicity are usually delayed. Nitrogen dioxide causes pulmonary toxicity, but symptoms are also delayed.

Peters JW. Hydrogen sulfide poisoning in a hospital setting. *JAMA*. 1981;246:1588-1589.

121.10 Answer: A. Silo-filler's disease occurs when oxides of nitrogen are generated during decomposition of silage during grain storage. If there is inadequate ventilation, then sudden depletion of oxygen and cardiac arrest occur. However, with incomplete ventilation, it leads to delayed-onset pulmonary toxicity. Nitrogen dioxide was responsible for many deaths in the Cleveland Clinic fire in 1929, which occurred from the burning of nitrocellulose radiographic films. Carbon dioxide would not lead to delayed shortness of breath. Delayed toxicity would also be unusual in carbon monoxide toxicity, except for xenobiotics that are metabolized to carbon monoxide, such as methylene chloride. Hydrogen sulfide is not classically the cause of toxicity in silo-related illnesses and is more often found in waste management and natural gas. *Claviceps purpurea* is a fungus that grows on rye and is associated with the development of ergot toxicity when ingested.

Douglas WW, et al. Silo-filler's disease. *Mayo Clin Proc.* 1989;64:291-304.

122

Carbon Monoxide

QUESTIONS

122.1. A 27-year-old man was brought to the emergency department after being found unresponsive at his work site. Prior to losing consciousness, he had an episode of vomiting and complained of blurred vision. He received 100% oxygen via a non-rebreather mask. Initial laboratory studies demonstrated a carboxyhemoglobin level (COHb) of 5.4%. Eight hours later, repeat laboratory studies are obtained and his COHb is 13.8%. What is the most likely explanation for this delayed rise in COHb?
A. Dichloromethane
B. Hydrogen sulfide
C. Hydrogen cyanide
D. Formaldehyde
E. Methyl isocyanate

122.2. A 16-year-old boy is brought into the hospital from an ice-skating rink after complaining of a headache. His initial COHb is 23%. He is placed on 100% oxygen via a non-rebreather mask. What is the approximate half-life of carbon monoxide (CO) on 100% oxygen?
A. 400-500 minutes
B. 250-300 minutes
C. 60-120 minutes
D. 20-30 minutes
E. 5-10 minutes

122.3. Which of the following options contributes to carbon monoxide (CO) toxicity?
A. CO binds weakly to hemoglobin
B. CO causes a rightward shift of the oxyhemoglobin dissociation curve

C. CO interferes with cellular respiration by binding to mitochondrial cytochrome oxidase
D. CO increases erythrocyte 2,3-bisphosphoglycerate (2,3-BPG)
E. CO increases offloading of oxygen from hemoglobin to tissues

122.4. Which of the following options is most predictive of developing delayed neuropsychiatric symptoms as a consequence of carbon monoxide (CO) exposure?
A. Loss of consciousness
B. Headache
C. Vomiting
D. Chest pain
E. Dysrhythmias

122.5. A 22-year-old, non-smoking woman presents to the emergency department from home with a chief complaint of a headache that has been persistent throughout the day. A carboxyhemoglobin (COHb) is 19%. The patient's neurologic examination is entirely within the normal limits. She has not had an episode of loss of consciousness. What is the most important next step in management?
A. Immediate transfer to a facility that has hyperbaric oxygen (HBO) capabilities
B. Contact the local fire department to inspect the home
C. Administration of 325 mg of aspirin
D. Order a brain magnetic resonance imaging (MRI)
E. Order an electrocardiogram (ECG)

122.6. A 7-day-old baby boy has a co-oximeter panel obtained as part of a sepsis evaluation. It results with a carboxyhemoglobin (COHb) of 8%. The patient is currently receiving oxygen via a ventilator and has been intubated for 48 hours. What is the most likely etiology for his elevated COHb?
A. Diarrhea leading to an elevated COHb
B. An inhaled anesthetic that is being degraded to carbon monoxide (CO)
C. A malfunctioning ventilator
D. Fetal hemoglobin being interpreted by the co-oximeter as COHb
E. Sulfhemoglobin being misinterpreted by the co-oximeter as CO as COHb

122.7. Which of the following organ systems is most sensitive to carbon monoxide toxicity?
A. Central nervous system
B. Pulmonary
C. Integumentary
D. Hepatobiliary
E. Kidney

122.8. In patients with severe carbon monoxide poisoning, which of the following areas of the brain is commonly abnormal on neuroimaging?

A. Substantia nigra
B. Pineal gland
C. Hypothalamus
D. Globus pallidus
E. Cerebellum

122.9. Which of the following options is associated with central neurologic injury in animal models of carbon monoxide (CO) poisoning?
A. Leukocyte adherence
B. Lysosomal degeneration
C. Hypertensive episode
D. Carboxyhemoglobin level at least 50%
E. Decrease in cerebral adenosine

122.10. A 42-year-old woman is found unresponsive in a car with the tail pipe obstructed and the motor running. Emergency medicine personnel provided her with oxygen therapy and 5 g of intravenous hydroxocobalamin. Upon arrival to the emergency department, her carboxyhemoglobin (COHb) level is 2.5%. Which of the following options is the best next step in management?
A. Repeat hydroxocobalamin
B. Sodium thiosulfate
C. Sodium nitrite
D. Methylene blue
E. Hyperbaric oxygen therapy

ANSWERS

122.1. Answer: A. Dichloromethane is another name for methylene chloride, a chemical that is used in the oil and gas industry. Like many other hydrocarbons, it leads to altered mental status that progresses to generalized anesthesia. This explains the patient's loss of consciousness that improved when he was no longer at the work site. Dichloromethane is metabolized by CYP2E1 to form carbon monoxide; because of this, a delayed rise in COHb occurs. In 2019, the US Environmental Protection Agency banned the use of methylene chloride in all paint strippers due to several fatalities.

Rioux JP, Myers RA. Hyperbaric oxygen for methylene chloride poisoning: Report on two cases. *Ann Emerg Med*. 1989;18:691-695.

Ahmed AE, et al. Halogenated methanes: Metabolism and toxicity. *Fed Proc*.1980;39:3150-3155.

Environmental Protection Agency. EPA bans consumer sales of methylene chloride paint removers, protecting public. https://www.epa.gov/newsreleases/epa-bans-consumer-sales-methylene-chloride-paint-removers-protecting-public. Accessed May 16, 2022.

122.2. Answer: C. The half-life of carbon monoxide (CO) while a patient is breathing room air is between 249 and 320 minutes. The half-life of CO is reduced to 74-131 minutes in patients breathing 100% oxygen. The CO half-life during hyperbaric oxygen therapy is 20-30 minutes. While the half-life is significantly decreased while receiving hyperbaric oxygen therapy, the actual reason to provide hyperbaric oxygen therapy is to protect against the delayed neurologic and psychiatric complications of CO poisoning.

Peterson JE, Stewart RD. Absorption and elimination of carbon monoxide by inactive young men. *Arch Environ Health*. 1970;21:165-171.

Weaver LK, et al. Carboxyhemoglobin half-life in carbon monoxide-poisoned patients treated with 100% oxygen at atmospheric pressure. *Chest*. 2000;117:801-808.

122.3. Answer: C. Carbon monoxide (CO) causes toxicity in a multifactorial manner. Not only does it bind more avidly to hemoglobin than oxygen, but it also causes a leftward shift of the oxyhemoglobin dissociation curve, further impairing oxygen delivery to tissue. There is also a decrease in erythrocyte 2,3-bisphosphoglycerate concentrations. While CO poisoning is often attributed to impaired oxygen delivery, this is insufficient to explain the toxicity. This is best illustrated by an animal model where five dogs inhaled CO and then five other dogs received transfused blood that contained CO bound to hemoglobin. While all the dogs that inhaled CO died, none of the dogs that were given transfused blood that contained CO bound to hemoglobin died. Both groups had similar COHb levels.

Roughton FJWD. The effect of carbon monoxide on the oxyhemoglobin dissociation curve. *Am J Physiol*. 1944;141:17-31.

Goldbaum LR, et al. Mechanism of the toxic action of carbon monoxide. *Ann Clin Lab Sci*. 1976;6:372-376.

122.4. Answer: A. Loss of consciousness in the acute phase of exposure to carbon monoxide is a risk factor for developing delayed neuropsychiatric symptoms. As COHb concentrations are used as a surrogate for toxicity, it is important to remember other factors when deciding what type of therapy to provide for a patient who has CO toxicity. Questions such as "soaking time" or duration of continuous exposure to CO as well as whether the patient had an episode of loss of consciousness during the exposure are very important prognostic signs. Loss of consciousness in the setting of CO exposure is an indication to perform hyperbaric oxygen therapy if it can be performed safely within 24 hours of exposure.

Weaver LK, et al. Carbon monoxide poisoning: Risk factors for cognitive sequelae and the role of hyperbaric oxygen. *Am J Respir Crit Care Med*. 2007;176:491-497.

122.5. Answer: B. While this patient's headache is likely caused by carbon monoxide (CO) toxicity, her neurologic examination shows no focal deficits and she did not have an episode of loss of consciousness; therefore, the appropriate next step in management would be oxygen via a 100% nonrebreather. However, the most important next steps are to ensure there are no other victims and that the patient is safe to return home. Contacting the local fire department or gas company to go to the patient's home will ensure that there are no other victims and will address the source of the toxicity. It is also important to have a working CO detector is installed in the home. While chronic CO exposure is associated with cardiac toxicity, the patient is not complaining of chest pain. Unless there is a concern for another etiology of this patient's headache, a brain MRI is not necessary to make this diagnosis.

Krenzelok EP, et al. Carbon monoxide . . . the silent killer with an audible solution. *Am J Emerg Med*. 1996;14:484-486.

122.6. Answer: D. Certain cooximeters give a falsely elevated COHb result when fetal hemoglobin is present. This is typically reported as between 6 and 8%. If an infant's COHb returns significantly higher than 10%, it is important to be certain that the baby does not have another etiology for the elevated COHb. Diarrhea is associated with an elevated methemoglobin in infants. While certain inhaled anesthetics are degraded to CO, this is much less likely in this patient as there is no anesthetic being administered.

Vreman HJ, et al. Interference of fetal hemoglobin with the spectrophotometric measurement of carboxyhemoglobin. *Clin Chem*. 1988;34:975-977.

122.7. Answer: A. The central nervous system is the most sensitive organ system to carbon monoxide toxicity. Headache, dizziness, and ataxia occur at concentrations as low as 15-20%. The cardiovascular system is also very sensitive to carbon monoxide toxicity. Troponin elevations develop even without any electrocardiographic changes. Takatsubo cardiomyopathy also occurs. Pulmonary toxicity is less common than central nervous system and cardiac toxicity. The other organ systems listed are not typically involved.

Weaver LK. Clinical practice. Carbon monoxide poisoning. *N Engl J Med*. 2009;360:1217-1225.

122.8. Answer: D: The globus pallidus and deep white matter are the most common areas showing low density on computed tomography (CT) scanning after consequential CO poisoning.

Choi IS, et al. Evaluation of outcome after acute carbon monoxide poisoning by CT. *J Korean Med Sci*. 1993;8:78-83.

Tom T, et al. Neuroimaging characteristics in carbon monoxide toxicity. *J Neuroimaging*. 1996;6:161-166.

122.9. Answer: A. Leukocyte adherence to brain microvasculature is an essential step that precedes lipid peroxidation of the brain in the rat models of serious CO toxicity. This is most pronounced in the hippocampus and corpus striatum. Animal models also have cell loss in the frontal lobe. These are areas of the brain that correspond to learning and memory.

Thom SR. Leukocytes in carbon monoxide-mediated brain oxidative injury. *Toxicol Appl Pharmacol*. 1993;123:234-247.

122.10. Answer: E. Hydroxocobalamin, a therapy for cyanide poisoning, negatively interferes with many laboratory values, including COHb. It is important to not be reassured by a low COHb level and to instead rely on the patient's history and physical examination. If possible, blood obtained prior to administration of hydroxocobalamin should be evaluated. This scenario is consistent with carbon monoxide toxicity, and the patient experienced an episode of loss of consciousness; therefore, hyperbaric therapy is indicated. This patient's prehospital COHb concentration was 34.9%.

Livshits Z, et al. Falsely low carboxyhemoglobin level after hydroxocobalamin therapy. *N Engl J Med.* 2012;367:1270-1271.

Cyanide and Hydrogen Sulfide

QUESTIONS

123.1. Ingestion of which of the following xenobiotics causes cyanide toxicity?
A. Methylene chloride
B. *Blighia sapida*
C. Acetone
D. Methyl isocyanate
E. Acetonitrile

123.2. A 27-year-old woman presents to the emergency department after an intentional overdose of "vitamin B_{17}." Which of the following laboratory abnormalities is most likely to occur?
A. Increased venous PO_2
B. Decreased venous lactate
C. Hypokalemia
D. Decreased venous PCO_2
E. Hyponatremia

123.3. Tapioca is a starch made from cassava (*Manihot esculenta*). Which of the following conditions occurs as a result of chronic ingestion of insufficiently processed cassava?
A. Pellagra
B. Scombroid
C. Botulism
D. Oral cancer
E. Konzo

123.4. A 22-year-old man is brought to the hospital after a house fire. He is hypotensive, tachycardic, and hypoxic with signs of smoke inhalation. In addition to supportive care, which of the following treatments is indicated immediately?

A. Hydroxocobalamin
B. Methylene blue
C. Dantrolene
D. Hyperbaric oxygen therapy
E. *N*-Acetylcysteine

123.5. Which of the following laboratory values is the most clinically relevant biomarker of cyanide toxicity?
A. Serum lactate
B. Whole blood cyanide
C. Serum thiocyanate
D. Serum potassium
E. Serum ammonia

123.6. Delayed neurologic sequelae from acute cyanide poisoning are most commonly due to lesions of which area(s) of the brain?
A. Vermis of the cerebellum
B. Basal ganglia
C. Reticular activating system
D. Temporal lobes of the cerebral cortex
E. Frontal lobes of the cerebral cortex

123.7. In patients with cyanide poisoning, which of the following mechanisms contributes to its toxicity?
A. Enhances *N*-methyl-D-aspartic acid (NMDA) receptor activity
B. Reversibly inhibits cytochrome c oxidase
C. Decreases glycine receptor activity
D. Uncouples oxidative phosphorylation
E. Blocks voltage-gated sodium channel blockade

123.8. Rescuers of victims of hydrogen sulfide poisoning often become victims themselves due to olfactory fatigue. At what atmospheric concentration does this typically occur?
   A. 1 part per million (ppm)
   B. 10 ppm
   C. 100 ppm
   D. 1,000 ppm
   E. 10,000 ppm

123.9. Which of the following exposures is a source of hydrogen sulfide?
   A. Decomposition of grain in silos (silo filler's disease)
   B. Combustion of silk
   C. Sewer gas
   D. Combining hypochlorite and ammonia
   E. Mercury refining

123.10. A school is evacuated due to a rotten egg smell. The fire department arrives but is unable to detect hydrogen sulfide using their "four-gas detection unit." Which of the following statements is most correct?
   A. Positive findings from the detector are reliable, whereas negative findings are not
   B. Negative findings from the detector are reliable, whereas positive findings are not
   C. Both positive and negative findings from the detector are reliable
   D. Air from the exposure site should be captured for confirmatory analysis
   E. Interpretation of detector results depends on clinical history, examination, and degree of suspicion

ANSWERS

123.1. Answer: E. Acetonitrile is a component of some artificial nail removers. It is metabolized by CYP2E1 to cyanide and causes severe toxicity, even after small unintentional ingestions. It is important to differentiate between nail remover and nail polish remover, the latter of which contains acetone and is a relatively benign ingestion. *Blighia sapida* is also known as ackee fruit; the unripe version contains hypoglycin A and leads to hypoglycemia. Although methyl isocyanate contains a cyanide moiety, metabolism does not release cyanide. Methyl isocyanate is primarily an ocular and pulmonary irritant that was responsible for the casualties in the Bhopal, India disaster. Methylene chloride is metabolized to carbon monoxide.

Caravati EM, Litovitz TL. Pediatric cyanide intoxication and death from an acetonitrile-containing cosmetic. *JAMA.* 1988;260:3470-3473.

123.2. Answer: A. Vitamin B_{17} is a misnomer, as it is not a vitamin. It is the name under which amygdalin, a cyanogenic glycoside, is sold. Cyanide is an irreversible cytochrome c oxidase inhibitor that prevents the transfer of high-energy electrons to O_2. Therefore, the PO_2 on the venous blood gas increases with progressive cyanide toxicity, provided respirations continue.

Klimmek R, et al. Cerebral blood flow, circulation, and blood homeostasis of dogs during slow cyanide poisoning and after treatment with 4-dimethylaminophenol. *Arch Toxicol.* 1982;50:65-76.

123.3. Answer: E. Konzo is a spastic paresis caused by the consumption of improperly processed *M. esculenta,* commonly known as cassava. Cassava contains linamarin, a cyanogenic glycoside. Epidemics of konzo occur in Africa and are typically driven by poverty and food shortages.

Tylleskär T, et al. Cassava cyanogens and konzo, an upper motoneuron disease found in Africa. *Lancet.* 1992;339:208-211.

123.4. Answer: A. Cyanide is a combustion product of polyurethane wool, synthetic rubber, and other materials. Cyanide toxicity should be suspected in patients who have hypotension, tachycardia, or an elevated lactate after being removed from a fire. Intravenous hydroxocobalamin should be administered in this patient and re-dosed if needed. While hyperbaric therapy might be necessary later as part of the management of carbon monoxide, treatment of the cyanide toxicity should be prioritized.

Borron SW, et al. Prospective study of hydroxocobalamin for acute cyanide poisoning in smoke inhalation. *Ann Emerg Med.* 2007;49:794-801.

123.5. Answer: A. Serum lactate is readily available in most clinical laboratories and is associated with life-threatening toxicity following ingested cyanide when elevated more than 8 mmol/L or life-threatening toxicity following inhaled cyanide when >10 mmol/L. In contrast, whole blood cyanide is not widely available or processed quickly enough to guide clinical care. Sodium thiocyanate is useful for confirming exposure but does not correlate well with symptoms.

Baud FJ, et al. Value of lactic acidosis in the assessment of the severity of acute cyanide poisoning. *Crit Care Med.* 2002;30:2044-2050.

123.6.   Answer: B. The basal ganglia, which is one of the most oxygen-sensitive areas of the brain, is the region of the brain that is most consistently injured following cyanide poisoning. Delayed sequelae include symptoms of parkinsonism.

Rosenberg NL, et al. Cyanide-induced parkinsonism: Clinical, MRI, and 6-fluorodopa PET studies. *Neurology.* 1989;39:142-144.

Uitti RJ, et al. Cyanide-induced parkinsonism: A clinicopathologic report. *Neurology.* 1985;35:921-925.

123.7.   Answer: A. In addition to inhibiting oxidative phosphorylation, cyanide directly activates the NMDA receptor, causing increased excitatory glutamatergic tone. This manifests as seizures acutely and contributes to delayed neurotoxicity.

Sun P, et al. Modulation of the NMDA receptor by cyanide: Enhancement of receptor-mediated responses. *J Pharmac Exp Ther.* 1997; 280:1341-1348.

123.8.   Answer: C. Olfactory fatigue occurs at 100-150 ppm. Coma occurs at >700 ppm. Thus, rescuers misperceive failure to smell rotten eggs as an indicator that it is safe to enter a contaminated area and potentially expose themselves further.

Beauchamp RO, et al. A critical review of the literature on hydrogen sulfide toxicity. *Crit Rev Toxicol.* 1984; 13:25-97.

Reiffenstein RJ, et al. Toxicology of hydrogen sulfide. *Annu Rev Pharmacol Toxicol.* 1992;32:109-134.

123.9.   Answer: C. Hydrogen sulfide is a by-product of industrial processes (paper mills, leather tanning, vulcanization of rubber, natural gas refining) and a natural product of bacterial decomposition of protein-containing substances (fish, sewage, manure) and of volcanoes, sulfur springs, and underground deposits of natural gas.

Centers for Disease Control and Prevention. Fatalities attributed to entering manure waste pits: Minnesota, 1992. *MMWR.* 1993;42:325-329.

Rorison DG, McPherson SJ. Acute toxic inhalations. *Emerg Med Clin North Am.* 1992;10:409-435.

123.10.   Answer: E. Many fire departments carry "four-gas detection units" to the site of potential hydrogen sulfide exposures. Four-gas detection units measure hydrogen sulfide by electrochemical sensors along with measurements of atmospheric oxygen concentration and the presence of explosive gases and carbon monoxide. False-negative readings occur when the gas has already dissipated, whereas false-positive readings occur in the presence of other chemicals (eg, mercaptans). Either can occur due to improper calibration or a malfunctioning device.

Ursulan S. Confined space entry and compliance. *Occup Health Saf.* 2009;78:32, 34-35.

Methemoglobin Inducers

124.1. Which of the following arterial blood gases is most consistent with methemoglobinemia?
A. pH 7.32/PCO_2 36/PO_2 250/SaO_2 99%
B. pH 6.89/PCO_2 98/PO_2 150/SaO_2 98%
C. pH 7.22/PCO_2 36/PO_2 400/SaO_2 86%
D. pH 7.39/PCO_2 66/PO_2 58/SaO_2 94%
E. pH 7.40/PCO_2 40/PO_2 100/SaO_2 98%

124.2. Which of the following statements best explains the mechanism by which oxidant stress leads to methemoglobinemia?
A. It causes the globin portion of hemoglobin to change its configuration
B. It causes the porphyrin ring to destabilize
C. It causes the iron in the center of the porphyrin ring to lose an electron
D. It causes the denaturation of protein in the red cell membrane with subsequent hemolysis
E. It causes an individual with glucose-6-phosphate dehydrogenase (G6PD) deficiency to undergo hemolysis

124.3. Which of the following options is expected to occur at a methemoglobin level of 15% in an otherwise healthy patient?
A. Shortness of breath
B. Cyanosis
C. Dizziness and fatigue
D. Coma or asystole
E. Headache and confusion

124.4. A 22-year-old man presents to the emergency department following an episode of loss of consciousness. On physical examination, he is cyanotic; however, he is awake and is speaking comfortably. His pulse oximeter has a reading of 86%, which does not improve with oxygen. Which amount of hemoglobin must exist in the Fe^{3+} state for a detectable cyanosis to be present?
A. 0.5 g/dL
B. 1.5 g/dL
C. 3 g/dL
D. 5 g/dL
E. 10 g/dL

124.5. A 36-year-old man presents to the emergency department with cyanosis after ingesting isobutyl nitrite. His methemoglobin level is 35%. As methylene blue is being administered, the patient's pulse oximeter reading drops to 64%. Which of the following courses of action is the most appropriate next step in the management of this patient?
A. Rapid sequence intubation
B. Administer intramuscular epinephrine
C. Administer inhaled albuterol
D. Administer a repeat dose of methylene blue
E. Observation alone

124.6. Which of the following best explains a pulse oximeter reading that is approximately 85% in patients who have methemoglobinemia?
   A. There is a disproportionate amount of hemoglobin in the deoxy state
   B. Patients develop pulmonary emboli because of a hypercoagulable state
   C. Methemoglobin binds 200 times more avidly to hemoglobin as compared to oxygen
   D. Methemoglobin causes the blood to have a bright red discoloration
   E. Methemoglobin has equal absorbance at both 660- and 940-nm wavelengths

124.7. A 42-year-old man presents to the emergency department with shortness of breath, chest pain, and fatigue. He is notably cyanotic with a pulse oximeter reading of 87%. His methemoglobin level is 32%. He has a past medical history of leprosy for which he is receiving treatment. His electrocardiogram is normal. Which of the following therapies should be added as part of this patient's treatment regimen?
   A. Hyperbaric oxygen therapy
   B. Exchange transfusion
   C. Cimetidine
   D. Hydroxocobalamin
   E. Sodium thiosulfate

124.8. A 15-day-old girl presents to the emergency department with vomiting and diarrhea. She is ill appearing; on examination, she has poor capillary refill and sunken fontanelles. A blood gas reveals that she has a methemoglobin level of 14%. Which of the following is the most appropriate next step in this patient's management?
   A. Methylene blue
   B. Vitamin C
   C. Cimetidine
   D. Fluid bolus
   E. Hydroxocobalamin

124.9. Which of the following options best explains why sulfhemoglobinemia is better tolerated than methemoglobinemia?
   A. There is a decreased affinity for oxygen in the unaltered hemoglobin
   B. Sulfhemoglobin is an extremely unstable compound
   C. Oxygen-carrying capacity is not reduced by sulfhemoglobinemia
   D. Sulfhemoglobin is usually treated with hyperbaric oxygen therapy
   E. Sulfhemoglobin produces less cyanosis than methemoglobinemia

124.10. Which of the following options is an adverse effect associated with high-dose methylene blue?
   A. Polycythemia
   B. Methemoglobinemia
   C. Purple-colored urine
   D. Flaccid paralysis
   E. Hypotension

ANSWERS

124.1. Answer: A. Patients with methemoglobinemia usually have a normal arterial PO_2 as methemoglobin does not interfere with the pulmonary function to deliver dissolved oxygen to the blood. In fact, often patients with methemoglobinemia have a very elevated arterial PO_2 as they are placed on oxygen therapy for a low pulse oximeter reading. The SaO_2 reported on a blood gas is a calculated oxygen saturation, utilizing the partial pressure of oxygen in the blood. Patients with methemoglobinemia have a saturation gap, wherein the oxygen saturation on the blood gas is normal while the oxygen saturation on pulse oximeter reading is depressed.

Singh S, et al. Dapsone-induced methemoglobinemia: "Saturation gap"-the key to diagnosis. *J Anaesthesiol Clin Pharmacol.* 2014;30:86-88.

124.2. Answer: C. A relatively small portion of the hemoglobin molecule is affected when methemoglobin is formed. The loss of an electron from the outer shell of iron in the center of the porphyrin ring profoundly alters oxygen affinity. Oxidant stress on the proteins in the red cell membrane causes hemolysis, but this is unrelated to methemoglobinemia.

Mansouri A, Lurie AA. Concise review: Methemoglobinemia. *Am J Hematol.* 1993;42:7-12.

124.3. Answer: B. Patients generally tolerate methemoglobin levels of 15% quite well, only exhibiting mild cyanosis. However, pre-existing disease such as anemia, pneumonia, or cardiovascular disease makes this level of methemoglobin of greater clinical significance.

Jaffe ER. It is bad to be blue. *N Engl J Med.* 1969;281:957-958.

124.4. Answer: B. Small amounts (1.5 g/dL) of oxidized hemoglobin (methemoglobin) produce a detectable cyanosis. It takes 5 g/dL of reduced hemoglobin (deoxygenated hemoglobin) to produce the same cyanosis. Sulfhemoglobin produces detectable cyanosis when just 0.5 g/dL is present.

Jafee ER. Methemoglobinemia in the differential diagnosis of cyanosis. *Hosp Pract.* 1985;20:92-110.

124.5. Answer: E. Methylene blue is a dye and will transiently alter pulse oximeter readings. Often during administration of methylene blue, the pulse oximeter reading will drop precipitously. If the medical team at the bedside is not prepared for this expected effect, it is very startling and leads to unnecessary treatments. It is important to evaluate the clinical status of the patient and not rely on a pulse oximeter reading in patients who either have methemoglobinemia or are being treated with methylene blue.

Kessler MR, et al. Spurious pulse oximeter desaturation with methylene blue injection. *Anesthesiology.* 1986;65:435-436.

124.6. Answer: E. Most pulse oximeters rely on two different wavelengths to determine the oxygen saturation. Dual wavelength pulse oximeters read absorbance of light at wavelengths of 660 and 940 nm, which efficiently separate oxyhemoglobin and deoxyhemoglobin. Methemoglobin absorption at these wavelengths is greater than that of either oxyhemoglobin or deoxyhemoglobin, leading to inaccurate oxygen saturation readings. Though 85% is often quoted as the value with which a typical patient with methemoglobinemia will present, this number varies depending on which instrument is used.

Barker SJ, et al. Measurement of carboxyhemoglobin and methemoglobin by pulse oximetry: A human volunteer study. *Anesthesiology.* 2006;105:892-897.

124.7. Answer: C. Dapsone is used in the treatment of leprosy. Dapsone is metabolized by CYP2C9 and CYP3A4 to a hydroxylamine metabolite, which leads to prolonged methemoglobinemia. Methemoglobinemia occurs both in therapeutic dosing as well as in overdose. Cimetidine is a competitive inhibitor of CYP450 and will reduce methemoglobin in therapeutic dosing by blocking metabolite formation. Caution is needed when cimetidine is added to a therapeutic regimen as it has many other medication interactions.

Kim YJ, et al. Difference of the clinical course and outcome between dapsone-induced methemoglobinemia and other toxic-agent-induced methemoglobinemia. *Clin Toxicol.* 2016;54:581-584.

Rhodes LE, et al. Cimetidine improves the therapeutic/toxic ratio of dapsone in patients on chronic dapsone therapy. *Br J Dermatol.* 1995;132:257-262.

124.8. Answer: D. This baby is ill appearing and is likely septic. NADH methemoglobin reductase activity is low in the first 4 months of life; therefore, infants are more susceptible to the development of methemoglobinemia caused by stressful events, such as sepsis. The most important management strategy in this patient is to ensure appropriate treatment of the underlying condition. As the patient's sepsis improves, her methemoglobin level will also resolve. Antidotal therapy is only indicated if the child does not improve after volume resuscitation and the methemoglobin persists.

Pollack ES, Pollack CV. Incidence of subclinical methemoglobinemia in infants with diarrhea. *Ann Emerg Med.* 1994;24:652-656.

Sager S, et al. Methemoglobinemia associated with acidosis of probable renal origin. *J Pediatr.* 1995;126:59-61.

Yano SS, et al. Transient methemoglobinemia with acidosis in infants. *J Pediatr.* 1982;100:415-418.

124.9. Answer: A. While the oxygen-carrying capacity of hemoglobin is reduced by sulfhemoglobinemia, unlike in methemoglobinemia, there is also a decreased affinity for oxygen in the remaining unaltered hemoglobin. This pushes the oxyhemoglobin dissociation curve to the right, makes oxygen more available to tissues, and reduces the clinical effect of sulfhemoglobin as compared to methemoglobin. Sulfhemoglobin is an extremely stable compound and is only eliminated when red blood cells are removed naturally from circulation. Sulfhemoglobin is treated by removing the offending xenobiotic that led to its formation. Sulfhemoglobin is a darker pigment than methemoglobin and produces cyanosis when only 0.5 g/dL of blood is affected.

Lu HC, et al. Pseudomethemoglobinemia: A case report and review of sulfhemoglobinemia. *Arch Pediatr Adolesc Med.* 1998;152:803-805.

Noor M, Beutler E. Acquired sulfhemoglobinemia an underreported diagnosis? *West J Med.* 1998;169:386-389.

124.10. Answer: B. Methylene blue causes paradoxical induction of methemoglobinemia when administered at high doses. This is likely due to an equilibrium between the direct oxidization of hemoglobin to methemoglobin by methylene blue and its ability to reduce methemoglobin to hemoglobin.

Methylene blue does not produce methemoglobinemia at standard treatment doses of 1-2 mg/kg. Methylene blue also causes hemolysis in high doses, causes green-colored urine, and is associated with an increased risk of developing serotonin toxicity. Rather than producing hypotension, methylene blue is used to treat hypotension, particularly in patients who have distributive shock.

Whitwam JG, et al. Potential hazard of methylene blue. *Anesthesiology*. 1979;34:181-182.

Bodansky O. Methemoglobinemia and methemoglobin-producing compounds. *Pharmacol Rev*. 1951;3:144-196.

Nanotoxicology

125.1. Which of the following statements is correct regarding the generation of nanoparticles?
A. Evaporation of ocean spray yields nanoparticles
B. Joint replacements resist the creation of endogenous nanoparticle wear debris
C. Naturally occurring nanoparticles occur during sublimation
D. The Ayurvedic medicine preparation, "swarna bhasma" (gold ash), is free of nanoparticles
E. Welding produces nanosized particles

125.2. Which of the following statements is a correct nanoparticle description?
A. Dendrimers are branched polymers with a central core, internal branching, and surface terminal groups
B. Fullerenes are silicon-based cages
C. Graphene contains multiple layers of single-carbon atoms
D. Micelles are homogenously hydrophilic globular vesicles
E. Quantum dots are semiconductor nanocrystals that exhibit a size-invariant fluorescence

125.3. Which of the following statements regarding nanoparticles and the central nervous system is correct?
A. Nanoparticles instilled in the olfactory bulb access the central nervous system
B. The blood–brain barrier excludes nanoparticles from the central nervous system
C. Polymer nanoparticles, quantum dots (QDs), carbon nanotubes, and cerium nanoparticles

decrease the rate of beta$_2$-microglobulin amyloid fibrillation
D. The intraperitoneal administration of nanoparticles prevents central nervous system injury
E. The toxicity of exposure to air pollution particles is confined to the pulmonary system

125.4. Which of the following statements regarding the cellular organelle toxicity of nanoparticles is correct?
A. Autophagosome induction by nanoparticles leads to apoptosis
B. Mammalian proteins resist nanoparticle degradation and unfolding
C. Nanoparticles induce dissipation of the mitochondrial membrane potential
D. The bilayer structure of lipid membranes prevents through-and-through hole formation and nanoparticle cutting
E. Tight junctions protect the cell nucleus from nanoparticle access

125.5. Which of the following statements regarding the photothermal effects of nanoparticles is correct?
A. Nanoparticle coatings are impervious to photolysis
B. Titanium dioxide (TiO_2) nanoparticles were removed from sunscreens
C. Type I photosensitized oxidation reactions involve generation of singlet oxygen ($^1O_2$)
D. Type II photosensitized oxidation reactions involve generation of free radicals
E. Visible light activates nanoparticles

125.6. Which of the following factors increases pulmonary toxicity from nanoparticle toxicity?
   A. Coating materials
   B. "Doping" (intentionally introduced impurities)
   C. High aspect ratios
   D. Lower surface area
   E. Neutral surface charge (zeta potential)

125.7. Inhalation of carbon nanotubes is associated with which of the following findings?
   A. Airway opening
   B. Alveolar wall thinning
   C. Asbestoslike effects
   D. Decreased inflammatory and oxidative stress biomarkers
   E. Granulomata regression

125.8. Which of the following nanotechnology regulatory guidelines is correct?
   A. The Environmental Protection Agency (EPA) regulates nanomaterials in food
   B. The Food and Drug Administration (FDA) requires manufacturers to disclose the use of nanotoxicology in medicines
   C. The National Institute for Occupational Safety and Health (NIOSH) considers carbon nanotubes to be a respiratory hazard

   D. The National Institute of Standards and Technology (NIST) is the lead federal agency for human nanomaterials environmental research
   E. US nanotechnology policy is guided by the 20th Century Nanotechnology Research and Development Act

125.9. Which of the following statements correctly describes nanoparticle reproductive effects?
   A. Bioaccumulation of nanoparticles up the food chain is not demonstrated
   B. Nanoparticles pass to daughter cells upon mammalian cell division
   C. The blood–testis barrier effectively excludes nanoparticles from the male reproductive tract
   D. The motility of human sperm cells permits evasion from damage from gold nanoparticles
   E. The placenta effectively excludes nanoparticles from the fetus

125.10. Cardiovascular toxicity of nanoparticles is mediated by which of the following options?
   A. Accelerated vascular thrombosis
   B. Arteriolar dilation
   C. Erythrocyte homeostasis
   D. Increased heart rate variability
   E. Platelet dispersion

ANSWERS

125.1. Answer: E. Combustion, cooking, discharge of munitions, or welding incidentally generate nanosized particles. "Natural" nanoparticles are generated from volcanic explosions, fires, ocean spray, sandstorms, soil, sediment weathering, and biomineralization processes. Evaporation is a phase transition from liquid to a gas or vapor. Sublimation is a phase transition from solid to gas. Joint and spinal implants produce nanosized particulate wear debris. "Swarna bhasma" contains nanosized colloidal gold.

Deguchi S, et al. Non-engineered nanoparticles of c60. *Sci Rep.* 2013;3:2094.

125.2. Answer: A. Dendrimers are branched polymers with a central core, variable internal branching, and surface terminal groups. Dendrons are wedge-shaped portions of dendrimers that contain an accessible reactive group. Graphene is a single layer of carbon atoms in a hexagonal lattice. Fullerenes are an allotrope (physical form) of carbon, resembling a cage or cylinder, which encloses additional atoms, ions, or molecular clusters. Quantum dots are semiconductor nanocrystals capable of size-dependent fluorescence (eg, red through violet) and a "tunable"

emission spectrum. Micelles are globular vesicles with both hydrophobic and hydrophilic zones composed of phospholipids, sphingolipids, and ceramides or other esters or polymers.

Agashe HB, et al. Investigations on biodistribution of technetium-99m-labeled carbohydrate-coated poly(propylene imine) dendrimers. *Nanomedicine.* 2007;3:120-127.

125.3. Answer: A. Nanoparticles access the central nervous system through retrograde neuronal transport from the olfactory bulb. Circulating nanoparticles also cross the blood–brain barrier after intravenous or intraperitoneal administration. Nanoparticles contribute to secondary excitatory neurotoxicity. Children and dogs exposed to air pollution show prefrontal white matter hyperintense brain lesions, and cardiac effects are also described. Polymer nanoparticles, quantum dots, carbon nanotubes, and cerium nanoparticles all greatly enhance the rate of beta$_2$-microglobulin amyloid fibrillation by decreasing the lag time for nucleation.

Tjalve H, Henriksson J. Uptake of metals in the brain via olfactory pathways. *Neurotoxicology.* 1999;20:181-195.

125.4. Answer: C. The mitochondrial toxicity from nanoparticles includes mitochondrial apoptosis, alterations in mitochondrial calcium concentrations, dissipation of the mitochondrial membrane potential, lipid membrane destruction, localization within the mitochondria, and mitochondrial DNA damage. The process of autophagy is characterized by autophagosome formation, followed by lysosome fusion, and autophagosome degradation by lysosomes. Nanoparticles lead to disruption and compromise integrity of biological membranes by causing holes in lipid bilayers, and graphene nanosheets cut cell membranes. Quantum dots localize rapidly and preferentially in the nucleus of human macrophages. Multiple nanoparticle types alter protein functions and induce unfolding and precipitation.

Lovric J, et al. Unmodified cadmium telluride quantum dots induce reactive oxygen species formation leading to multiple organelle damage and cell death. *Chem Biol.* 2005;12:1227-1234.

125.5. Answer: E. Visible light activates nanoparticles. This is used medicinally as the basis of efficacy of action of liposomal verteporfin, which is activated by light at 689 nm. Photolytic conditions degrade nanoparticle coatings and expose toxic cores. Type I photosensitized oxidation reactions involve generation of free radicals. Type II photosensitized oxidation reactions involve generation of singlet oxygen ($^1O_2$). Titanium dioxide (TiO_2) nanoparticles are common is sunscreens and cosmetics.

Wielgus A, et al. Phototoxicity and cytotoxicity of fullerol in human retinal pigment epithelial cells. *Toxicol Appl Pharmacol.* 2010;242:79.

125.6. Answer: C. A high aspect ratio is thought to contribute to nanoparticle pulmonary toxicity, including penetration of the alveolar wall and visceral pleura. Nanoparticles have an increased surface area compared to bulk materials. Coating materials shield toxicity of core compounds or alternatively possess inherent toxicity. Contaminants introduce or mitigate toxicity. Doping improves biocompatibility. Both positive and negative charged particles and increased charge density are associated with toxicity.

Donaldson K, Poland CA. Nanotoxicity: Challenging the myth of nano-specific toxicity. *Curr Opin Biotechnol.* 2013;24:724-734.

125.7. Answer: C. Carbon nanotubes produce a variety of adverse effects in animal models, including upper airway mechanical blockage, occlusive airway granulomata, macrophage uptake and intermacrophage carbon bridges, abnormal macrophage mitoses, type I pulmonary epithelial cell damage, lymphocytic proliferation, multifocal granulomatas, aggregation in alveolar spaces and interstitium, increased inflammatory and oxidative stress biomarkers,

fibrinogenic reactions, alveolar wall thickening, bronchiolar epithelial cell hypertrophy, peribronchial inflammation, and asbestoslike, length-dependent effects.

Lynch RM, et al. Assessing the pulmonary toxicity of single-walled carbon nanohorns. *Nanotoxicology.* 2007;1:157.

125.8. Answer: C. NIOSH considers carbon nanotubes and nanofibers to be potential respiratory toxins. The FDA does not regulate "nanotechnology" per se and has no regulatory definitions of "nanotechnology" or related terms. The FDA is not always aware when nanotechnology is used, particularly if no nano-related medicinal claims are made. The EPA coordinates human nanomaterials environmental research. The 21st Century Nanotechnology Research and Development Act guides US nanotechnology policy.

President's Council of Advisors on Science and Technology. *Report to the President and Congress on the Fourth Assessment of the National Nanotechnology Initiative.* Washington, DC: Executive Office of the President; 2012.

125.9. Answer: B. Nanoparticles breach the blood–testis barrier and locate in the testes. Gold nanoparticles penetrate human sperm cells, causing fragmentation and dysmotility. Other nanoparticles, particularly multiwalled carbon nanotubes (MWCNTs), single-walled carbon nanotubes (SWCNTs), and TiO_2 nanoparticles, cross the placenta. TiO_2 nanoparticles bioaccumulate up the food chain (by a factor of >100% in certain species).

Mattheakis LC, et al. Optical coding of mammalian cells using semiconductor quantum dots. *Anal Biochem.* 2004;327:200-208.

125.10. Answer: A. Engineered and combustion-derived carbon nanoparticles (MWCNTs, SWCNTs, and mixed carbon nanoparticles) stimulate human platelet aggregation, activate glycoprotein IIb/IIIa, and accelerate the rate of vascular thrombosis. Multiple metal nanoparticles (iron, copper, gold, cadmium sulfide) induce dose-dependent platelet aggregation through the P2Y12 ADP receptor. Heart rate variability provides a measure of cardiac autonomic control; a decrease predicts death in patients with prior myocardial infarction. Nanoparticle aerosols display systemic impaired endothelium-dependent arteriolar dilation, direct vasoconstriction, and decreases in nitric oxide bioavailability by increasing local reactive oxidative and nitrosative species. Multiple nanoparticle types adversely affect erythrocyte morphology, causing deformation and hemolysis.

Radomski A, et al. Nanoparticle-induced platelet aggregation and vascular thrombosis. *Br J Pharmacol.* 2005;146:882-893.

QUESTIONS

126.1. Adequate skin decontamination of nerve agents and sulfur mustard is safely accomplished with which of the following substances?
A. Copper chloride
B. Hydrochloric acid
C. Selenious acid
D. Sodium hydroxide
E. Water

126.2. Appropriate treatment for a chemical warfare agent that produces muscle fasciculations following dermal exposure includes which of the following antidotes?
A. Atropine
B. Dimercaprol
C. Hydroxocobalamin
D. Naloxone
E. Sodium bicarbonate

126.3. Sulfur mustard cross-links purine bases via which of the following mechanisms?
A. Acetylation
B. Alkylation
C. Glucuronidation
D. Methylation
E. Sulfonation

126.4. Dimercaprol was developed as a specific antidote for which of the following xenobiotics?
A. Bis-(2-chloroethyl) sulfide
B. Chloroacetophenone
C. 2-Chlorovinyldichloroarsine
D. Dichloroformoxime
E. Diphenylaminechlorarsine

126.5. Delayed acute respiratory distress syndrome (ARDS) occurs following exposure to which of the following chemical warfare agents?
A. Carfentanil
B. Chlorine
C. Isopropyl-methylphosphonofluoridate
D. Lysergic acid diethylamide
E. 3-Quinuclidinyl benzilate

126.6. Lung injury caused by phosgene is mediated in part by which of the following acids?
A. Carbonic acid
B. Hydrochloric acid
C. Nitric acid
D. Phosphoric acid
E. Sulfuric acid

126.7. Exposure to *o*-chlorobenzilidene malononitrile results in which of the following symptoms?
A. Defecation
B. Fasciculation
C. Lacrimation
D. Putrification
E. Urination

126.8. Which of the following xenobiotics is added as a warning agent during sulfuryl fluoride fumigation?
A. Ammonia
B. Chloropicrin
C. Hydrogen sulfide
D. Methane
E. Sulfur dioxide

126.9. Poisoning with 3-quinuclidinyl benzilate would be expected to induce which of the following eye findings?
A. Corneal ulceration
B. Lacrimation
C. Melioidosis
D. Miosis
E. Mydriasis

126.10. Exposure to which of the following chemical warfare agents produces symptoms most rapidly?
A. Chlorine
B. Lewisite
C. Phosgene
D. Phosgene oxime
E. Sulfur mustard

ANSWERS

126.1. Answer: E. Copious and rapid washing is more important than the choice of decontamination solution. A 1:10 solution of household bleach (sodium hypochlorite) in water that produces a 0.5% hypochlorite solution is reported as a method to decontaminate sulfur mustard. However, sodium hypochlorite takes 15-20 minutes to inactivate chemical compounds; therefore, rapid washing with water is still superior. The other chemicals listed are either ineffective or corrosive.

> Macintyre AG, et al. Weapons of mass destruction events with contaminated casualties: Effective planning for health care facilities. *JAMA.* 2000;283:242-249.

126.2. Answer: A. The presence of fasciculations suggests nerve agent poisoning. Atropine and oximes are nerve agent antidotes. Dimercaprol is a specific antidote for Lewisite. Hydroxocobalamin is a specific antidote for cyanide. Naloxone would be an antidote for fentanyl derivatives. Inhaled (nebulized) sodium bicarbonate is used to treat chlorine gas inhalation.

> Holstege CP, et al. Chemical warfare nerve agent poisoning. *Crit Care Clin.* 1997;13:923-942.

126.3. Answer: B. Sulfur mustard and vesicants cross-link purine bases via alkylation. This causes damage to DNA strands. Nitrogen mustards derive their antineoplastic properties by the same mechanism.

> Dacre JC, Goldman M. Toxicology and pharmacology of the chemical warfare agent sulfur mustard. *Pharmacol Rev.* 1996;48:289-326.

126.4. Answer: C. 2-Chlorovinyldichloroarsine is the chemical name for Lewisite. Britain developed British anti-Lewisite (BAL, dimercaprol) as a specific antidote. Bis-(2-chloroethyl) sulfide is the chemical name for sulfur mustard. Chloroacetophenone (CN) is a riot control agent. Dichloroformoxime is the chemical name for phosgene oxime. It does not have a specific antidote. Diphenylaminechlorarsine is the chemical name for Adamsite, an emetic.

> Sidell FR, et al. Vesicants. In: Sidell FR, et al, eds. *Medical Aspects of Chemical and Biological Warfare.* Washington, DC: Office of the Surgeon General; 1997:197-228.

126.5. Answer: B. The "pulmonary irritants"—chlorine, phosgene, and diphosgene—all cause delayed ARDS. Carfentanil produces immediate central nervous system (CNS) and respiratory depression. Isopropyl-methylphosphonofluoridate (sarin) causes muscarinic, nicotinic, and immediate CNS effects. Lysergic acid diethylamide (LSD) produces CNS effects. 3-Quinuclidinyl benzilate (BZ) produces antimuscarinic effects.

> Urbanetti JS. Toxic inhalational injury. In: Sidell FR, et al, eds. *Medical Aspects of Chemical and Biological Warfare.* Washington, DC: Office of the Surgeon General; 1997:247-270.

126.6. Answer: B. Phosgene forms hydrochloric acid and an amide upon reaction with amine groups. Because phosgene is nonirritating and poorly water soluble, this reaction occurs deep in the alveoli.

> Russell D, et al. Clinical management of casualties exposed to lung damaging agents: A critical review. *Emerg Med J.* 2006;23:421-424.

126.7. Answer: C. *o*-Chlorobenzilidene malononitrile (CS tear gas), along with 1-chloroacetophenone (CN), dibenzo[*b,f*][1,4] oxazepine (CR), and *trans*-8-methyl-*N*-vanillyl-6-noneamide (OC, capsaicin pepper spray), are riot control agents, also known as "lacrimators" for their prominent symptom.

> Sidell FR. Riot control agents. In: Sidell FR, et al, eds. *Medical Aspects of Chemical and Biological Warfare.* Washington, DC: Office of the Surgeon General; 1997:307-324.

126.8. Answer: B. Chloropicrin, a lacrimator, is used as a warning agent for structures undergoing fumigation to prevent unintended human exposure. Ammonia is a pulmonary irritant, but it is not used as a warning agent. Hydrogen sulfide is a mitochondrial cytochrome oxidase inhibitor.

Methane gas is flammable and odorless. Sulfur dioxide is an air pollutant.

TeSlaa G, et al. Chloropicrin toxicity involving animal and human exposure. *Vet Hum Toxicol*. 1986;28:323-324.

126.9. Answer: E. 3-Quinuclidinyl benzilate (BZ, QNB) is an antimuscarinic agent that produces mydriasis. Melioidosis is an infectious disease caused by the biological warfare agent *Burkholderia pseudomallei*. Nerve agents usually cause miosis. Chloropicrin is an example of a lacrimator.

Ketchum JS, Sidell FR. Incapacitating agents. In: Sidell FR, et al, eds. *Medical Aspects of Chemical and Biological Warfare*. Washington, DC: Office of the Surgeon General; 1997:287-305.

126.10. Answer: D. Although grouped with "vesicants," phosgene oxime produces dermal symptoms immediately (erythema and hives). This occurs more rapidly than with exposure to Lewisite or sulfur mustard. The acute respiratory distress syndrome (ARDS) that develops following chlorine or phosgene exposures occurs in a delayed manner.

Sidell FR, et al. Vesicants. In: Sidell FR, et al, eds. *Medical Aspects of Chemical and Biological Warfare*. Washington, DC: Office of the Surgeon General; 1997:197-228.

Biological Weapons

QUESTIONS

127.1. Raxibacumab, used as a therapy for anthrax, targets which of the following sites?
A. Adenylate cyclase
B. Edema factor
C. Lethal factor
D. Protective antigen
E. Tumor necrosis factor alpha

127.2. Which of the following statements regarding pneumonic plague is correct?
A. It has the lowest mortality rate compared to other forms of plague
B. It is reliably prevented by vaccination
C. It is transmissible among humans
D. It manifests 7-10 days after exposure
E. It results in enlarged regional lymph nodes

127.3. Mediastinal lymphadenopathy is consistent with inhalational exposure to which of the following?
A. *Clostridium botulinum* toxin
B. *Francisella tularensis*
C. Trichothecene mycotoxin
D. Ricin
E. Staphylococcal enterotoxin B

127.4. Which of the following options is the most potent [lowest LD_{50} (mg/kg)]?
A. Ciguatoxin
B. *Clostridium botulinum* toxin
C. O-Ethyl-S-(2-diisopropylaminoethyl)-methylphosphonothiolate (VX)
D. Ricin
E. Tetrodotoxin

127.5. Smallpox is prevented by postexposure inoculation within 2-3 days with which of the following vaccines?
A. Vaccinia
B. Varicella
C. Variola
D. Virgaviridae
E. Viridans

127.6. Which of the following options is a complication of the smallpox vaccination?
A. Gastritis
B. Hepatitis
C. Myopericarditis
D. Phlebitis
E. Urethritis

127.7. Which of the following statements regarding staphylococcal enterotoxin B is correct?
A. It binds to neutrophils
B. It is cultured from *Staphylococcus epidermidis*
C. It mimics food poisoning upon ingestion
D. It produces dermal necrosis
E. It suppresses immune function

127.8. Poisoning by which of the following biologics produces a syndrome clinically similar to acute radiation poisoning?
A. Botulinum toxin
B. Brucellosis
C. Staphylococcal enterotoxin B
D. Trichothecene mycotoxin
E. Tularemia

127.9. Which of the following statements regarding ricin toxicity is correct?
   A. It depends on cell binding and entry facilitated by the A chain
   B. It is mediated by ribosome inactivation
   C. It is preventable through vaccination
   D. It is treated with doxycycline
   E. Toxicity occurs rapidly (seconds to minutes)

127.10. Which of the following statements regarding Q (query) fever is correct?
   A. It produces illness within hours
   B. It naturally infects sheep
   C. It requires multiple organisms to produce clinical illness
   D. It responds poorly to tetracyclines
   E. It results from an undetermined etiology

ANSWERS

127.1. Answer: D. Raxibacumab is a human monoclonal antibody that prevents protective antigen from binding to the host cell. It is approved for the treatment of inhalational anthrax. Edema factor complexes with protective antigen to form edema toxin, which functions as a calmodulin-dependent adenylate cyclase. Lethal factor complexes with protective antigen to form lethal toxin, which stimulates macrophages to release tumor necrosis factor alpha and interleukin-1 beta.

> Kummerfeldt CE. Raxibacumab: Potential role in the treatment of inhalational anthrax. *Infect Drug Resist.* 2014;7:101-109.

127.2. Answer: C. Pneumonic plague, unlike anthrax, is capable of human-to-human transmission. It is a pulmonary infection that is caused by *Yersinia pestis*. It has the highest mortality rate among the bubonic, septicemic, and pneumonic forms of plague, with an incubation period of 2-3 days. Vaccination has no demonstrable efficacy against pneumonic plague. Bubonic plague results in enlarged regional lymph nodes.

> Franz DR, et al. Clinical recognition and management of patients exposed to biological warfare agents. *JAMA.* 1997;278:399-411.

127.3. Answer: B. *Francisella tularensis* is the causative agent of tularemia. Typhoidal (pneumonic) tularemia is the most serious form and causes infiltrates, mediastinal lymphadenopathy, and pleural effusions. The other choices do not usually produce adenopathy. Inhalational anthrax also causes a mediastinitis; diagnostic imaging demonstrates a widened mediastinum from enlarged hilar lymph nodes as well as pleural effusions.

> Dennis DT, et al. Tularemia as a biological weapon: Medical and public health management. *JAMA.* 2001;285:2763-2773.

127.4. Answer: B. *Clostridium botulinum* toxin is the most potent of the listed xenobiotics. It is one of the high-risk biological warfare agents as it is easily disseminated and could cause high mortality.

> Centers for Disease Control and Prevention. Biological and chemical terrorism: Strategic plan for preparedness and response. *MMWR Morbid Mortal Wkly Rep.* 2000;49(RR04):1-14.

127.5. Answer: A. The vaccinia virus (derived from cowpox) protects against smallpox. Varicella causes chicken pox and zoster. Variola is the name for the virus that causes smallpox. Viridans are streptococci that cause infections, including pneumonia and sepsis. Virgaviridae are non-enveloped, positive-strand RNA viruses that infect plants.

> Wittek R. Vaccinia immune globulin: Current policies, preparedness, and product safety and efficacy. *Int J Infect Dis.* 2006;10:193-201.

127.6. Answer: C. Complications of smallpox vaccination include generalized vaccinia, progressive vaccinia, erythema multiforme, encephalitis, myopericarditis, and eczema vaccinatum.

> Wittek R. Vaccinia immune globulin: Current policies, preparedness, and product safety and efficacy. *Int J Infect Dis.* 2006;10:193-201.

127.7. Answer: C. Staphylococcal enterotoxin B (SEB) produced from *Staphylococcus aureus* mimics food poisoning upon ingestion. As a "superantigen," SEB stimulates helper T cells and immune function to induce cytokine release.

> Ulrich RG, et al. Staphylococcal enterotoxin B and related pyrogenic toxins. In: Sidell FR, et al, eds. *Medical Aspects of Chemical and Biological Warfare.* Washington, DC: Office of the Surgeon General; 1997:621-630.

127.8. Answer: D. Trichothecene mycotoxin produces a syndrome known as alimentary toxic aleukia, which is clinically similar to acute radiation poisoning, with gastrointestinal findings, bone marrow suppression, and dermal effects. Botulinum toxin produces flaccid paralysis. Tularemia infection results in ulceroglandular and typhoidal presentations. Staphylococcal enterotoxin B produces acute gastroenteritis as well as fibrous interstitial pneumonia. Brucellosis produces a nonspecific febrile illness resembling influenza.

> Bennett JW, Klich M. Mycotoxins. *Clin Microbiol Rev.* 2003;16:497-516.

127.9. Answer: B. Ricin depurinates a specific adenine of the 28S ribosomal RNA. Ricin consists of two protein chains; the B chain facilitates cell binding and entry of the A chain into cells. The A chain is responsible for the inhibition of protein synthesis. There is no effective vaccine. Treatment is supportive. Depending upon the route, symptoms occur over hours to days.

Audi J, et al. Ricin poisoning: A comprehensive review. *JAMA*. 2005; 294:2342-2351.

127.10. Answer: B. Q fever is caused by the rickettsia bacteria *Coxiella burnetii*, an intracellular bacterium. Natural reservoirs are sheep, cattle, and goats. A single inhaled organism may produce clinical illness. Patchy pulmonary infiltrates occur in approximately half of cases. Therapy is with either tetracycline or doxycycline. The incubation time for Q fever is 10-40 days.

Franz DR, et al. Clinical recognition and management of patients exposed to biological warfare agents. *JAMA*. 1997;278:399-411.

QUESTIONS

128.1. Survivors of the atomic bomb blast in Nagasaki had an increased incidence of developing which of the following conditions?
A. Thyroid disease
B. Pancreatic carcinoma
C. Lung carcinoma
D. Osteogenic sarcoma
E. No significant increase in disease

128.2. A 47-year-old man presents to the emergency department following an incident at a nuclear power plant. Which of the following findings confers the worst prognosis?
A. Lymphocyte count 2×10^9/L
B. A temperature of 100.4 °F (38 °C)
C. More than 10 episodes of diarrhea per day
D. A blood pressure of 90/60 mmHg
E. Patchy, dry skin with associated desquamation

128.3. Residential radon exposures are associated with which of the following malignancies?
A. Bone cancer
B. Breast cancer
C. Lung cancer
D. Hematologic cancer
E. Intestinal cancer

128.4. Radium incorporation among women employed as watch-dial painters before 1930 resulted in a higher mortality from which of the following cancers?
A. Lung cancer
B. Bone cancer
C. Hematologic cancer
D. Breast cancer
E. Colon cancer

128.5. Elimination of incorporated radioactive cesium-137 is enhanced by which of the following antidotes?
A. Prussian blue
B. Succimer (DMSA)
C. British anti-Lewisite (BAL)
D. Calcium disodium edetate
E. 4,5-Dihydroxy-1,3-benzenedisulfonic acid (Tiron)

128.6. A 62-year-old man presents to the emergency department with neck pain, On physical examination, his submandibular glands are enlarged bilaterally. Which of the following medications was the patient exposed to?
A. Diethylenetriamine pentaacetate (DTPA)
B. Potassium iodide
C. Prussian blue
D. Calcium disodium edetate
E. Dimercaptosuccinic acid (succimer)

128.7. A single, whole-body irradiation at which of the following doses is likely to be immediately fatal?
A. 10 rad
B. 100 rad
C. 500 rad
D. 10 Gy
E. 100 Gy

128.8. Which of the following options is the most useful chelator following acute uranium poisoning?
A. Prussian blue
B. Dimercaptosuccinic acid (succimer)
C. British anti-Lewisite (BAL)
D. Calcium disodium edetate
E. 4,5-Dihydroxy-1,3-benzenedisulfonic acid (Tiron)

128.9. A 43-year-old man presents to the hospital with nausea and vomiting. He is treated with antiemetics and hydration and is discharged home. Three days later, he returns to the emergency department with continued vomiting and abdominal pain. On examination, he is lying on the bed with a blanket covering the lower half of his body. Over the course of the next 22 days, he develops alopecia, weight loss, hypotension, kidney failure, and leukopenia. Which of the following xenobiotics was he poisoned with?

A. Ricin
B. Novichok
C. Thallium
D. Polonium
E. *Gelsemium*

128.10. When compared to control populations, children born to survivors of atomic bombings at Hiroshima and Nagasaki who ***were not*** exposed in utero had an increased risk of developing which of the following diseases?
A. Leukemia
B. Thyroid disease
C. Developmental delay
D. Microcephaly
E. No discernible increase in disease

ANSWERS

128.1. Answer: A. A dose–response relationship was established between radiation exposure in Nagasaki and thyroid disease. Survivors had a high incidence of thyroid cancer, adenomatous goiter, adenoma, solid nodules, and nodules without histologic diagnosis. The concave shape to the dose–response curve suggests an unclear relationship with relatively low-dose radiation.

Nagataki S, et al. Thyroid diseases among atomic bomb survivors in Nagasaki. *JAMA*. 1994;272:364-370.

128.2. Answer: C. More than 10 episodes of diarrhea assigns an organ system dysfunction of 4 on a scale of 1-4, yielding a response category (RC) of 4, which is the worst prognostic category. Answer choice A is degree 1; answer choice B is degree 2; answer choice C is degree 3; and answer choice E is degree 2. The RC grade suggests which level of care the person requires.

Dainiak N, et al. Literature review and global consensus on management of acute radiation syndrome affecting nonhematopoietic organ systems. *Disaster Med Public Health Prep*. 2011;5:183-201.

128.3. Answer: C. Radon is the only gaseous radioactive uranium daughter. People with exposure to radioactive uranium-238 (through mining or residential exposure) inhale radioactive radon-222, which results from decay of the uranium. The radon then irradiates their lungs, resulting in an increased risk of pulmonary carcinoma.

Pershagen G, et al. Residential radon exposure and lung cancer in Sweden. *N Engl J Med*. 1994;330:159-164.

128.4. Answer: B. A relative mortality ratio from bone cancer of >80 occurred in this cohort of women. Smaller increases in other malignancies also occurred. External exposure to radium is generally considered benign because alpha emissions do not penetrate skin. When ingestion occurred, as these workers licked their paint brushes, radium was selectively incorporated into bone, where years of exposure resulted in an increased incidence of malignant transformation.

Polednak AP, et al. Mortality among women first employed before 1930 in the US radium dialpainting industry. *Am J Epidemiol*. 1978;107:179-194.

128.5. Answer: A. Approximately 250 people were exposed to radioactive cesium in 1987 in Goiania, Brazil, following inappropriate disposal of a medical cesium source that was scavenged and dispersed. In vitro studies show good binding between cesium and Prussian blue. In vivo studies in survivors demonstrated that Prussian blue reduces the half-life of cesium by 32%.

Dresow B, et al. In vivo binding of radiocesium by two forms of Prussian blue and by ammonium iron hexacyanoferrate(II). *J Toxicol Clin Toxicol*. 1993;31:563-569.

Lipsztein JL, et al. Studies of Cs retention in the human body related to body parameters and Prussian blue administration. *Health Physics*. 1991;60:57-61.

128.6. Answer: B. Sialadenitis, also known as iodide mumps, is inflammation of the salivary glands that occurs rarely following exposure to iodine-containing medication, such as potassium iodide. Interestingly, this also occurs after exposure to contrast media that contains iodide. The exact mechanism is currently unknown. Treatment is usually supportive care, and symptoms typically resolve entirely.

Carter JE. Iodide "mumps". *N Engl J Med*. 1961;264:987-988.

Drori A, Yosha-Orpaz L. Case 277: Iodide mumps. *Radiology*. 2020;295: 490-494.

128.7. Answer: E. Total body radiation doses of >1,000 rad (10 Gy) are usually fatal, but with a delay of 1-2 weeks. Patients die of gastrointestinal fluid loss, bleeding, and subsequent infection. Doses >10,000 rad (100 Gy) are immediately fatal, and result from cerebral edema.

Fry RJM, Fry SA. Health effects of ionizing radiation. *Med Clin North Am*. 1990;74:475-488.

128.8. Answer: E. In an animal model, Tiron, or gallic acid, substantially increased uranium elimination. The time to onset of therapy is critical; there is no increased elimination when delays exceed 4 hours. In other models, diethylenetriamine pentaacetic acid (DTPA) is an effective chelator. Traditional chelators such as BAL, succimer, calcium disodium edetate, and Prussian blue have no utility in uranium toxicity.

Domingo JL, et al. Effectiveness of chelation therapy with time after acute uranium intoxication. *Fund Appl Toxicol*. 1990;14:88-95.

128.9. Answer: D. This case scenario is based on the poisoning of Alexander Litvinenko, a former Soviet KGB operative who was poisoned with polonium. Initially, physicians thought that he was poisoned with thallium. However, photos that were circulated at the time of his illness showed a man who was laying on the stretcher, comfortably tolerating a blanket covering the lower half of his body. This made thallium a less likely culprit as patients have a very painful neuropathy and are described as not being able to tolerate even a sheet over them.

McFee RB, Leikin JB. Death by polonium-210: Lessons learned from the murder of former Soviet spy Alexander Litvinenko. *Semin Diagn Pathol*. 2009;26:61-67.

128.10. Answer: E. Children exposed in utero to radiation from atomic bombs have a higher incidence of developmental delay and microcephaly. However, first-generation offspring of bomb survivors who were not exposed in utero have no increased incidence of cancer or these other disorders.

Yoshimoto Y. Cancer risk among children of atomic bomb survivors: A review of RERF epidemiologic studies. *JAMA*. 1990;264:596-600.

Poison Prevention and Education

129.1. Which of the following options pertains directly to the United States (US) program for "Healthy People 2020" health goals for the nation?
A. Defining standards of poison control centers
B. Developing community-based public education programs
C. Distributing home safety equipment
D. Reducing fatal and nonfatal poisonings
E. Decreasing the number of pesticide ingestions

129.2. Which of the following options was the first poison prevention legislation event?
A. National Poison Prevention Week
B. The Poison Prevention Packaging Act
C. The Toxic Household Products Act
D. The Poison Control Center Enhancement and Awareness Act
E. The World Health Organization International Programme on Chemical Safety Poison Prevention and Management

129.3. Which of the following options is most important in preventing poisoning in children under 5 years of age?
A. Never leaving the child alone for >5 minutes
B. Keeping products in their original containers
C. Keeping plants out of reach
D. Using child-resistant containers for all products
E. Posting the poison control center number on all telephones

129.4. Which of the following statements about health literacy is most appropriate?
A. The font, size, and color are most important
B. The graphics and layout are most important
C. Tenth-grade reading level is the target level
D. Health literacy encompasses the ability to read, count, and understand
E. Warnings on medications are the most valuable

129.5. Which of the following options is correct regarding planning for multicultural population poison education programs in the United States?
A. Language is more important than culture
B. Most immigrant populations use the poison control centers
C. Most poison control centers are too expensive
D. Qualitative research is more valuable than quantitative research in identifying cultural issues in immigrant communities
E. Herbal preparations are rarely used by second-generation immigrant families

129.6. Which of the following choices is the most common taste-averse xenobiotic added to household products?
A. Denatonium benzoate
B. Sodium bicarbonate
C. Sodium chloride
D. Isopropyl alcohol
E. Methyl mercaptan

129.7. Which of the following phone numbers is the toll-free phone number for all US poison control centers?

A. 212-764-7667
B. 212-222-1222
C. 800-222-1222
D. 800-777-7777
E. 800-764-7667

129.8. Which of the following is an important poison prevention tip?

A. Keep food and nonfood items together
B. Remove products from their original containers
C. A carbon monoxide detector in the kitchen is sufficient
D. Ensure lots of plants are present in the home
E. Program the poison control center number in to all cell phones

129.9. Which of the following statements best describes the role of promotoras?

A. Community health workers who work in hard-to-reach communities
B. Pharmaceutical representatives sent to hospitals
C. Poison center specialists who manage initial phone consultations
D. Practitioners of alternative medicine
E. Toxicologists who have specialty training in herbal supplements

129.10. Which of the following statements best describes what is meant by self-efficacy?

A. A psychological pattern in which individuals doubt their skills, talents, or accomplishments
B. A motivation to achieve something based on one's own enthusiasm
C. The individual's belief that they will be able to accomplish the task requested
D. When an individual takes either active or passive steps to prevent themselves from reaching their goals
E. A person who earns an income by contracting with a business directly

ANSWERS

129.1. Answer: D. "Healthy People 2020" is a US federal program that outlines the health goals for the nation. Two objectives in the Injury and Violence Prevention (IVP) section relate to poison prevention. IVP-9 is to reduce poisoning deaths, and IVP-10 is to reduce nonfatal poisoning.

Healthy People 2020. http://www.healthypeople.gov/2020/default.aspx. Accessed May 16, 2022.

129.2. Answer: A. In 1961, President Kennedy signed Public Law 87-319 designating the third week of March as Poison Prevention Week. The Poison Prevention Packaging Act was passed in 1970. In 1995, the Toxic Household Products Act in Oregon mandated that aversive agents be added to methanol and ethylene glycol. In 2000, the Poison Control Center Enhancement and Awareness Act legislated nationwide access and the toll-free number (800-222-1222). The WHO Programme for Poison Safety was established 2012.

Swartz MK. Poison prevention. *J Pediatr Health Care.* 1993;7:143-144.

129.3. Answer: D. Ongoing parent education regarding child-resistant containers (an engineering approach) is the most effective of the poison prevention approaches listed. All the choices are useful but only have limited realistic benefit for the inquisitive child.

Gibbs L, et al. Understanding parental motivators and barriers to uptake of child poison safety strategies: A qualitative study. *Inj Prev.* 2005;11:373-377.

129.4. Answer: D. Health literacy is defined as the degree to which individuals have the capacity to obtain, process, and understand basic health information and services needed to make appropriate health decisions. Health numeracy is a distinct component of health literacy. Font, size, color, graphics, layout, and warnings are important but do not achieve the desired goals. Sixth-grade literacy is a goal for all labels.

Nelson W, et al. Clinical implications of numeracy: Theory and practice. *Ann Behav Med.* 2008;35:261-274.

US Department of Health and Human Services. *National Action Plan to Improve Health Literacy.* Washington, DC Office of Disease Prevention and Health Promotion; 2010.

129.5. Answer: D. Language and culture must be addressed when planning community-based programs. Poison centers must increase community penetrance to reach out to their non–English-speaking community members.

Albertson TE, et al. Regional variations in the use and awareness of the California Poison Control System. *J Toxicol Clin Toxicol.* 2004;42:625-633.

Vassilev ZP, et al. Assessment of barriers to utilization of poison control centers by Hispanic/Latino populations. *J Toxicol Environ Health A.* 2006;69:1711-1718.

129.6. Answer: A. Denatonium benzoate, commonly known as Bitrex, is one of the most bitter-tasting xenobiotics known. The bitter taste is detected at concentrations as low as 50 parts per billion. Taste aversion therapy is only partially effective in minimizing toxic ingestions and should not be substituted for other poison prevention modalities.

Rodgers GC Jr, Tenenbein M. The role of aversive bittering agents in the prevention of pediatric poisonings. *Pediatrics.* 1994;93:68-69.

Klein-Schwartz W. Denatonium benzoate: review of efficacy and safety. *Vet Hum Toxicol.* 1991;33:545-547.

Berning CK, Griffith JF, Wild JE. Research on the effectiveness of denatonium benzoate as a deterrent to liquid detergent ingestion by children. *Fundam Appl Toxicol.* 1982;2:44-48.

129.7. Answer: C. In 2001, the toll-free phone number 800-222-1222 was established for all US poison control centers. Callers are connected to poison control centers based on area code and telephone number exchange. This single universal number standardized awareness programs across communities.

Woolf AD, et al. Preserving the United States's poison control system. *Clin Toxicol (Phila).* 2011;49:284-286.

129.8. Answer: E. Important poison prevention tips include: programming the poison control center number in to all cell phones; identifying poisons both inside and outside the home; keeping poisons out of reach of children in a locked cabinet; keeping products in their original containers; never keeping food and nonfood items together; installing carbon monoxide detectors throughout the home; keeping plants out of reach of children and pets; and using child-resistant containers.

Liller KD, et al. Evaluation of a poison prevention lesson for kindergarten and third grade students. *Inj Prev.* 1998;4:218-221.

129.9. Answer: A. Promotoras are native Spanish-speaking community health workers who are involved in health promotion, especially in hard-to-reach communities in the United States. They are trained to advocate, promote health, and be culturally aware of the communities they serve.

Crosslin KL, et al. Acculturation in Hispanics and childhood poisoning: are medicines and household cleaners stored properly? *Accid Anal Prev.* 2011;43:1010-1014.

129.10. Answer: C. Self-efficacy is the individual's belief that he or she will be able to accomplish the task requested. Both the health belief model and the social cognitive theory incorporate self-efficacy and are used when designing poison prevention interventions and mass media campaigns.

Randolph W, Viswanath K. Lessons learned from public health mass media campaigns: marketing health in a crowded media world. *Annu Rev Public Health.* 2004;25:419-437.

QUESTIONS

130.1. Which of the following statements is most representative of the American Association of Poison Control Centers (AAPCC) National Poison Data System (NPDS)?
A. NPDS data correlate well with fatal poisoning cases from medical examiners
B. NPDS data correlate well with hospital discharge data for poisoning admission
C. NPDS data correlate well with substance abuse data from the Drug Abuse Warning Network (DAWN)
D. NPDS data correlate well with occupational exposures reported to legislative authorities
E. None of the above

130.2. Appropriate use of the telephone services provided by poison centers is demonstrated to do which of the following?
A. Reduce mortality from childhood poisoning
B. Reduce mortality from intentional adult exposures
C. Prevent unnecessary utilization of health care services
D. Prevent recurrent poisoning in the home
E. Reduce morbidity following a known toxic exposure

130.3. Which of the following statements is true of poisoning epidemiology?
A. Poisoning is the most frequent cause of injury-related fatalities in the United States
B. Poisoning is the third most frequent cause of injury-related fatalities in the United States

C. Poisoning is the fifth most frequent cause of injury-related fatalities in the United States
D. Poisoning is the 10th most frequent cause of injury-related fatalities in the United States
E. Poisoning fatality is so uncommon that it is not listed in the top 10 causes of either all fatalities or injury-related fatalities in the United States

130.4. For a xenobiotic to be classified as "nontoxic," which of the following factors is required?
A. The exposure must be intentional
B. The exposed individual must have mild symptoms
C. The route of exposure must be unknown
D. Multiple products must be involved
E. The product must be identified

130.5. As of 2020, the national average cost of a US poison center responding to a single phone call is closest to which amount?
A. $3.50
B. $35.00
C. $350.00
D. $10.00
E. $100.00

130.6. What is the most important principle in poison prevention?
A. Identify the pathology
B. Restore health
C. Identify the risk
D. Promote individual service
E. Identify clinical intervention

130.7. Which of the following options best describes the "*Pollyanna phenomenon*"?
  A. Overreporting of new events and underreporting of common events
  B. Confounding an exposure with an ingestion
  C. Assuming that children who were managed at home had good outcomes
  D. A bias resulting from incomplete inclusion of medical examiner deaths
  E. Newer poison center staff are more likely to refer patients to hospitals

130.8. Which of the following options represents a common strategy advocated to help prevent poisoning?
  A. All xenobiotics should be transferred out of their original containers
  B. Unused portions of prescription medication should be saved for future use
  C. Xenobiotics should be stored in a cabinet under the sink
  D. Adults should not take their medication in front of children
  E. It is acceptable for xenobiotics to be stored in a car glove compartment

130.9. Which of the following options is a reasonable goal to improve poisoning epidemiology?
  A. Rely on a single method of reporting
  B. Encourage optional reporting of exposures
  C. Remove unconfirmed exposures from the database
  D. Allow rapid access to translational services
  E. Separate American Association of Poison Control Centers (AAPCC) database from other databases

130.10. Which of the following US federal- or state-funded agencies is *least* successful in preventing occupational illnesses and collecting data on occupational exposures?
  A. National Institute for Occupational Safety and Health (NIOSH)
  B. Occupational Safety and Health Administration (OSHA)
  C. The Agency for Toxic Substances and Disease Registry (ATSDR)
  D. Local state occupational reporting systems
  E. Poison control centers (PCCs)

ANSWERS

130.1. Answer: E. Multiple comparisons of National Poison Data System (NPDS) data with other existing databases clearly demonstrate that these systems fail to agree and that, under most circumstances, NPDS underreports cases of significant exposure.

Blanc PD, Olson KR. Occupationally related illness reported to a regional poison control center. *Am J Public Health.* 1986;76:1303-1307.

Chafee-Bahamon C, et al. Patterns in hospitals' use of a regional poison information center. *Am J Public Health.* 1983;73:396-400.

Linakis JG, Frederick KA. Poisoning deaths not reported to the regional poison control center. *Ann Emerg Med.* 1993;22:42-48.

130.2. Answer: C. Although it would be nice to think that utilization of poison services reduces morbidity and mortality following exposure, and this might be the case, the data only support that because many exposures are unlikely to result in toxicity. Timely use of poison centers prevents unnecessary use of ambulances and emergency departments by assuring parents that their children are unlikely to become ill and by providing appropriate follow-up.

Chafee-Bahamon C, Lovejoy FH. Effectiveness of a regional poison center in reducing excess emergency room visits for children's poisonings. *Pediatrics.* 1983;72:164-169.

130.3. Answer: A. Poisoning ranks first as a cause of injury-related fatalities in the United States, surpassing death related to motor vehicle collisions.

Bernard SJ, et al. Fatal injuries among children by race and ethnicity— United States, 1999-2002. *MMWR Surveill Summ.* 2007;56:1-16.

130.4. Answer: E. In order for a xenobiotic to be classified as nontoxic, the exposure must be unintentional. The exposed individual must be free of symptoms. Only a single product must be involved. The route of exposure should be defined because some xenobiotics are toxic by one route but not another. In addition to the factors listed in the answer, the ingested quantity should be known and the exposed individuals must be available for follow-up. Unless all of these factors are met, the exposure should not be immediately labeled nontoxic.

Mofenson HC, et al. Ingestions considered nontoxic. *Emerg Med Clin North Am.* 1984;2:159-174.

130.5. Answer: B. The average cost is approximately $35 for a US poison center to answer a single call. When compared to the price of an ambulance response, emergency department visit, or visit to a physician's office, this value is clearly justified.

Youniss J, et al. Characterization of US poison centers: A 1998 survey conducted by the American Association of Poison Control Centers. *Vet Hum Toxicol.* 2000;42:43-53.

130.6. Answer: C. Approaches to curative and preventive medicine are complementary. Preventive medicine emphasizes identifying the risk and reducing the risk (shift in norm) to a population. Behavioral and social interventions predominate in preventative medicine. Curative medicine emphasizes identifying pathology, restoring health, promoting individual service. Clinical intervention predominates in curative medicine.

Fineberg HV. The paradox of disease of prevention. *JAMA.* 2013; 310:83-90.

130.7. Answer: A. There are many intrinsic limitations to poison control center data. The Pollyanna phenomenon is a form of reporting bias that describes the observation that calls to the poison center are more frequent when a new drug or outbreak occurs and are less frequent when more common ingestions occur or as physicians become more familiar with the management of the a novel xenobiotic.

Hamilton RJ, Goldfrank LR. Poison center data and the Pollyanna phenomenon. *J Toxicol Clin Toxicol.* 1997;35:21-23.

130.8. Answer: D. All xenobiotics should be kept in their original containers. Xenobiotics should never be stored in unlocked cabinets under the sink. Xenobiotics should never be left in an unlocked glove compartment. Unused portions of prescription medication should be discarded or returned to the pharmacy. Adults should not take their medication in front of children, as this will limit imitative behavior.

Lovejoy FH Jr, et al. Poison centers, poison prevention, and the pediatrician. *Pediatrics.* 1994;94:220-224.

130.9. Answer: D. Goals for improving poisoning epidemiology data include allowing rapid access to translation services, creating multiple methods of reporting, creating a category for unconfirmed exposures in the database, establishing a public health legistation requiring professional reporting of exposure, and integrating the AAPCC database with other databases.

American Academy of Clinical Toxicology. Facility assessment guidelines for regional toxicology treatment centers. American Academy of Clinical Toxicology. *J Toxicol Clin Toxicol.* 1993;31:211-217.

130.10. Answer: E. Legislation for options A-D requires mandatory reporting in some instances and offers workers protection for voluntary reporting. There are significant discrepancies betweeen PCC reporting and state and national occupational injury reporting.

Blanc PD, et al. Occupational illness and poison control centers. Referral patterns and service needs. *West J Med.* 1990;152:181-184.

Bresnitz EA. Poison Control Center follow-up of occupational disease. *Am J Public Health.* 1990;80:711-712.

Principles of Occupational Toxicology: Diagnosis and Control

QUESTIONS

131.1. A 42-year-old photographer complains of visual difficulties, fatigue, anxiety, and inability to hold a camera steady for the last several weeks. Which of the following occupational exposures is most likely to be responsible for his symptoms?
A. Nitric acid
B. Mercuric oxide
C. Silver nitrate
D. Sulfur dioxide
E. Formaldehyde

131.2. Which of the following options would be considered evidence supporting work-relatedness of occupational disease?
A. Unknown exposure to a causative xenobiotic
B. Only a single worker who is presenting with symptoms
C. No clear temporality of the symptoms with the exposure
D. Absence of a nonoccupational etiology
E. Easily treated because employees continue to be exposed at work

131.3. Which of the following US organizations places legal responsibility for providing a safe and healthy workplace on the employer?
A. OSHA
B. JC
C. HIPAA
D. EMTALA
E. EPA

131.4. The Superfund Act was enacted by the United States Congress in 1980. This law created a tax on the chemical and petroleum industries and provided broad federal authority to respond directly to releases or threatened releases of hazardous xenobiotics that might endanger public health or the environment. Which of the following options is the official name for the Superfund Act?
A. Toxic Substances Control Act
B. Hazardous and Solid Waste Amendments
C. Resource Conservation and Recovery Act
D. Americans with Disabilities Act
E. Comprehensive Environmental Response, Compensation, and Liability Act

131.5. Which of the following metabolites of benzene is measured in the urine as part of occupational biological monitoring?
A. Phenol
B. Toluene
C. Benzoic acid
D. Mandelic acid
E. Hippuric acid

131.6. Which of the following ocular effects is associated with occupational exposure to ethylene oxide?
A. Hyphema
B. Cataract formation
C. Conjunctivitis
D. Lid edema
E. Chalazion formation

131.7. A 22-year-old man presents to the emergency department with myalgias, fevers, chills, chest pain, and dyspnea. Several of his co-workers at his construction site experience similar symptoms at the start of every week. The patient has a normal chest radiograph. Which of the following exposures best explains his symptoms?
A. Zinc oxide
B. Hexavalent chromium
C. Cadmium
D. Inorganic mercury
E. Arsine gas

131.8. A 57-year-old man presents to the emergency department with symptoms consistent with parkinsonism. On occupational history, he states that he worked as a welder for many years. Which of the following occupational exposures best explains his presentation?

A. Chromium
B. Arsenic
C. Lead
D. Mercury
E. Manganese

131.9. Which of the following exposures poses the greatest chronic health hazard?
A. Inhalation of zinc welding fumes
B. Ingestion of clay dusts
C. Inhalation of clay dust
D. Skin contact with concentrated nitric acid
E. Topical exposure to trivalent chromium

131.10. Which of the following exposures causes the most severe eye injuries in farmers?
A. Anhydrous ammonia
B. Carbamates
C. Gasoline
D. Hydraulic fluid
E. Grain dust

ANSWERS

131. Answer: B. This patient is presenting with erethism, visual complaints, and tremor because of occupational exposure to mercuric oxide. Mercury was used in the development of photographic film. These symptoms are characteristic of chronic inorganic mercury poisoning.

Sunderman FW. Perils of mercury. *Ann Clin Lab Sci.* 1988;18:89-101.

131.2. Answer: D. Evidence that supports work-relatedness of an occupational disease includes known or documented exposure to a causative xenobiotic; symptoms consistent with those previously reported from exposure to the suspected xenobiotic; suggestive or diagnostic physical signs; similar problems in coworkers; temporal relationship of complaints to related work; confirmatory environmental or biologic monitoring data; scientific biologic plausibility; absence of nonoccupational etiology; and resistance to maximum medical therapy because employees continue to be exposed at work.

Burgess WA. *Recognition of Health Hazards in Industry: A Review of Materials and Processes.* 2nd ed. New York, NY: Wiley; 1995.

131.3. Answer: A. The Occupational Safety and Health Administration (OSHA) places legal responsibility for providing a safe and healthy workplace on the employer. The Joint Commission (JC) is an organization that provides voluntary certification that places no legal responsibility on the employer. Health Insurance Portability and Accountability Act (HIPAA)

protects patients' privacy and allows patients the ability to transmit information from one site to another if they change their health care providers. The Emergency Medical Treatment and Labor Act (EMTALA) ensures that patients who are in active labor or who have a critical illness and present to an emergency department are cared for regardless of their insurance status, this prevents the inappropriate transfer of patients from private institutions to public safety net hospitals. The Environmental Protection Agency (EPA) has the ability to track at least 75,000 industrial xenobiotics currently produced or imported into the United States. The EPA screens these xenobiotics and is able to require reporting or testing of those that pose an environmental or human health hazard. The EPA can ban the manufacture and import of xenobiotics that pose an unreasonable risk.

https://www.osha.gov/node/999880441. Accessed August 10, 2021.

131.4. Answer: E. The Comprehensive Environmental Response, Compensation, and Liability Act (CERCLA) is commonly known as the Superfund Act. CERCLA established prohibitions and requirements concerning closed and abandoned hazardous waste sites, provided for liability of persons responsible for releases of hazardous waste at these sites, and established a trust fund to provide for cleanup when no responsible party could be identified.

https://www.epa.gov/superfund/superfund-cercla-overview. Accessed August 10, 2021.

131.5. Answer: A. Urinary phenol is used as a biologic marker for benzene exposure. Urinary hippuric acid is used as a marker of toluene exposure. Urinary mandelic acid is used as marker of styrene exposure.

Rainsford SG, Davies TA. Urinary excretion of phenol by men exposed to vapour of benzene: A screening test. *Br J Ind Med*. 1965;22:21-26.

131.6. Answer: B. Prolonged exposure to ethylene oxide is associated with the development of cataracts. While lid and conjunctival irritation is possible at high concentrations, these concentrations are rarely, if ever, attained and maintained long enough during routine use to result in these effects. Hyphema is almost exclusively related to direct ocular trauma. Chalazions do not generally form in response to chemical irritation.

Bihari V, et al. Occupational health hazards among operating room personnel exposed to anesthetic gases: A review. *J Environ Pathol Toxicol Oncol*. 1994;13:213-219.

Richmond GW. An evaluation of possible effects on health following exposure to ethylene oxide. *Arch Environ Health*. 1985;40:20-24.

131.7. Answer: A. This patient is presenting with metal fume fever. This is a benign process that occurs following exposure to zinc oxide. Patients present with myalgias, fevers, chills, chest pain, and dyspnea that are often worse on the first day of the work week and get better as the week progresses, which is why this disease is also known as Monday morning ague. Most patients are managed as outpatients with supportive care alone.

El Safty A, et al. Zinc toxicity among galvanization workers in the iron and steel industry. *Ann N Y Acad Sci*. 2008;1140:256-262.

131.8. Answer: E. Manganese accumulates in the basal ganglia and is associated with occupational parkinsonism. Welders, miners, and other workers exposed to manganese are at risk of developing this. This diagnosis is best confirmed using a T1 hyperintensity magnetic resonance imaging (MRI) of the brain.

Josephs KA, et al. Neurologic manifestations in welders with pallidal MRI T1 hyperintensity. *Neurology*. 2005;64:2033-2039.

131.9. Answer: C. Chronic inhalation of clay dust causes silicosis. Ingestion is not a hazard. Inhalation of zinc fumes causes metal fume fever, an acute illness that does not appear to have any long-term effects. Concentrated nitric acid is corrosive and is an acute health hazard. Topical exposure to hexavalent, not trivalent, chromium is associated with long-term toxicity. Trivalent chromium is not readily absorbed.

Rushton L. Chronic obstructive pulmonary disease and occupational exposure to silica. *Rev Environ Health*. 2007;22:255-272.

131.10. Answer: A. Anhydrous ammonia is used as a fertilizer to increase nitrogen concentrations in the soil. It is extremely caustic to the eye, and severe eye injuries, including blindness, occur rapidly.

Helmers S, et al. Ammonia injuries in agriculture. *J Iowa Med Soc*. 1971;36:271-280.

Hazardous Materials Incident Response

132.1. What is the federal agency responsible for the management of hazardous materials (HAZMAT) incidents in the United States?
A. National Incident Management System
B. Pipeline and Hazardous Materials Safety Administration
C. Environmental Protection Agency
D. Federal Emergency Management Agency
E. There is no federal agency; individual states manage their own HAZMAT incidents

132.2. What does the color blue indicate on a National Fire Protection Association placard?
A. Flammability
B. Chemical form (solid, liquid, gas, or aerosol)
C. Health hazard
D. Reactivity
E. Personal protective equipment requirement

132.3. What is the most common route of exposure at hazardous materials (HAZMAT) incidents?
A. Dermal
B. Intentional ingestion
C. Inhalational
D. Open wound contamination
E. Unspecified/insufficient information recorded

132.4. What hazardous material control zone corresponds to contamination reduction?
A. Hot zone
B. Support zone
C. Cold zone
D. Warm zone
E. Staging zone

132.5. What Environmental Protection Agency level of personal protective equipment offers the highest respiratory protection but only skin splash protection?
A. Level A
B. Level B
C. Level C
D. Level D
E. Level E

132.6. When should Environmental Protection Agency level D personal protective equipment be used?
A. When the highest level of protection for skin, eyes, and respiratory system is required
B. When splash protection is required but not respiratory protection
C. When there is a high level of respiratory tract protection required but less skin protection required
D. When there is no significant chemical respiratory, skin, or splash protection required
E. At a radioactive incident

132.7. When should the United States National Fire Protection Association guidelines for hazardous materials be used?
A. Only at fire scenes
B. They do not meet OSHA requirements and should not be used
C. At any hazardous materials incident
D. Only in prehospital incidents
E. They are guidelines to be used only by specialized firefighters

132.8. According to the United States National Incident Management System, what are the four subsections of the incident command system?

    A. Operations, planning, logistics, and finance and administration

    B. Operations, planning, logistics, and administration

    C. Operations, planning, medical, and administration

    D. Operations, planning, medical, and finance and administration

    E. Operations, planning, medical, and logistics

132.9. How should medical personnel respond to a mass casualty hazardous materials incident?

    A. Respond to their respective health care institutions

    B. Respond to the incident site

    C. Respond to the incident site only if they hold a medical license in that state

    D. Respond to the closest emergency medical services location

    E. Never; they only should report to their next scheduled shift

132.10. Multiple patients present to the emergency department after being exposed to an anhydrous ammonia spill. What risk do they present to health care workers?

    A. Primary contamination

    B. Secondary contamination

    C. Tertiary contamination

    D. No risk if the health care workers wear Level D protection

    E. No risk regardless of the level of protection

ANSWERS

132.1. Answer: D. The Federal Emergency Management Agency (FEMA) is the lead federal emergency management agency in the United States. FEMA is also responsible for hazardous materials incidents in the United States.

Federal Emergency Management Agency. 2018-2022 Strategic Plan Federal Emergency Management Agency. https://www.fema.gov/sites/default/files/2020-03/fema-strategic-plan_2018-2022.pdf. Accessed May 19, 2022.

132.2. Answer: C. The blue quadrant indicates health hazard. The other categories on the placard include red (flammability), white (other information), and yellow (reactivity).

National Fire Protection Association. NFPA 704 Standard System for the Identification of the Hazards of Materials for Emergency Response 2022. Quincy, MA: National Fire Protection Association; 2020.

132.3. Answer: C. Inhalation is the most common route of exposure at hazardous materials incidents.

Kales SN, et al. Injuries caused by hazardous materials accidents. *Ann Emerg Med.* 1997;30:598-603.

132.4. Answer: D. The warm zone corresponds to contamination reduction. The hot zone corresponds to exclusion and the cold zone to support. The warm zone also contains the access corridor, where victims, hazardous materials technicians, and equipment are decontaminated as they move out of the hot zone.

US Environmental Protection Agency. Safety zones. https://www.epa.gov/emergency-response/safety-zones. Accessed May 19, 2022.

132.5. Answer: B. Level A provides the highest level of both respiratory and skin (clothing) protection and provides vapor protection to the respiratory tract, mucous membranes, and skin. This level of personal protective equipment is airtight, and a breathing apparatus must be worn under the suit. Level B provides the highest level of respiratory protection and skin splash protection by using chemical-resistant clothing. It does not provide skin vapor protection but does provide respiratory tract vapor protection. Level C should be used when the type of airborne xenobiotic is known, its concentration is measurable, the criteria for using air-purifying respirators are met, and skin and eye exposures are unlikely. Level C has a lower level of respiratory protection than A or B. Level D is basically a regular work uniform. It provides no respiratory protection and minimal skin protection. Level E does not exist.

US Department of Labor Occupational Safety and Health Administration. 1910.120 App B - General description and discussion of the levels of protection and protective gear. 1994. https://www.osha.gov/laws-regs/regulations/standardnumber/1910/1910.120AppB. Accessed May 19, 2022.

132.6. Answer: D. Level D protection is the lowest level of protection and should be worn when there is no chemical protection required.

US Department of Labor Occupational Safety and Health Administration. 1910.120 App B - General description and discussion of the levels of protection and protective gear. 1994. https://www.osha.gov/laws-regs/regulations/standardnumber/1910/1910.120AppB. Accessed May 19, 2022.

132.7. Answer: C. National Fire Protection Association guidelines meet OSHA standards and are used at any hazardous materials incident.

National Fire Protection Association Technical Committee on Hazardous Materials Response Personnel. NFPA 473 Standard for Competencies for EMS Personnel Responding to Hazardous Materials Incidents. Quincy, MA: National Fire Protection Association; 1997.

National Fire Protection Association Technical Committee on Hazardous Materials Response Personnel. NFPA 472 Standard on Professional Competence of Responders to Hazardous Materials Incidents. Quincy, MA: National Fire Protection Association; 2002.

132.8. Answer: A. The four subsections of the incident command system are operations, planning, logistics, and finance and administration. The operations section controls the organizational efforts to reach incident management objectives and directs resources. The planning section supports the incident action planning process, collects and analyzes information, and tracks resources. The logistics section arranges for resources and services. The finance and administration section monitors costs related to the incident.

Federal Emergency Management Agency. *National Incident Management System*. 3rd ed. 2017. https://www.fema.gov/sites/default/files/2020-07/fema_nims_doctrine-2017.pdf. Accessed May 19, 2022.

132.9. Answer: A. Unsolicited medical personnel at the scene of a hazardous materials incident, although well intentioned, risk harming the coordinated response and are liable to interfere with operational efforts. Medical personnel should respond only to their own health care institution.

Unsolicited medical personnel volunteering at disaster scenes. *Ann Emerg Med*. 2018;71:e41.

132.10. Answer: B. Anhydrous ammonia potentially causes secondary contamination to health care workers from adherent liquids if the patient is not adequately decontaminated. Secondary contamination is caused by solids, liquids, and aerosols. Anhydrous ammonia causes ocular, respiratory, gastrointestinal, and skin irritation. At significant concentrations, it leads to severe pulmonary edema and death.

Larson TC, et al. Threat of secondary chemical contamination of emergency departments and personnel: An uncommon but recurrent problem. *Disaster Med Public Health Prep*. 2016;10:199-202.

National Research Council (US) Committee on Acute Exposure Guideline Levels. Acute Exposure Guideline Levels for Selected Airborne Chemicals: Volume 6. Washington, DC: National Academies Press; 2008. 2, Ammonia Acute Exposure Guideline Levels. https://www.ncbi.nlm.nih.gov/books/NBK207883/. Accessed May 19, 2022.

Risk Assessment and Risk Communication

133.1. A deterministic toxicity assessment is which of the following options?
A. Multifactorial
B. Probabilistic
C. Related to carcinogenesis
D. Dose dependent
E. Transgenerational

133.2. Refined and improved risk assessment is based on accumulating knowledge in a polarized debate. Which of the following options represents the best explanation of the Kehoe principle?
A. Define whether a substance is harmful before permitting its use
B. Permit continued utilization of a product until definitive evidence of harm is demonstrated
C. The uncertainty of a threat should be minimized if the financial benefits to continued use are substantial
D. Define the cost to society before any change in use or application is decided
E. Ensure a substance is beneficial before permitting its use

133.3. Which of the following options is a component of a risk assessment?
A. Hazard identification
B. Exposure pathway
C. Modifying factors
D. Toxicity assessment
E. All of the above

133.4. The recommended dietary consumption of fish by pregnant women is based on what data?
A. Outcome limits from randomized controlled human studies
B. The highest observed adverse effect level (HOAEL)
C. The no observed adverse effect level (NOAEL)
D. Limiting exposure to arsenobetaine
E. The use of no uncertainty factors

133.5. Which of the following factors would improve the acceptability of a perceived risk?
A. Human made
B. Not associated with a trusted source
C. Unfamiliar
D. Voluntary
E. Unfairly distributed throughout the population

133.6. Which of the following principles will enhance risk communication from the poison control center?
A. Dictating care to the caller
B. Reactionary planning
C. Involving the individual as a partner
D. Not interpreting for an individual whose preferred language is not English.
E. Minimizing the risk and lying to assuage concerns

133.7. Which of the following options is an advantage in achieving effective risk communication?
A. First-time poison control center use
B. Inadequate response to prior question
C. Appreciation of cultural differences
D. Limited science comprehension
E. Loss of credibility

133.8. Many individuals at a school complained of odor-triggered nonspecific symptoms, such as dizziness, nausea, and palpitations. Symptoms spread, even occurring in some individuals after removal from the building. No plausible scenario that would account for significant symptoms could be identified. Which of the following best explains what occurred at this school?
A. Chlorine toxicity
B. Phosgene toxicity
C. Metal fume fever
D. Tricresyl phosphate (aerotoxic syndrome)
E. Mass psychogenic illness

133.9. A certified specialist in poison information (CSPI) is able to make a risk assessment that a certain exposure is benign or minimally toxic as long as which of the following characteristics is true?

A. A CSPI does have confidence in the caller
B. The risk of adverse reactions is acceptable to both the CSPI and caller
C. The ingestion was of a benign xenobiotic in a suicidal ingestion
D. Small ingestions are benign; however, the worst potential effects are life threatening
E. The specialist is unable to make a reasonable estimation of maximum amount involved

133.10. Effective risk communication depends on defining which of the following factors?
A. Magnitude of the risk
B. Urgency of the risk
C. Applicability of the risk categorization
D. Uncertainties of the risk
E. All of the above

ANSWERS

133.1. Answer: D. A toxicity assessment evaluates both deterministic and stochastic effects. Deterministic effects are dose dependent and usually result in acute or chronic injury, while stochastic effects are multifactorial and probabilistic and are predominantly related to carcinogenesis and developmental or transgenerational in impact.

Calabrese EJ, Baldwin LA. The frequency of U-shaped dose response in the toxicological literature. *Toxicol Sci.* 2001;62:330 338.

133.2. Answer: B. The Kehoe principle is best summarized as "prove something is harmful before excluding a product with known benefits because of concern about potential unproven future adverse effects." It is the opposite of the precautionary principle (a risk exists until otherwise proven).

Martuzzi M, Tickner JA, eds. *The Precautionary Principle: Protecting Public Health, the Environment and the Future of Our Children.* Budapest, Hungary: Fourth Ministerial Conference on Environment and Health, World Health Organization; 2004. http://www.euro.who.int.ezproxy.med .nyu.edu/__data/assets/pdf_file/0003/91173/E83079.pdf. Accessed May 19, 2022.

Teeguarden JG, Hanson-Drury S. A systematic review of bisphenol A "low dose" studies in the context of human exposure: A case for establishing standards for reporting "low-dose" effects of chemicals. *Food Chem Toxicol.* 2013;62:935-948.

133.3. Answer: E. Risk assessment is the process of determining the likelihood of toxicity for an individual or group after a perceived exposure to a xenobiotic. When available, a published body of knowledge should be applied to some components of risk characterization or assessment.

Agency for Toxic Substance and Disease Registry. *Public Health Assessment Guidance Manual (2005 update) 2005.* https://www.atsdr.cdc .gov/hac/PHAManual/toc.html. Accessed May 19, 2022.

Environmental Protection Agency. Risk assessment website portal. http://www.epa.gov/risk. Accessed May 19, 2022.

133.4. Answer: C. Differentiating public health from individual risk assessment is very difficult and usually done by the Environmental Protection Agency (EPA) and other regulatory and advisory organizations to achieve a meaningful translation of knowledge. The recommended dietary consumption of fish by pregnant women is based on outcome limits in animal models—the lowest observed adverse effect level (LOAEL) as well as the no observed effect level (NOEL) no observed adverse effect level (NOAEL). The recommended dietary consumption is based on limiting exposure to methylmercury and polychlorinated biphenyls. In contrast, arsenobetaine is a benign form of arsenic. There are also uncertainty factors (usually multiples of 10, added to account for variability between humans and research data) built into the recommendations.

Agency for Toxic Substance and Disease Registry. Toxicological profile for mercury. http://www.atsdr.cdc.gov/toxprofiles/tp.asp?id=115&tid=24. Accessed August 4, 2021.

133.5. Answer: D. Factors that improve acceptability of a perceived risk include natural products, associated with a trusted source, familiar information, voluntary involvement, potentially beneficial, statistically a low likelihood, shared by all, and affecting adults.

Fischhoff B, et al. *Acceptable Risk*. Cambridge, MA: Cambridge University Press; 1981.

133.6. Answer: C. Involving the individual as a partner, care planning, listening carefully to patient concerns, honesty, openness, working with credible sources, meeting the needs of the media, and speaking clearly and compassionately improve risk communication. It is also important that an interpreter is utilized if a patient's primary language is not English.

Covello V, Allen F. *Seven Cardinal Rules of Risk Communication*. Washington, DC: US Environmental Protection Agency, Office of Policy Analysis; 1988.

133.7. Answer: C. All the listed options affect appropriate risk assessment and effective risk communication: nature of previous encounter, lack of prior health care–patient relationship, inadequate response to a prior question, the provision of information contrary to popular understanding, loss of credibility, lack of appreciation of individual or cultural differences, and incomplete comprehension of science or statistics.

Fischhoff B, et al. *Acceptable Risk*. Cambridge, MA: Cambridge University Press; 1981.

133.8. Answer: E. This case is an example of a mass psychogenic illness and highlights the practical difficulties involved in a risk assessment. The fear-arousal cycle triggers a multitude of "medically unexplained symptoms" and precipitates maladaptive thoughts, feelings, and behaviors that characterize somatic symptom disorder. A similar phenomenon occurs among certain first responders who are exposed to fentanyl topically and develop symptoms that are not consistent with the exposure.

Black D, Murray V. Mass psychogenic illness attributed to toxic exposure at a high school. *N Engl J Med*. 2000;342:1674.

133.9. Answer: B. A joint position statement released by the American Association of Poison Control Centers, the American Academy of Clinical Toxicology, and the American College of Medical Toxicology states that a CSPI is able to make a risk assessment that an exposure is benign or minimally toxic only if the following characteristics are true: (1) The information specialist has confidence in the accuracy of the history obtained and the ability to communicate effectively with the caller. (2) The information specialist has confidence in the identity of the products or substances and a reasonable estimation of the maximum amount involved in the exposure. (3) The risks of adverse reactions or expected effects are acceptable to both the poison specialist and the caller based on available medical literature. (4) The exposure does not require a health care referral because the worst potential effects are benign and self-limited. If a person ingests a xenobiotic in a suicide attempt, they should immediately be referred to the hospital regardless of how benign the xenobiotic is.

McGuigan MA. Guideline Consensus Panel. Guideline for the out-of-hospital management of human exposures to minimally toxic substances. *J Toxicol Clin Toxicol*. 2003;41:907-917.

133.10. Answer: E. Effective risk communication must address several questions. The appropriate process is to first obtain the best information regarding the identification of the xenobiotic and the nature of the exposure and then to convey the magnitude of the risk, the urgency of the risk, the applicability of the risk categorization, the uncertainties of the risk, and any available management options.

Robertson WO. Poison center data and the Pollyanna phenomenon disputed. *J Toxicol Clin Toxicol*. 1998;36:139-141.

Medication Safety and Adverse Drug Events

QUESTIONS

134.1. Which of the following medication classes is most associated with medication errors?
A. Anticoagulants
B. Antihistamines
C. Antilipemics
D. Thyroid medications
E. Vitamins

134.2. The greatest number of errors resulting in preventable adverse drug events occur at which of the following points of time?
A. Dispensing phase
B. Documentation phase
C. Monitoring phase
D. Prescribing stage
E. Transcribing stage

134.3. Which of the following statements best describes pediatric adverse medication events?
A. They are more likely to involve academic or pediatric emergency departments
B. They are more likely to involve anticoagulants
C. They are more likely to involve rectal medication administration
D. They are more likely to involve children in general hospital wards
E. They are more likely to involve incorrect dosing

134.4. Which of the following factors contributes to medication errors in geriatric patients?
A. Age between 50 and 65 years
B. Cognitive preservation

C. Medication deprescribing
D. Physiological preservation
E. Medical comorbidities

134.5. Beers Criteria is a tool to determine which of the following risks?
A. Bleeding risk
B. Ethanol use
C. In-hospital ethanol withdrawal risk
D. Medication prescribing risk
E. Sedation risk

134.6. Which of the following factors positively affects human performance?
A. Care transition
B. Cognitive loading
C. Distraction
D. Experience
E. Fatigue

134.7. Which of the following choices is an information technology (IT) or computerized provider order entry (CPOE) solution that decreases medication errors?
A. Automated dispensing cabinet (ADC) override
B. Barcode medication administration
C. Bulk dose dispensing
D. Downtime processes
E. Multiple medication alerts

134.8. Which of the following options is an effective response to medication error?
A. Blaming individuals
B. Employment termination
C. Malpractice litigation
D. Systems evaluation
E. Unstructured analysis

134.9. Best practices for medication orders include use of which of the following options?
A. Abbreviations for efficiency
B. Handwritten orders

C. Indications for utilization
D. "Trailing zeros" for clarity
E. Verbal orders for flexibility

134.10. Clinical pharmacists increase which of the following events?
A. Adverse medication errors
B. Length of stay
C. Medication costs
D. Medication reconciliation
E. Readmissions

ANSWERS

134.1. Answer: A. Drugs that are most associated with medication errors include anticoagulants. Other medications with a high incidence of medication errors are antidiabetics, corticosteroids, chemotherapeutics, electrolyte salts, immune modulators, nonsteroidal anti-inflammatory drugs (including salicylates), opioids, and sedatives. Extra care is required when prescribing and reconciling these medications.

Santell JP, et al. Medication errors: Experience of the United States Pharmacopeia (USP) MEDMARX reporting system. *J Clin Pharmacol.* 2003;43:760-767.

Poudel DR, et al. Burden of hospitalizations related to adverse drug events in the USA: A retrospective analysis from large inpatient database. *Pharmacoepidemiol Drug Saf.* 2017;26:635-641.

134.2. Answer: D. The greatest number of preventable adverse drug events occurs at the prescribing stage. Emergency department errors most commonly occur in either the prescribing or administering phase. Although electronic ordering helps eliminate some of these errors, it introduces the potential for different types of errors.

Bates DW, et al. Relationship between medication errors and adverse drug events. *J Gen Intern Med.* 1995;10:199-205.

Patanwala AE, et al. A prospective observational study of medication errors in a tertiary care emergency department. *Ann Emerg Med.* 2010;55:522-526.

134.3. Answer: E. Incorrect dosing is the most commonly reported error. Errors occur more commonly in nonacademic or rural emergency departments (EDs) compared with academic or pediatric EDs. Antimicrobials and intravenous fluid errors are most common. Weight-based dose-related errors occur more often in children. Hospitalized children experience more medication errors than adults,

and those in intensive care units (ICUs) are at higher risk compared to children not in the ICU.

Crowley E, et al. Medication errors in children: A descriptive summary of medication error reports submitted to the United States Pharmacopeia. *Curr Ther Res Clin Exp.* 2001;26:627-640.

Kaushal R, et al. Medication errors and adverse drug events in pediatric inpatients. *JAMA.* 2001;285:2114-2120.

134.4. Answer: E. Age greater than 65 years increases risk of complications. Medical comorbidities, and thus multiple medications, increase potential errors and interactions. Frailty and cognitive decline put patients at risk for self-administration errors. Elders living in assisted-living facilities suffer from inadequate oversight and poorly trained staff.

Gurwitz JH, et al. Incidence and preventability of adverse drug events among older persons in the ambulatory setting. *JAMA.* 2003;289:1107-1116.

134.5. Answer: D. Beers Criteria is a tool to determine appropriate medication prescribing in geriatric patients. The HAS-BLED tool stratifies the risk of bleeding with anticoagulation. The AUDIT-C and CIWA-Ar, and other tools, are used to assess at-risk alcohol use and withdrawal risk. Screening, brief intervention, referral, and treatment (SBIRT) is used to screen and reduce alcohol use in light or moderate drinkers. The Aldrete and aRASS scores are used to monitor sedation.

American Geriatric Society 2015 Beers Criteria Update Expert Panel. American Geriatrics Society 2015 updated Beers Criteria for potentially inappropriate medication use in older adults. *J Am Geriatr Soc.* 2015;63:2227-2246.

134.6. Answer: D. Major factors that adversely affect human performance include diminished motivation and morale, distractions, fatigue, transitions of care, increased cognitive load, inexperience, interruptions, poor workplace ergonomics, and sleep deprivation or debt. Increased experience positively affects human performance.

Fahrenkopf AM, et al. Rates of medication errors among depressed and burnt out residents: Prospective cohort study. *BMJ.* 2008;336:488-491.

Patanwala AE, et al. A prospective observational study of medication errors in a tertiary care emergency department. *Ann Emerg Med.* 2010;55:522-526.

134.7. Answer: B. Barcoding for the dispensing and administration of patient-specific medication reduces errors. The ability to override automated dispensing cabinets (ADCs) increases errors. Excessive alerts cause alert fatigue and bypassing of alerts. Downtime processes circumvent computerized provider order entry (CPOE) protections.

Morriss FH Jr, et al. Effectiveness of a barcode medication administration system in reducing preventable adverse drug events in a neonatal intensive care unit: A prospective cohort study. *J Pediatr.* 2009;154:363-368.

134.8. Answer: D. A structured approach, through techniques such as root cause analysis, clinical incident analysis, failure mode and effect analysis, and Lean Six Sigma (LSS), is an effective response to medication errors. Blame, personal litigation, and individual terminations are counterproductive.

Vincent C, et al. How to investigate and analyse clinical incidents: Clinical risk unit and association of litigation and risk management protocol. *BMJ.* 2000;320:777-781.

134.9. Answer: C. Providers should indicate the reason a medication is prescribed. Use of abbreviations should be limited, trailing zeros should be eliminated, and verbal orders should be rare. Computerized provider order entry (CPOE) should be utilized to eliminate unclear handwritten orders.

Peth HA Jr. Medication errors in the emergency department: A systems approach to minimizing risk. *Emerg Med Clin North Am.* 2003;21:141-158.

134.10. Answer: D. Clinical pharmacists improve medication reconciliation and are available for medication questions, discussion, and consultation. They also decrease adverse medication errors, length of stay, medication costs, and readmissions.

Cunningham KJ. Analysis of clinical interventions and the impact of pediatric pharmacists on medication error prevention in a teaching hospital. *J Pediatr Pharmacol Ther.* 2012;17:365-373.

Kwan JL, et al. Medication reconciliation during transitions of care as a patient safety strategy: A systematic review. *Ann Intern Med.* 2013;158:397-403.

QUESTIONS

135.1. Which of the following xenobiotics resulted in the passage of the Food, Drug, and Cosmetic Act of 1938?
A. Diethylene glycol
B. Oxalic acid
C. Sodium hydroxide
D. Thalidomide
E. Tri-*ortho*-cresylphosphate

135.2. The Drug Amendments of 1962 to the Federal Food, Drug, and Cosmetic Act (Kefauver-Harris Act of 1962) required drug manufacturers or sponsors to perform which of the following actions?
A. Demonstrate cost effectiveness
B. Demonstrate effectiveness of existing drugs on the market
C. Demonstrate noninferiority compared to existing drugs
D. Perform studies in claimed indication in pediatric patients
E. Submit a new drug application prior to initiating clinical studies in humans

135.3. Which of the following statements best describes the Dietary Supplement Health and Education Act (DSHEA) of 1994?
A. Authorized the US Food and Drug Administration (FDA) to require dietary supplements to demonstrate proof of safety and efficacy for functional claims
B. Ensured rigorous premarketing testing of dietary supplements

C. Permitted marketing of dietary supplements with functional claims of "supporting health"
D. Prohibited pediatric functional claims
E. Required manufacturers to demonstrate safety for United States distribution

135.4. The Animal Efficacy Rule (Animal Rule) of 2002 permitted the United States (US) Food and Drug and Administration (FDA) to extend approval to products used to treat serious or life-threatening conditions caused by exposure to biologic, chemical, radiologic, or nuclear substances based on which of the following options?
A. Efficacy in human volunteers
B. In silico efficacy
C. In vitro efficacy
D. Safety in animals
E. Safety in healthy human volunteers

135.5. A phase 1 study is designed to test which of the following options?
A. The efficacy of a drug candidate in humans with a mild or early form of the disease
B. The efficacy of a drug candidate in the patient population for whom the drug is intended in a large-scale study
C. The initial efficacy of a drug candidate in animals
D. The safety of a cancer chemotherapeutic candidate in oncology patients
E. The safety of a drug candidate in humans with advanced disease

135.6. A diagnosis of an adverse drug event would be best supported by an occurrence at which point in time?
- A. Antecedent to exposure to the suspect drug
- B. In the setting of multiple possible etiologies
- C. Upon drug rechallenge
- D. Upon placebo administration
- E. With drug underdosing

135.7. Which of the following statements regarding post-marketing surveillance is correct?
- A. Establishing causality is required to submit a MedWatch report
- B. Hospital information technology systems actively report adverse drug events to the MedWatch systems
- C. Premarketing clinical studies are adequate to detect rare adverse drug events
- D. Most reports in the FDA Adverse Event Reporting System (FAERS) come from manufacturers
- E. The number of serious adverse events reported to MedWatch continues to decrease

135.8. Which of the following pharmaceuticals was removed from the US market due to significant drug-drug interactions?
- A. Cerivastatin
- B. Mibefradil
- C. Phenacetin
- D. Rapacuronium
- E. Tegaserod

135.9. Which of the following pharmaceuticals was removed from the United States (US) market due to drug-related prolongation of the QT interval?
- A. Astemizole
- B. Gatifloxacin
- C. Pemoline
- D. Pergolide
- E. Valdecoxib

135.10. Which of the following statements is correct?
- A. The most common regulatory action taken by the US Food and Drug Administration (FDA) is to require a boxed warning (a "black box" warning) in the prescribing information
- B. A boxed warning removes marketing approval for certain populations
- C. FDA drug approval preempts legal action (tort action against a product's manufacturer)
- D. The FDA requires implementation of restricted availability measures for certain drugs
- E. FDA regulatory action precludes manufacturers from filing suit against the FDA to fight or delay the planned action against the product

ANSWERS

135.1. Answer: A. The Massengil pharmaceutical company used diethylene glycol (DEG) in their elixir of sulfanilamide, which resulted in >100 deaths, and gave rise to the passage of the Food, Drug, and Cosmetic Act that helped to establish the US Food and Drug Administration. Oxalic acid, sodium hydroxide, and other caustic exposures led to passage of the 1927 Federal Caustic Poison Act. The thalidomide disaster led to the Kefauver-Harris Act of 1962. Tri-*ortho*-cresylphosphate (TOCP) contaminated ethanolic extracts of Jamaican ginger ("ginger jake").

Geiling EHK, Cannon PR. Pathological effects of elixir of sulfanilamide (diethylene glycol) poisoning: A clinical and experimental correlation - final report. *JAMA*. 1938;111:919-926.

135.2. Answer: E. The Kefauver-Harris Act required demonstration that the drug was effective for the condition that it was being marketed to treat. It also required submission of an investigational new drug (IND) application prior to initiating studies in humans, as well as adequate directions for safe usage of the drug. It did not require comparison to existing therapies, either in efficacy or cost. The act did not apply retroactively to drugs already marketed. The Pediatric Research Equity Act of 2003 required pediatric studies for claimed indications.

Beninger P. Pharmacovigilance: An overview. *Clin Ther*. 2018;40: 1991-2004.

135.3. Answer: C. The Dietary Supplement Health and Education Act removed from FDA the authority to require proof of safety or efficacy prior to marketing of products considered dietary supplements (including herbal remedies). The burden of proof of safety and efficacy was removed from the manufacturer and required the FDA to demonstrate that a product was unsafe to prevent sale and distribution in the United States.

Pawar RS, Grundel E. Overview of regulation of dietary supplements in the USA and issues of adulteration with phenethylamines (PEAs). *Drug Test Anal*. 2017;9:500-517.

135.4. Answer: E. The Animal Rule allows a sponsor to establish product efficacy in a validated animal model and then provide human safety data from healthy human volunteers. This was done to preclude exposure of humans to toxic biologic, chemical, radiologic, or nuclear substances. Safety in animal studies (preclinical testing) is required prior to study in humans in general. In vitro and in silico testing alone does not support drug approval.

Snoy PJ. Establishing efficacy of human products using animals: The US food and drug administration's "animal rule". *Vet Pathol.* 2010;47:774-778.

135.5. Answer: D. Safety in animal studies (preclinical testing) is required prior to study in humans (pre–investigational new drug). Phase 1 studies test a small number of participants with the primary aim of determining the safety and toxicity of the drug. Phase 1 studies are conducted in healthy volunteer participants, with the exception that only patients with cancer are enrolled in phase 1 studies for cancer chemotherapeutics. Phase 2 clinical testing is designed to determine the potential efficacy of the drug candidate in humans, usually at varying levels of exposure to the drug candidate. Phase 3 clinical drug studies usually involve large-scale clinical trials in the actual, or close to the actual, patient population for whom the drug is intended. "Phase 4" involves postmarketing surveillance.

https://www.fda.gov/patients/drug-development-process/step-3-clinical-research. Accessed August 3, 2021.

135.6. Answer: C. Questions to assist in determining an adverse drug event (ADE) include the following: Was the event appropriate in presentation relative to the exposure? Has the suspected ADE been previously reported? Was excessive exposure to the drug reported? Are there other more likely etiologies? Was there an appropriate response to cessation of a suspect drug (de-challenge)? What was the patient's response to rechallenge?

Edwards IR, Aronson JK. Adverse drug reactions: Definitions, diagnosis, and management. *Lancet.* 2000;356:1255-1259.

135.7. Answer: D. The MedWatch system is based on spontaneous reporting of adverse drug events (ADEs). Approximately 95% of reports in FAERS come from the mandatory reporting from pharmaceutical manufacturers. Establishing causality is not required to submit a MedWatch report. Serious adverse events reported to MedWatch continue to increase, although the quality is limited. Premarketing clinical studies (phases 1, 2, and 3) are usually inadequate to detect rare ADEs, incorrectly diagnosed ADEs, or ADEs that result from a drug interaction.

https://www.fda.gov/drugs/surveillance/questions-and-answers-fdas-adverse-event-reporting-system-faers. Accessed August 3, 2021.

135.8. Answer: B. Mibefradil was responsible for multiple drug-drug interactions that ultimately led to its removal from the US market. Cerivastatin was associated with rhabdomyolysis. Phenacetin was associated with kidney damage. Rapacuronium caused bronchospasm and unexplained deaths. The US Food and Drug Administration (FDA) removed tegaserod due to possible adverse cardiovascular effects but subsequently approved its reintroduction.

SoRelle R. Withdrawal of Posicor from market. *Circulation.* 1998;98:831-832.

135.9. Answer: A. Terfenadine (Seldane), astemizole (Hismanal), and cisapride (Propulsid) were removed from the US market due to drug-related prolongation of the QT interval. Because of this finding in the 1990s, the FDA now requires a thorough QT study (TQT) for all new molecular entities. Gatifloxacin was removed for hypoglycemia. Pemoline was removed for liver toxicity. Pergolide was removed due to risk of serious damage to the heart valves. Valdecoxib increased the risk of adverse cardiovascular events in short-term coronary artery bypass surgery (CABG) trials and was associated with reports of serious and potentially life-threatening skin reactions.

Malik M, et al. Thorough QT studies: Questions and quandaries. *Drug Saf.* 2010;33:1-14.

135.10. Answer: D. For certain drugs, the FDA requires implementation of restricted availability measures to permit continued availability of the drug, but only with specified restrictions, such as Risk Evaluation and Mitigation Strategies (REMS) programs (eg, for clozapine, isotretinoin, lenalidomide, and vigabatrin). The most common regulatory action taken by the FDA is modification of the drug label. A black box warning is the most serious warning placed in the prescribing information of a drug but does not preclude use. US FDA approval does not preclude legal challenges against the manufacturer (*Wyeth v. Levine*). While manufacturers often voluntarily cease to market a specific drug after notification by the FDA that regulatory action is being initiated to remove a specific drug from the market, the FDA itself sometimes has to remove a drug from the market through due process legal proceedings in the courts.

https://www.fda.gov/drugs/drug-safety-and-availability/risk-evaluation-and-mitigation-strategies-rems. Accessed August 3, 2021.

International Perspectives on Medical Toxicology

QUESTIONS

136.1. Which of the following xenobiotics is the most common cause of fatality in low to middle income countries?
A. Snake bites
B. Arsenic
C. Pesticides
D. Benzodiazepines
E. Chloroquine

136.2. Which of the following options is considered a reason for the exceptionally high fatality rate of poisoning in low to middle income countries?
A. Limited public health education about poisoning
B. Unlimited exposure to the most highly toxic chemicals
C. Limited access to quality medical care
D. Medical toxicology is frequently an unrecognized specialty
E. All of the above

136.3. Which of the following options is the most consequential cause for the higher fatality rate of pesticide poisoning in low to middle income countries?
A. The intrinsic lethality of available pesticides
B. The number of different pesticides available
C. The quality of the safety packaging of pesticides
D. The rural community use of pesticides
E. The ease of drinking these compounds

136.4. Snake envenomation is a significant problem in low to middle income countries. As of 2009, how large is the maximum estimated problem?
A. 500,000 envenomings and 100,000 deaths
B. 750,000 envenomings and 100,000 deaths
C. 1,000,000 envenomings and 90,000 deaths
D. 1,400,000 envenomings and 90,000 deaths
E. 1,800,000 envenomings and 90,000 deaths

136.5. Which of the following options is true regarding traditional medicine use in low- to middle-income countries?
A. Traditional medicines are less cost effective than Western medicine
B. Western medicine has more sociocultural preference
C. Patients understand the risk of natural products
D. There is an easy accessibility of doctors in low- to middle-income countries
E. Traditional medicine is one of the most common causes of death from acute poisoning in low- to middle-income countries

136.6. What xenobiotic is used commonly in drug-facilitated robbery on public transportation in multiple countries?
A. Cardioactive steroids
B. Scopolamine
C. Benzodiazepines
D. Toxic alcohols
E. Fentanyl

136.7. Plants are common causes of poisoning in low to middle income countries. Which of the following options is a correct combination of a plant and its toxic ingredient?
A. *Thevetia peruviana* and digoxin
B. *Gloriosa superba* and colchicine
C. *Datura stramonium* and podophyllin
D. *Ricinus communis* and abrin
E. *Blighia sapida* and oleandrin

136.8. In 2012, authorities in Pakistan temporarily closed a drug company that was dispensing isosorbide mononitrate free of charge to patients with heart conditions. At least 120 people died because of a serious error in the manufacturing, which led to a contamination. Patients presented initially with a rapid drop of their white blood cell counts. Which of the following contaminants led to this disaster?
A. Melamine
B. Pyrimethamine
C. Colchicine
D. Diethylene glycol
E. Methyl isocyanate

136.9. Which of the following options is most effective in the hierarchical strategy to reduce pesticide mortality in low to middle income countries?
A. Isolate people from the hazard
B. Label products and train applicators
C. Reduce use through improved equipment
D. Promote the use of personal protective equipment
E. Ban the most highly toxic pesticides

136.10. Which of the following options is the most common household xenobiotic associated with serious childhood unintentional poisoning in low- to middle-income communities?
A. Cleansing products
B. Rat poisons
C. Insecticides
D. Cosmetics
E. Kerosene

ANSWERS

136.1. Answer: C. Of the xenobiotics cited, pesticides are the most common cause of poisoning fatalities. At least 150,000 people die each year from acute pesticide poisoning. Ground water arsenic is associated with innumerable poisonings that result in chronic disease. Non fatal poisoning from contaminated foods and industrial waste also exceptionally common.

Gunnell D, et al. The global distribution of fatal pesticide self-poisoning: Systematic review. *BMC Public Health*. 2007;7:357.

Kasturiratne A, et al. The global burden of snakebite: A literature analysis and modelling based on regional estimates of envenoming and deaths. *PLoS Med*. 2008;5:e218.

136.2. Answer: E. All of these factors, in addition to limited diagnostic and treatment centers, limited availability of antidotes, and limited equipment such as ventilators and intensive care units, contribute to a high case-fatality rate.

Brown NI. Consequences of neglect: Analysis of the sub-Saharan African snake antivenom market and the global context. *PLoS Negl Trop Dis*. 2012;6:e1670.

136.3. Answer: A. All of these answers are in part correct. The major difference is that in low to middle income

countries there is continued use of pesticides that are listed among the extremely hazardous, and highly hazardous groups. The diversity of the pesticides is enormous, and many are currently banned in high-income countries while they remain available in low- to middle-income countries. Most products have readily available access without child-resistant packaging.

Eddleston M, et al. Deliberate self-harm in Sri Lanka: An overlooked tragedy in the developing world. *BMJ*. 1998;317:133-135.

Eddleston M, et al. Pesticide poisoning in the developing world—a minimum pesticides list. *Lancet*. 2002;360:1163-1167.

136.4. Answer: E. These rough estimates demonstrate the enormous morbidity and mortality associated with snake envenomations. Mortality is greatly due to reliance on traditional healers, tourniquet use, incision, and lack of adequate or accessible antivenoms and health care.

Harrison R, et al. Snake envenoming: A disease of poverty. *PLoS Negl Trop Dis*. 2009;3:e569.

Kasturiratne A, et al. The global burden of snakebite: A literature analysis and modelling based on regional estimates of envenoming and deaths. *PLoS Med. 2008*;5:e218.

136.5. Answer: E. Traditional medicine used to treat or prevent health problems is widespread. Traditional medicine encompasses a wide variety of spiritual, religious, or physical manipulation therapies often including administration of herbal remedies orally, topically, or via enema. Reasons that patients prefer traditional medicine over Western medicine include financial considerations, sociocultural preferences, the belief that traditional medicines are safer than Western medicine, and mistrust and lack of accessibility of doctors. Traditional medicines are among the most common causes of admission and death from acute poisoning in low- to middle-income countries.

Galvão TF, et al. Impact of a poison control center on the length of hospital stay of poisoned patients: Retrospective cohort. *Sao Paulo Med J.* 2011;129:23-29.

Hughes GD, et al. The prevalence of traditional herbal medicine use among hypertensives living in South African communities. *BMC Complement Altern Med.* 2013;13:38.

Tagwireyi D, et al. Traditional medicine poisoning in Zimbabwe: Clinical presentation and management in adults. *Hum Exp Toxicol.* 2002;21:579-586.

136.6. Answer: C. Criminal poisoning is a common problem in South Asia, particularly in Bangladesh and Pakistan. Benzodiazepines are frequently employed.

Khan T, et al. Drugs-facilitated street and travel related crimes: A new public health issue. *Gomal J Med Sci.* 2014;12:205-209.

Majumder MM, et al. Criminal poisoning of commuters in Bangladesh: Prospective and retrospective study. *Forensic Sci Int.* 2008;180:10-16.

136.7. Answer: B. There are numerous poisonous plants throughout the world used as abortifacients, for recreation, for homicide, and for self-harm. *Gloriosa superba* contains colchicine. *Thevetia peruviana* contains oleandrin. *Datura stramonium* contains scopolamine. *Ricinus communis* contains ricin. *Blighia sapida* contains hypoglycin.

Mendis S. Colchicine cardiotoxicity following ingestion of *Gloriosa superba* tubers. *Postgrad Med J.* 1989;65:752-755.

Premaratna R, et al. Gloriosa superba poisoning mimicking an acute infection—a case report. *BMC Pharmacol Toxicol.* 2015;16:27.

136.8. Answer: B. Pyrimethamine, an antimalarial that is associated with leukopenia, was found as a contaminant in isosorbide mononitrate tablets in Pakistan. More than nine million tablets of isosorbide mononitrate were produced by Efroze Chemical at its factory in Karachi. This episode led to reforms within the Pakistani health services and systems.

Arie S. Contaminated drugs are held responsible for 120 deaths in Pakistan. *BMJ.* 2012;34:e951.

136.9. Answer: E. While all the listed efforts have been utilized to reduce pesticide mortality, answer choices A-D are minor compared to eliminating the most highly toxic pesticides. Administrative controls are the least efficacious.

Roberts DM, et al. Influence of pesticide regulation on acute poisoning deaths in Sri Lanka. *Bull World Health Organ.* 2003;81:789-798.

136.10. Answer: E. Kerosene remains among the most common childhood poisonings in low- to middle-income communities. The events are reminiscent of the kerosene epidemic of the first half of the 20th century in America.

Bond GR, et al. A clinical decision rule for triage of children under 5 years of age with hydrocarbon (kerosene) aspiration in developing countries. *Clin Toxicol.* 2008;46:222-229.

Keka A, et al. Acute poisoning in children; changes over the years, data of pediatric clinic department of toxicology. *J Acute Dis.* 2014;3:56-58.

Manzar N, et al. The study of etiological and demographic characteristics of acute household accidental poisoning in children—a consecutive case series study from Pakistan. *BMC Pediatr.* 2010;10:28.

Principles of Epidemiology and Research Design

137

QUESTIONS

137.1. Which of the following options best describes the Grading of Recommendations, Assessment, Development, and Evaluation (GRADE) framework?
  A. It provides a mathematical method for assessing the degree of consensus
  B. It provides a framework for communicating the strength of evidence
  C. It provides a checklist to help write more reproducible guidelines
  D. It provides an organized flow sheet to describe how articles are included in a systematic review
  E. It provides an organized flow sheet to describe how patients are included in a research study

137.2. Which of the following options best describes the Bradford Hill Criteria?
  A. They are a scientific method used to rate the quality of research
  B. They are a set of questions used to help determine consensus
  C. They are a scientific method to determine the best statistical test to analyze data
  D. They are a set of questions to help determine causation between events
  E. They are a scientific method to determine if data are best fit as a normal distribution

137.3. Which of the following options best describes the difference between a case-control study and a cohort study?
  A. Cohort studies are always retrospective in nature
  B. Well-designed case-control studies assign causation

  C. Case-control studies are valuable for evaluating rare events
  D. Case-control studies follow patients from exposure to illness
  E. Cohort studies start with an outcome of interest

137.4. Which of the following options best describes odds ratio and relative risk?
  A. Odds ratio is typically used for cohort studies
  B. The relative risk is a mathematic approximation of the odds ratio
  C. The odds ratio and the relative risk are essentially the same estimation in different study designs
  D. The odds ratio approximates the relative risk when an outcome is rare
  E. The odds ratio is a better description of the true strength of association

137.5. Sensitivity is best defined as which of the following options?
  A. The prevalence of positive tests among diseased individuals
  B. The prevalence of negative tests among diseased individuals
  C. The prevalence of disease in patients who test positive
  D. The absence of disease in patients who test negative
  E. A measure of the ability of a test to provide the same answer when repeated

137.6. Specificity is best defined as which of the following options?

A. The prevalence of positive tests among diseased individuals

B. The prevalence of negative tests among nondiseased individuals

C. The prevalence of disease in patients who test positive

D. The absence of disease in patients who test negative

E. A measure of the ability of a test to provide the same answer when repeated

137.7. Positive predictive value is best defined as which of the following options?

A. The prevalence of positive tests among diseased individuals

B. The prevalence of negative tests among nondiseased individuals

C. The prevalence of disease in patients who test positive

D. The absence of disease in patients who test negative

E. A measure of the ability of a test to provide the same answer when repeated

137.8. Negative predictive value is best defined as which of the following options?

A. The prevalence of positive tests among diseased individuals

B. The prevalence of negative tests among nondiseased individuals

C. The prevalence of disease in patients who test positive

D. The absence of disease in patients who test negative

E. A measure of the ability of a test to provide the same answer when repeated

137.9. Which of the following options is an example of a type 2 statistical error?

A. An interim analysis of a study found a statistical difference on the first few patients that ultimately turned out to be wrong

B. A study concluded that there was no difference but did not include enough data to be sure that the null hypothesis could not be rejected

C. Analysis of a randomized controlled trial discovered that randomization left the two study groups different in important baseline characteristics

D. A randomized controlled trial produced different results when the intention-to-treat analysis was compared to analysis by actual treatment

E. Study investigators have reason to believe that blinding was improperly concealed

137.10. Which of the following options is an example of a type 1 statistical error?

A. An interim analysis of a study found a statistical difference on the first few patients that ultimately turned out to be wrong

B. A study concluded that there was no difference but did not include enough data to be sure that the null hypothesis could not be rejected

C. Analysis of a randomized controlled trial discovered that randomization left the two study groups different in important baseline characteristics

D. A randomized controlled trial produced different results when the intention-to-treat analysis was compared to analysis by actual treatment

E. Study investigators have reason to believe that blinding was improperly concealed

ANSWERS

137.1. Answer: B. The Grading of Recommendations, Assessment, Development, and Evaluation (GRADE) Working Group provides a framework for assessing and communicating levels of scientific evidence. Typically, evidence is divided into four levels of quality (high, moderate, low, very low) based on predefined reproducible methods. This allows readers of systematic reviews and meta-analyses to better understand the basis for practice recommendations. Choice A refers to techniques such as the Rand/UCLA method. Choice C refers to the AGREE checklist. Choices D and E refer to the PRIMA and CONSORT tools, respectively.

Kavanagh BP. The GRADE system for rating clinical guidelines. *PLoS Med.* 2009;6:e1000094.

137.2. Answer: D. The Bradford Hill Criteria were proposed in 1965 as a set of questions to help determine if there was a causal link between observations. Questions include items such as strength of relationship, consistency, temporality, and biological plausibility. The more items that are fulfilled, the more likely there is a causal relationship between observed events.

Hill AB. The environment and disease: Association or causation? *Proc R Soc Med*. 1965;58:295-300.

137.3. **Answer: C.** Both case-control and cohort studies are examples of observational studies and, as such, suggest associations but are generally insufficiently robust to assign causation. A case-control study is a retrospective analysis of patients separated by outcome of interest. Since the outcome is defined, this study type is very useful for rare events. In contrast, a cohort study begins with an exposure and follows patients until an outcome develops.

Gamble J. An Introduction to the fundamentals of cohort and case–control studies. *Can J Hosp Pharm*. 2014;67:366-372.

Song JW, Chung KC. Observational studies: Cohort and case-control studies. *Plast Reconstr Surg*. 2010;126:2234-2242.

137.4. **Answer: D.** The relative risk represents a prospective analysis of events in a cohort study. Since many studies are retrospective, an odds ratio is the more appropriate measure. When event rates are small, the odds ratio tends to approximate the relative risk well.

Schmidt CO, Kohlmann T. When to use the odds ratio or the relative risk? *Int J Public Health*. 2008;53:165-167.

137.5. **Answer: A.** The sensitivity of a test is best defined as the prevalence of positive tests among diseased individuals. It is calculated by dividing true-positive (TP) tests by the sum of TP plus false-negative (FN) tests: TP/(TP + FN). In doing so, it only looks at the sum of diseased individuals. Choice B is specificity, choice C is positive predictive value, choice D is the negative predictive value, and choice E is precision.

Buderer NM. Statistical methodology: I. Incorporating the prevalence of disease into the sample size calculation for sensitivity and specificity. *Acad Emerg Med*. 1996;3:895-900.

137.6. **Answer: B.** Specificity is the prevalence of negative tests among nondiseased individuals. It is calculated by dividing true-negative (TN) tests by the sum of TN plus false-positive (FP) tests: TN/(TN + FP). Choice A is sensitivity, choice C is positive predictive value, choice D is the negative predictive value, and choice E is precision.

Buderer NM. Statistical methodology: I. Incorporating the prevalence of disease into the sample size calculation for sensitivity and specificity. *Acad Emerg Med*. 1996;3:895-900.

137.7. **Answer: C.** The positive predictive value is defined as the prevalence of disease in patients who test positive. It is determined from all the positive tests as follows: true positives/(true positives + false positives). Choices A and B are sensitivity and specificity, respectively; choice D is the negative predictive value; and choice E is precision.

Buderer NM. Statistical methodology: I. Incorporating the prevalence of disease into the sample size calculation for sensitivity and specificity. *Acad Emerg Med*. 1996;3:895-900.

137.8. **Answer: D.** The negative predictive value is defined as the absence of disease in patients who test negative. It is determined from all the negative tests as follows: true negatives/(true negatives + false negatives). Choices A and B are sensitivity and specificity, respectively; choice C is the positive predictive value; and choice E is precision.

Buderer NM. Statistical methodology: I. Incorporating the prevalence of disease into the sample size calculation for sensitivity and specificity. *Acad Emerg Med*. 1996;3:895-900.

137.9. **Answer: B.** Type 2 (or beta) statistical error occurs when a study that fails to find a difference is underpowered to be certain of its findings. A sample size calculation should be done before the study is started to assure that an adequate number of events is recorded. A power analysis will drive that calculation and can be done post hoc to assess a completed study.

Banerjee A, et al. Hypothesis testing, type I and type II errors. *Ind Psychiatry J*. 2009;18:127-131.

137.10. **Answer: A.** Type 1 (or alpha) statistical error occurs when a study wrongfully rejects the null hypothesis. This sometimes occurs during interim analyses of larger studies. It would be correct, under most circumstances, to continue the study to the targeted sample size to assure that the findings are correct.

Banerjee A, et al. Hypothesis testing, type I and type II errors. *Ind Psychiatry J*. 2009;18:127-131.

Risk Management and Legal Principles

QUESTIONS

138.1. Which of the following options is included in the definition of informed consent?
- A. The patient must comprehend the risks of not receiving treatment
- B. Suicidal patients are allowed to refuse definitive interventions
- C. Informed consent must be obtained in all situations, including emergent presentations
- D. The patient must comprehend exceptionally rare risks not commonly known to the medical community
- E. Personal autonomy can be overridden by a physician if they are acting in the best interest of a patient

138.2. A 27-year-old man presents to the emergency department after being found naked in the street. He is confused and combative. The patient is declining all medical intervention and is attempting to leave the hospital. Which of the following interventions should the emergency physician perform next?
- A. Review the hospital policy on refusal of treatment
- B. Allow the patient to leave the emergency department
- C. Restrain the patient
- D. Contact the risk management department
- E. Contact a family member

138.3. A 67-year-old man is refusing care in the emergency department. Which of the following interventions is reasonable to perform next?

- A. Consult psychiatry to assess for capacity
- B. Contact the risk management department
- C. Honor the patient's right to refuse treatment without further inquiry
- D. Temporarily detain the patient while assessing the patient's understanding of the necessity for treatment
- E. Notify hospital police that the patient needs to be detained and restrained

138.4. It is acceptable to discharge a patient with an elevated blood alcohol concentration in which of the following scenarios?
- A. A patient with alcohol use disorder who is clinically sober with an ethanol concentration of 200 mg/dL (43.4 mmol/L) who is walking home
- B. A 2-year-old boy who has an ethanol concentration of 80 mg/dL (17.4 mmol/L) to the care of his parents
- C. A patient who is ambulating steadily with an ethanol concentration of 100 mg/dL (21.7 mmol/L) who is intending to drive home
- D. A clinically intoxicated 22-year-old-woman into the care of a man who was with her on a first date
- E. A 32-year-old man who is slurring his speech and has obvious signs of head trauma but who is accompanied by his family who are sober

138.5. A 29-year-old woman is brought in by police because they had witnessed her ingesting several drug packets. The patient is awake and alert and is declining further medical evaluation. Which of the following is a reasonable treatment approach in this patient?

A. Sedate patient to obtain blood work as incarcerated patients do not have capacity

B. If the police have a warrant, physicians are required to perform an endoscopy and submit over any drug packets

C. Admit the patient for observation, but respect her wishes to not perform a physical examination

D. Call the patient's family to obtain consent

E. Discharge the patient immediately to police custody

138.6. A 27-year-old man is stopped by police for a concern of driving while intoxicated. Which of the following options is true regarding performing an ethanol breath test (EBT) in the United States?

A. Only a control must be performed prior to breath alcohol analysis

B. A control analysis is performed on a liquid ethanol sample of known concentration prior to an EBT

C. A 20-minute window of alcohol deprivation is required prior to an EBT

D. Any police officer is able to perform an EBT

E. EBT results are not admissible in court

138.7. Which of the following options is required to constitute a medical malpractice case in the United States?

A. A limited amount of evidence that deviation from accepted practice occurred

B. It is unnecessary that a patient–physician relationship was established prior to the case

C. A negligent act occurred, even if it did not proximately cause the patient's injury

D. A patient dies despite a physician performing standard care

E. An act of omission occurred prior to the patient's injury

138.8. Which of the following options should alert a physician that their colleague is hiding a substance use disorder?

A. Multiple tattoos

B. Working an isolated night schedule

C. Drinking several drinks of alcohol at an annual holiday party

D. Multiple sick call activations in a short period of time

E. Frequently sending text messages and invitations to social events to work colleagues

139.9. A 27-year-old physician presents to the emergency department clinically intoxicated. Which of the following options violates the US Health Insurance Portability and Accountability Act (HIPAA)?

A. Reporting the ingestion to the poison control center

B. A pharmacist in the hospital accesses the chart to dispense thiamine

C. A health care clearinghouse accesses the patient's records to create a bill

D. An adverse medication reaction that occurs as part of her care is reported to MedWatch

E. Her close friend, who is an emergency physician at the hospital, accesses her chart to ensure that she gets appropriate care

138.10. A 22-year-old man presents to the emergency department in respiratory arrest following an intentional overdose of methadone. Following intravenous administration of naloxone, the patient wakes up agitated and demands to be discharged immediately. Which of the following management strategies would be the best treatment strategy in this patient?

A. Allow the patient to immediately leave the emergency department

B. Discharge the patient with a take-home naloxone kit

C. Administer naltrexone and then discharge the patient

D. Temporarily restrain the patient and hold in the emergency department

E. Administer a dose of methadone to treat his withdrawal

ANSWERS

138.1. Answer: A. The basic elements of informed consent include an explanation of the treatment or the procedure, disclosure of alternative choices to the proposed intervention, a discussion of the relevant risks, benefits, and uncertainties associated with each alternative, and disclosure of the likely outcome with the various treatment options, including the choice of no treatment. Suicidal patients are deemed to not have capacity and, in most states, are unable to refuse definitive interventions. Informed consent is implied in emergent presentations in which immediate, life-saving procedures are needed. It is not necessary for patients to understand exceptionally rare risks not commonly known in the medical community. Personal autonomy cannot be overridden by a physician, even if they believe they are acting in the best interest of the patient.

Walter P. The doctrine of informed consent: To inform or not to inform? *St John's Law Rev.* 1997;71:543-589.

138.2. Answer: C. This patient is presenting with obvious signs of impairment, and it is not safe to allow this patient to be discharged from the emergency department at this time. The ability of a hospital to retain and physically restrain a person who has an altered level of consciousness for evaluation and emergency intervention is generally well supported by state statutes and case law. The use of restraints should be reserved for patients who have life-threatening conditions with impaired judgement and an inability to understand the consequences of their actions. Physical restraints should be used for the shortest possible time and are usually replaced by sedation. While reviewing the hospital policy on refusal of treatment, contacting risk management, and contacting a family member are often reasonable later in the care of this patient, the immediate next step involves restraining the patient so further medical evaluation is performed.

Gatter R. Informed consent law and the forgotten duty of physician inquiry. *Loyola Univ Chicago Law J.* 1999;31:557-597.

138.3. Answer: D. Patients who are refusing further care in the emergency department should be temporarily detained to further understand the reason for their refusal. A Jehovah's Witness patient will often refuse a blood transfusion, even if their life is in jeopardy. It is not necessary to consult psychiatry to assess all patients for capacity. Depending on what else is going on in the patient's presentation, contacting risk management is reasonable; however, this is rare, and the first step is to assess why the patient is refusing care. Physically restraining a patient should be reserved only for patients who have a condition that is imminently life-threatening and are unable to comprehend the consequences of their actions. Often, verbal de-escalation and open communication are sufficient to assess whether a patient has capacity and to calm most agitated patients.

Schloendorff v Society of New York Hospital, 211 NY 125, 105, NE (1914).

138.4. Answer: A. Patients with an alcohol use disorder are often clinically sober despite elevated ethanol concentrations, and it is reasonable to discharge these patients when they are clinically sober as opposed to waiting until their blood ethanol concentration drops below a certain value, as these patients are likely to develop alcohol withdrawal despite being at concentrations that are above the *per se* legal limit for driving in the US. It is prudent, however, to ensure that, despite apparent clinical sobriety, the patient will not be driving. Children, especially young children, should be admitted overnight for observation when they present with an elevated ethanol concentration as they have a risk of developing hypoglycemia due to their limited glycogen stores. Furthermore, investigation to evaluate for potential abuse or neglect is indicated. It is best to observe patients who are intoxicated until they are sober or until a trusted family member or friend is available to take them home. As the relationship is not clearly established with this young woman in choice D, it would be best to not discharge her into his care. Patients who present with alcohol intoxication and have concomitant signs of head trauma should be evaluated for underlying signs of intracranial injury that mimics clinical intoxication.

Davis AR, Lipson AH. Central nervous system tolerance to high blood alcohol levels. *Med J Aust.* 1986;144:9-12.

138.5. Answer: C. Patients who are under police custody continue to have capacity to refuse medical interventions and maintain the right to choose a personal course of medical treatment. If this person had an altered mental status or had respiratory depression, the physician would need to perform emergent procedures. It is not appropriate to sedate this patient to perform blood work or an invasive procedure without this patient's consent as this would be assault. It is not appropriate to bypass this patient's autonomy and contact the family to obtain consent. As this patient was witnessed to ingest drug packets and rupture could be life-threatening, it would not be appropriate to immediately discharge the patient to police custody. It is reasonable to admit the patient for observation alone; that way, if the patient develops signs of toxicity from a leaking drug packet, then the physician would be able to intervene at that time and perform life-saving procedures.

https://leginfo.legislature.ca.gov/faces/billTextClient.xhtml?bill_id=201520160AB1423. Accessed August 4, 2021.

138.6. Answer: C. A 15- to 20-minute window of complete alcohol deprivation (including no vomiting or belching) is required prior to performing an ethanol breath test. Any ethanol in the mouth will lead to a false elevation in the result. Ethanol breath tests are admissible in court, but to be admissible, they need to be performed by a trained and certified operator. Both a blank and a control analysis need to be performed prior to a breath alcohol analysis. A control analysis is performed on a gas ethanol sample of known

Harding P, Zettl JR. Methods for breath analysis. In: Garriott JC, ed. *Garriott's Medicolegal Aspects of Alcohol.* Tucson, AZ: Lawyers and Judges Publishing Company, Inc; 2008:229-253.

concentration. Drunk driving laws vary from state to state in the United States and among countries. Clinicians should be aware of their local laws.

138.7. Answer: E. For a case to constitute a medical malpractice case in the United States, there needs to be a preponderance of evidence that deviation from accepted practice occurred. A physician–patient relationship needs to have been established. A negligent act or an act of omission has to occur as a proximate cause of the patient's injury. Even if a patient dies or has a bad outcome, as long as the physician followed accepted practice, that does not necessarily constitute a malpractice case.

Vialva v City of New York, 118 AD 2d. 701, 499, NY 2d 977 (2nd Dept 1986).

138.8. Answer: D. Often health care workers are very adept at hiding a substance use disorder until it becomes severe. Signs that should alert a physician that their colleague is hiding a substance use disorder include deteriorating social and interpersonal behaviors, inaccessibility to patients and staff, frequent conflicts with staff members, unexplained absenteeism, and frequent moves to different jobs and locations. Multiple tattoos, earrings, and choice of dress do not point to a substance use disorder and imply a bias. Working an isolated night schedule is a personal preference and does not mean a physician has a substance use disorder. If a health care worker is neither working nor on call, ethanol is legal, and drinking several drinks at an isolated social event does not imply a substance use disorder.

Sudan R, Seymour K. The impaired surgeon. *Surg Clin North Am.* 2016;96:89-93.

138.9. Answer: E. HIPAA was enacted by the US Congress in 1996 to increase the portability of health insurance and to allow employees to maintain insurance when they switch jobs.

However, the Privacy Rule of HIPAA is the most publicized part of this act. There are stringent rules that protect a patient's medical records and who is able to access their chart. Only health care workers who are actively managing a patient's care should access a patient's chart. Even if a person is a close friend and is accessing a chart to help, that violates the patient's privacy. Reporting an ingestion to the poison control center is not a violation of HIPAA and is, in fact, legally required in certain states. A pharmacist dispensing thiamine is part of the patient's care. A health care clearinghouse is able to access a patient's medical records to create a bill, and this does not violate HIPAA. Reporting an adverse medication reaction to MedWatch also does not violate the HIPAA Privacy Rule.

Health Insurance Portability and Accessibility Act of 1996, Pub No L104-191, 110, Stat 1936 (1996). See also 45 CFR 160, 164 (2002).

138.10. Answer: D. Methadone is a long-acting opioid, and naloxone usually works for approximately 30-45 minutes. As the opioid this patient ingested is in the patient's system for much longer than the antidote, there is a real concern that this patient will leave the hospital and develop recurrent respiratory arrest. Allowing the patient to immediately leave the emergency department is not prudent. Often, verbal de-escalation is sufficient to convince patients to remain in the emergency department for longer observation. Rarely, it is necessary to temporally restrain a patient and hold them until the opioid is no longer in their system. While eventually ensuring that the patient is discharged with a naloxone kit is appropriate, that should only be performed when the medical risk of the acute opioid overdose has resolved. Naltrexone should not be given to a patient who has a recent opioid overdose as naltrexone puts patients at risk of developing life-threatening precipitated opioid withdrawal. Administering a dose of methadone would not be correct in this patient as the naloxone will wear off and he will now have an even greater quantity of long-acting opioids in his system.

Vilke GM, et al. Assessment for deaths in out-of-hospital heroin overdose patients treated with naloxone who refuse transport. *Acad Emerg Med.* 2003;10:893-896.

Medicolegal Interpretive Toxicology

139

QUESTIONS

139.1. A 27-year-old asymptomatic man states that he was poisoned by brodifacoum. Blood work is performed, and he has an elevated international normalized ratio (INR) of 2.2. Which of the following options demonstrates the most likely preanalytical factor that could affect the interpretation of these results?
A. The specimen was drawn in a collection tube that contains a preservative
B. The specimen tube was not filled completely
C. Ethanol-based swabs were used to clean the skin prior to administration
D. There was a significant ingestion of green leafy vegetables
E. The specimen was drawn off an intravenous line as opposed to a direct blood draw

139.2. A murder victim has significant opioid concentrations detected in his postmortem bile. He has a negligible concentration of opioids in his blood. Which of the following best explains this finding?
A. The person injected heroin immediately prior to his death
B. The person was poisoned with large amounts of morphine in his food
C. The person took too many of his prescribed oxycodone
D. The person had systemic absorption from a topically applied opioid
E. This finding provides no interpretive data

139.3. The appropriate chain of evidence for a blood specimen collection includes which of the following options?
A. No one can see the blood specimen being drawn
B. Only key personnel involved in the handling of the specimen must be identified
C. An intoxicated patient cannot have a blood specimen drawn, even if they assent to the procedure
D. Specimens are admissible in court if a break in custody occurs if that break is documented
E. Every individual who handles the specimen should sign the accompanying document

139.4. A 27-year-old man presents to the emergency department with suspected cocaine use. His urine drug screen is negative. Which of the following options would still be consistent with a true-negative result?
A. Analysis of the urine sample > 12 hours after specimen collection
B. Addition of bleach, glutaraldehyde, or ammonia to the specimen
C. Substitution of the patient's urine with the urine of an animal or another person
D. Ingestion of baking soda or vinegar before urination
E. Presence of cocaine at concentrations below assay detection limits

139.5. A 29-year-old man is brought into the emergency department after sustaining a gunshot wound to the chest and subsequently dies. His urine drug screen is positive for benzodiazepines, and a toxicologist is called to assist with interpretation of the results. Which of the following options best explains this finding?
  A. The benzodiazepines contributed to this patient dying
  B. The results are a false positive from a cross-reaction
  C. The urine was from another patient
  D. The results are due to post-mortem redistribution
  E. The urine drug screen is irrelevant to this person's death

139.6. Which of the following options is correct regarding hair testing for medicolegal interpretive toxicology?
  A. Hair should be collected immediately following exposure
  B. Only hair from the scalp is accurate
  C. The root ends should be identified by tying with a string or wrapping with a foil
  D. Rinsing the hair prior to testing is contraindicated as it invalidates results
  E. Two to three strands of hair are sufficient for testing

139.7. A 45-year-old man is found dead in his basement. A vitreous potassium is performed and results at 11 mmol/L. Which of the following best explains this finding?
  A. The patient died from rhabdomyolysis
  B. This specimen has significant hemolysis

  C. This is consistent with severe digoxin toxicity
  D. A vitreous to serum potassium ratio is diagnostic
  E. This vitreous potassium is within normal limits

139.8. Which of the following options best describes the Mellanby effect?
  A. When the kinetics of a certain xenobiotic switches from being first order to zero order
  B. The clinical effect of ethanol intoxication is greater during the absorptive phase than the elimination phase
  C. The effect of the xenobiotic continues or occasionally increases even as the serum concentration decreases
  D. The dose makes the poison
  E. A dose–response effect that results in a J-shaped curve

139.9. Which of the following compartments is expected to contain the highest concentration of phencyclidine during acute toxicity?
  A. Intravascular
  B. Skin
  C. Muscle
  D. Central nervous system
  E. Bone

139.10. Which of the following pieces of information should be gathered to accurately interpret analytical findings?
  A. Individual history
  B. Medical history
  C. Cohabitants
  D. Recent activity
  E. All of the above

ANSWERS

139.1 Answer: B. Major sources of error in analytical toxicology are based not on laboratory error, but on preanalytical issues, which are defined as those events that affect an analytical result prior to the specimen arriving at the laboratory. The INR is measured in blood drawn in a collection tube that contains 3.2% buffered sodium citrate. As such, incomplete filling of the specimen tube leads to a falsely elevated INR.

https://www.labcorp.com/resource/blood-specimens-coagulation. Accessed August 12, 2021.

139.2. Answer: E. Certain xenobiotics that are eliminated fecally, like opioids, accumulate in the bile. Therefore, opioids remain in the bile after clearance from the blood. Concentrations in the bile are difficult to interpret as the presence of a xenobiotic does not necessarily provide temporal information for an exposure.

Pounder DJ, Jones GR. Post-mortem drug redistribution—a toxicological nightmare. *Forensic Sci Int.* 1990;45:253-263.

139.3. Answer: E. The appropriate chain of evidence for blood specimen collection must be maintained in order for the results to be admissible in court. The specimen must be obtained in full view of a witness. Any person in the United States who operates a motor vehicle is considered to have consented to a test to determine alcohol or drug ingestion. Every person involved in the handling of the specimen must be identified. Each step of the process and transport of the specimen must be documented without a break in the custody of the specimen. Every individual who handles the specimen should sign the accompanying document.

Smith ML, et al. Quality assurance in drug testing laboratories. *Clin Lab Med*. 1990;10:503-516.

139.4.　Answer: A. Most drugs are stable in the urine; therefore, analysis performed > 12 hours after collection should still be accurate. The chances of a false-negative urine drug test are increased by ingestion of weak acids or bases, dilution of specimens, adulteration of samples with one or more interfering substances, or substitution of one specimen for another.

Mikkelson SL, Ash KO. Adulterants causing false negatives in illicit drug testing. *Clin Chem*. 1988;34:2333-2336.

139.5.　Answer: E. Urine drug screens need to be interpreted in conjunction with a patient's current presentation. While this patient's urine drug screen is likely a true positive, it only indicates that he had been exposed to benzodiazepines at some point in the last few days. It does not necessarily correspond to current toxicity, and it certainly has no relevance in a patient who sustained a lethal gunshot wound.

Moeller KE, et al. Clinical interpretation of urine drug tests: What clinicians need to know about urine drug screens. *Mayo Clin Proc*. 2017;92:774-796.

139.6.　Answer: C. Hair testing provides an alternative specimen that has a longer window of detection. Analytical precautions, such as rinsing procedures, are used to minimize some concerns with hair testing. Waiting 1-3 months before collecting hair will capture the potential exposure period in growing hair. Collection of hair should be from the posterior vertex of the head; however, virtually any other source of hair is also acceptable for testing, including pubic and axillary hair, although they do have limitations, including shorter growth rates. About a pencil thickness worth of hair should be clipped as closely to the scalp as possible. The root ends should be identified either by tying with string or wrapping in foil.

Dolan K, et al. An overview of the use of urine, hair, sweat and saliva to detect drug use. *Drug Alcohol Rev*. 2004;23:213-217.

139.7.　Answer: E. A vitreous potassium of < 15 mmol/L is normal. The postmortem interval affects the vitreous potassium. Normal postmortem vitreous concentrations are as follows: chloride, 105-135 mmol/L; sodium, 135-150 mmol/L; and urea nitrogen, 8-20 mmol/L.

Collins K. Postmortem vitreous analyses. Medscape. http://emedicine.medscape.com/article/1966150-overview. Accessed March 12, 2014.

139.8.　Answer: B. The Mellanby effect is also known as acute tolerance. The central nervous system effects of ethanol intoxication are typically more pronounced on the ascending portion of the ethanol kinetic curve than on the descending side due to acute tolerance. The clinical effect of intoxication is greater during the absorptive arm of the kinetic curve than on the elimination arm, even though the same blood ethanol concentration is measured in both kinetic phases. Choice A describes Michaelis-Menten kinetics. Choice C describes hysteresis. Choice D is a classic quote attributed to Paracelsus. Choice E describes hormesis.

Garriott JC, Manno JE. Pharmacology and toxicology of ethyl alcohol. In: Garriott JC, ed. *Garriott's Medicolegal Aspects of Alcohol*. 5th ed. Tucson, AZ: Lawyers and Judges Publishing Company, Inc; 2008:25-46.

139.9.　Answer: D. The concentration of phencyclidine (PCP) in the central nervous system, as evidenced by the cerebral spinal fluid concentrations, is four times greater than in the plasma. Phencyclidine is extremely lipophilic and would not be expected to be found in greater concentrations in the bone, muscle, or skin compartments.

Jackson EJ. Phencyclidine pharmacokinetics after a massive overdose. *Ann Intern Med*. 1989;111:613-615.

139.10.　Answer: E. Important aspects of the case history need to be ascertained to accurately interpret analytic finding. This includes the individual history, including age, gender, and hobbies; the patient's medical history; the patient's recent activity; and the timing of when the event occurred. How much time passed between the event and specimen collection should also be evaluated. Documentation of cohabitants, including their vocations and medication, in addition to a description of the scene, the position and description of the body, and any notes and journals are also useful to accurately interpret any analytic findings.

Flanagan RJ, Connally G. Interpretation of analytical toxicology results in life and at postmortem. *Toxicol Rev*. 2005;24:51-62.

QUESTIONS

140.1. In the first 3 days after death, which of the following biochemical values remains relatively stable in the blood?
A. Aspartate aminotransferase
B. Sodium
C. Ammonia
D. Cholinesterases
E. Glucose

140.2. A 41-year-old woman has died of suspected streptozocin toxicity. Rapid sampling of glucose from which of the following sites is most likely to provide supportive information?
A. Vitreous humor
B. Femoral blood
C. Right heart blood
D. Cerebrospinal fluid
E. Bile

140.3. A 44-year-old woman is found dead at home after not being seen for 4 days. She has a history of depression and was on a stable dose of amitriptyline for many years. Site investigation shows no evidence of foul play, and a medication bottle is found and contains an amount of amitriptyline consistent with use as prescribed. Although a forensic autopsy in unable to find a cause of death, toxicology analysis of right heart blood reveals an amitriptyline concentration of 1,200 ng/mL (4,326 nmol/L) and a nortriptyline concentration of 800 ng/mL (3,038 nmol/L). The therapeutic range for the combined concentrations is reported in a reference of up to 200 ng/mL. Which of the following statements best explains these findings?

A. The patient was chronically overmedicated and ultimately died
B. The patient stored up her pills and took an acute overdose
C. Postmortem redistribution increased the concentration in the blood
D. Proximity to the stomach led to a massive rise in postmortem blood from the last pill ingested
E. She was poisoned from another source of medication

140.4. The body of an adult man of unknown age is found badly decomposed in a field. Which of the following samples might provide the most useful toxicologic analysis to support a diagnosis of acute overdose or poisoning by homicide?
A. Bone
B. Dirt surrounding the body
C. Plants growing next to the body
D. Fingernails
E. Pupal casings left from flies that consumed the body

140.5. A 60-year-old man is found dead in his car with a suicide note. Based on the note and a scene investigation, it is estimated that he has been dead for >24 hours. He had access to glyburide, metformin, spironolactone, and oxycodone. Which of the following results would be most likely to support a toxicologic cause of death?
A. A vitreous glucose of 9 mg/dL (0.5 mmol/L)
B. A blood carboxyhemoglobin of 48%
C. A blood lactate concentration of 22 mmol/L
D. An oxycodone concentration three times greater than the reported upper limit of therapeutic in femoral blood
E. A blood potassium concentration of 12 mEq/L

140.6. A 66-year-old woman with end-stage kidney disease and metastatic cancer is found dead at home after a 1-day diarrheal illness. The patient was maintained only on an opioid for chronic pain and a beta adrenergic antagonist for hypertension. A local coroner decides that the death was natural, and no autopsy is performed. After the body was taken to a funeral home, embalmed, and buried, a family member claims the decedent was poisoned by her husband to collect her life insurance. A court orders that the body is exhumed 10 days later. Which of the following toxicologic results is expected to be reliable?

   A. A vitreous methanol concentration determined by gas chromatography
   B. An immunoassay of muscle for digoxin
   C. Hair for thallium
   D. Nails for arsenic
   E. Vitreous colchicine by gas chromatography–mass spectroscopy

140.7. After cremation, which of the following toxicologic analyses is still possible?

   A. Cocaine
   B. Lead
   C. Phenobarbital
   D. Cyanide
   E. Ethyl glucuronide

140.8. The body of a badly decomposed adult man is found floating in a river. Which of the following findings is most supportive of a diagnosis of postmortem ethanol formation?

   A. Ethanol in the vitreous but not in the urine or the blood
   B. Ethanol in the urine but not in the vitreous or the blood
   C. Ethanol in the blood but not in the urine or the vitreous
   D. Ethanol in the blood and urine but not in the vitreous
   E. Ethanol in the vitreous and urine but not in the blood

140.9. A 64-year-old man with a history of diabetes, hypertension, kidney disease, and hyperlipidemia is maintained on a stable dose of nortriptyline for neuropathic pain. He is found dead in his bed with no apparent cause. The local coroner certifies that the death was due to natural causes and the body is embalmed and prepared for burial. A family member is concerned and petitions a judge who orders toxicologic testing, which returns showing amitriptyline but no nortriptyline. The family begins legal proceedings against the pharmacy for dispensing the wrong medication. Which of the following events is most likely?

   A. The family is correct; the pharmacy dispensed amitriptyline instead of nortriptyline
   B. All of the nortriptyline was metabolized to amitriptyline before death
   C. All of the nortriptyline was metabolized to amitriptyline during the postmortem interval
   D. Formaldehyde converted nortriptyline to amitriptyline
   E. Nortriptyline was metabolized to amitriptyline by bacterial decomposition

140.10. A 22-year-old man was brought to the hospital after being found wildly agitated. He had a history of substance use disorder and schizophrenia. He was noncompliant with his psychiatric medication and had a previous admission for acute cocaine toxicity. On arrival, the patient had the following vital signs: blood pressure, 80/40 mmHg; pulse, 188 beats/min; respirations, 26 breaths/min; and core temperature, 109.6 °F (43.1 °C). Despite intubation, sedation, rapid cooling, and volume resuscitation, the patient died the day after presentation of disseminated intravascular coagulopathy, shock, and cerebral edema. The medical examiner requests residual antemortem blood as part of the forensic analysis. Only a sample of spun serum was available for testing. Standard toxicology testing performed 5 days after death reveals the presence of benzodiazepines, benzoyl ecgonine, delta-9-tetrahydrocannabinol but no cocaine is detected. Which of the following statements best explains these findings?

   A. The patient used marijuana and cocaine in the recent past, but neither is likely responsible for the acute hyperthermia
   B. Marijuana likely contributed to an agitated delirium and hyperthermia
   C. Primary psychiatric agitation is excluded by the drug use
   D. The toxicology testing likely missed the responsible drug
   E. Parent cocaine that was present antemortem was metabolized to benzoyl ecgonine in the serum as it waited for analysis

ANSWERS

140.1. Answer: D. In the early postmortem interval, defined as the first 3 days after death, there are many biochemical changes in the blood and some values increase (aspartate aminotransferase, ammonia), some values decrease (glucose, sodium), and a few others remain stable, such as cholinesterases.

Spitz WU, ed. *Spitz's and Fischer's Medicolegal Investigation of Death.* Springfield, IL: Charles C. Thomas; 1993.

140.2. Answer: A. Streptazocin leads to destruction of pancreatic beta islet cells with resultant hyperglycemia. Glucose rapidly falls in most compartments during the postmortem interval, as red blood cells and ultimately bacteria consume remaining stores. However, the vitreous humor is a relatively protected environment, and the expected hyperglycemia would likely persist.

Choo-Kang E, et al. Vitreous humor analytes in assessing the postmortem interval and the antemortem clinical status. *West Med J.* 1983;32:23-26.

Daae LN, et al. Determination of glucose in human vitreous humor. *J Legal Med.* 1978;80:287-290.

140.3. Answer: C. Postmortem redistribution is more common with xenobiotics with large volumes of distribution and results from release into the extracellular space. Blood concentrations rapidly rise over a few hours, as in the case of cyclic antidepressants, potentially leading to a false conclusion.

Apple FS, Bandt CM. Liver and blood postmortem tricyclic antidepressant concentrations. *Am J Clin Pathol.* 1988;89:794-796.

140.4. Answer: E. Insects, such as the common blow fly, are attracted to the smell of dead tissue and lay eggs there. The larva that hatch feed off of the cadaver, and when they pupate, they leave casings around the body that are used for toxicologic analysis. Although bone and fingernails persist in decomposed bodies, their toxicologic analysis is more likely to be reflective of chronic exposures than acute toxicity.

Amendt J, et al. Forensic entomology. *Naturwissenschaften.* 2004; 91:51-56.

Goff ML, Lord WD. Entomotoxicology. A new area for forensic investigation. *Am J Forensic Med Pathol.* 1994;15:51-57.

140.5. Answer: B. Because of the strong affinity of carbon monoxide for hemoglobin, the carboxyhemoglobin concentration remains stable for an extensive period postmortem. Concentrations of glucose fall, even in vitreous humor, and concentrations of potassium and lactate rise because of anaerobic glycolysis and cell lysis. While postmortem analysis of opioids provides reproducible results, no postmortem test can assess tolerance. Someone who is dependent on opioids survives concentrations far more than those reported with short-term therapy.

Kunsman GW, et al. Carbon monoxide stability in stored postmortem blood samples. *J Anal Toxicol.* 2000;24:572-578.

140.6. Answer: E. When a body is prepared for burial and embalmed, many subsequent sources for toxicologic analysis are lost. While hair and nails are used to assess chronic exposure, it is unlikely that there is any deposition immediately after an overdose. In a patient with chronic kidney disease, an immunoassay might falsely identify an endogenous digoxinlike substance. Interestingly, there is at least one reported false-positive methanol test that resulted from formalin exposure during the embalming process. As the patient had no reason to be on colchicine, the finding of colchicine in the vitreous fluid would be highly suspicious, especially given that colchicine toxicity presents as severe diarrhea. Colchicine is known to enter the eye following oral administration.

Lemor M, et al. Oral colchicine for the treatment of experimental traction retinal detachment. *Arch Ophthalmol.* 1986;10:1226-1229.

Caughlin J. An unusual source for postmortem findings of methyl ethyl ketone and methanol in two homicide victims. *Forensic Sci Int.* 1994;67:27-31.

140.7. Answer: B. Cremation is a highly destructive process that leaves a fine powder residue. Most organics will be destroyed by the high temperatures used, but there is some evidence to support metal testing of cremated remains.

Barry M. Metal residues after cremation. *BMJ.* 1994;308:390.

140.8. Answer: C. As the body putrefies, bacteria begin to ferment available carbohydrate sources into ethanol. The net result is that blood ethanol concentrations rise postmortem and are elevated even when no ethanol was consumed. Bacterial purification is less likely to occur in the vitreous and urine. Since ingested alcohol that reaches the blood appears in the urine quite rapidly, the finding of ethanol in the blood but not in either the urine or the vitreous is suggestive of postmortem ethanol formation.

Kugelberg FC, Jones AW. Interpreting results of ethanol analysis in postmortem specimens: A review of the literature. *Forensic Sci Int.* 2007;165:10-29.

O'Neal CL, Poklis A. Postmortem production of ethanol and factors that influence interpretation: A critical review. *Am J Forensic Med Pathol.* 1996;17:8-20.

140.9. Answer: D. Normal metabolism demethylates amitriptyline to nortriptyline and not the reverse. These reactions cannot occur in either the postmortem interval or by bacterial decomposition. In fixed tissue or blood that is contaminated, the formaldehyde rapidly methylates nortriptyline to amitriptyline.

Dettling RJ, et al. The production of amitriptyline from nortriptyline in formaldehyde-containing solutions. *J Anal Toxicol.* 1990;14:325-326.

Winek CL, et al. The study of tricyclic antidepressants in formalin fixed human liver and formalin solutions. *Forensic Sci Int.* 1993;61:175-183.

140.10. Answer: E. The conversion of cocaine to benzoyl ecgonine occurs both by enzymatic metabolism by plasma cholinesterase and nonenzymatic hydrolysis. Both reactions will continue to occur in vitro in serum that is free of all cellular elements. While the presence of benzoyl ecgonine confirms cocaine use, it is insufficient to confirm acute cocaine toxicity.

Tardiff K, et al. Analysis of cocaine positive fatalities. *J Forensic Sci.* 1989;34:53-63.

Stewart DJ, et al. Hydrolysis of cocaine in human plasma by cholinesterase. *Life Sci.* 1977;20:1557-1563.